competishun
Power of real gurus

AF657232

NEET (UG)

BIOLOGY

Team Competishun

Published by :

Invincible Publication Pvt. Ltd.

INVINCIBLE
Publication Private Limited

Published by

Invincible Publication Pvt. Ltd.

201A, SAS Tower, Sector 38, Gurugram – 122003
Phone: +91-124-4034247, +91 9599066061
www.invinciblepublishers.com

NEET (UG) BIOLOGY

First Edition 2024

This edition can be exported from India only by Invincible Publication.

ISBN-13 : 978-93-58866-70-4

Invincible Publication Pvt. Ltd.

Sales Office : 4760-61/23, Basement, Pratap Street, Ansari Road,

Daryaganj, New Delhi - 110002

Phone: +91-11-40198405

Email: invinciblepublishers@gmail.com

CONTENT

Chapter : 1

THE LIVING WORLD

WHAT IS LIVING ?

1. Which one of the following aspects is an exclusive characteristic of living things? ***(Mains 2011)***

(a) Isolated metabolic reactions occur in vitro.
(b) Increase in mass from outside only.
(c) Perception of events happening in the environment and their memory.
(d) Increase in mass by accumulation of material both on surface as well as internally.

2. The living organisms can be unexceptionally distinguished from the non-living things on the basis of their ability for ***(2007)***

(a) interaction with the environment and progressive evolution
(b) reproduction
(c) growth and movement
(d) responsiveness to touch.

3. Biological organisation starts with ***(2007)***

(a) cellular level
(b) organismic level
(c) atomic level
(d) submicroscopic molecular level.

DIVERSITY IN THE LIVING WORLD

4. Select the correctly written scientific name of Mango which was first described by Carolus Linnaeus. ***(2019)***

(a) Mangifera indica
(b) Mangifera indica Car. Linn.
(c) Mangifera indica Linn.
(d) Mangifera indica

5. Which of the following is against the rules of ICB N? ***(Odisha NEET 2019)***

(a) Hand written scientific names should be underlined.
(b) Every species should have a generic name and a specific epithet.
(c) Scientific names are in Latin and should be italicized.
(d) Generic and specific names should be written starting with small letters.

6. Nomenclature is governed by certain universal rules. Which one of the following is contrary to the rules of nomenclature? ***(NEET-I 2016)***

(a) The names are written in Latin and are italicised.
(b) When written by hand the names are to be underlined.
(c) Biological names can be written in any language.
(d) The first word in a biological name represents the genus name and the second is a specific epithet.

7. ICBN stands for ***(2007)***

(a) International Code of Botanical Nomenclature
(b) International Congress of Biological Names
(c) Indian Code of Botanical Nomenclature
(d) Indian Congress of Biological Names.

8. Biosystematics aims at ***(2003)***

(a) the classification of organisms based on broad morphological characters
(b) delimiting various taxa of organisms and establishing their relationships
(c) the classification of organisms based on their evolutionary history and establishing their phylogeny on the totality of various parameters from all fields of studies
(d) identification and arrangement of organisms on the basis of their cytological characteristics.

9. The book 'Genera Plantarum' was written by **(1999)**
(a) Engler and Prantl
(b) Bentham and Hooker
(c) Bessey
(d) Hutchinson.

10. Linnaeus is credited with **(1993)**
(a) binomial nomenclature
(b) theory of biogenesis
(c) discovery of microscope
(d) discovery of blood circulation.

11. Linnaeus evolved a system of nomenclature called **(1990)**
(a) mononomial (b) vernacular
(c) binomial (d) polynomial.

12. The term "New Systematics" was introduced by **(1988)**
(a) Bentham and Hooker
(b) Linnaeus
(c) Julian Huxley
(d) A.P. de Candolle.

TAXONOMIC CATEGORIES

13. In the taxonomic categories which hierarchial arrangement in ascending order is correct in case of animals? **(2022)**
(a) Kingdom, Phylum, Class, Order, Family, Genus, Species
(b) Kingdom, Class, Phylum, Family, Order, Genus, Species
(c) Kingdom, Order, Class, Phylum, Family, Genus, Species
(d) Kingdom, Order, Phylum, Class, Family, Genus, Species

14. Which one of the following belongs to the Family Muscidae? **(2021)**
(a) House fly (b) Fire fly
(c) Grasshopper (d) Cockroach

15. Match column I with column II for housefly classification and select the correct option using the codes given below. **(NEET-II 2016)**

Column I	Column II
A. Family	(i) Diptera
B. Order	(ii) Arthropoda
C. Class	(iii) Muscidae
D. Phylum	(iv) Insecta

(a) A-(iii), B-(i), C-(iv), D-(ii)
(b) A-(iii), B-(ii), C-(iv), D-(i)
(c) A-(iv), B-(iii), C-(ii), D-(i)
(d) A-(iv), B-(ii), C-(i), D-(iii)

16. Study the four statements (A-D) given below and select the two correct ones out of them. **(NEET-II 2016)**
A. Definition of biological species was given by Ernst Mayr.
B. Photoperiod does not affect reproduction in plants.
C. Binomial nomenclature system was given by R.H. Whittaker.
D. In unicellular organisms, reproduction is synonymous with growth.
The two correct statements are
(a) B and C (b) C and D
(c) A and D (d) A and B.

17. The common characteristics between tomato and potato will be maximum at the level of their **(Karnataka NEET 2013)**
(a) family (b) order
(c) division (d) genus.

18. Which one of the following organisms is scientifically correctly named, correctly printed according to the International Rules of Nomenclature and correctly described? **(Mains 2012)**
(a) *Musca domestica* - the common house lizard, a reptile
(b) *Plasmodium falciparum* - a protozoan pathogen causing the most serious type of malaria.
(c) *Felis tigris* - the Indian tiger, well protected in Gir forests.
(d) E.coli - full name Entamoeba coli, a commonly occurring bacterium in human intestine.

19. Which one of the following animals is correctly matched with its particular taxonomic category? ***(2011)***
(a) Tiger - tigris, species
(b) Cuttlefish - mollusca, class
(c) Humans - primata, family
(d) Housefly - Musca, order

20. Species are considered as ***(2003)***
(a) real basic units of classification
(b) the lowest units of classification
(c) artificial concept of human mind which cannot be defined in absolute terms
(d) real units of classification devised by taxonomists.

21. Which of the following is less general in characters as compared to genus? ***(2001)***
(a) Species (b) Division
(c) Class (d) Family

22. 'Taxon' is the unit of a group of ***(1996)***
(a) order (b) taxonomy
(c) species (d) genes.

23. Sequence of taxonomic categories is ***(1992)***
(a) class-phylum-tribe-order-family-genus–species
(b) division-class-family-tribe-order-genus–species
(c) division-class-order-family-tribe-genus–species.
(d) phylum-order-class-tribe-family -genus–species.

24. A group of plants or animals with similar traits of any rank is ***(1992,1991)***
(a) species (b) genus
(c) order (d) taxon.

25. A taxon is ***(1992,1990)***
(a) a group of related families
(b) a group of related species
(c) a type of living organisms
(d) a taxonomic group of any ranking.

26. Basic unit or smallest taxon of taxonomy/classification is ***(1990)***
(a) species (b) kingdom
(c) family (d) variety.

ANSWER KEY

1.	(c)	2.	(d)	3.	(d)
4.	(c)	5.	(d)	6.	(c)
7.	(a)	8.	(c)	9.	(b)
10.	(a)	11.	(c)	12.	(c)
13.	(*)	14.	(a)	15.	(a)
16.	(c)	17.	(a)	18.	(b)
19.	(a)	20.	(a)	21.	(a)
22.	(b)	23.	(c)	24.	(d)
25.	(d)	26.	(a)		

HINTS & EXPLANATIONS

1. (c) **2. (d)**

3. (d) : Molecular assemblies are large organised sets of molecular units that make up parts of organelles. For example, one common macromolecular assembly is the microtubule which is important in forming structure in the cell related to maintaining the cell structure or related to cell movement. The cell (plasma) membrane surrounds many organelles and the cell is a highly organised molecular assembly.

4. (c) : According to binomial nomenclature, the first word denoting the genus starts with a capital letter while the specific epithet starts with a small letter. E.g., scientific name of mango is *Mangifera indica*. Name of the author appears after the specific epithet, i.e., at the end of biological name and is written in an abbreviated form, e.g., *Mangifera indica* Linn. It indicates that this species was first described by Linnaeus.

5. (d) : According to International Code for Botanical Nomenclature (ICBN) the first word denoting the genus starts with a capital letter while the specific epithet starts with a small letter.

6. **(c) :** Biological names are derived either from Latin language or are latinised. This is because Latin language is a dead language and therefore it will not change in form or spellings with the passage of time.

7. **(a) :** The International Code of Botanical Nomenclature (ICBN) is a set of rules and recommendations dealing with the formal botanical names given to plant. The foundations of ICBN are given in book written by C. Linnaeus named Philosophia Botanica. It is independent of zoological nomenclature.

8. **(c) :** Biosystematics is the study of identification, nomenclature, classification and relationships amongst living beings. In other words, it is the study of diversity of organisms, their comparative and evolutionary relationships based on comparative anatomy, ecology, physiology, biochemistry and other fields.

9. **(b) :** Bentham and Hooker in their monumental work Genera Plantarum (1862-1883) have provided elaborate keys for the easy identification of 202 natural orders and genera.

10. **(a) :** Binomial nomenclature was first given by C. Linnaeus (1735) in his book "Systema Naturae" and later in "Species Plantarum" (1753). He used two latin words for any organism, the first being generic name and the second is specific name. The generic name begins with capital letter and the species name with small letter.

11. **(c) :**

12. **(c) :** The term "New Systematics", was given by Julian Huxley (1940). This classification takes into account the cytological, morphological, genetical, anatomical, palynological and physiological characters.

13. **(*) :** (None of the options is correct) : Hierarchy of categories is the classification of organisms in a definite sequence of categories (taxonomic categories) in a descending order starting from Kingdom and reaching upto Species or an ascending order from Species to Kingdom. The number of similar characters of categories decreases from lowest rank (Species) to highest rank (Kingdom). The taxonomic hierarchy includes seven obligate categories-Kingdom, Division or Phylum, Class, Order, Family, Genus and Species.

14. **(a) :** Housefly (Musea domestica) belongs to Family Muscidae.

15. **(a)**

16. **(c) :** Photoperiod affects flowering and reproduction in plants. Binomial nomenclature system was given by Carolus Linnaeus.

17. **(a) :** Potato (Solanum tuberosum) and tomato (Lycopersicum esculentum) both belong to Family Solanaceae, which is commonly called as the "potato family". Many plants belonging to this family are sources of vegetables, fruits, etc.

18. **(b) :** Plasmodium falciparum is a protozoan parasite, one of the species of Plasmodium that causes malaria in humans. Being digenetic, its life cycle is complete in two hosts - man and mosquito.

19. **(a)**

20. **(a) :** Species is a natural population or group of natural populations of individuals which are genetically distinct and reproductively isolated with similar essential morphological traits. Species is also a genetically closed system because its members do not interbreed with members of other species.

21. (a) : A taxonomic hierarchy is the sequence of arrangement of taxonomic categories in a descending order during the classification of an organism. There are seven obligate categories - kingdom, division, class, order, family, genus and species. Species is the lowest category while kingdom is the highest category. The number of common characters is maximum in case of organisms placed in the lowest category. Number of common characters decreases with the rise in category. Species are the smallest group of individuals which can be recognized by ordinary methods as groups and which are consistently and persistently different from other groups because their characters are less general.

22. (b) : Taxon refers to all the categories in the taxonomic hierarchy. It may be a kingdom, class, order, family, genus or species. It is any level of grouping of organisms. Each of these categories has been divided further into intermediate categories like subkingdom, subdivision, superclass, subgenus, subspecies, etc.

23. (c) : Tribe is a taxon between family and genus.

24. (d) : A taxon (plural taxa) or taxonomic unit, is a name designating an organism or group of organisms. A taxon is assigned a rank and can be placed at a particular level in a systematic hierarchy reflecting evolutionary relationships.

25. (d)

26. (a) : Basic unit or smallest taxon of taxonomy/classification is species. Species is a group of individuals that resemble one another in all essential morphological and reproductive characters so that they are able to interbreed freely and produce fertile offspring.

Chapter : 02

BIOLOGICAL CLASSIFICATION

INTRODUCTION

1. Five kingdom system of classification suggested by R.H. Whittaker is not based on ***(2014)***
   (a) presence or absence of a well defined nucleus
   (b) mode of reproduction
   (c) mode of nutrition
   (d) complexity of body organisation.

2. Maximum nutritional diversity is found in the group ***(2012)***
   (a) fungi (b) animalia
   (c) monera (d) plantae.

3. In the five kingdom classification, Chlamydomonas and Chlorella have been included in ***(Mains 2012)***
   (a) protista (b) algae
   (c) plantae (d) monera.

4. In which kingdom would you classify the archaea and nitrogen-fixing organisms, if the five kingdom system of classification is used? ***(2003)***
   (a) Plantae (b) Fungi
   (c) Protista (d) Monera

5. In five kingdom system, the main basis of classification is ***(2002)***
   (a) structure of nucleus
   (b) mode of nutrition
   (c) structure of cell wall
   (d) asexual reproduction.

6. In the five kingdom system of classification, which single kingdom out of the following can include blue-green algae, nitrogen fixing bacteria and methanogenic archaebacteria? ***(1998)***
   (a) Plantae (b) Protista
   (c) Monera (d) Fungi

7. BGA (blue green algae) are included in which of the following groups? ***(1996)***
   (a) Bryophytes (b) Prokaryotes
   (c) Protista (d) Fungi

8. An important criterion for modern day classification is ***(1991)***
   (a) resemblances in morphology
   (b) anatomical and physiological traits
   (c) breeding habits
   (d) presence or absence of notochord.

KINGDOM MONERA

9. Given below are two statements: ***(2022)***

   Statement I: Mycoplasma can pass through less than 1 micron filter size.

   Statement II : Mycoplasma are bacteria with cell wall.

   In the light of the above statements, choose the most appropriate answer from the options given below.
   (a) Both Statement I and Statement II are correct
   (b) Both Statement I and Statement II are incorrect
   (c) Statement I is correct but Statement II is incorrect
   (d) Statement I is incorrect but Statement II is correct

10. Match the organisms in column-I with habitats in column-II. ***(Odisha NEET 2019)***

Column-I	Column-II
A. Halophiles	(i) Hot springs
B. Thermoacidophiles	(ii) Aquatic environment
C. Methanogens	(iii) Guts of ruminants
D. Cyanobacteria	(iv) Salty area

Select the correct answer from the options given below.
(a) A-(iv), B-(i), C-(iii), D-(ii)
(b) A-(i), B-(ii), C-(iii), D-(iv)
(c) A-(iii), B-(iv), C-(ii), D-(i)
(d) A-(ii), B-(iv), C-(iii), D-(i)

11. Which of the following are found in extreme saline conditions? ***(2017)***
(a) Eubacteria (b) Cyanobacteria
(c) Mycobacteria (d) Archaebacteria

12. Which among the following are the smallest living cells, known without a definite cell wall, pathogenic to plants as well as animals and can survive without oxygen? ***(2017)***
(a) Pseudomonas (b) Mycoplasma
(c) Nostoc (d) Bacillus

13. Which of the following components provides sticky character to the bacterial cell? ***(2017)***
(a) Nuclear membrane
(b) Plasma membrane
(c) Glycocalyx
(d) Cell wall

14. DNA replication in bacteria occurs ***(2017)***
(a) within nucleolus
(b) prior to fission
(c) just before transcription
(d) during S phase.

15. Methanogens belong to ***(NEET-II 2016)***
(a) eubacteria (b) archaebacteria
(c) dinoflagellates (d) slime moulds.

16. The primitive prokaryotes responsible for the production of biogas from the dung of ruminant animals, include the ***(NEET-I 2016)***
(a) methanogens (b) eubacteria
(c) halophiles (d) thermoacidophiles.

17. Archaebacteria differ from eubacteria in ***(2014)***
(a) cell membrane structure
(b) mode of nutrition
(c) cell shape
(d) mode of reproduction.

18. Which of the following are likely to be present in deep sea water? ***(2013)***
(a) Blue-green algae (b) Saprophytic fungi
(c) Archaebacteria (d) Eubacteria

19. Pigment containing membranous extensions in some cyanobacteria are ***(2013)***
(a) pneumatophores (b) chromatophores
(c) heterocysts (d) basal bodies.

20. The cyanobacteria are also referred to as ***(2012)***
(a) protists (b) golden algae
(c) slime moulds (d) blue green algae.

21. The most abundant prokaryotes helpful to humans in making curd from milk and in production of antibiotics are the ones categorised as ***(2012)***
(a) cyanobacteria (b) archaebacteria
(c) chemosynthetic autotrophs
(d) heterotrophic bacteria.

22. In eubacteria, a cellular component that resembles eukaryotic cell is ***(2011)***
(a) plasma membrane
(b) nucleus
(c) ribosomes (d) cell wall.

23. Some hyperthermophilic organisms that grow in highly acidic (pH-2) habitats belong to the two groups ***(2010)***
(a) eubacteria and archaea
(b) cyanobacteria and diatoms
(c) protists and mosses
(d) liverworts and yeasts.

24. Select the correct combination of the statements (i-iv) regarding the characteristics of certain organisms. ***(Mains 2010)***
(i) Methanogens are archaebacteria which produce methane in marshy areas.
(ii) Nostoc is a filamentous blue-green alga which fixes atmospheric nitrogen.
(iii) Chemosynthetic autotrophic bacteria synthesize cellulose from glucose.

(iv) Mycoplasma lack a cell wall and can survive without oxygen.

The correct statements are

(a) (ii) and (iii) (b) (i),(ii) and (iii)
(c) (ii), (iii) and (iv) (d) (i), (ii) and (iv).

25. Bacterial leaf blight of rice is caused by a species ***(2008)***
(a) Alternaria (b) Erwinia
(c) Xanthomonas (d) Pseudomonas.

26. Thermococcus, Methanococcus and Methanobacterium exemplify ***(2008)***
(a) bacteria whose DNA is relaxed or positively supercoiled but which have a cytoskeleton as well as mitochondria
(b) bacteria that contain a cytoskeleton and ribosomes
(c) archaebacteria that contain protein homologous to eukaryotic core histones
(d) archaebacteria that lack any histones resembling those found in eukaryotes but whose DNA is negatively supercoiled.

27. In the light of recent classification of living organisms into three domains of life (bacteria, archaea and eukarya), which one of the following statements is true about archaea? ***(2008)***
(a) Archaea completely differ from both prokaryotes and eukaryotes.
(b) Archaea completely differ from prokaryotes.
(c) Archaea resemble eukarya in all respects.
(d) Archaea have some novel features that are absent in other prokaryotes and eukaryotes.

28. Which one of the following statements about mycoplasma is wrong? ***(2007)***
(a) They are pleomorphic.
(b) They are sensitive to penicillin.
(c) They cause diseases in plants.
(d) They are also called PPLO.

29. Curing of tea leaves is brought about by the activity of ***(2006)***
(a) fungi (b) bacteria
(c) mycorrhiza (d) viruses.

30. All of the following statements concerning the actinomycetous filamentous soil bacterium Frankia are correct except that Frankia ***(2005)***
(a) can induce root nodules on many plant species
(b) can fix nitrogen in the free-living state
(c) cannot fix specialized vesicles in which the nitrogenase is protected from oxygen by a chemical barrier involving triterpene hopanoids
(d) like Rhizobium, it usually infects its host plant through root hair deformation and stimulates cell proliferation in the host's cortex.

31. For retting of jute the fermenting microbe used is ***(2005)***
(a) methanophilic bacteria
(b) butyric acid bacteria
(c) Helicobacter pylori
(d) Streptococcus lactin.

32. Basophilic prokaryotes ***(2005)***
(a) grow and multiply in very deep marine sediments
(b) occur in water containing high concentrations of barium hydroxide
(c) readily grow and divide in sea water enriched in any soluble salt of barium
(d) grow slowly in highly alkaline frozen lakes at high altitudes.

33. Which statement is correct for bacterial transduction? ***(2002)***
(a) Transfer of some genes from one bacteria to another bacteria through virus.
(b) Transfer of genes from one bacteria to another bacteria by conjugation.
(c) Bacteria obtained its DNA directly from mother cell.
(d) Bacteria obtained DNA from other external source.

34. In bacteria, plasmid is ***(2002)***
(a) extra chromosomal material
(b) main DNA
(c) non functional DNA
(d) repetitive gene

35. Organisms which obtain energy by the oxidation of reduced inorganic compounds are called ***(2002)***
(a) photoautotrophs
(b) chemoautotrophs
(c) saprozoic
(d) coproheterotrophs.

36. What is true for archaebacteria? ***(2001)***
(a) All halophiles (b) All photosynthetics
(c) All fossils (d) Oldest living beings

37. Difference in Gram positive and Gram negative bacteria is due to ***(2001)***
(a) cell wall (b) cell membrane
(c) ribosome (d) cytoplasm.

38. Transfer of genetic information from one bacterium to another in the transduction process is through ***(1998)***
(a) bacteriophages released from the donor bacterial strain
(b) another bacterium having special organ for conjugation
(c) physical contact between donor and recipient strains
(d) conjugation between opposite strain bacterium.

39. A bacterium divides every 35 minutes. If a culture containing 10^5 cells per mL is grown for 175 minutes, what will be the cell concentration per mL after 175 minutes? ***(1998)***
(a) 35×10^5 cells (b) 32×10^5 cells
(c) 175×10^5 cells (d) 85×10^5 cells

40. The DNA of E.coli is ***(1998)***
(a) double stranded and linear
(b) double stranded and circular
(c) single stranded and linear
(d) single stranded and circular.

41. The main role of bacteria in the carbon cycle involves ***(1998)***
(a) chemosynthesis
(b) dig estion or breakdown of organic compounds
(c) photosynthesis
(d) assimilation of nitrogenous compounds.

42. A few organisms are known to grow and multiply at temperatures of 100 – 105°C. They belong to ***(1998)***
(a) thermophilic sulphur bacteria
(b) hot spring blue-green algae
(c) methanogenic archaebacteria
(d) marine archaebacteria.

43. The hereditary material present in the bacterium E.coli is ***(1997)***
(a) single-stranded DNA
(b) double-stranded DNA
(c) DNA
(d) RNA.

44. Which type of DNA is found in bacteria? ***(1996)***
(a) Circular free DNA
(b) Membrane bound DNA
(c) Straight DNA
(d) Helical DNA

45. Many blue-green algae occur in thermal springs (hot-water springs). The temperature tolerance of these algae have been attributed to their ***(1994)***
(a) mitochondrial structure
(b) importance of homopolar bonds in their proteins
(c) cell wall structure
(d) modern cell organization.

46. Organisms, which fix atmospheric nitrogen in the soil, fall under the category of ***(1994)***
(a) bacteria (b) green algae
(c) soil fungi (d) mosses.

47. Transduction in bacteria is mediated by ***(1994)***
(a) plasmid vectors (b) phage vectors
(c) cosmids (d) F-factors.

48. Genophore/bacterial genome or nucleoid is made of ***(1993)***
(a) histones and non-histones
(b) RNA and histones
(c) a single double stranded DNA
(d) a single stranded DNA.

49. Escherichia coli is used extensively in biological research as it is ***(1993)***
(a) easily cultured
(b) easily available
(c) easy to handle
(d) easily multiplied in host.

50. Bacteria lack alternation of generation because there is ***(1992, 1991)***
(a) neither syngamy nor reduction division
(b) distinct chromosomes are absent
(c) no conjugation
(d) no exchange of genetic material.

51. Name the organisms which do not derive energy directly or indirectly from sun. ***(1991)***
(a) Chemosynthetic bacteria
(b) Pathogenic bacteria
(c) Symbiotic bacteria
(d) Mould

52. The main difference in Gram (+)ve and Gram (-) ve bacteria resides in their ***(1990)***
(a) cell wall (b) cell membrane
(c) cytoplasm (d) flagella.

53. Which one belongs to Monera? ***(1990)***
(a) Amoeba (b) Escherichia
(c) Gelidium (d) Spirogyra

KINGDOM PROTISTA

54. Which of the following is a correct statement? ***(2022)***
(a) Cyanobacteria are a group of autotrophic organisms classified under Kingdom Monera.
(b) Bacteria are exclusively heterotrophic organisms.
(c) Slime moulds are saprophytic organisms classified under Kingdom Monera.
(d) Mycoplasma have DNA, Ribosome and cell wall

55. Which of the following organisms are known as chief producers in the oceans? **(2018)**
(a) Dinoflagellates (b) Diatoms
(c) Cyanobacteria (d) Euglenoids

56. Ciliates differ from all other protozoans in***(2018)***
(a) using flagella for locomotion
(b) having a contractile vacuole for removing excess water
(c) using pseudopodia for capturing prey
(d) having two types of nuclei.

57. Select the wrong statement. ***(NEET-II 2016)***
(a) The walls of diatoms are easily destructible.
(b) 'Diatomaceous earth' is formed by the cell walls of diatoms.
(c) Diatoms are chief producers in the oceans.
(d) Diatoms are microscopic and float passively in water.

58. Chrysophytes, Euglenoids, Dinoflagellates and Slime moulds are included in the Kingdom ***(NEET-I 2016)***
(a) Fungi (b) Animalia
(c) Monera (d) Protista.

59. In which group of organisms the cell walls form two thin overlapping shells which fit together? ***(2015)***
(a) Dinoflagellates (b) Slime moulds
(c) Chrysophytes (d) Euglenoids

60. Which one of the following organisms is not an eukaryote? ***(2011)***
(a) Paramecium caudatum
(b) Escherichia coli
(c) Euglena viridis
(d) Amoeba proteus

61. Which one of the following is a slime mould? ***(2007)***
(a) Physarum (b) Thiobacillus
(c) Anabaena (d) Rhizopus

62. Auxospores and hormogonia are formed, respectively, by ***(2005)***
(a) some diatoms and several cyanobacteria
(b) some cyanobacteria and many diatoms
(c) several cyanobacteria and several diatoms
(d) several diatoms and a few cyanobacteria.

63. When a fresh-water protozoan possessing a contractile vacuole, is placed in a glass containing marine water, the vacuole will ***(2004)***
(a) increase in number
(b) disappear
(c) increase in size
(d) decrease in size.

64. The chief advantage of encystment of an Amoeba is ***(2003)***
(a) the ability to survive during adverse physical conditions
(b) the ability to live for sometime without ingesting food
(c) protection from parasites and predators
(d) the chance to get rid of accumulated waste products.

65. In which of the following animals dimorphic nucleus is found? ***(2002)***
(a) Amoeba proteus
(b) Trypanosomagambiense
(c) Plasmodium vivax
(d) Paramecium caudatum

66. In protozoa like Amoeba and Paramecium, the organ for osmoregulation is ***(2002)***
(a) contractile vacuole (b) mitochondria
(c) nucleus (d) food vacuole.

67. Which of the following organisms possesses characteristics of a plant and an animal? ***(1995)***
(a) Euglena (b) Paramecium
(c) Bacteria (d) Mycoplasma

68. The function of contractile vacuole, in protozoa, is ***(1995)***
(a) osmoregulation (b) reproduction
(c) locomotion (d) digestion of food.

69. In Amoeba and Paramecium osmoregulation occurs through ***(1991)***
(a) pseudopodia (b) nucleus
(c) contractile vacuole (d) general surface.

70. Plasmodium, the malarial parasite, belongs to class ***(1990)***
(a) sarcodina (b) ciliata
(c) sporozoa (d) dinophyceae.

71. Which is true about Trypanosoma? ***(1990)***
(a) Polymorphic (b) Monogenetic
(c) Facultative parasite (d) Non-pathogenic

72. Genetic information in Paramecium is contained in ***(1990)***
(a) micronucleus
(b) macronucleus
(c) both micronucleus and macronucleus
(d) mitochondria.

73. Trypanosoma belongs to Class ***(1989)***
(a) Sarcodina (b) Zooflagellata
(c) Ciliata (d) Sporozoa.

KINGDOM FUNGI

74. Which of the following statements is correct? ***(2021)***
(a) Some of the organisms can fix atmospheric nitrogen in specialised cells called sheath cells.
(b) Fusion of two cells is called karyogamy.
(c) Fusion of protoplasms between two motile or non-motile gametes is called plasmogamy.
(d) Organisms that depend on living plants are called saprophytes.

75. Which of the following statements is incorrect? ***(2019)***

(a) Yeasts have filamentous bodies with long thread like hyphae.

(b) Morels and truffles are edible delicacies.

(c) Claviceps is a source of many alkaloids and LSD.

(d) Conidia are produced exogenously and ascospores endogenously.

76. Match column -I with column - II.

Column-I		Column-II	
(A)	Saprophyte	**(i)**	Symbiotic association of fungi with plant roots
(B)	Parasite	**(ii)**	Decomposition of dead organic materials
(C)	Lichens	**(iii)**	Living on living plants or animals
(D)	Mycorrhiza	**(iv)**	Symbiotic association of algae and fungi

Choose the correct answer from the options given below. ***(2019)***

	A	**B**	**C**	**D**
(a)	(ii)	(iii)	(iv)	(i)
(b)	(ii)	(ii)	(iii)	(iv)
(c)	(iii)	(ii)	(i)	(iv)
(d)	(ii)	(i)	(iii)	(iv)

77. Which among the following is not a prokaryote? ***(2018)***

(a) Saccharomyces (b) Mycobacterium

(c) Nostoc (d) Oscillatoria

78. After karyogamy followed by meiosis, spores are produced exogenously in ***(2018)***

(a) Neurospora (b) Alternaria

(c) Agaricus (d) Saccharomyces.

79. Which one of the following is wrong for fungi? ***(NEET-II 2016)***

(a) They are eukaryotic.

(b) All fungi possess a purely cellulosic cell wall.

(c) They are heterotrophic.

(d) They are both unicellular and multicellular.

80. Which one of the following statements is wro ng? ***(NEET-I 2016)***

(a) Eubacteria are also called false bacteria.

(b) Phycomycetes are also called algal fungi.

(c) Cyanobacteria are also called blue-green algae.

(d) Golden algae are also called desmids.

81. One of the major components of cell wall of most fungi is ***(NEET-I 2016)***

(a) cellulose (b) hemicellulose

(c) chitin (d) peptidoglycan.

82. The imperfect fungi which are decomposers of litter and help in mineral cycling belong to ***(2015)***

(a) Phycomycetes (b) Ascomycetes

(c) Deuteromycetes (d) Basidiomycetes.

83. Choose the wrong statement. ***(2015)***

(a) Morels and truffles are poisonous mushrooms.

(b) Yeast is unicellular and useful in fermentation.

(c) Penicillium is multicellular and produces antibiotics.

(d) Neurospora is used in the study of biochemical genetics.

84. Which one of the following matches is correct? ***(2015 Cancelled)***

(a)	Mucor	Reproduction by conjugation	Ascomycetes
(b)	Agaricus	Parasitic fungus	Basidiomycetes
(c)	Phytophthora	Aseptate mycelium	Basidiomycetes
(d)	Alternaria	Sexual reproduction absent	Deuteromycetes

85. Which one of the following fungi contains hallucinogens? ***(2014)***
(a) Morchella esculenta
(b) Amanita muscaria
(c) Neurospora sp.
(d) Ustilago sp.

86. Which one of the following is true for fungi? ***(Karnataka NEET 2013)***
(a) They lack a rigid cell wall.
(b) They are heterotrophs.
(c) They lack nuclear membrane.
(d) They are phagotrophs.

87. The pathogen Microsporum responsible for ringworm disease in humans belongs to the same kingdom of organisms as that of ***(Mains 2011)***
(a) Taenia, a tapeworm
(b) Wuchereria, a filarial worm
(c) Rhizopus, a mould
(d) Ascaris, a round worm.

88. Single-celled eukaryotes are included in ***(2010)***
(a) protista (b) fungi
(c) archaea (d) monera.

89. Membrane-bound organelles are absent in ***(2010)***
(a) Saccharomyces (b) Streptococcus
(c) Chlamydomonas (d) Plasmodium.

90. Black (stem) rust of wheat is caused by ***(Mains 2010)***
(a) Alternaria solani (b) Ustilago nuda
(c) Puccinia graminis
(d) Xanthomonas oryzae.

91. Which one is the wrong pairing for the disease and its causal organism? ***(2009)***
(a) Black rust of wheat-Puccinia graminis
(b) Loose smut of wheat-Ustilago nuda
(c) Root knot of vegetables-Meloidogyne sp.
(d) Late blight of potato-Alternaria solani

92. Which pair of the following belongs to basidiomycetes? ***(2007)***
(a) Puffballs and Claviceps
(b) Peziza and stink horns
(c) Morchella and mushrooms
(d) Birds nest fungi and puffballs

93. Which of the following environmental conditions are essential for optimum growth of Mucor on a piece of bread? ***(2006)***
A. Temperature of about 25°C
B. Temperature of about 5°C
C. Relative humidity of about 5%
D. Relative humidity of about 95%
E. A shady place
F. A brightly illuminated place
Choose the answer from the following options.
(a) B, C and F only (b) A, C and E only
(c) A, D and E only (d) B, D and E only

94. Which fungal disease spreads by seed and flowers? ***(2002)***
(a) Loose smut of wheat
(b) Corn smut
(c) Covered smut of barley
(d) Soft rot of potato

95. Which of the following secretes toxins during storage conditions of crop plants? ***(2002)***
(a) Aspergillus (b) Penicillium
(c) Fusarium (d) Colletotrichum

96. Black rust of wheat is caused by ***(2000)***
(a) Puccinia (b) Ustilago
(c) Albugo (d) Phytophthora.

97. Mycorrhiza is correctly described as ***(1996)***
(a) parasitic association between roots and some fungi
(b) symbiotic relationship between fungi and roots of some higher plants
(c) symbiosis of algae and fungi
(d) relation of ants with the stem of some trees.

98. The black rust of wheat is a fungal disease caused by ***(1995)***

(a) Albugo candida
(b) Puccinia graminis tritici
(c) Melampsora lini
(d) Claviceps purpurea.

KINGDOM PLANTAE

99. Select the wrong statement. ***(2018)***

(a) Cell wall is present in members of fungi and plantae.
(b) Mushrooms belong to basidiomycetes.
(c) Pseudopodia are locomotory and feeding structures in sporozoans.
(d) Mitochondria are the powerhouse of the cell in all kingdoms except monera.

100. Cell wall is absent in ***(2015)***

(a) Mycoplasma (b) Nostoc
(c) Aspergillus (d) Funaria.

101. True nucleus is absent in ***(2015 Cancelled)***

(a) Vaucheria (b) Volvox
(c) Anabaena (d) Mucor.

102. Nuclear membrane is absent in ***(2012)***

(a) Penicillium (b) Agaricus
(c) Volvox (d) Nostoc.

103. Absorptive heterotrophic nutrition is exhibited by ***(1990)***

(a) algae (b) fungi
(c) bryophytes (d) pteridophytes.

KINGDOM ANIMALIA

104. Pick up the wrong statement. ***(2015)***

(a) Some fungi are edible.
(b) Nuclear membrane is present in Monera.
(c) Cell wall is absent in Animalia.
(d) Protists have photosynthetic and heterotrophic modes of nutrition.

105. Which one of the following living organisms completely lacks a cell wall? ***(2014)***

(a) Cyanobacteria (b) Sea-fan (Gorgonia)
(c) Saccharomyces (d) Blue-green algae

VIRUSES, VIROIDS, PRIONS AND LICHENS

106. Which of the following is correct about viroids? ***(2020)***

(a) They have RNA with protein coat.
(b) They have free RNA without protein coat.
(c) They have DNA with protein coat.
(d) They have free DNA without protein coat.

107. Mad cow disease in cattle is caused by an organism which has **(Odisha NEET 2019)**

(a) inert crystalline structure
(b) abnormally folded protein
(c) free RNA without protein coat
(d) free DNA without protein coat.

108. Which of the following statements is incorrect? ***(2019)***

(a) Prions consist of abnormally folded proteins.
(b) Viroids lack a protein coat.
(c) Viruses are obligate parasites.
(d) Infective constituent in viruses is the protein coat.

109. Viroids differ from viruses in having ***(2017)***

(a) DNA molecules without protein coat
(b) RNA molecules with protein coat
(c) RNA molecules without protein coat
(d) DNA molecules with protein coat.

110. Which of the following statements is wrong for viroids? ***(NEET-I 2016)***

(a) They cause infections.
(b) Their RNA is of high molecular weight.
(c) They lack a protein coat.
(d) They are smaller than viruses.

111. Select the wrong statement. ***(2015)***

(a) The term 'contagium vivum fluidum' was coined by M. W. Beijerinck.
(b) Mosaic disease in tobacco and AIDS in human being are caused by viruses.
(c) The viroids were discovered by D.J. Ivanowsky.
(d) W.M. Stanley showed that viruses could be crystallised.

112. Which of the following shows coiled RNA strand and capsomeres? ***(2014)***

(a) Polio virus (b) Tobacco mosaic virus

(c) Measles virus (d) Retrovirus

113. Viruses have ***(2014)***

(a) DNA enclosed in a protein coat

(b) prokaryotic nucleus

(c) single chromosome

(d) both DNA and RNA.

114. Which statement is wrong for viruses? ***(2012)***

(a) All are parasites.

(b) All of them have helical symmetry.

(c) They have ability to synthesize nucleic acids and proteins.

(d) Antibiotics have no effect on them.

115. Which one single organism or the pair of organisms is correctly assigned to its or their named taxonomic group? ***(2012)***

(a) Paramecium and Plasmodium belong to the same kingdom as that of Penicillium.

(b) Lichen is a composite organism formed from the symbiotic association of an algae and a protozoan.

(c) Yeast used in making bread and beer is a fungus.

(d) Nostoc and Anabaena are examples of protista.

116. Virus envelope is known as ***(2010)***

(a) capsid (b) virion

(c) nucleoprotein (d) core.

117. Given below is the diagram of a bacteriophage. In which one of the options all the four parts A, B, C and D are correct? ***(Mains 2010)***

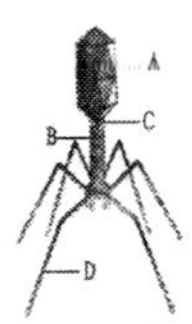

	A	B	C	D
(a)	Tail fibres	Head	Sheath	Collar
(b)	Sheath	Collar	Head	Tail fibres
(c)	Head	Sheath	Collar	Tail fibres
(d)	Collar	Tail fibres	Head	Sheath

(Mains 2010)

	A	B	C	D
(a)	Tail fibres	Head	Sheath	Collar
(b)	Sheath	Collar	Head	Tail fibres
(c)	Head	Sheath	Collar	Tail fibres
(d)	Collar	Tail fibres	Head	Sheath

118. T.O. Diener discovered a ***(2009)***

(a) free infectious DNA

(b) infectious protein

(c) bacteriophage

(d) free infectious RNA.

119. There exists a close association between the alga and the fungus within a lichen. The fungus ***(2005)***

(a) provides protection, anchorage and absorption for the algae

(b) provides food for the alga

(c) fixes the atmospheric nitrogen for the alga

(d) releases oxygen for the alga.

120. Which of the following statements is not true for retroviruses? ***(2004)***

(a) DNA is not present at any stage in the life cycle of retroviruses.

(b) Retroviruses carry gene for RNA-dependent DNA polymerase.

(c) The genetic material in mature retroviruses is RNA.

(d) Retroviruses are causative agents for certain kinds of cancer in man.

121. Viruses that infect bacteria multiply and cause their lysis, are called ***(2004)***

(a) lysozymes (b) lipolytic

(c) lytic (d) lysogenic.

122. Lichens are well known combination of an alga and a fungus where fungus has ***(2004)***

(a) a saprophytic relationship with the alga

(b) an epiphytic relationship with the alga

(c) a parasitic relationship with alga

(d) a symbiotic relationship with alga.

123. Which one of the following statements about viruses is correct? ***(2003)***
(a) Viruses possess their own metabolic system.
(b) All viruses contain both RNA and DNA.
(c) Viruses are obligate parasites.
(d) Nucleic acid of viruses is known as capsid.

124. Viruses are no more "alive" than isolated chromosomes because ***(2003)***
(a) they require both RNA and DNA
(b) they both need food molecules
(c) they both require oxygen for respiration
(d) both require the environment of a cell to replicate.

125. Cauliflower mosaic virus contains ***(2001)***
(a) ss RNA (b) ds RNA
(c) ds DNA (d) ss DNA.

126. Viruses possess ***(1997)***
(a) ribosomes to synthesize protein
(b) organelle for its vital mechanism
(c) either DNA or RNA
(d) none of these.

127. Most of the lichens consist of ***(1997)***
(a) green algae and ascomycetes
(b) brown algae and higher plant
(c) blue green algae and basidiomycetes
(d) red algae and ascomycetes.

128. What is the genetic material in influenza virus? ***(1996)***
(a) Double helical DNA
(b) RNA
(c) Single helix DNA
(d) None of these

129. Which one of the following statement about lichens is wrong? ***(1996)***
(a) These grow very rapidly (2 cm per day).
(b) They show fungal and algal symbiotic relationships.
(c) Some of its species are eaten by reindeers.
(d) These are pollution indicators.

130. Tobacco mosaic virus (TMV) genes are ***(1994)***
(a) single stranded RNA
(b) double stranded DNA
(c) proteinaceous
(d) double stranded RNA.

131. Organisms which are indicator of SO_2 pollution of air ***(1992)***
(a) mosses (b) lichens
(c) mushrooms (d) puffballs.

132. Lichens indicate SO_2 pollution because they ***(1989)***
(a) show association between algae and fungi
(b) grow faster than others
(c) are sensitive to SO2
(d) flourish in SO_2 rich environment.

ANSWER KEY

1.	(a)	2.	(c)	3.	(a)	4.	(d)	5.	(b)	6.	(c)	7.	(b)
8.	(b)	9.	(c)	10.	(a)	11.	(d)	12.	(b)	13.	(c)	14.	(b)
15.	(b)	16.	(a)	17.	(a)	18.	(c)	19.	(b)	20.	(d)	21.	(d)
22.	(a)	23.	(a)	24.	(d)	25.	(c)	26.	(c)	27.	(d)	28.	(b)
29.	(b)	30.	(b)	31.	(b)	32.	(a)	33.	(a)	34.	(a)	35.	(b)
36.	(d)	37.	(a)	38.	(a)	39.	(b)	40.	(b)	41.	(b)	42.	(a)
43.	(b)	44.	(a)	45.	(b)	46.	(a)	47.	(b)	48.	(c)	49.	(a)
50	(a)	51.	(a)	52.	(a)	53.	(b)	54.	(a)	55.	(b)	56.	(d)
57.	(a)	58.	(d)	59.	(c)	60.	(b)	61.	(a)	62.	(d)	63.	(d)
64.	(a)	65	(d)	66.	(a)	67.	(a)	68.	(a)	69.	(c)	70.	(c)
71.	(a)	72.	(a)	73.	(b)	74.	(c)	75.	(a)	76.	(a)	77.	(a)
78.	(c)	79.	(b)	80.	(a)	81.	(c)	82.	(c)	83.	(a)	84.	(d)
85.	(b)	86.	(b)	87.	(c)	88.	(a)	89.	(b)	90.	(c)	91.	(d)
92.	(d)	93.	(c)	94.	(a)	95	(a,b)	96.	(a)	97.	(b)	98.	(b)
99.	(c)	100.	(a)	101	(c)	102.	(d)	103.	(b)	104.	(b)	105.	(b)
106.	(b)	107.	(b)	108.	(d)	109.	(c)	110	(b)	111	(c)	112.	(b)
113.	(a)	114.	(b)	115.	(c)	116.	(a)	117.	(c)	118.	(d)	119.	(a)
120.	(a)	121.	(c)	122.	(d)	123	(c)	124.	(d)	125.	(c)	126.	(c)
127.	(a)	128.	(b)	129.	(a)	130.	(a)	131.	(b)	132.	(c)		

HINTS & EXPLANATIONS

1. (a) : R.H. Whittaker considered complexity of cell structure and structural (body) organisation, mode of nutrition, mode of reproduction and phylogenetic relationships for the five kingdom system of classification.

2. (c) : Compared to many other group, monerans (bacteria) show the most extensive metabolic diversity. Some of the bacteria are autotrophic, i.e, they synthesize their own food from inorganic substrates. They may be photosynthetic autotrophic or chemosynthetic autotrophic. The vast majority of bacteria are heterotrophs, i.e., they do not synthesize their own food but depend on other organisms or on dead organic matter for food.

3. (a) : In order to develop phylogenetic classification, R.H. Whittaker (1969), an American taxonomist, divided all the organisms into five kingdoms. Whittaker has used five criteria for delimiting the different kingdoms. (i) Complexity of cell structure, prokaryotic and eukaryotic (ii) Complexity of body structure or structural organization, unicellular and multicellular. (iii) Mode of nutrition which is divergent in multicellular kingdoms. (iv) Ecological life style like producers (plantae), decomposers (fungi) and consumers (animalia), (v) Phylogenetic relationship. When such characteristics were considered, the fungi were placed in a separate kingdom Kingdom Fungi. All prokaryotic organisms were grouped together under

Kingdom Monera and the unicellular eukaryotic organisms were placed in Kingdom Protista. Kingdom Protista has brought together Chlamydomonas, Chlurellu (ealler placed in Algae within Plants añd both having cell walls) with Paramecium and Amoeba (which were earlier placed in the animal kingdom which lack cell wall). It has put together organisms which, in earlier classifications, were placed in different kingdoms. This happened because the criteria for classification has changed.

4. **(d)** : The Kingdom Monera includes all prokaryotes. They are basically unicellular. The archaea and nitrogen-fixing organisms are placed under monera. All others fungi, plantae, protists and animalia are eukaryotic.

5. **(b) :** Whittaker's system is based on the following three criteria -

   - complexity of cell structure
   - complexity of the body organization
   - mode of nutrition.

   On the basis of these criteria, Whittaker divided organisms into five kingdoms. These five kingdoms are monera, protista, algae, fungi and animalia. In the five kingdom classification, all prokaryotes have been placed in Kingdom Monera, all unicellular eukaryotes in Kingdom Protista, Fungi (except slime moulds and water moulds) in their separate Kingdom while Kingdom Plantae and Kingdom Animalia have been retained for multicellular, autotrophic and multicellular holozoic organisms respectively.

6. **(c)** R.H. Whittaker had proposed a five kingdom system of biological classification in 1969. It is based on complexity of cell structure, body organization and mode of nutrition. The Kingdom Monera includes all prokaryotes. The blue-green algae, nitrogen fixing bacteria and methanogenic archaebacteria are all unicellular prokaryotes so they are included in the Kingdom Monera.

7. **(b)**

8. **(b)**

9. **(c)** Mycoplasma are organisms that completely lack a cell wall. They are the smallest living cells that can penetrate a 0.2 mu m rated filter.

10. **(a)**

11. **(d)** Ilalophiles, a type of archaebacteria, usually occur in extreme saline conditions like salt pans, salt beds and salt marshes.

12. **(b)** Mycoplasmas are the smallest living cells, known without a definite cell wall. They are pathogenic to both plants and animals and can survive without oxygen.

13. **(c)** Glycucalyx is the outermost mucilage layer of the cell envelope which consists of non-cellulosic polysaccharides with or without proteins. It gives sticky character to the cell.

14. **(b)** DNA replicates in bacteria just before they divide by fission.

15. **(b)** Methanogens belong to archaebacteria. They include methane producing genera such as Methanobacillus and Methanothrix. Methanogens are obligate anaerobes found in oxygen-deficient environments, such as marshes, swamps, sludge (formed during sewage treatment) and the digestive systems of ruminants. Mostly they obtain their energy by reducing carbon dioxide and oxidising hydrogen, with the production of methanc.

16. **(a)**

17. **(a):** The archaebacteria are the 'ancient' bacteria that include extremophiles like methanogens, halophiles and thermophiles. They represent some of the most ancient of life forms that

persist today. They have both eubacterial and eukaryotic characters besides the features unique to them. Their mode of reproduction, nutrition and cell shape and size resembles a typical eubacteria. Their cell walls are made of a variety of polymers, but do not contain peptidoglycan unlike eubacteria. Lipids of their cytoplasmic membranes are either linked unlike eubacteria which contain glycerol ester lipids in their cell membrane.

18. **(c):** Archaebacteria belong to a group of prokaryotic organisms called Monera. These include the methanogens, which produce methane; the thermoacidophilic bacteria, which live in extremely hot and acidic environments (such as hot springs); and the halophilic bacteria, which can only function at high salt concentrations and are abundant in the world's oceans.

19. **(b):** Chromatophore is a pigmented lamellar or vesicular structure that can be isolated from disrupted photosynthetic bacteria or cyanobacteria. Their plasma membrane may be projected in folds into the cytoplasm forming lamellae that have, therefore, double unit-membrane structure. The pigments and most of the enzymes required for the light-induced electron transport and phosphorylation processes of photosynthesis, are located in the plasma membrane and lamellae.

20. **(d):** Cyanobacteria consist of two groups of photosynthetic eubacteria: the blue-green bacteria (formerly known as blue-green algae, or cyanophyta), which comprise the vast majority of members and the grass-green bacteria, or chloroxybacteria.

21. **(d):** Maximum number of antibiotics are produced by mycelial bacteria known as actinomycetes and most of the actinomycetes are saprotrophic (heterotrophic). Lactic acid bacteria that are used in preparation of curd are also heterotrophic ones.

22. **(a):** Plasma membrane of eubacteria resembles plasma membrane of eukaryotic cell. But nucleus, ribosomes and cell wall are little different in eukaryotic cell in their structure and organization from eubacterial cell.

23. **(a):** There are two major groups of monerans archaebacteria (ancient bacteria) and eubacteria (true bacteria). Eubacteria is of further two types - bacteria and cyanobacteria. Thermoacidophiles are a type of archaebacteria which live in extremely acidic environment (pH-2) that have extremely high temperatures (upto 110°C). They are found in hot sulphur springs. Some of the eubacteria are also famous for living under the most hostile environment like salt pans, petroleum pans, spilled oil, hot springs, sulphur springs, snow, etc.

24. **(d):** Chemosynthetic autotrophic bacteria oxidise various inorganic substances such as nitrates, nitrites and ammonia and use the released energy for their ATP production. They play a great role in recycling nutrients like nitrogen, phosphorus, iron and sulphur.

25. **(c):** Bacterial leaf blight of rice is caused by Xanthomonas oryzae a bacterium which is gram-negative, aerobic, capsulated and motile with a single polar flagellum.

26. **(c):** Thermococcus, Methanococcus and Methanobacterium are examples of archaebacteria which are characterized by a unique cell wall that lack peptidoglycan and consist of polysaccharides and protein and closely resemble the eukaryotic cell in the mechanism of protein synthesis, structural protein and RNA compliments of the ribosomes.

27. (d): Archaebacteria represent a cell type that seems to possess the characteristics of both prokaryotes as well as eukaryotes. In size, the archaebacteria are about 1μm in diameter, the size of typical prokaryotes lack membranebound organelles, nuclear bodies are not bound by nuclear membranes as it is in eukaryotes and ribosomes are 70S, the size of those found in typical prokaryotes. They have unique cell wall that lacks peptidoglycan, closely resemble the eukaryotic cells in the mechanisms of protein synthesis, structural proteins. Archaebacteria also possess unique characteristic found in neither eukaryotes nor prokaryotes. For example, their membrane contain branched chain lipids with other. This enables them to tolerate extremes of heat and pH.

28. (b): Mycoplasma are small, unicellular, (non-motile) prokaryotic organisms. They are pleomorphic. Therefore they are known as pleuro pneumonia like organisms (PPLO). They lack cell wall. It contains cytoplasm, ribosomes and DNA. They are inhibited by tetracyclines but insensitive to penicillin. They cause various diseases.

29. (b): Curing is a process done to add special flavour and taste in tea leaves. It is also done for tobacco. In this process after harvesting the cured leaves are hung in shade and are permitted for the action of bacteria. The curing of tea leaves is done by Micrococcus candidans. Micrococcus is a gram positive aerobic bacterium which is a member of micrococcaceae.

30. (b): Frankia, is a nitrogen fixing symbiotic bacteria. It induces root nodules just like Rhizobium. It is associated symbiotically with the root nodules of several non-legume plants like Casuarina, Alnus, Rubus, etc. It cannot fix nitrogen in free state.

31. (b): Retting is the process of separating fibres that are held together in close association using a variety of bacteria. Fibres of jute are held together in close association and they are separated by the action of butyric acid bacteria, e.g., Clostridium butyricum. These plants are immersed in water so that they absorb water and swell. Due to the activity of bacteria, the pectic substances of middle lamella are hydrolysed and the fibres are separated. These separated fibres are used in making of ropes and sacks.

32. (a): Basophilic prokaryotes are facultatively anaerobic bacteria. They grow and multiply in very deep marine sediments. Most basophiles grow better at a pH of 8.5 or higher.

33. (a): In transduction, genetic material of one bacterial cell goes to other bacterial cell by agency of bacteriophages or phages (viruses, infecting bacteria).

Transduction was first of all reported in Salmonella typhimurium by Zinder and Lederberg (1952).

Transduction is used for gene mapping and analysis in bacteria and also for strain construction.

34. (a) In addition to the nucleoid, bacterial cytoplasm normally contains many small, separate pieces of DNA, called plasmids. These circular DNA units are $1 / 100$ the size of the main nuclear DNA (nucleoid) and are also not enclosed in a membrane structure. When found in cytoplasm, entirely independent of the bacterial chromosome, they replicate autonomously. Sometimes it becomes integrated into the main DNA and replicates with it. During conjugation, the plasmids, sometimes called episomes, help in the transfer of the genetic material between different bacteria. It may carry some genes of resistance to a variety of antibiotics.

35. (b): Chemoautotrophs are organisms that are capable of manufacturing their organic food utilising chemical energy released in oxidation of some inorganic substances. The process of manufacture of food in such organisms is called chemosynthesis. It includes some aerobic bacteria. Photoautotroph obtain energy for their synthesis of food from light.

Fungi living on dead or decaying plant or animal remains and also growing on dung of herbivores are saprophytes.

36. (d): Archaebacteria are believed to have originated at a time when there were extreme conditions in the biosphere. Even today they are found in environments where other kinds of bacteria cannot survive. So they are considered to be the oldest of the living fossils, e.g., Methanobacterium, Methanococcus, etc.

All of them are not halophiles. Only some forms like Halobacterium, Halococcus can survive under extreme saline conditions. All of them are not fossils because many forms are still surviving and flourishing.

37. (a) : Using Gram stain, developed by Danish physician, Christian Gram in 1884, two kinds of bacteria were noted those species of bacteria that are decolorized by alcohol are called Gram negative and those that retain the stain are called Gram positive. This property of bacteria is related with the structure and compositional differences between the walls of gram positive and gram negative forms. In the cell wall of Gram+ve bacteria, both horizontal and vertical peptide linkages are present, due to which mesh is dense and hence the stain does not come out. Further outer layer of cell wall of Gram +ve bacteria is made of teichoic acid. In the cell wall of Gram-ve bacteria, either horizontal or vertical peptide linkage are present, due to which mesh is loose and hence stain comes out. Further outermost layer of cell wall of Gram-ve bacteria is made of lipopolysaccharides.

38. (a): Transduction is the phenomenon of transfer of genetic material from one bacterial cell to another through the agency of virus. The viruses carry a segment of DNA from one host and infect another host which is different from the first one, the latter may inherit some of the properties of the former host due to transfer of DNA segment through infecting phage.

39. (b): A bacterium divides every 35 minutes.

$\therefore$ In 175 minutes it would be $2^{175/35}$ times $= 2^5$ times.

$\therefore$ In 175 minutes 10^5 bacterium cells would be $= 2^5 \times 10^5 = 32 \times 10^5 / mL$.

40. (b) : E. coli is a Gram-negative, rod shaped, motile or non-motile bacteria. E. coli contains a double stranded DNA as its genetic material. The DNA is not associated with any histone proteins so it is referred to as naked DNA. This DNA is circular with no free ends.

41. (b): Bacteria are responsible for maintaining the conditions of life as the earth by virtue of their powers of decomposition of plant and animal bodies by which the limited supply of CO_2 available for photosynthesis is replenished. Thus, they act as decomposers in the carbon cycle. Bacteria mainly function as decomposers in the carbon cycle.

42. (a): Thermoacidophiles (temperature and acid loving) archaebacteria are found in hot sulphur springs. Although they are microscopic, single-celled organisms, they flourish under conditions which would kill higher organisms. These are aerobic bacteria and have the capacity to oxidize sulphur to H_2SO_4 at high temperature and high acidity (pH = 2.0). Some of them are also able to reduce sulphur to H_2S under anaerobic conditions. As a rule, they grow best between 80° C and 100°C and several species do not grow below 80° C.

43. (b)

44. (a): Bacterial cells do not have nucleus. Nuclear material of bacteria lies free in the cell in the form of an irregular, thin fibrillar and circular single molecule of DNA called nucleoid or chromatin body.

45. (b)

46. (a): A few free living bacteria are able to pick up dinitrogen from the soil atmosphere and convert it into organic nitrogenous materials like amino acids, e.g., Azotobacter. Symbiotic nitrogen fixing bacteria of the genus Rhizobium occur in the root nodules of a number of legumes. Root nodules containing symbiotic nitrogen bacteria also occur in Casuarina and Alnus. Leaf nodules containing such bacteria are found in Ardisia. Many cyanobacteria (blue-green algae) fix atmospheric nitrogen due to presence of heterocysts.

47. (b)

48. (c): Bacteria has no nuclear membrane hence it is called as nucleoid. The genetic material is referred to as genophore. Genophore is the bacterial chromosome. It has a double stranded circular supercoiled DNA. DNA has about 10,000 genes in E.coli. Double stranded DNA in bacteria is without histones.

49. (a): E. coli bacteria acts as a human symbionts and it is found in human intestine, synthesize vitamin K and B and also help in food fermentation. It is easily cultured in any nutrient medium in the laboratory.

50. (a): In sexual reproduction, syngamy and meiotic division takes place but in bacteria, during sexual reproduction there is no formation of gametes hence no syngamy and reduction division occurs, bacteria lack alternation of generation. Conjugation and exchange of genetic material takes place in bacteria.

51. (a): Chemosynthetic bacteria do not derive energy directly or indirectly from sun. The source of energy of these bacteria is inorganic substances. They utilise the energy liberated by oxidation of inorganic compounds and synthesize organic compounds.

52. (a)

53. (b): All prokaryotic organisms come under Kingdom Monera. Escherichia coli is a bacterium. Monera includes bacteria, mycoplasmas, cyanobacteria (blue green algae) and actinomycetes.

54. (a): Some of bacteria are autotrophic and vast majority are heterotrophic. Slime moulds are classified under Kingdom Protista. Mycoplasma completely lack a cell wall.

55. (b): Diatoms are the most common form of phytoplankton in the ocean. They have the pigment chlorophyll which helps in photosynthesis. Since, they are the primary producers of the aquatic food chain and the marine ecosystem depends on them. They are called chief producers in the oceans.

56. (d): Ciliates differ from other protozoans in having two types of nuclei : macronucleus and micronucleus (nuclear dimorphism). E.g., Paramecium has macronucleus which controls metabolic activities as well as growth and micronucleus that takes part in reproduction.

57. (a): Diatoms are marine or freshwater unicellular organisms which have cell walls (frustules) composed of pectin impregnated with silica and consisting of two halves, one overlapping the other. The siliceous frustules of diatoms do not decay easily.

58. (d): Protista is a kingdom of unicellular eukaryotic organisms. It includes photosynthetic protists (dinoflagellates, chrysophytes and euglenoids), consumer-decomposer protists (slime moulds) and protozoan protists.

59.(c) :Chrysophytes include diatoms and desmids. The body of diatoms is covered by a transparent siliceous shell (silica deposited in cell wall) known as frustule. The frustule is made of two valves, epitheca and hypotheca, which fit together like a soap box.

60. (b): Escherichia coli (bacterium) is not an example of eukaryotic cell. It is a typical example of prokaryotic cell.

61. (a): Slime moulds are peculiar protists that normally take the form of amoebae, but under certain conditions develop fruiting bodies that release spores, superficially similar to the sporangia of fungi. The order physarales include Physarum species. The fruiting bodies (sporangia) are characterized by the presence of abundant amount of calcium salt. The order comprises 142 species which are placed under 12 genera. Physarum polycephalum is the best known. The somatic phase is multinucleate, diploid holocarpic plasmodium which is the product of syngamy.

62. (d): Until 1907, auxospore formation was regarded as asexual process but now it is considered as an act of sexual process. The auxospores may be autogamous, isogamous, anisogamous or oogamous. Their pattern of formation differs in pennate and centric diatoms.

Formation of hormogonia is the common method of reproduction in Nostoc which are produced by accidental breaking of trichome into several pieces. It may also be formed by death and decay of ordinary intercalary cells. Soon, the hormogonium escapes from mucilage and grows into a new filament and then into a new colony.

63. (d): Amoeba is a fresh water protozoan containing contractile vacuole that is meant for osmoregulation. When Amoeba is placed in a marine water, then the water from the contractile vacuole will move out resulting in decrease in size of it. Contractile vacuole will increase in size if it is placed in hypotonic solution. Water will enter into contractile vacuole, thus increasing its size and ultimately it will burst and disappear.

64. (a): Amoeba forms a cyst and reproduces by multiple fission, during adverse environmental conditions. The animal secretes a three-layered, protective, chitinous cyst around it and becomes inactive. Inside the cyst, the nucleus repeatedly divides to form several daughter nuclei, which arrange themselves near the periphery. Each daughter nucleus becomes enveloped by a small amount of cytoplasm, thus forming a daughter Amoeba, called amoebula or pseudopodiospore. When favourable conditions arrive, the cyst breaks off liberating the young pseudopodiospores, each with fine pseudopodia. They feed and grow rapidly to become adults and lead an independent life.

65. (d): Dimorphic nucleus means two types of nuclei are present in P. caudatum - large macronucleus and small micronucleus. The macronucleus is roughly kidney-shaped and with inconspicuous nuclear membrane. Macronucleus is the somatic or vegetative nucleus and controls the day-to-day metabolic activities of the cell. The micronucleus is lodged in a depression on the surface of the macronucleus. It is usually spherical, with a nuclear membrane and with diploid number of chromosomes. It controls the reproductive activities of the organism. Amoeba, Trypanosoma and Plasmodium have only one nucleus.

66. (a): The function of contractile vacuole is osmoregulatory. Water in freshwater protozoan enters the organism by endosmosis during feeding. If the organism does not possess a mechanism to get rid of this excess water, it will swell to the point of rupture and dissolution. The mechanism which is assumed to effect water regulation is the contractile vacuole. The vacuole periodically increases in volume (diastole) to get filled with water and contracts (systole) to discharge its water content to the surrounding environment.

67. (a): Euglena possesses the characteristics of both plant and animal. It has chlorophyll, thus it is autotrophic like plants. In contrast to this, it has flagellated locomotion like animals.

68. (a)

69. (c): In Amoeba and Paramecium, osmoregulation occurs through contractile vacoule. Osmoregulation is a phenomenon in which contractile vacuole plays an important role in maintaining the water balance of the cell. Paramecium contains two contractile vacuoles which have fixed position. One contractile vacuole is present near the anterior end while another is present towards posterior end of the body. Each contractile vacuole is surrounded by 5-12 radial canals. Excess of water is transferred from the cytoplasm to the radial canals. The latter pour water into the contractile vacuole. The contractile vacuole expels water outside the body. Thus the contractile vacuoles and radial canals are for osmoregulation. In Amoeba the endoplasm, at its posterior end, contains a single, clear rounded and pulsating contractile vacuole, filled with a watery fluid and enclosed by a unit membrane. Surrounding this membrane is a region containing many tiny feeder vacuoles and mitochondria. It helps in the osmoregulatory and excretory activities of the animal.

70 (c)

71. (a): Trypanosoma is polymorphic, i.e., it has more than one form. It has at least four forms that are recognized on the basis of the positions of kinetoplast and blepharoplast and the course taken by the flagellum. Two or more such forms occur either in one or both the hosts in the life cycles of various species of Trypanosoma. These forms are

(i) Leishmanial (amastigote) : Round or oval form with a nucleus, blepharoplast and kinetoplast. Flagellum reduced and fibril-like, embedded in cytoplasm.

(ii) Leptomonad (promastigote) : Body elongate, nucleus large and anteriorly located blepharoplast and kinetoplast. Flagellum short and unattached.

(iii) Crithidial (epimastigote) : Body elongate blepharoplast and kinetoplast placed immediately anterior to nucleus. Undulating membrane inconspicuous.

(iv) Trypanosomid (trypomastigote) : Body elongate and slender. Blepharoplast and kinetoplast situated at or near posterior end. Undulating membrane conspicuous.

Trypanosoma is digenetic, i.e., it completes its life cycle in two hosts. It is an obligate parasite and is pathogenic.

72. (a): Paramecium contains a single large macronucleus and one small micronucleus. The macronucleus controls metabolism such as feeding and maintenance, whereas the micronucleus takes an important role in reproduction and stores genetic information, hence it is also termed as reproductive nucleus whereas macronucleus is termed as vegetative nucleus.

73. (b)

74. (c) : Some of the cyanobacteria like Nostoc can fix nitrogen in specialised cells called heterocysts. Fusion of two nuclei is called karyogamy. Organisms that depend on living plants and animals are called parasites.

75 (a) : Yeast is a non-mycelial unicellular ascomycetes fungus.

76. (a)

77. (a) : Saccharomyces, i.e., yeast is a eukaryote unicellular fungus. Prokaryotes include bacteria (Mycobacterium), cyanobacteria (Nostoc and Oscillatoria), mycoplasma and archaebacteria.

78. (c) : In Agaricus, (member of Basidiomycetes), basidium commonly produces four meiospores or basidiospores exogenously. Neurospora (member of Ascomycetes) produces ascospores, endogenously inside the fruiting body, ascus. Alternaria (member of Deuteromycetes) does not produce any sexual spores. Saccharomyces (member of Ascomycetes) produces ascospores endogenously.

79. (b) : Cell wall in fungi is composed of chitin, a polysaccharide comprising N-acetyl-D-glucosamine (a derivative of glucose).

80.(a) : Eubacteria are also called true bacteria.

81. (c) : Fungal cell wall contains chitin or fungal cellulose along with other polysaccharides, proteins, lipids and a number of other substances.

82. (c) : Deuteromycetes are the imperfect fungi which include all those fungi in which sexual stage is either absent or not known. Some members are saprophytes or parasites while a large number of them are decomposers of litter and help in mineral cycling. E.g., Colletotrichum, Helminthosporium, etc.

83. (a) : Morels are Ascomycetes with edible ascocarps that have fleshy sponge-like conical cap or pileus and a stalk like stipe, e.g., Morchella esculenta. Truffles are also edible members of Ascomycetes with tuber-like subterranean ascocarps that are often dug out with the help of trained dogs and pigs, e.g., Tuber aestivum.

84. (d) : Alternaria is a Deuteromycetes member which are also known as fungi imperfecti. Their perfect stages (sexually reproducing stages) are either absent or not known. Now, Alternaria belongs to Ascomycetes.

85. (b) : Amanita muscaria is a member of Class Basidiomycetes. It is a poisonous mushroom and has hallucinogenic properties. It produces a toxic alkaloid, muscarine, which mimics the effects of acetylcholine and binds to muscarinic receptors as well as ibotenic acid which also binds to different receptors. This leads to excitation of neurons bearing these receptors and hence hallucinations.

86. (b) : Fungi are achlorophyllous, heterotrophic, spore forming, non-vascular, eukaryotic organisms which often contain chitin or fungal cellulose in their walls. Hence, their cell wall is rigid.

87.(c) : The pathogen Microsporum is genus of Kingdom Fungi that causes diseases of skin and hair in humans and animals like dog, cat, monkey.

Ringworm is caused by the dermatophyte fungi- species of Microsporum, Trichophyton and Epidermophyton.

Rhizopus, a black bread mould belongs to group zygomycetes of Kingdom Fungi.

88. (a) : Protista include all unicellular and colonial eukaryotes except those of green and red algae. The protistan cells aretypicallyeukaryotichaving membranebound organelles like mitochondria, chloroplasts, Golgi bodies, endoplasmic reticulum, nucleus, etc. Protista is commonly known as kingdom of unicellular eukaryotes. Kingdom Fungi contains achlorophyllous, spore producing, heterotrophic, multicellular or multinucleate eukaryotic organisms (unicellular yeasts are also included amongst fungi because their sexual reproduction is similar to that of some fungi). Monerans are basically unicellular prokaryotes. Archaea (ancient bacteria) are also a type of monerans which live in primitive environment like high temperature, high salt content, acidic pH, etc.

89. (b) : Streptococcus is a bacteria which is included under Kingdom Monera. Monerans have prokaryotic cell organisation in which membrane bound organelles like mitochondria, E.R., Golgi bodies, etc., are absent. All the other three i.e., Sacharomyces (a fungus), Chlamydomonas (an algae) and Plasmodium (a protozoan protist) are eukaryotes containing true membrane bound organelles.

90. (c) : Black stem rust is caused by Puccinia graminis tritici. The genus Puccinia includes 700 species, which cause rust diseases of many economic plants such as wheat, barley, oats, etc.

91. (d) : Late blight of potato disease is caused by Phytophthora infestans. It is a phycomycetes fungus. Alternaria solani is the causal organism of early blight of potato disease.

92. (d) : The Cyathus is known as bird's nest fungi, and Lycoperdon is called puffballs. Both these fungi belong to the group of club fungi or basidiomycetes. These fungi produce spores inside club shaped fruit bodies called basidium. Typically basidium has 4 basidiospores produced exogenously. Peziza, Morchella and Claviceps belong to ascomycetes (produce ascospores in ascocarps). Mushroom are basidiomycetes fungi.

93. (c) : Mucor is a filamentous fungus found in the humus of soil decaying fruits, vegetables. It is commonly known as black mould. Most of the Mucor sp. are unable to grow at 37° C and the strains isolated from human infections are usually one of the few thermotolerant Mucor sp. Colonies of Mucor grow rapidly at 25-30° C, humidity about 90-95 % and quickly cover the surface of the agar. It requires moist and shady place for its growth. Many sp. of Mucor are responsible for causing rotting of fruit and vegetables. A few sp. e.g., Mucor pusillus are pathogenic to man.

94. (a) : Loose smut of wheat infects the healthy wheat plants at the time of flowering. Here chlamydospores, from smutted heads (blown by the wind) germinate on the stigmas and produce infection threads, infecting the ovaries and stigma. Ultimately, the fungus continues to grow within the embryo, as the seed matures. With the germination of these infected seeds, internal dormant fungal mycelium resumes its activity again. In covered smut of Barley, fungal spores are liberated out only by rupturing the wall of the grains, specially at the time of threshing. This type of infection takes place during the young seedling stage. Seedling infection occurs in covered smut of Barley. Shoot infection occurs in corn smut.

95. (a,b) : Penicillium and Aspergillus both produce toxins in stored seeds and grains. Aspergillus produces aflatoxin in fruits, vegetables, food grains and seeds, etc. Penicillium produces yellow rice toxins in rice, barley and corns.

96. (a) : Black stem rust is caused by Puccinia graminis tritici. The genus Puccinia includes 700 species, which cause rust diseases of many economic plants such as wheat, barley, oats, etc.

97. (b) : Association between roots of higher plants, e.g., pine, birch and fungal hyphae is called mycorrhiza. It exhibits the phenomenon of symbiosis. Here both the organisms in association are mutually benefitted. In this, fungal hyphae take nutrition from the plant and in return increase surface area for absorption of water and minerals for the plant.

98. (b) : Puccinia graminis tritici belongs to basidiomycotina and causes black rust of wheat. It is internal obligate parasite. It is found everywhere, where wheat is grown. The teleutospores of the fungus causes the rust. They are produced inside teleutosori. These telia form elongated, dark brown to black pustules on the surface of stems and leaves of the wheat. Albugo candida causes white rust of crucifers. Melampsora lini causes linseed rust. Claviceps purpurea causes ergot of Graminae.

99. (c) : Pseudopodia is the locomotory organ in amoeboid protozoans, e.g., Amoeba. Flagellated protozoans possess flagella for locomotion, e.g, Trypanosoma. In sporozoans, locomotory organelles (cilia, flagella, pseudopodia, etc.) are absent, e.g., Plasmodium. Ciliated protozoans possess cilia as locomotory organelles, e.g., Paramecium.

100. (a) : Mycoplasma (Kingdom-Monera) are the simplest and smallest free living prokaryotes which are devoid of a cell wall. Plasma membrane forms the outer boundary of the cell of mycoplasma. Nostoc is a cyanobacterium (Kingdom- Monera), in which cell wall comprises of peptidoglycans. Aspergillus is a fungus (Kingdom-Fungi) in which cell wall is mainly made of chitin. Funaria is a bryophyte (Kingdom-Plantae) in which cell wall is cellulosic in nature.

101. (c) : Anabaena is a prokaryotic organism. It is a cyanobacteria (blue-green algae) which belongs to Kingdom Monera. Like all other prokaryotes, it lacks a true nucleus and other cell organelles.

102. (d) : Penicillium and Agaricus are fungi while Volvox is an alga. All three are eukaryotes thus have a membrane bound nucleus. Nostoc is a cyanobacterium, i.e., prokaryote, so it lacks true nucleus, thus nuclear membrane is absent.

103. (b) : The true fungi or the eumycetes are special types of achlorophyllous thallophytic organisms living a parasitic or a saprophytic mode of existence; they are always heterophytes and never autophytes. They depend on others for food, but all other groups as algae, bryophytes and pteridophytes are chlorophyll containing green plants that are autotrophic.

104. (b) : Kingdom Monera consists of prokaryotic organisms, characterised by absence of nuclear envelope around nucleus and absence of membrane-bound cell organelles.

105. (b) : Gorgonia (sea-fan) is an animal belonging to Phylum Coelenterata. All animals lack cell wall.

106. (b) : Viroids are free RNA particles that lack protein coat. They are infectious agents smaller than viruses.

107. (b)

108. (d) : Infective constituent in the viruses is the genetic material, i.e., either DNA or RNA.

109. (c) :

110. (b) : RNA of viroid has low molecular weight.

111. (c) : Viroids are infectious RNA particles which were discovered by T.O. Diener (1971). These are devoid of protein coat and cause diseases in plants only, e.g., potato spindle tuber, chrysanthemum stunt, etc.

112. (b) Tobacco mosaic virus is a RNA virus that causes tobacco mosaic disease. It has single stranded coiled RNA molecule as its genetic material a part of which hangs outside the protein coat. Protein coat consists of approximately 2130 capsomeres which are helically arranged to form a hollow cylinder of about 4 nm diameter.

113. (a) Viruses are nucleoprotein entities which are able to utilize synthetic machinery of a living cell of the host organism for its multiplication which does not involve growth and division. They have either RNA or DNA as genetic material and a protein coat.

114. (b) In viruses, three architectural forms are found helical (elongated body, e.g., TMV), cuboidal (short broad body with rhombic, rounded, polyhedral shape, e.g.. poliovirus) and binal (with both cuboidal and helical parts, e.g., T_2 phage).

115. (c) Yeast is a group of unicellular fungi of the class ascomycetes. They occur as single cell or as a group or chain of cells. Yeast of the genus Saccharomyces ferments sugar and are used to make bread and beer.

116. (a) The nucleic acid of a virus is surrounded by a protein coat called the capsid. The capsid is composed of protein subunits called capsomeres. In some viruses, the capsid is covered by an envelope, which usually consists of some combination of lipids, proteins and carbohydrates.

117. (c)

118. (d)

119. (a) Lichens are peculiar dual organisms produced by the intimate association of two organisms: a fungus and an alga. The association between the two organisms is symbiosis. Both the organisms are mutually benefitted in this association and are dependent on each other. The algal cell photosynthesizes with the help of chloroplast. Therefore lichens are autotrophic. A part of these manufactured carbohydrates are used by the alga in its nutrition, the rest is supplied to the fungal partner. The fungus in turn provides water and nutrients which it absorbs from the soil using the rhizoidal hyphae. Thus both the partners get benefitted from each other. The algal partner is called phycobiont and the fungal partner is called mycobiont.

120. (a) Retroviruses contain RNA as genetic material and this RNA is converted to DNA using enzyme reverse transcriptase.

121. (c) Viruses like bacteriophage T4 undergo lytic cycle that involves lysis of bacteria. The replication cycle of bacteriophage T4 consists of following phases -

(i) Adsorption of the phage to bacterial or host cell. Then the viral genetic material penetrates into the host cell.

(ii) Eclipse period involves the synthesis of new

phage DNA and proteins.

(iii) Maturation involves the assembly of phage DNA into the protein coat.

(iv) Lysis of host cell occurs and releases infective progeny phases.

122. (d)

123. (c) Viruses contain a protein coat known as capsid which encloses a single type of nucleic acid, either RNA or DNA. They do not have enzymes for protein synthesis. They multiply only inside the living host cell and for multiplication they take over the machinery of the host cell. Thus viruses are obligatory intercellular parasites. They lack cell division and enzymes for protein synthesis. They do not have cell organelles like mitochondria, Golgi complex, lysosomes, ribosomes, etc., so they cannot live or reproduce separately.

124. (d)

125. (c) Cauliflower mosaic virus contain dsDNA. It is circular and shows semidiscontinuous type of replication.

126. (c) Viruses always contain only a single kind of nucleic acid. It can be either DNA or RNA. The nucleic acid may occur as single or double strands.

127. (a) Lichens are peculiar dual organisms produced by the intimate association of two organisms - a fungus and an alga. The association between the two organisms is called symbiosis. On the basis of fungal partner, lichens are of two types :

(i) Ascolichens: In which ascomycetes member is the fungal partner. Further in ascolichens, algal partner is mostly member of green algae and rarely blue-green algae.

(ii) Basidiolichens : Where basidiomycetes member is fungal partner. In them algal partner is generally blue-green algae. In 80% cases algal partner is member of green algae or chlorophyceae and in 20% cases, blue-green algae or myxophyceae.

Important members of green algae found in lichens are: Trebouxia, Pleurococcus, Trentepohlia and Cladophora.

128. (b) Influenza viruses are spherical in shape measuring about 800–1200Å in diameter. It has a protein capsid that encloses a single stranded RNA. The single stranded RNA is generally linear and constitutes about 10% of the virus particle. RNA is genetic material in other viruses like poliomyelitis, foot and mouth disease virus and tobacco mosaic virus, etc.

129. (a) Lichens grow by extending their thallus outwards from either tips or edges. They grow very slowly. Rates of growth can vary from 0.5 mm per year to 500 mm per year. This slow growth rate equates with their long life.

130. (a) Tobacco Mosaic Virus is a ribovirus and contains single stranded RNA.

131. (b) Lichens are found in Arctic Tundra region where no other plant can grow. Lichens prefer to grow in pollution free environment. They are often used as a indicator of pollution and also they are very sensitive to SO2. They are first to die in a polluted environment (more SO2).

132. (c)

Chapter : 03

PLANT KINGDOM

INTRODUCTION

1. Phylogenetic system of classification is based on **(2009)**
(a) morphological features
(b) chemical constituents
(c) floral characters
(d) evolutionary relationships.

2. Phenetic classification of organisms is based on **(2004,2003)**
(a) observable characteristics of existing organisms
(b) the ancestral lineage of existing organisms
(c) dendrogram based on DNA characteristics
(d) sexual characteristics.

3. A system of classification, in which a large number of traits are considered, is **(1999)**
(a) natural system
(b) phylogenetic system
(c) artificial system
(d) synthetic system.

4. Phylogenetic classification is one which is based on **(1994)**
(a) overall similarities
(b) utilitarian system
(c) habits of plants
(d) common evolutionary descent.

5. System of classification used by Linnaeus was **(1989)**
(a) natural system
(b) artificial system
(c) phylogenetic system
(d) asexual system.

6. Artificial system of classification was first used by **(1989)**
(a) Linnaeus (b) De Candolle
(c) Pliny the Edler (d) Bentham and Hooker.

7. Classification given by Bentham and Hooker is **(1988)**
(a) artificial (b) natural
(c) phylogenetic (d) numerical.

ALGAE

8. Which of the following is incorrectly matched? **(2022)**
(a) Ectocarpus - Fucoxanthin
(b) Ulothrix - Mannitol
(c) Porphyra - Floridean starch
(d) Volvox - Starch

9. Hydrocolloid carrageen is obtained from **(2022)**
(a) Chlorophyceae and Phaeophyceae
(b) Phaeophyceae and Rhodophyceae
(c) Rhodophyceae only
(d) Phaeophyceae only.

10. Which of the following algae produce Carrageen? **(2021)**
(a) Blue-green algae(b) Green algae
(c) Brown algae(d) Red algae

11. Which of the following algae contains mannitol as reserve food material? **(2021)**
(a) Ulothrix (b) Ectocarpus
(c) Gracilaria (d) Volvox

12. Floridean starch has structure similar to **(2020)**
(a) starch and cellulose
(b) amylopectin and glycogen
(c) mannitol and algin
(d) laminarin and cellulose.

13. Which of the following pairs is of unicellular algae? **(2020)**
(a) Laminaria and Sargassum
(b) Gelidium and Gracilaria
(c) Anabaena and Volvox
(d) Chlorella and Spirulina

14. An example of colonial alga is ***(2017)***
(a) Volvox (b) Ulothrix
(c) Spirogyra (d) Chlorella.

15. Which one of the following statements is wrong? ***(NEET-II 2016)***
(a) Algae increase the level of dissolved oxygen in the immediate environment.
(b) Algin is obtained from red algae, and carrageenan from brown algae.
(c) Agar-agar is obtained from Gelidium and Gracilaria.
(d) Laminaria and Sargassum are used as food.

16. Which one of the following statements is wrong? ***(2015 Cancelled)***
(a) Chlorella and Spirulina are used as space food.
(b) Mannitol is stored food in Rhodophyceae.
(c) Algin and carrageenan are products of algae.
(d) Agar-agar is obtained from Gelidium and Gracilaria.

17. Male gametes are flagellated in ***(2015 Cancelled)***
(a) Ectocarpus (b) Spirogyra
(c) Polysiphonia (d) Anabaena.

18. Which one of the following is wrong about Chara? ***(2014)***
(a) Upper oogonium and lower round antheridium
(b) Globule and nucule present on the same plant
(c) Upper antheridium and lower oogonium
(d) Globule is male reproductive structure

19. Which one of the following shows isogamy with non-flagellated gametes? ***(2014)***
(a) Sargassum (b) Ectocarpus
(c) Ulothrix (d) Spirogyra

20. Select the wrong statement. ***(2013)***
(a) In oomycetes, female gamete is smaller and motile, while male gamete is larger and nonmotile.
(b) Chlamydomonas exhibits both isogamy and anisogamy and Fucus shows oogamy.
(c) Isogametes are similar in structure, function and behaviour.
(d) Anisogametes differ either in structure, function or behaviour.

21. Isogamous condition with non-flagellated gametes is found in ***(2013)***
(a) Volvox (b) Fucus
(c) Chlamydomonas (d) Spirogyra.

22. Monoecious plant of Chara shows occurrence of ***(2013)***
(a) upper antheridium and lower oogonium on the same plant
(b) upper oogonium and lower antheridium on the same plant
(c) antheridiophore and archegoniophore on the same plant
(d) stamen and carpel on the same plant.

23. Which one of the following is wrongly matched? ***(Karnataka NEET 2013)***
(a) Spirogyra - Motile gametes
(b) Sargassum - Chlorophyll
(c) Basidiomycetes - Puffballs
(d) Nostoc - Water blooms

24. Algae have cell wall made up of ***(2010)***
(a) cellulose, galactans and mannans
(b) hemicellulose, pectins and proteins
(c) pectins, cellulose and proteins
(d) cellulose, hemicellulose and pectins.

25. Mannitol is the stored food in ***(2009)***
(a) Porphyra (b) Fucus
(c) Gracilaria (d) Chara.

26. If you are asked to classify the various algae into distinct groups, which of the following characters you should choose? ***(2007)***
(a) Nature of stored food materials in the cell
(b) Structural organization of thallus
(c) Chemical composition of the cell wall
(d) Types of pigments present in the cell

27. Sexual reproduction in Spirogyra is an advanced feature because it shows ***(2003)***
(a) different sizes of motile sex organs
(b) same size of motile sex organs
(c) morphologically different sex organs
(d) physiologically differentiated sex organs.

28. A student observed an algae with chlorophyll a, d and phycoerythrin, it should belong to ***(2000)***
(a) Phaeophyta (b) Rhodophyta
(c) Chlorophyta (d) Bacillariophyta.

29. Ulothrix can be described as a ***(1998)***
(a) filamentous alga lacking flagellated reproductive stages
(b) membranous alga producing zoospores
(c) filamentous alga with flagellated reproductive stages
(d) non-motile colonial alga lacking zoospores.

30. An alga, very rich in protein, is ***(1997)***
(a) Chlorella (b) Nostoc
(c) Spirogyra (d) Ulothrix.

31. Ulothrix filaments produce **(1997)**
(a) heterogametes (b) basidiospores
(c) isogametes (d) anisogametes.

32. Brown algae is characterised by the presence of ***(1997)***
(a) fucoxanthin (b) haematochrome
(c) phycocyanin (d) phycoerythrin.

33. The pyrenoids are made up of ***(1995)***
(a) proteinaceous centre and starchy sheath
(b) core of nucleic acid surrounded by protein sheath
(c) core of protein surrounded by fatty sheath
(d) core of starch surrounded by sheath of protein.

34. In Chlorophyceae, the mode of sexual reproduction is **(1994)**
(a) isogamy (b) anisogamy
(c) oogamy (d) all of these.

35. Pyrenoids are the centres for formation of ***(1993)***
(a) Porphyra (b) enzymes
(c) fat (d) starch.

36. Chloroplast of Chlamydomonas is ***(1993)***
(a) stellate (b) cup-shaped
(c) collar-shaped (d) spiral.

37. In Ulothrix/Spirogyra, reduction division (meiosis) occurs at the time of ***(1993)***
(a) gamete formation
(b) zoospore formation
(c) zygospore germination
(d) vegetative reproduction.

38. The common mode of sexual reproduction in Chlamydomonas is ***(1991)***
(a) isogamous (b) anisogamous
(c) oogamous (d) hologamous.

BRYOPHYTES

39. Given below are two statements : ***(2023)***
One is labelled as Assertion (A) and the other is labelled as Reason (R).

Assertion (A): The first state of gametophyte in the life cycle of moss is protonema stage.

Reason (R) : Protonema develops directly from spores produced in capsule.

In the light of the above statements, choose the most appropriate answer from the options given below:

(a) (A) is correct but (R) is not correct.
(b) (A) is not correct but (R) is correct.
(c) Both (A) and (R) are correct and (R) is the correct explanation of (A).
(d) Both (A) and (R) are correct but (R) is not the correct explanation of (A).

40. Gemmae are present in ***(2021)***
(a) some liverworts (b) mosses
(c) pteridophytes (d) some gymnosperms.

41. Which one is wrongly matched? ***(2018)***
(a) Uniflagellate gametes - Polysiphonia
(b) Biflagellate zoospores - Brown algae
(c) Gemma cups - Marchantia
(d) Unicellular organism - Chlorella

42. Which of the following is responsible for peat formation? ***(2014)***
(a) Marchantia (b) Riccia
(c) Funaria (d) Sphagnum

43. Which one of the following is common to multicellular fungi, filamentous algae and protonema of mosses? ***(2012)***
(a) Diplontic life cycle
(b) Members of Kingdom Plantae
(c) Mode of nutrition
(d) Multiplication by fragmentation

44. Examine the given figure and select the correct option giving all the four parts (A, B, C and D) rightly identified. ***(Mains 2011)***

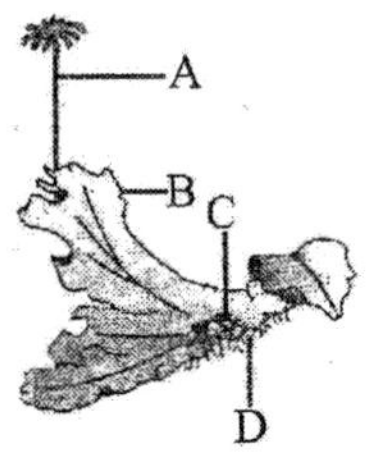

	A	B	C	D
(a)	Archego-niophore	Female thallus	Gemma cup	Rhizoids
(b)	Archego-niophore	Female thallus	Bud	Foot
(c)	Seta	Sporo-phyte	Proto nema	Rhizoids
(d)	Antherid-iophore	Male-thallus	Globule	Roots

45. Spore dissemination in some liverworts is aided by ***(2007)***
(a) indusium (b) calyptra
(c) peristome teeth (d) elaters.

46. Peat moss is used as a packing material for sending flowers and live plants to distant places because ***(2006)***
(a) it serves as a disinfectant
(b) it is easily available
(c) it is hygroscopic
(d) it reduces transpiration.

47. In a moss, the sporophyte ***(2006)***
(a) manufactures food for itself, as well as for the gametophyte
(b) is partially parasitic on the gametophyte
(c) produces gametes that give rise to the gametophyte
(d) arises from a spore produced from the gametophyte.

48. Bryophytes comprise ***(1999)***
(a) dominant phase of gametophyte which produces spores
(b) small sporophyte phase and generally parasitic on gametophyte
(c) sporophyte is of longer duration
(d) dominant phase of sporophyte which is parasitic.

49. Which of the following is true about bryophytcs? ***(1999)***
(a) They are thalloid.
(b) They posses archegonia.
(c) They contain chloroplast.
(d) All of these

50. Bryophytes are dependent on water, because ***(1998)***
(a) water is essential for their vegetative propagation
(b) the sperms can easily reach upto egg in the archegonium
(c) archegonium has to remain filled with water for fertilization
(d) water is essential for fertilization for their homosporous nature.

51. Bryophytes can be separated from algae, because they ***(1997)***
(a) possess archegonia
(b) contain chloroplast
(c) are thalloid forms
(d) have no conducting tissue.

52. The plant body of moss (Funaria) is ***(1995)***
(a) completely sporophyte
(b) predominantly gametophyte with sporophyte
(c) completely gametophyte
(d) predominantly sporophyte with gametophyte.

53. In bryophytes *(1994)*
(a) both generations are independent
(b) gametophytes are dependent upon sporophytes
(c) sporophytes complete their life cycle
(d) sporophytes are dependent upon gametophytes.

54. Protonema occurs in the life cycle of *(1993, 1990)*
(a) Riccia (b) Funaria
(c) Anthoceros (d) Spirogya.

55. Bryophytes are amphibians because *(1991)*
(a) they require a layer of water for carrying out sexual reproduction
(b) they occur in damp places
(c) they are mostly aquatic
(d) all the above.

56. Moss peristome takes part in *(1990)*
(a) spore dispersal (b) photosynthesis
(c) protection (d) absorption.

PTERIDOPHYTES

57. Genera like Selaginella and Salvinia produce two kinds of spores. Such plants are known as *(2021)*
(a) Air currents carry the pollen
(b) homosorus
(c) heterosorus
(d) homosporous.

58. Strobili cones are found in *(2020)*
(a) Salvinia (b) Pteris
(c) Marchantia (d) Equisetum.

59. In bryophytes and pteridophytes, transport of male gametes requires *(NEET-I 2016)*
(a) birds (b) water
(c) wind (d) insects.

60. Syngamy can occur outside the body of the organism in *(Karnataka NEET 2013)*
(a) mosses (b) algae
(c) ferns (d) fungi.

61. The plant body is thalloid in *(Karnataka NEET 2013)*
(a) Sphagnum (b) Salvinia
(c) Marchantia (d) Funaria.

62. Compared with the gametophytes of the bryophytes, the gametophytes of vascular plants tend to be *(2011)*
(a) smaller but to have larger sex organs
(b) larger but to have smaller sex organs
(c) larger and to have larger sex organs
(d) smaller and to have smaller sex organs.

63. Archegoniophore is present in *(2011)*
(a) Marchantia (b) Chara
(c) Adiantum (d) Funaria.

64. Selaginella and Salvinia are considered to represent a significant step toward evolution of seed habit because *(Mains 2011)*
(a) female gametophyte is free and gets dispersed like seeds
(b) female gametophyte lacks archegonia
(c) megaspores possess endosperm and embryo surrounded by seed coat
(d) embryo develops in female gametophyte which is retained on parent sporophyte.

65. Which one of the following is considered important in the development of seed habit? *(2009)*
(a) Heterospory
(b) Haplontic life cycle
(c) Free-living gametophyte
(d) Dependent sporophyte

66. Which one of the following is heterosporous? *(2008)*
(a) Adiantum (b) Equisetum
(c) Dryopteris (d) Salvinia

67. In the prothallus of a vascular cryptogam, the antherozoids and eggs mature at different times. As a result *(2007)*
(a) there is high degree of sterility
(b) one can conclude that the plant is apomictic
(c) self fertilization is prevented
(d) there is no change in success rate of fertilization.

68. Plants reproducing by spores such as mosses and ferns are grouped under the general term ***(2003)***
(a) cryptogams (b) bryophytes
(c) sporophytes (d) thallophytes.

69. In ferns, meiosis takes place at the time of ***(2000)***
(a) spore formation (b) spore germination
(c) gamete formation
(d) antheridia and archegonia formation.

70. Dichotomous branching is found in ***(1999)***
(a) liverworts (b) pteridophytes
(c) fern (d) Funaria.

71. The walking fern is so named because ***(1998)***
(a) it propagates vegetatively by its leaf tips
(b) it knows how to walk by itself
(c) its spores are able to walk
(d) it is dispersed through the agency of walking animals.

72. Which of the following plant kingdom is called 'amphibians'? ***(1996)***
(a) Pteridophyta (b) Thallophyta
(c) Tracheophyta (d) Bryophyta

73. Pteridophytes differ from bryophytes and thallophytes in having ***(1993)***
(a) vascular tissues
(b) motile antherozoids
(c) archegonia
(d) alternation of generations.

74. Pteridophytes differ from mosses/bryophytes in possessing ***(1993)***
(a) independent gametophyte
(b) well developed vascular system
(c) archegonia
(d) flagellate spermatozoids.

75. The plant group that produces spores and embryo but lacks vascular tissues and seeds is ***(1992)***
(a) Pteridophyta (b) Rhodophyta
(c) Bryophyta (d) Phaeophyta.

76. Sperms of both Funaria and Pteris were released together near the archegonia of Pteris. Only its sperms enter the archegonia as ***(1989)***
(a) Pteris archegonia repel Funaria sperms
(b) Funaria sperms get killed by Pteris sperms
(c) Funaria sperms are less mobile
(d) Pteris archegonia release chemical to attract its sperms.

77. Evolutionary important character of Selaginella is ***(1989)***
(a) heterosporous nature
(b) rhizophore
(c) strobili (d) ligule.

GYMNOSPERMS

78. Given below are two statements :
One is labelled as Assertion (A) and the other is labelled as Reason (R).

Assertion (A) : In gymnosperms, the pollen grains are released from the microsporangium and carried by air currents.

Reason (R) : Air currents carry the pollen grains to the mouth of the archegonia where the male gametes are discharged and pollen tube is not formed. ***(2023)***

In the light of the above statements, choose the correct answer from the options given below :

(a) (A) is true but (R) is false.
(b) (A) is false but R is true.
(c) Both (A) and (R) are true and (R) is the correct explanation of (A).
(d) Both (A) and (R) are true but (R) is not the correct explanation of A.

79. Which of the following plants is monoecious? ***(2021)***
(a) Cycas circinalis
(b) Carica papaya
(c) Chara
(d) Marchantia polymorpha

80. Which of the following statements is correct? ***(2018)***

(a) Ovules are not enclosed by ovary wall in gymnosperms.
(b) Selaginella is heterosporous, while Salvinia is homosporous.
(c) Horsetails are gymnosperms.
(d) Stems are usually unbranched in both Cycas and Cedrus.

81. Select the mismatch. ***(2017)***

(a) Cycas- Dioecious
(b) Salvinia- Heterosporous
(c) Equisetum- Homosporous
(d) Pinus - Dioecious

82. Conifers are adapted to tolerate extreme environmental conditions because of ***(NEET-II 2016)***

(a) broad hardy leaves
(b) superficial stomata
(c) thick cuticle
(d) presence of vessels.

83. Select the correct statement. ***(NEET-I 2016)***

(a) Sequoia is one of the tallest trees.
(b) The leaves of gymnosperms are not well adapted to extremes of climate.
(c) Gymnosperms are both homosporous and heterosporous.
(d) Salvinia, Ginkgo and Pinus all are gymnosperms.

84. In which of the following, gametophyte is not independent free living? ***(2015 Cancelled)***

(a) Pteris (b) Pinus
(c) Funaria (d) Marchantia

85. Read the following five statements (λ to E) and select the option with all correct statements.

A. Mosses and lichens are the first organisms to colonise a bare rock.
B. Selaginella is a homosporous pteridophyte.
C. Coralloid roots in Cycas have VAM.
D. Main plant body in bryophytes is gametophytic, whereas in pteridophytes it is sporophytic.
E. In gymnosperms, male and female gametophytes are present within sporangia located on sporophyte. ***(2015 Cancelled)***

(a) A, D and E (b) B, C and E
(c) A, C and D (d) B, C and D

86. Which one is a wrong statement? ***(2015)***

(a) Haploid endosperm is typical feature of Gymnosperms.
(b) Brown algae have chlorophyll a and c and fucoxanthin.
(c) Archegonia are found in Bryophyta, Pteridophyta and Gymnosperms.
(d) Mucor has biflagellate zoospores.

87. Read the following statements (A – E) and answer the question which follows them. ***(2013)***

(A) In liverworts, mosses and ferns gametophytes are free-living.
(B) Gymnosperms and some ferns are heterosporous.
(C) Sexual reproduction in Fucus, Volvox and Albugo is oogamous.
(D) The sporophyte in liverworts is more elaborate than that in mosses.
(E) Both, Pinus and Marchantia are dioecious.
How many of the above statements are correct?

(a) Three (b) Four
(c) One (d) Two

88. What is common in all the three, Funaria, Dryopteris and Ginkgo? ***(Karnataka NEET 2013)***

(a) Presence of archegonia
(b) Well developed vascular tissues
(c) Independent gametophyte
(d) Independent sporophyte

89. Which one of the following is a correct statement? ***(2012)***
(a) Pteridophyte gametophyte has a protonemal and leafy stage.
(b) In gymnosperms, female gametophyte is freeliving.
(c) Antheridiophores and archegoniophores are present in pteridophytes.
(d) Origin of seed habit can be traced in pteridophytes.

90. Cycas and Adiantum resemble each other in having ***(2012)***
(a) seeds (b) motile sperms
(c) cambium (d) vessels.

91. Read the following five statements (A - E) and answer as asked next to them. ***(Mains 2012)***
(A) In Equisetum, the female gametophyte is retained on the parent sporophyte.
(B) In Ginkgo, male gametophyte is not independent.
(C) The sporophyte in Riccia is more developed than that in Polytrichum.
(D) Sexual reproduction in Volvox is isogamous.
(E) The spores of slime moulds lack cell walls.
How many of the above statements are correct?
(a) Two (b) Three (c) Four (d) One

92. Examine the figures A, B, C and D. In which one of the four options all the items A, B, C and D are correct? ***(Mains 2010)***

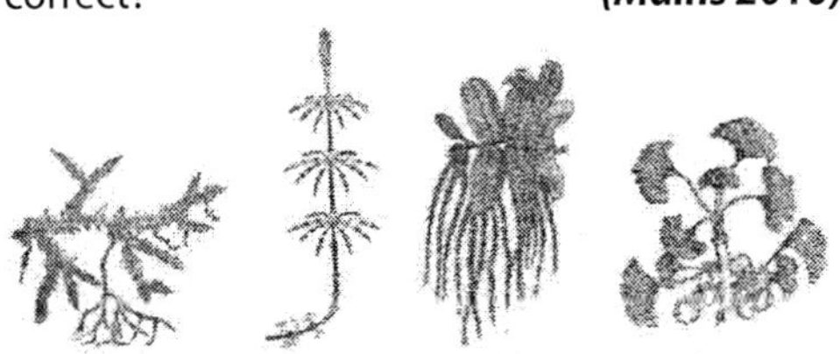

A B C D

	A	B	C	D
(a)	Chara	Marchanta	Fucus	Pinus
(b)	Equisetum	Ginkgo	Selaginella	Lycopodium
(c)	Selaginella	Equisetum	Salvinia	Ginkgo
(d)	Funaria	Adiantum	Salvinia	Riccia

93. Which one of the following is a vascular cryptogam? ***(2009)***
(a) Ginkgo (b) Marchantia
(c) Cedrus (d) Equisetum

94. In which one of the following male and female gametophytes do not have free living independent existence? ***(2008)***
(a) Polytrichum (b) Cedrus
(c) Pteris (d) Funaria

95. In gymnosperms, the pollen chamber represents ***(2007)***
(a) a cavity in the ovule in which pollen grains are stored after pollination
(b) an opening in the megagametophyte through which the pollen tube approaches the egg
(c) the microsporangium in which pollen grains develop
(d) a cell in the pollen grain in which the sperms are formed.

96. Flagellated male gametes are present in all the three of which one of the following sets? ***(2007)***
(a) Zygnema, Saprolegnia and Hydrilla
(b) Fucus, Marsilea and Calotropis
(c) Riccia, Dryopteris and Cycas
(d) Anthoceros, Funaria and Spirogyra

97. Which one of the following pairs of plants are not seed producers? ***(2003)***
(a) Fern and Funaria
(b) Funaria and Ficus
(c) Ficus and Chlamydomonas
(d) Funaria and Pinus

98. Which one of the following is a living fossil? ***(2004)***
(a) Cycas (b) Moss
(c) Saccharomyces (d) Spirogyra

99. Which one of the following is categorised under living fossils? ***(2003)***
(a) Pinus (b) Cycas
(c) Selaginella (d) Metasequoia

100. Cycas has two cotyledons but not included in angiosperms because of ***(2001)***
(a) naked ovules (b) seems like monocot
(c) circinate ptyxis (d) compound leaves.

101. In which of the following would you place the plants having vascular tissue lacking seeds? ***(1999)***
(a) Pteridophytes (b) Gymnosperms
(c) Algae (d) Bryophytes

102. The endosperm of gymnosperm is ***(1999)***
(a) diploid (b) polyploid
(c) triploid (d) haploid.

103. Which one of the following statements about Cycas is incorrect? ***(1998)***
(a) It has circinate vernation.
(b) Its xylem is mainly composed of xylem vessel.
(c) Its roots contain some blue-green algae.
(d) It does not have a well organized female flower.

104. Multicellular branched rhizoids and leafy gametophytes are the characteristics of ***(1997)***
(a) some bryophytes (b) pteridophytes
(c) all bryophytes (d) gymnosperms.

105. A gymnospermic leaf carries 16 chromosomes. The number of chromosomes in its endosperm will be ***(1996)***
(a) 12 (b) 8 (c) 16 (d) 24

106. Which one is the most advanced from evolutionary view point? ***(1993)***
(a) Selaginella (b) Funaria
(c) Chlamydomonas (d) Pinus

107. Resin and turpentine are obtained from ***(1992)***
(a) Cycas (b) Pinus
(c) Cedrus (d) Abies.

108. In Pinus, the pollen grain has 6 chromosomes then in its endosperm will have ***(1992)***
(a) 12 (b) 18 (c) 6 (d) 24

109. A plant having seeds but lacking flowers and fruits belongs to ***(1992)***
(a) pteridophytes (b) mosses
(c) ferns (d) gymnosperms.

110. A plant in which sporophytic generation is represented by zygote is ***(1992)***
(a) Pinus (b) Selaginella
(c) Chlamydomonas (d) Dryopteris.

111. In Pinus/gymnosperms, the haploid structure are ***(1989)***
(a) megaspore, endosperm and embryo
(b) megaspore, pollen grain and endosperm
(c) megaspore, integument and root
(d) pollen grain, leaf and root.

112. In Pinus/Cycas/gymnosperms, the endosperm is ***(1988)***
(a) triploid (b) haploid
(c) diploid (d) tetraploid.

ANSWER KEY

1.	(d)	2.	(a)	3.	(a)	4.	(d)	5.	(b)	6.	(a)	7.	(b)
8.	(b)	9.	(c)	10.	(d)	11.	(b)	12.	(b)	13.	(d)	14.	(a)
15.	(b)	16.	(b)	17.	(a)	18.	(c)	19.	(d)	20.	(a)	21.	(d)
22.	(b)	23.	(a)	24.	(a)	25.	(b)	26.	(d)	27.	(d)	28.	(b)
29.	(c)	30.	(a)	31.	(c)	32.	(a)	33.	(a)	34.	(d)	35.	(d)
36.	(b)	37.	(c)	38.	(a)	39.	(c)	40.	(a)	41.	(a)	42.	(d)
43.	(d)	44.	(a)	45.	(d)	46.	(c)	47.	(b)	48.	(b)	49.	(d)
50.	(b)	51.	(a)	52.	(b)	53.	(d)	54.	(b)	55.	(a)	56.	(a)
57.	(a)	58.	(d)	59.	(b)	60.	(b)	61.	(c)	62.	(d)	63.	(a)
64.	(d)	65.	(a)	66.	(d)	67.	(c)	68.	(a)	69.	(a)	70.	(a)
71.	(a)	72.	(d)	73.	(a)	74.	(b)	75.	(c)	76.	(d)	77.	(a)
78.	(a)	79.	(c)	80.	(a)	81.	(d)	82.	(c)	83.	(a)	84.	(b)
85.	(a)	86.	(d)	87.	(a)	88.	(a)	89.	(d)	90.	(b)	91.	(d)
92.	(c)	93.	(d)	94.	(b)	95.	(c)	96.	(c)	97.	(a)	98.	(a)
99.	(b)	100.	(a)	101.	(a)	102.	(d)	103.	(b)	104.	(a)	105.	(b)
106.	(d)	107.	(b)	108.	(c)	109.	(d)	110.	(c)	111.	(b)	112.	(b)

HINTS & EXPLANATIONS

1. **(d)** Phylogenetic system or classification is based on evolutionary sequence as well as the genetic relationship among the living beings. Engler and Prantl's System of Classification was jointly proposed in Die Naturlichen Pflanzenfamilien in 1892. It is the first phylogenetic system of classification which includes all the plants from algae to angiosperms arranged in an evolutionary sequence from simplicity to complexity.

2. **(a)** Phenetic classification is a type of numerical taxonomy. In this type of classification the organisms are arranged according to overall similarity of existing organisms based on available characters. It is also called Adansonian taxonomy because the same was first attempted by Adanson (1763), of course on the basis of external traits only. Numerical taxonomy evolved around 1950. It has received impetus with the availability of calculating machines and computers. In numcrical taxonomy as many characters as possible are employed for evaluating degree of similarity and difference. All characteristics used in analysis are given equal weightage and importance. A proper selection of characters, their organisation and analysis in the light of current knowledge is key to success of this method. A lot of subjectivity can creep in depending upon the judgement of the biosystematist. No weightage is given to the quantity of the character present.

3. **(a)** There are three systems of classification - artificial, natural and phylogenetic. In the natural system of classification the organisms are

arranged on the basis of all known taxonomic characters instead of one or first few. These include morphological, anatomical, cytological, physiological and biochemical characters of the organisms. The artificial system is based on one or a few characters that are easily observable. The phylogenetic system tries to organize organisms on the basis of their genetic and phylogenetic relationships besides taxonomic characters.

4. **(d)** Phylogenetic systems of classification bring out evolutionary relationships of organisms. Phylogenetic systems of classification came into existence after acceptance of doctrine of evolution and natural selection propounded by Charles Darwin in his book "On the origin of Species" by means of Natural Selection. Darwin had put forward the view that the present day plants/animals originated from some ancestral ones after undergoing some periodical changes. So the phylogenetic classification is based on the evolutionary descent of a group of organisms and the relationships are depicted through a phylogram and a cladogram.

5.**(b)** Linnaeus put forward an "Artificial system" of plant classification which was based on sexual characters like cryptogamia, monoecia, monandria, diandria, polyandria, etc. It is commonly also called as sexual system of plant classification.

6. **(a)** Artificial system of classification was first used by Linnaeus.

7. **(b)** Classification given by Bentham and Hooker is Natural System. Monocots were placed after dicots; closely related families were separated; gymnosperms were placed between dicots and monocots.

8.**(b)** Ulothrix is a member of chlorophyceae. The stored food material in Ulothrix is starch. Mannitol is stored food material for members of phaeophyceae.

9. **(c)** Hydrocolloid carrageen is obtained from rhodophyceae alga Chondrus crispus.

10. **(d)** Carrageen obtained from red algae Chondrus crispus and used as pharmaceutical emulsifier, cleaning agent and in textile, leather and brewing industry.

11. **(b)** Mannitol is reserve food material in phaeophyceae, e.g., Ectocarpus.

12. **(b)** In Rhodophyceae, food is stored as floridean starch which is very similar to amylopectin and glycogen in structure.

13. **(d)** Gelidium, Gracilaria, Laminaria and Sargassum are multicellular. Anabaena is filamentous blue green algae. Volvox is colonial.

14. **(a)**

15. **(b)** Alginic acid is obtained from brown algae whereas carrageenan is obtained from red algae.

16. **(b)** Laminarin and mannitol are food reserves of brown algae or Phaeophyceae. Rhodophycean algae store food in the form of floridean starch.

17. **(a)** Ectocarpus produces biflagellate gametes. Anabaena is a cyanobacteria and does not reproduce sexually. Spirogyra produces non-flagellated male gamete during conjugation, where entire cell content functions as gamete. Polysiphonia also produces non-flagellated spermatia.

18. **(c)** All species of Chara reproduce sexually and show highly advanced oogamy. The sex organs are the most distinctive features of the Order Charales and are the most complicated among the thallophytes. Male and female gametangia are called antheridia and oogonia respectively. Male fructification (cluster of antheridia) is

called globule and the female is nucule. They are borne at the nodes of short branches, globule towards lower side and nuculc (fcmale structure) towards upper side.

19. **(d)** Sexual reproduction in algae takes place through fusion of two gametes. In Spirogyra, the gametes are similar in size (isogamy) and non-flagellated (non-motile).

20. **(a)** In oomycetes, like other oogamous organisms female gamete is large and non-motile, while male gamete is small and motile.

21. **(d)** Chlamydomonas has flagellated gametes which are similar or dissimilar in size. In Volvox and Fucus, nonmotile female gametes and motile male gametes are produced (oogamy). Spirogyra has gametes that are similar in size (isogamous) and are non-flagellated.

22. **(b)**

23. **(a)** In Spirogyra, gametes are non-motile and sexual reproduction takes place by conjugation. Sargassum belongs to Phaeophyceae group of algae. They are commonly called as 'brown algae' and contain photosynthetic pigments chlorophyll a and c. Puffballs are Basidomycetes with a stalked rounded structure that sends out puffs of spores, e.g., Lycoperdon oblongisporum. Nostoc is a colonial cyanobacterium. It enriches its habitat with nitrogen by fixing atmospheric nitrogen and also causes water bloom.

24. **(a)** Majority of algae (eukaryotes) possess a definite cell wall containing cellulose and other carbohydrates. In algal cell wall, different chemical components are present which vary widely among different groups (e.g., xylan, mannan, galactan, alginic acid, silica, agar, pectin, carrageenin, etc.). Cell wall of blue-green algae is made up of micro-peptides (proteins). This micro-peptide is not found in eukaryotic algae.

25. **(b)** Fucus is a brown algae, that belongs to Class Phaeophyta. In this alga the accumulation product of photosynthesis is D-mannitol (a sugar alcohol) and the reserve food material is laminarin.

26. **(d)** Algae are a group of chlorophyllous, nonvascular plants with thallose plant body. Different algae show different pigments present in the cell like chlorophyll - a, b, xanthophylls, carotenes, etc. These pigments provide the base for classification of various groups of algae into different classes. Members of Chlorophyceae possess chlorophyll-a, b pigments, Bacillariophyceae contains diatomin pigment whereas that of Phaeophyceae has fucoxanthin, Rhodophyceae has r-phycocyanin and r-phycoerythrin and cyanophyceae has phycobilin pigment.

27. **(d)** Spirogyra is a freshwater green alga which belongs to Class Chlorophyceae. The sexual reproduction in Spirogyra is called conjugation. It involves the fusion of two morphologically identical but physiologically dissimilar nonciliated gametes.

For development of gametes, some of the cells start to act like male and female gametangia in which the cell contents become separated from the cell wall, shrink and ultimately forms gametes. The fusion of these gametes takes place by scalariform conjugation or lateral conjugation.

28. **(b)** The algal Class Rhodophyceae contains a red pigment (r-phycoerythrin) and a blue pigment (r-phycocyanin) in the chromatophores.

These pigments can utilize those wavelengths of light (blue-green region of spectrum, i.e., 480-520 nm) that are not absorbed by chlorophyll. This enables red algae to grow at greater depths than other plants (upto 300 ft. below water). In addition to these, chl. a, chl. d, carotenes and xanthophylls are present.

In phaeophyceae chromatophores are yellowish brown in colour possessing xanthophylls in abundance.

Bacillariophyceae are called 'diatoms' due to presence of an accessory brown pigment called 'diatomin', other pigments are chl. a, chl. c (but not chl. b), carotenes and xanthophylls.

In chlorophyceae colouring pigments are just like higher plants, i.e., chl. a, chl. b, xanthophylls and carotenes.

29. **(c)** Ulothrix is a green filamentous alga, belonging to Class Chlorophyceae. The plant body is an unbranched filament consisting of numerous cylindrical cells joined end to end. Under favourable conditions, each cell produces zoospores except holdfast. These zoospores are of two types macrozoospores and microzoospores. The macrozoospores are larger in size and are quadriflagellate and the microzoospores are smaller zoospores which may be biflagellate or quadrifagelleate. Under unfavourable conditions, nonmotile mitospores called aplanospores are produced. Sexual reproduction in Ulothrix is of isogamous type. The isogametes fuse to form a quadriflagellate zygospore which after meiosis forms 16 aplanospores or zoospores.

30. **(a)** Chlorella is a unicellular green alga that contains high percentage of proteins, lipids and most of the known vitamins (carotene, riboflavin, vitamin B12, choline, etc.) and grows more quickly than Porphyra, so scientists are doing research to obtain food from it. The nutritional value is comparable to the mixture of soybeans and spinach.

31. **(c)** Ulothrix belongs to Class Chlorophyceae of Division Thallophyta. The plant body consists of an unbranched filament, consisting of numerous cylindrical cells joined end to end. It is heterothallic and sexual reproduction is of isogamous type. Except holdfast each cell of the filament can give rise to 64 to 128 gametes. The gametes are similar in size, shape and other features. So these gametes are called isogametes. When two gametes of (+) and (-) strain come together they fuse and a quadriflagellate zygospore is formed.

32. **(a)** Brown algae are the members of the Class Phaeophyceae. Their chromatopores are ellipsoidal or discoid. They contain chlorophyll a, chl c, b and c-carotenes and xanthophyll pigments (e.g., lutein, flavoxanthin, violaxanthin). They also contain large amount of a brown pigment fucoxanthin which masks the green colour of chlorophyll pigment. This gives characteristic brown colour to these plants, hence the name brown algae.

33. **(a)** Pyrenoids are found in many bryophytes and algae. They are small, spherical bodies found in the cytoplasm of a plant cell. They are rich in proteins and are surrounded by a starch sheath.

34. **(d)**

35. **(d)** Pyrenoids are the centres for formation of starch. There are present in chloroplast and are proteinaceous in nature covered by starch plate. They synthesize and store starch in them.

36. **(b)** Chloroplast in Chlamydomonas is cup-shaped. It is one celled structure whereas stellate, spiral and collar shaped chloroplasts are present in Zygnema, Spirogyra and Ulothrix respectively.

37. **(c)** In Ulothrix/Spirogyra reduction division (meiosis) occurs at the time of zygospore formation. Plant body of Ulothrix and Spirogyra, is gametophytic (haploid), they produce zoogametes (n) which fuses to form zygosporic (2n) diploid, which is a resting spore. Onset of favourable condition zygospore undergoes reductional division, or meiosis to produce zoo-meiospores.

38. (a) In Chlamydomonas sexual reproduction takes place through isogamy, anisogamy, and oogamy. Isogamy i.e., the fusion of similar gametes is the common mode of sexual reproduction in it. Anisogamy is fusion of morphologically similar but physiologically different cells. Oogamy is fusion of different gametes.

39. (c) The predominant stage of the life cycle of a moss is the gametophyte which consists of two stages - protonema stage and leafy stage. The first stage is the protonema stage, which develops directly from a spore. The spore are formed after meiosis in capsule.

40. (a) In some liverworts like Marchantia, special structures called gemmae are present for asexual reproduction.

41. (a) A non-motile male gamete or spermatium is the characteristic feature of Polysiphonia.

42. (d) Among the bryophytes Sphagnum accounts by far the most important place economically. It is popularly called bog moss or peat moss. It is perennial and its growth continues year after year. Older portions undergo death but do not decompose due to secretion of acid that accounts for the antibacterial and antifungal actions. The increasing mass of dead remains accumulate year after year and form a compact dark coloured mass rich in carbon which is called peat. Peat is used as fuels. Paraffin, acetic acid, peat tar and ammonia are formed as byproducts of peat obtained for industrial uses.

43. (d) Algae and moss are included in plant kingdom while fungi constitute a separate kingdom. Among them, mosses invariably show diplontic life cycle while others may or may not. Algae and moss are autotrophic while fungi are heterotrophs. But they all show multiplication by fragmentation.

44. (a) The given figure is of female thallus of Marchantia (bryophyte) in which A, B, C and D are archegoniophore, female thallus, gemma cup and rhizoids respectively.

45. (d) An elater is a cell (or structure attached to a cell) that is hygroscopic and therefore will change shape in response to changes in moisture in the environment. Elaters come in a variety of forms, but are always associated with plant spores. In plants that do not have seeds, they function in dispersing the spores to a new location. In the liverworts, elaters are cells that develop in the sporophyte alongside the spores. They are complete cells, usually with helical thickenings at maturity that respond to moisture content. In most liverworts, the elaters are unattached, but in some leafy species (such as Frullania) a few elaters will remain attached to the inside of the sporangium (spore capsule). The elaters by hygroscopic movement help in spore dispersal.

46. (c) The partially decomposed Sphagnum mass accumulates to form compressed mass called peat, which after drying is used as coal. So, it is also called peat moss. Sphagnum has the capacity to retain water for long periods and thus it is used to cover plant roots during transportation.

47. (b)

48. (b) In bryophytes the main plant body is gametophytic which is independent and may be thallose (no differentiation in root, stem and leaves) e.g., Riccia, Marchantia, Anthoceros, etc. or foliose (having leafy axis) e.g., Sphagnum, Funaria, etc. The gametophyte bears the sex organs antheridium and archegonium. Sexual reproduction is of oogamous type. It forms zygote that gives rise to the sporophytic phase. It is differentiated into foot, seta and capsule. The capsule produces spores after meiosis that again gives rise to gametophytic phase. The sporophyte is partially or fully dependent upon the gametophyte and is of shorter duration.

49. (d) Bryophytes are green photosynthetic and thalloid structures where the plant body lacks true root, stem and leaves. Instead of roots, rhizoids are present for attachment and absorption purpose. They have motile sperms and so they need water for fertilization. Archegonia evolved for the first time in bryophytes in the plant kingdom. It is a flask shaped structure with swollen base called venter and upper elongated neck. The venter contains a venter canal cell and an egg cell. It is surrounded by one celled thick sterile jacket layer.

50. (b) Bryophytes are called amphibians of plant kingdom because they complete their vegetative phase on land but water is necessary for their reproductive phase. Water helps in maturation and dehiscence of sex organs in bryophytes. It also helps in the transfer of sperms to the archegonium that make water essential for completion of life cycle of bryophytes.

51. (a) Bryophytes and algae are both autotrophic, plant body thallus like and devoid of vascular tissues. Instead of roots, rhizoids are present for attachment and absorption purpose. Both algae and bryophytes have motile sperms and need water for fertilization. But bryophytes can be separated from algae because archegonium originated for the first time in bryophytes in plant kingdom. It is a flask shaped structure with swollen base called venter and upper elongated neck. The venter contains a venter canal cell and an egg cell. It is surrounded by one celled thick sterile jacket layer. In algae sex organs are non-jacketed and unicellular.

52. (b) Funaria is known as common moss or green moss. The plant body is foliose that consists of stem axis which bears many leaves and instead of roots, rhizoids are present. It is gametophytic (n) and independent. It bears antheridia and archegonia on the same plant but on different branches.

After fertilization the zygote (2n) divides to form the sporophyte which consists of foot, seta and capsule. The basal foot is embedded in the apex of female branch. It absorbs nutrients and provides support for the sporophyte. Inside the capsule haploid spores are produced as a result of meiosis. Thus again the gametophytic phase starts. So the gametophytic phase is the dominant phase of the life cycle of Funaria.

53. (d)

54. (b) Protonema occurs in the life cycle of Funaria. The spore is the first cell of gametophytic generation and it germinates to form a filamentous branched alga like structure called protonema. If gives rise to new plant.

55. (a)

56. (a) Moss peristome is present in capsule and takes part in spore dispersal. The hygroscopic action of peristomial teeth help in the removal of operculum. The lengthening and shortening of peristomial teeth help in the dispersal of spores. The inner peristome acts as a sieve allowing only a few spores to escape at a time.

57. (a) Genera like Selaginella and Salvinia which produce two kinds of spores, macro (large) and micro (small) spores, are known as heterosporous.

58. (d) The sporophytes of pteridophytes bear sporangia that are subtended by leaf-like appendages called sporophylls.

In some cases sporophylls may form distinct compact structures called strobili or cones, e.g., Selaginella, Equisetum.

59. (b) The sperms of bryophytes and pteridophytes are flagellated and hence require an external supply of water to reach archegonia.

60. (b) Syngamy is the complete and permanent fusion of male and female gametes to form the zygote. When fertilization occurs outside the body of the organism, this type of gametic fusion is called external fertilization or external syngamy. In majority of algae, external fertilization occurs.

61. (c) Sphagnum and Funaria belong to Class Bryopsida of Division Bryophyta. They are typically mosses. The plant body has radial symmetry and is essentially leafy.

Salvinia belongs to Division Pteridophyta. It has a sporophyte plant body with true leaves, stem and roots. Marchantia belongs to Class Hepaticopsida of Division Bryophyta. They are also called liverworts. The plant body is a dorsoventrally flattened thallus.

62.(d) In bryophytes, the dominant phase of life cycle is gametophytic plant body. In contrast, vascular plants have sporophytic plant body in most of their life cycle and reduced, smaller gametophyte which have smaller sex organs.

63.(a) Marchantia is a dioecious plant. Male plants bear antheridiophores and female plants bear archegoniophores. Antheridiophores consists of a stalk and a disc like portion called receptacle. Archegoniophore is composed of a stalk and disc like receptacle at its distal end.

64. (d) In majority of the pteridophytes all the spores are of similar kinds; such plants are called homosporous. Genera like Selaginella and Salvinia which produce two kinds of spores, macro (large) and micro (small) spores, are known as heterosporous. The megaspores and microspores germinate and give rise to female and male gametophytes, respectively. The female gametophytes in these plants are retained on the parent sporophytes for variable periods. The development of the zygotes into young embryos take place within the female gametophytes. This event is a precursor to the seed habit considered an important step in evolution.

65. (a) The differentiation of spores into microspores and megaspores and their dependence on the parent sporophyte for the nutrition, are certain features in the life cycle of Selaginella, which have been considered as the essential pre-requisties for the formation of seeds, characteristic of spermatophytes. It is generally agreed, that the seed plants arose from the heterosporous vascular plants that instead of discharging the megaspore acquired the habit of retaining it within the megasporangium.

66. (d) The sporophyte of pteridophyte produces meiospores inside sporangia, which may be homosporous (e.g., Equisetum, Adiantum, Dryopteris, etc.) or heterosporous (e.g., Salvinia, Selaginella etc.).

67. (c) In prothallus of vascular cryptogams the antherozoids and eggs mature at different times. The spores on germination gives rise to prothallus. The antherozoids are biflagellated or multiflagellated. The egg is produced inside the venter, water is essential for fertilization and it is always crossfertilization. Self fertilization is prevented.

68.(a) Eichler divided Plant Kingdom into two subkingdoms - Cryptogamae and Phanerogamae. All plants without flowers and seeds are included in the sub-kingdom Cryptogamae whereas Phanerogamae includes plants which bear flowers and seeds.

Cryptogams are further classified into three divisions: Thallophyta, Bryophyta and Pteridophyta.

Spore bearing plants such as mosses and ferns belong to cryptogams because instead of reproducing by flowers and seeds they reproduce by means of spores.

69. (a) A fern plant body is sporophytic (2n) and is differentiated into roots, stems and leaves. On the ventral surface of leaves sporangia are borne in a group called sori. Inside the sporangium are present the spores which are formed by reduction division. Thus the spores produced are haploid in nature and germinate to produce a prothallus that represents the gametophytic generation. Antheridium and archegonium are borne on this prothallus. Thus, meiosis takes place at the stage of spore formation.

70.(a) Dichotomous branching is characteristic feature of liverworts, e.g., Riccia, Marchantia, Pellia, etc. It is a primitive form of branching. It is also called forked branching. In liverworts the thallus is flat and dorsiventral and dichotomously branched. The thallus has a notch at the anterior end. At the base of the notch, there is a growing point consisting of a single apical cell. It divides repeatedly to form two branches of the same size.

71.(a) Walking fern is named so because when its leaf tips come in contact with soil, form new plants as adventitious buds develop at leaf tips. This helps in the spread of fern over a large soil surface and thus the name 'walking fern'.

72.(d) Bryophytes are called amphibians of plant kingdom because they complete their vegetative phase on land but water is necessary for their reproductive phase. Water helps in maturation and dehiscence of sex organs in bryophytes. It also helps in the transfer of sperms to the archegonium that make water essential for completion of life cycle of bryophytes.

73.(a) Pteridophytes differs from bryophytes and thallophytes in having well developed vascular tissue system. Vascular tissues plays an important role in conducting water and food materials to the plants. Whereas these are absent in bryophytes and thallophytes.

74. (b)

75. (c) Bryophytes are the plants which produces spores and embryos but they do not has vascular tissue system. While rhodophytes and phaeophytes are algae and produces spores (no embryos) only and pteridophytes produces spores, embryo and well developed vascular tissue system.

76. (d) Sperms of both Funaria and Pteris were released together near the archegonia. But only the sperms of Pteris enter the archegonia, as Pteris archegonia releases a chemical malic acid to attract its sperms for fertilization.

77. (a) Evolutionary important character of Selaginella is heterosporous nature. Selaginella produces two types of spores microspores and megaspores. Heterospory in the life cycle of Selaginella leads to the formation of seed habit.

78. (a) In gymnosperms, the male and the female gametophytes do not have an independent free-living existence. They remain within the sporangia retained on the sporophytes. The pollen grain is released from the microsporangium. They are carried in air currents and come in contact with the opening of the ovules borne on megasporophylls. The pollen tube carrying the male gametes grows towards archegonia in the ovules and discharge their contents near the mouth of the archegonia. Following fertilisation, zygote develops into an embryo and the ovules into seeds.

79. (c) Chara is an example of monoecious plant as both male sex organ (antheridium) and female sex organ (archegonium) are present on the same plant.

80.(a) Gymnosperms have naked ovule. Selaginella and Salvinia both produce two kinds of spores, macro (large) and micro (small) hence, called heterosporous. Equisetum (horse tail, scouring rush) is a pteridophyte. Stems are branched in Cedrus but unbranched in Cycas.

81. (d) Pinus is a monoecious plant, i.e., in Pinus the male and female cones or strobili are borne on the same plant.

82.(c) Needle like leaves with thick cuticle and sunken stomata are xerophytic adaptations of conifers for tolerating extreme environmental conditions.

83.(a) Sequoia sempervirens is the tallest gymnosperm. The leaves of gymnosperms are well adapted to extremes of climate. This is the reason for gymnosperm to flourish in cold areas where instead of rain, snow is the source of water. Gymnosperms are heterosporous, i.e., produce two different kinds of spores-microspores and megaspores. Salvinia is an aquatic pteridophyte.

84. (b) In gymnosperms (like Pinus), the male and female gametophyte do not have an independent free living existence. They remain within the sporangia retained on the sporophytes, i.e., female gametophyte (within megasporangium) and male gametophyte (within microsporangium).

85. (a) Selaginella is a heterosporous pteridophyte. Coralloid roots of Cycas harbour blue green algae like Nostoc, Anabaena and are not a type of VAM (vesicular arbuscular mycorrhiza) which is a symbiotic association with fungus.

86. (d) Mucor is a member of Zygomycetes (the conjugation fungi) in which motile cells, e.g., zoospores, planogametes, etc., are absent. Asexual reproduction takes place by the formation of nonmotile mitospores called sporangiospores. Sexual reproduction takes place by the formation of non-motile zygospores.

87. (a)

88.(a) In Funaria (Bryophyta), Dryopteris (Pteridophyta) and Ginkgo (Gymnosperm) female sex organ archaegonium is formed. Funaria lacks independent sporophyte and vascular tissues while independent gametophyte is absent in Ginkgo.

89. (d) In majority of the pteridophytes all the spores are of similar kinds; such plants are called homosporous. Genera like Selaginella and Salvinia which produce two kinds of spores, macro (large) and micro (small) spores, are known as heterosporous. The megaspores and microspores germinate and give rise to female and male gametophytes, respectively. The female gametophytes in these plants are retained on the parent sporophytes for variable periods. The development of the zygotes into young embryos take place within the female gametophytes. This event is a precursor to the seed habit considered an important step in evolution.

90. (b) Cycas is agymnosperm and Adiantum is a pteridophyte. Cambium and seeds are absent in pteridophytes, while vessels are absent in both of these two groups. Both Cycas and Adiantum resemble each other in having multi-ciliated sperms.

91.(d) Equisetum is a pteridophyte and in pteridophytes, the main plant body is a sporophyte which is differentiated into true root, stem and leaves. Gametophytes are small or inconspicuous and free living, mostly photosynthetic thalloid called prothallus.

Riccia is a liverwort and Polytrichum is a moss. The sporophyte in mosses is more elaborate than that in liverworts.

Volvox shows oogamous type of sexual reproduction, i.e., fusion between one large, non motile (static) female gamete and a smaller, motile male gamete.

During unfavourable conditions, the slime mould differentiates and forms fruiting bodies bearing spores at their tips. The spores possess true walls. They are extremely resistant and survive for many years, even under adverse conditions.

92. (c) A - Selaginella

B - Equisetum

C - Salvinia

D - Ginkgo

93.(d) Pteridophytes are known as vascular cryptogams (Gk kryptos = hidden + gamos = wedded). They reproduce by spores rather than seeds. They are the first vascular land plant. The pteridophyte Equisetum belongs to the Class Sphenophyta. All vegetative parts of it possess vascular tissues (i.e., hadrome equivalent to xylem and leptome equivalent to phloem) organised in definite groups of steles.

94. (b) In gymnosperm (like Cedrus) the male and female gametophyte do not have an independent free living existence. They remain within the sporangia retained on the sporophytes i.e., female gametophyte with megasporangium and male gametophyte within microsporangium.

95. (c) In gymnosperms, pollen chamber represents the microsporangium in which pollen grains develop. The microspore is generally a globular sac like structure having large number of microspores. The microspores are also termed as pollen grains.

96. (c) Flagellated male gametes are mostly seen in lower groups of plants like algae, bryophytes, pteridophytes. It is also seen in certain gymnosperms like Cycas. The bryophytes like Riccia have the male gametes which are biflagellate.

97.(a) Seed producing plants belong to Spermatophyta. It includes gymnosperms and angiosperms. Seed habit or seed formation originated in gymnosperms. It requires the retention of megasporangium or the only on the parent plant and non-shedding of megaspore, development of integument and in site formation of female gametophyte. All these features developed in gymnosperms and angiosperms. Thallophytes, bryophytes and pteridophytes lack these features and thus do not reproduce by producing seeds.

Fern and Funaria belong to pteridophytes and bryophytes respectively so they do not reproduce by producing seeds.

98.(a) Cycas and Ginkgo are often considered as the living fossil because they are one of the few representative of once a large group of plants (which was once a well flourished group) and possess traits of extinct pteridosperms and other gymnosperms.

99. (b)

100.(a) Cycas belongs to Order Cycadales of gymnosperms because it has naked seed. It is not enclosed inside a fruit. It does not have double fertilization and so the endosperm formed is haploid in nature and not triploid. So it is not included in angiosperms as they have ovules. (or seeds) produced inside fruit. This is the main difference between gymnosperms and angiosperms.

101. (a) Algae, bryophyte and pteridophyte are cryptogams, but out of them algae and bryophytes are lower cryptogams and do not possess vascular tissue (xylem and phloem), whereas in pteridophytes, vascular tissue system is well developed and so these are higher cryptogams or vascular cryptogams. The term cryptogams means that these plants reproduce by means of spores and do not produce seeds.

The vascular tissue of pteridophytes is well developed. They contain both xylem and phloem. In xylem, vessels are absent and in phloem companion cells are absent.

So pteridophytes or vascular cryptogams are a group of seedless vascular plants, that have successfully invaded the land and reproduce by means of spores. Gymnosperms are naked seed bearing plants called phanerogams.

102. (d) The endosperm of gymnosperms is haploid. It is a pre-fertilisation tissue and is equivalent to female gametophyte, hence it is haploid in nature but in angiosperms, it is postfertilization tissue and is generally triploid in nature.

103. (b) Cycas belongs to Order Cycadales of gymnosperms. Its leaves show circinate vernation, i.e., the leaves are coiled in young stage. The coralloid roots in Cycas arise from the lateral branches of the normal roots and contain blue-green algae like Nostoc and Anabaena. A well developed flower like that of angiosperms is absent in Cycas. It has compact cones containing microsporophylls and megasporophylls. The megaspores are loosely arranged on the megasporophyll. The male cone is a compact structure. Vessels in xylem are absent and it contains only tracheids for conduction of water.

104. (a) The Division Bryophyta includes three Classes Hepaticopsida, Anthocerotopsida and Bryopsida. The members of Hepaticopsida and Anthocerotopsida have a thallose plant body which is dorsiventrally differentiated and dichotomously branched. On the ventral surface unicellular or multicellular rhizoids are present. The member of Bryopsida have a main plant body that has a leafy gametophore made up of an axis having spirally arranged leaves. The rhizoids are multicellular and branched, e.g., Sphagnum, Funaria, Riccia, Anthoceros. So only few member of bryophytes have leafy gametophytes.

105. (b) Gymnosperms show distinct alternation of generations. The sporophytic phase is dominant. The sporphyte is differentiated into root, stem and leaves. So the number of chromosomes in a leaf cell is diploid (2n),(2n = 16). Double fertilization is absent in gymnosperms. The endosperm develops before fertilization directly from the megaspore. So the number of chromosomes in endosperm will be 8(n = 8).

106. (d) Pinus is more advanced from the evolutionary point of view. It is a gymnosperm (Phanerogams) having well developed vascular conducting system and bears seeds. While others Selaginella, Funaria and Chlamydomonas do not bear seeds.

107. (b) Resins and turpentine are obtained from Pinus which is gymnospermic plant. Cycas is an ornamental plant. Paper and Canada balsam are obtained from Abies and timber is obtained from Cedrus deodara.

108. (c) In Pinus, if the pollen grain has 6 chromosomes then in its endosperm will also have 6 chromosomes as endosperm and pollen grains are both haploid structures.

109.(d) A plant having seed but lacking flowers and fruit belongs to gymnosperms. Gymnosperms are vascular land plants and bears seeds which are naked i.e., ovules not enclosed in the ovary. Hence, flowers are absent.

110. (c) A plant in which sporophytic generation is represented by zygote is Chlamydomonas. It is a type of algae that has gametophytic plant body (haploid). It reproduce sexually by gametes which are isogametes that fuses to produce diploid zygote which is the only sporophytic generation.

111. (b) In Pinus/gymnosperms, endosperm is produced before fertilization and hence it is haploid. Megaspore and pollen grains are structures of male gametophytes and it is also haploid.

112. (b)

Chapter : 04 ANIMAL KINGDOM

BASIS OF CLASSIFICATION

1. Radial symmetry is not found in adults of phylum ***(2023)***
(a) Coelenterata (b) Echinodermata
(c) Ctenophora (d) Hemichordata

2. Consider following features. ***(2019)***
(A) Organ system level of organisation
(B) Bilateral symmetry
(C) True coelomates with segmentation of body
Select the correct option of animal groups which possess all the above characteristics.
(a) Annelida, Mollusca and Chordata
(b) Annelida, Arthropoda and Chordata
(c) Annelida, Arthropoda and Mollusca
(d) Arthropoda, Mollusca and Chordata

3. Which of the following animals are true coelomates with bilateral symmetry? ***(Odisha NEET 2019)***
(a) Adult Echinoderms (b) Aschelminthes
(c) Platyhelminthes (d) Annelids

4. Which one of the following kinds of animals are triploblastic? ***(2010)***
(a) Flatworms (b) Sponges
(c) Ctenophores (d) Corals

5. Which one of the following statements about certain given animals is correct? ***(2010)***
(a) Roundworms (Aschelminthes) are pseudocoelomates.
(b) Molluscs are acoelomates.
(c) Insects are pseudocoelomates.
(d) Flatworms (Platyhelminthes) are coelomates.

6. Which one of the following groups of animals is bilaterally symmetrical and triploblastic? ***(2009)***
(a) Aschelminthes (roundworms)
(b) Ctenophores
(c) Sponges
(d) Coelenterates (cnidarians)

7. Metameric segmentation is the characteristic of ***(2006)***
(a) mollusca and chordata
(b) platyhelminthes and arthropoda
(c) echinodermata and annelida
(d) annelida and arthropoda.

8. The animals with bilateral symmetry in young stage and radial pentamerous symmetry in the adult stage, belong to the Phylum ***(2004)***
(a) Annclida (b) Mollusca
(c) Cnidaria (d) Echinodermata.

9. Which of the following animals have scattered cells with cell - tissue grade organisation? ***(2000)***
(a) Sponge (b) Hydra
(c) Liver fluke (d) Ascaris

10. Coelom is found between ***(1996)***
(a) body wall and ectoderm
(b) ectoderm and endoderm
(c) mesoderm and body wall (endoderm)
(d) mesoderm and ectoderm.

11. Besides annelida and arthropoda, the metamerism is exhibited by ***(1995)***
(a) mollusca (b) acanthocephala
(c) cestoda (d) chordata.

CLASSIFICATION OF ANIMALS

12. The unique mammalian characteristics are ***(2023)***
(a) hairs, pinna and indirect development
(b) pinna, monocondylic skull and mammary glands
(c) hairs, tympanic membrane and mammary glands
(d) hairs, pinna and mammary glands.

13. Select the correct statements with reference to chordates. ***(2023)***

A. Presence of a mid-dorsal, solid and double nerve cord.

B. Presence of closed circulatory system.

C. Presence of paired pharyngeal gill slits

D. Presence of dorsal heart

E. Triploblastic pseudocoelomate animals.
Choose the correct answer from the options given below:

(a) B, D and E only (b) C, D and E only
(c) A, C and D only (d) B and C only

14. Exoskeleton of arthropods is composed of ***(2022)***

(a) cutin (b) cellulose
(c) chitin (d) glucosamine.

15. In which of the following animals, digestive tract has additional chambers like crop and gizzard? ***(2022)***

(a) Corvus, Columba, Chameleon
(b) Bufo, Balaenoptera, Bangarus
(c) Catla, Columba, Crocodilus
(d) Pavo, Psittacula, Corvus

16. Given below are two statements: one is labelled as Assertion (A) and the other is labelled as Reason(R).

Assertion (A) : All vertebrates are chordates but all chordates are not vertebrates.

Reason (R): Notochord is replaced by vertebral column in the adult vertebrates.

In the light of the above statements, choose appropriate answer from the options given below. ***(2022)***

(a) Both (A) and (R) are correct and (R) is the correct explanation of (A)
(b) (A) is correct but (R) is not correct
(c) (A) is not correct but (R) is correct
(d) Both (A) and (R) are correct but (R) is incorrect explanation of (A)

17. Match the following ***(2021)***

List - I	List - II
(p) Physalia	(i) Pearl oyster
(q) Limulus	(ii) Portuguese man of war
(r) Ancylostoma	(iii) Living fossil
(s) Pinctada	(iv) Hookworm

Choose the correct answer from the options given below.

	p	q	r	s
(a)	(i)	(iv)	(iii)	(ii)
(b)	(ii)	(iii)	(i)	(iv)
(c)	(iv)	(i)	(iii)	(ii)
(d)	(ii)	(iii)	(iv)	(i)

18. Which one of the following organisms bears hollow and pneumatic long bones? ***(2021)***

(a) Ornithorhynchus (b) Neophron
(c) Hemidactylus (d) Macropus

19. Read the following statements. ***(2021)***

(A) Metagenesis is observed in helminths.

(B) Echinoderms are triploblastic and coelomate animals.

(C) Round worms have organ-system level of body organization.

(D) Comb plates present in ctenophores help in digestion.

(E) Water vascular system is characteristic of echinoderms.

Choose the correct answer from the options given below.

(a) (B), (C) and (E) are correct
(b) (C), (D) and (E) are correct
(c) (A), (B) and (C) are correct
(d) (A), (D) and (E) are correct

20. Match List- I with List- II. ***(2021)***

List - I	List - II
(p) Metamerism	(i) Coelenterata
(q) Canal system	(ii) Ctenophora
(r) Comb plates	(iii) Annelida
(s) Cnidoblasts	(iv) Porifera

Choose the correct answer from the options given below.

	p	q	r	s
(a)	(iv)	(i)	(ii)	(iii)
(b)	(iv)	(iii)	(i)	(ii)
(c)	(iii)	(iv)	(i)	(ii)
(d)	(iii)	(iv)	(ii)	(i)

21. Bilaterally symmetrical and acoelomate animals are exemplified by ***(2020)***

(a) ctenophora (b) platyhelminthes
(c) aschelminthes (d) annelida.

22. Match the following columns and select the correct option. ***(2020)***

Column-I	Column-II
(A) 6-15 pairs of gill slits	(i) Trygon
(B) Heterocercal caudal fin	(ii) Cyclostomes
(C) Air bladder	(iii) Chondrichthyes
(D) Poison sting	(iv) Osteichthyes

	(A)	(B)	(C)	(D)
(a)	(ii)	(iii)	(iv)	(i)
(b)	(iii)	(iv)	(i)	(ii)
(c)	(iv)	(ii)	(iii)	(i)
(d)	(i)	(iv)	(iii)	(ii)

23. Which of the following statements are true for the Phylum Chordata? ***(2020)***

(A) In Urochordata, notochord extends from head to tail and it is present throughout their life.

(B) In Vertebrata, notochord is present during the embryonic period only.

(C) Central nervous system is dorsal and hollow.

(D) Chordata is divided into 3 subphyla : Hemichordata, Tunicata and Cephalochordata.

(a) (D) and (C) (b) (C) and (A)
(c) (A) and (B) (d) (B) and (C)

24. Match the following columns and select the correct option. (2020)

Column-I	Column-II
(A) Gregarious, polyphagous pest	(i) Asterias
(B) Adult with radial symmetry and larva with bilateral symmetry	(ii) Scorpion
(C) Book lungs	(iii) Ctenoplana
(D) Bioluminescence	(iv) Locusta

	(A)	(B)	(C)	(D)
(a)	(i)	(iii)	(ii)	(iv)
(b)	(iv)	(i)	(ii)	(iii)
(c)	(iii)	(ii)	(i)	(iv)
(d)	(ii)	(i)	(iii)	(iv)

25. Match the following organisms with respective characteristics. ***(2019)***

(A) Pila (i) Flame cells
(B) Bombyx (ii) Comb plates
(C) Pleurobrachia (iii) Radula
(D) Taenia (iv) Malpighian tubules

Select the correct option from the following.

	(A)	(B)	(C)	(D)
(a)	(iii)	(ii)	(iv)	(i)
(b)	(iii)	(ii)	(i)	(iv)
(c)	(iii)	(iv)	(ii)	(i)
(d)	(ii)	(iv)	(iii)	(i)

26. Match the following genera with their respective phylum. ***(Odisha NEET 2019)***

(1) Ophiura	(i) Mollusca
(2) Physalia	(ii) Platyhelminthes
(3) Pinctada	(iii) Echinodermata
(4) Planaria	(iv) Coelenterata

Select the correct option.
(a) (1)-(iv), (2)-(i), (3)-(iii), (4)-(ii)
(b) (1)-(iii), (2)-(iv), (3)-(i), (4)-(ii)
(c) (1)-(i), (2)-(iii), (3)-(iv), (4)-(ii)
(d) (1)-(iii), (2)-(iv), (3)-(ii), (4)-(i)

27. Which of the following animals does not undergo metamorphosis? ***(2018)***
(a) Earthworm (b) Tunicate
(c) Moth (d) Starfish

28. Identify the vertebrate group of animals characterised by crop and gizzard in its digestive system. ***(2018)***
(a) Amphibia (b) Reptilia
(c) Aves (d) Osteichthyes

29. Which one of these animals is not a homeotherm? ***(2018)***
(a) Macropus (b) Chelone
(c) Camelus (d) Psittacula

30. Important characteristic that hemichordates share with chordates is ***(2017)***
(a) ventral tubular nerve cord
(b) pharynx with gill slits
(c) pharynx without gill slits
(d) absence of notochord.

31. Which among these is the correct combination of aquatic mammals? ***(2017)***
(a) Dolphins, Seals, Trygon
(b) Whales, Dolphins, Seals
(c) Trygon, Whales, Seals
(d) Seals, Dolphins, Sharks

32. Which of the following represents order of 'Horse'? ***(2017)***
(a) Perissodactyla (b) Caballus
(c) Ferus (d) Equidae

33. In case of poriferans, the spongocoel is lined with flagellated cells called ***(2017)***
(a) oscula (b) choanocytes
(c) mesenchymal cells (d) ostia.

34. Choose the correct statement. ***(NEET-II 2016)***
(a) All mammals are viviparous.
(b) All cyclostomes do not possess jaws and paired fins.
(c) All reptiles have a three-chambered heart.
(d) All pisces have gills covered by an operculum.

35. Which one of the following characteristics is not shared by birds and mammals? ***(NEET-I 2016)***
(a) Viviparity
(b) Warm blooded nature
(c) Ossified endoskeleton
(d) Breathing using lungs

36. Which of the following characteristic features always holds true for the corresponding group of animals? ***(NEET-I 2016)***

(a)	Possess a mouth with an upper and a lower jaw	Chordata
(b)	3-chambered heart with one incompletely divided ventricle	Reptilia
(c)	Cartilaginous endoskeleton	Chondrichthyes
(d)	Viviparous	Mammalia

37. Which of the following features is not present in the Phylum Arthropoda? ***(NEET-I 2016)***
(a) Parapodia
(b) Jointed appendages
(c) Chitinous exoskeleton
(d) Metameric segmentation

38. Body having meshwork of cells, internal cavities lined with food filtering flagellated cells and indirect development are the characteristics of Phylum ***(2015)***
(a) Mollusca (b) Protozoa
(c) Coelenterata (d) Porifera.

39. Metagenesis refers to ***(2015)***

(a) occurrence of a drastic change in form during post-embryonic development

(b) presence of a segmented body and parthenogenetic mode of reproduction

(c) presence of different morphic forms

(d) alternation of generation between asexual and sexual phases of an organism.

40. A jawless fish, which lays eggs in fresh water and whose ammocoetes larvae after metamorphosis return to the ocean is ***(2015)***

(a) Neomyxine (b) Petromyzon

(c) Eptatretus (d) Myxine:

41. Which of the following endoparasites of humans does show viviparity? ***(2015 Cancelled)***

(a) Trichinella spiralis

(b) Ascaris lumbricoides

(c) Ancylostoma duodenale

(d) Enterobius vermicularis

42. Which of the following represents the correct combination without any exception? ***(2015 Cancelled)***

	Characteristics	**Class**
(a)	Sucking and circular mouth; jaws absent, integument without scales; paired appendages	Cyclostomata
(b)	Body covered with feathers; skin moist and glandular, fore- limbs form wings; lungs with air sacs.	Aves
(c)	Mammary gland; hair on body; pinnae; two pairs of limbs.	Mammalia
(d)	Mouth ventral; gills without operculum; skin with placoid scales; persistent notochord.	Chondrichthyes

43. Which of the following animals is not viviparous? ***(2015 Cancelled)***

(a) Platypus (b) Whale

(c) Flying fox (Bat) (d) Elephant

44. Which of the following characteristics is mainly responsible for diversification of insects on land ? ***(2015 Cancelled)***

(a) Exoskeleton (b) Eyes

(c) Segmentation (d) Bilateral symmetry

45. Select the taxon mentioned that represents both marine and fresh water species. ***(2014)***

(a) Echinoderms (b) Ctenophora

(c) Cephalochordata (d) Cnidaria

46. Planaria possesses high capacity of ***(2014)***

(a) metamorphosis (b) regeneration

(c) alternation of generation

(d) bioluminescence.

47. A marine cartilaginous fish that can produce electric current is ***(2014)***

(a) Pristis (b) Torpedo

(c) Trygon (d) Scoliodon.

48. Which of the following are correctly matched with respect to their taxonomic classification? ***(2013)***

(a) House fly, butterfly, tse-tse fly, silver fish -Insecta

(b) Spiny anteater, sea urchin, sea cucumber - Echinodermata

(c) Flying fish, cuttle fish silver fish - Pisces

(d) Centipede, millipede, spider, scorpion - Insecta

49. Which group of animals belong to the same phylum? ***(2013)***

(a) Prawn, Scorpion, Locusta

(b) Sponge, Sea anemone, Starfish

(c) Malarial parasite, Amoeba, Mosquito

(d) Earthworm, Pinworm, Tapeworm

50. Match the name of the animal (column I), with one characteristic (column II) and the phylum/class (column III) to which it belongs. ***(2013)***

	Column I	Column II	Column III
(a)	Limulus	Body covered by chitinous exoskeleton	Pisces
(b)	Adamsia	Radially symmetrical	Porifera
(c)	Petromyzon	Ectoparasite	Cyclostomata
(d)	Ichthyophis	Terrestrial	Reptilia

51. One of the representatives of Phylum Arthropoda is ***(2013)***
(a) puffer fish (b) flying fish
(c) cuttle fish (d) silver fish.

52. The characteristics of Class Reptilia are ***(Karnataka NEET 2013)***
(a) body covered with moist skin which is devoid of scales, the ear is represented by a tympanum, alimentary canal, urinary and reproductive tracts open into a common cloaca
(b) fresh water animals with bony endoskeleton, airbladder to regulate buoyancy
(c) marine animals with cartilaginous endoskeleton, body covered with placoid scales
(d) body covered with dry and cornified skin, scales over the body are epidermal, they do not have external ears.

53. Which one of the following groups of animals reproduces only by sexual means? ***(Karnataka NEET 2013)***
(a) Cnidaria (b) Porifera
(c) Protozoa (d) Ctenophora

54. Which one of the following animals is correctly matched with its one characteristic and the taxon?
Animal Characteristic Taxon ***(Karnataka NEET 2013)***

	Animal	Characteristic	Taxon
(a)	Millipede	Ventral nerve cord	Arachnida
(b)	Sea anemone	Triploblastic	Cnidaria
(c)	Silver fish	Pectoral and pelvic fins	Chordata
(d)	Duckbilled platypus	Oviparous	Mammalia

55. Sharks and dogfishes differ from skates and rays because ***(Karnataka NEET 2013)***
(a) gill slits are ventrally placed
(b) head and trunk are widened considerably
(c) distinct demarcation between body and tail
(d) their pectoral fins distinctly marked off from cylindrical bodies.

56. In which one of the following, the genus name, its two characters and its phylum are not correctly matched, whereas the remaining three are correct? ***(2012)***

(a)	Pila	(i) Body segmented (ii) Mouth with radula	Mollusca
(b)	Asterias	(i) Spiny skinned (ii) Water vascular system	Echinodermata
(c)	Sycon	(i) Pore bearing (ii) Canal system	Porifera
(d)	Periplaneta	(i) Jointed appendages (ii) Chitinous exoskeleton	Arthropoda

57. Which one of the following pairs of animals are similar to each other pertaining to the feature stated against them? ***(Mains 2012)***
(a) Pteropus and Ornithorhynchus - Viviparity
(b) Garden lizard and crocodile - Three chambered heart
(c) Ascaris and Ancylostoma - Metameric segmentation
(d) Sea horse and flying fish - Cold blooded (poikilothermal)

58. Which one of the following categories of animals, is correctly described with no single exception in it? ***(Mains 2012)***

(a) All reptiles possess scales, have a three chambered heart and are cold blooded (poikilothermal).

(b) All bony fishes have four pairs of gills and an operculum on each side.

(c) All sponges are marine and have collared cells.

(d) All mammals are viviparous and possess diaphragm for breathing.

59. What will you look for to identify the sex of the following? ***(2011)***

(a) Female Ascaris-sharply curved posterior end

(b) Male frog- a copulatory pad on the first digit of the hind limb

(c) Female cockroach-anal cerci

(d) Male shark-claspers borne on pelvic fins

60. Which one of the following groups of animals is correctly matched with its characteristic feature without any exception? ***(2011)***

(a) Reptilia : possess 3-chambered heart with an incompletely divided ventricle

(b) Chordata : possess a mouth with an upper and a lower jaw

(c) Chondrichthyes : possess cartilaginous endoskeleton

(d) Mammalia : give birth to young ones

61. In which one of the following the genus name, its two characters and its class/phylum are correctly matched? ***(2011)***

	Genus name	Two characters	Class/Phylum
(a)	Ascaris	(i) Body segmented (ii) Males and females distinct	Annelida
(b)	Salamandra	(i) A tympanum represents ear (ii) Fertilization is external	Amphibia
(c)	Pteropus	(i) Skin possesses hair (ii) Oviparous	Mammalia
(d)	Aurelia	(i) Cnidoblasts (ii) Organ level of organization	Coelenterata

62. Which one of the following statements is totally wrong about the occurrence of notochord, while the other three are correct? ***(Mains 2011)***

(a) It is present only in larval tail in ascidian.

(b) It is replaced by a vertebral column in adult frog.

(c) It is absent throughout life in humans from the very beginning.

(d) It is present throughout life in Amphioxus.

63. The figures (A–D) show four animals. Select the correct option with respect to a common characteristic of two of these animals. ***(Mains 2011)***

(a) 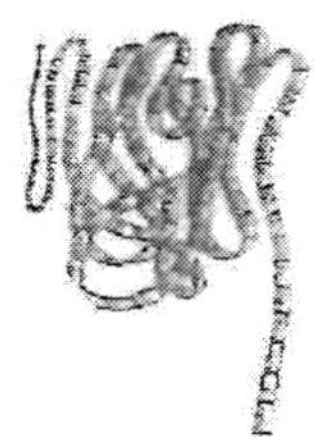

(b) 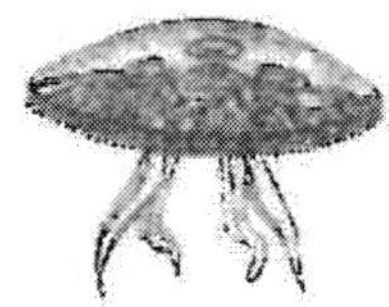

(c) 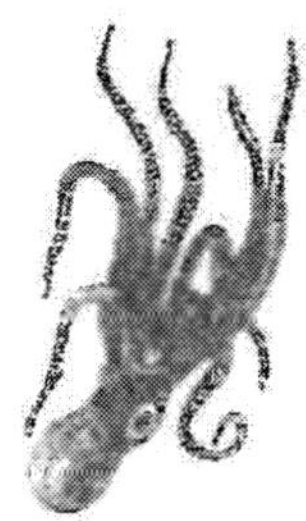

(d) 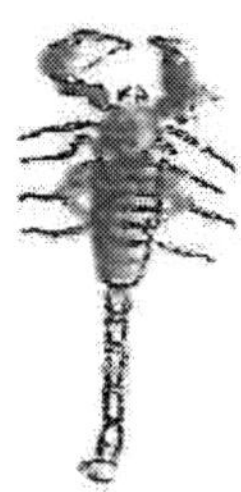

(a) (A) and (D) respire mainly through body wall.

(b) (B) and (C) show radial symmetry.

(c) (A) and (B) have cnidoblasts for selfdefence.

(d) (C) and (D) have a true coelom.

64. One example of animals having a single opening to the outside that serves both as mouth as well as anus is ***(2010)***

(a) Octopus (b) Asterias

(c) Ascidia (d) Fasciola.

65. Which one of the following statements about all the four of Spongilla, leech, dolphin and penguin is correct? ***(2010)***

(a) Penguin is homoiothermic while the remaining three are poikilothermic.

(b) Leech is a fresh water form while all others are marine.

(c) Spongilla has special collared cells called choanocytes, not found in the remaining three.

(d) All are bilaterally symmetrical.

66. In which one of the following organisms its excretory organs are correctly stated? ***(Mains 2010)***

(a) Humans - Kidneys, sebaceous glands and tear glands

(b) Earthworm - Pharyngeal, integumentary and septal nephridia

(c) Cockroach - Malpighian tubules and enteric caeca

(d) Frog - Kidneys, skin and buccal epithelium

67. Crocodile and penguin are similar to whale and dogfish in which one of the following features? ***(Mains 2010)***

(a) Possess a solid single stranded central nervous system

(b) Lay eggs and guard them till they hatch

(c) Possess bony skeleton

(d) Have gill slits at some stage

68. Which one of the following pairs of animals comprises 'jawless fishes'? ***(2009)***

(a) Mackerals and rohu

(b) Lampreys and hag fishes

(c) Guppies and hag fishes

(d) Lampreys and eels

69. Which one of the following in birds, indicates their reptilian ancestry? ***(2008)***

(a) Two special chambers crop and gizzard in their digestive tract

(b) Eggs with a calcareous shell

(c) Scales on their hind limbs

(d) Four-chambered heart

70. Ascaris is characterized by ***(2008)***

(a) presence of true coelom but absence of metamerism

(b) presence of true coelom and metamerism (metamerisation)

(c) absence of true coelom but presence of metamerism

(d) presence of neither true coelom nor metamerism.

71. Which one of the following groups of three animals each is correctly matched with their one characteristic morphological feature? ***(2008)***

	Animals	**Morphological features**
(a)	Scorpion, spider, cockroach	- Ventral solid central nervous system
(b)	Cockroach, locust, Taenia	- Metameric segmentation
(c)	Liver fluke, sea anemone, sea cucumber	- Bilateral symmetry
(d)	Centipede, prawn, sea urchin	- Jointed appendages

72. Which one of the following phyla is correctly matched with its two general characteristics? ***(2008)***

(a) Echinodermata - pentamerous radial symmetry and mostly internal fertilization

(b) Mollusca-normally oviparous and development through a trochophore or veliger larva

(c) Arthropoda - body divided into head, thorax and abdomen and respiration by tracheae

(d) Chordata - notochord at some stage and separate anal and urinary openings to the outside.

73. Which one of the following is not a characteristic of Phylum Annelida? ***(2008)***

(a) Pseudocoelom

(b) Ventral nerve cord

(c) Closed circulatory system

(d) Segmentation

74. Which of the following pairs are correctly matched? ***(2007)***

	Animals	Morphological features
(i)	Crocodile	- 4-chambered heart
(ii)	Sea urchin	- Parapodia
(iii)	Obelia	- Metagenesis
(iv)	Lemur	- Thecodont

(a) (ii), (iii) and (iv) (b) only (i) and (iv)
(c) only (i) and (ii) (d) (i), (iii) and (iv)

75. Which one of the following is a matching pair of a body feature and the animal possessing it? ***(2007)***
(a) Ventral central nervous system - Leech
(b) Pharyngeal gill slits absent in embryo - Chamaeleon
(c) Ventral heart - Scorpion
(d) Post-anal tail - Octopus

76. What is common between parrot, platypus and kangaroo? ***(2007)***
(a) Toothless jaws
(b) Functional post-anal tail
(c) Ovoparity
(d) Homoiothermy

77. What is true about Nereis, scorpion, cockroach and silver fish? ***(2007)***
(a) They all possess dorsal heart.
(b) None of them is aquatic.
(c) They all belong to the same phylum.
(d) They all have jointed paired appendages.

78. Biradial symmetry and lack of cnidoblasts are the characteristics of ***(2006)***
(a) Hydra and starfish
(b) Starfish and sea anemone
(c) Ctenoplana and Beroe
(d) Aurelia and Paramecium.

79. Two common characters found in centipede, cockroach and crab are ***(2006)***
(a) book lungs and antennae
(b) compound eyes and anal cerci
(c) jointed legs and chitinous exoskeletôn
(d) green gland and tracheae.

80. In which one of the following sets of animals do all the four give birth to young ones? ***(2006)***
(a) Kangaroo, hedgehog, dolphin, Loris
(b) Lion, bat, whale, ostrich
(c) Platypus, penguin, bat, hippopotamus
(d) Shrew, bat, cat, kiwi

81. Which one of the following is a matching set of a phylum and its three examples? ***(2006)***
(a) Porifera - Spongilla, Euplectella, Pennatula
(b) Cnidaria - Bonellia, Physalia, Aurelia
(c) Platyhelminthes - Planaria, Schistosoma, Enterobius
(d) Mollusca - Loligo, Teredo, Octopus

82. What is common about Trypanosoma, Noctiluca, Monocystis and Giardia? ***(2006)***
(a) These are all parasities.
(b) These are all unicellular protists.
(c) They have flagella.
(d) They produce spores.

83. In contrast to annelids the platyhelminthes show ***(2005)***
(a) absence of body cavity
(b) bilateral symmetry
(c) radial symmetry
(d) presence of pseudocoel.

84. From the following statements select the wrong one. ***(2005)***
(a) Prawn has two pairs of antennae.
(b) Nematocysts are characteristics of the Phylum Cnidaria.
(c) Millepedes have two pairs of appendages in each segment of the body.
(d) Animals belonging to Phylum Porifera are marine and fresh water.

85. Which one of the following characters is not typical of the Class Mammalia? ***(2005)***
(a) Thecodont dentition
(b) Alveolar lungs
(c) Ten pairs of cranial nerves
(d) Seven cervical vertebrae

86. In arthropoda, head and thorax are often used to form cephalothorax, but in which one of the following classes, is the body divided into head thorax and abdomen? ***(2004)***
(a) Insecta
(b) Myriapoda
(c) Crustacea
(d) Arachnida and crustacea

87. Presence of gills in the tadpole of frog indicates that ***(2004)***
(a) fish were amphibious in the past
(b) fish evolved from frog-like ancestors
(c) frogs will have gills in future
(d) frogs evolved from gilled ancestors.

88. One of the following is a very unique feature of the mammalian body ***(2004)***
(a) homeothermy
(b) presence of diaphragm
(c) four chambered heart
(d) rib cage.

89. Sycon belongs to a group of animals, which are best described as ***(2003)***
(a) unicellular or acellular
(b) multicellular without any tissue organization
(c) multicellular with a gastrovascular system
(d) multicellular having tissue organization, but no body cavity.

90. Which one of the following is a matching pair of an animal and a certain phenomenon it exhibits? ***(2003)***
(a) Pheretima - Sexual dimorphism
(b) Musca - Complete metamorphosis
(c) Chameleon - Mimicry
(d) Taenia - Polymorphism

91. Given below are four matchings of an animal and its kind of respiratory organ: ***(2003)***
(A) Silver fish - Trachea
(B) Scorpion - Book lung
(C) Sea squirt - Pharyngeal slits
(D) Dolphin - Skin

The correct matchings are
(a) (A) and (B) (b) (A), (B) and (C)
(c) (B) and (D) (d) (C) and (D).

92. In which of the following animals nerve cell is present but brain is absent? ***(2002)***
(a) Sponge (b) Earthworm
(c) Cockroach (d) Hydra

93. In which of the following, notochord is present in embryonic stage? ***(2002)***
(a) All chordates (b) Some chordates
(c) Vertebrates (d) Non chordates

94. In which of the following animals, haemocyanin pigment is found? ***(2001)***
(a) Annelida (b) Echinodermata
(c) Insecta (d) Mollusca

95. In which of the following animals post anal tail is found? ***(2001)***
(a) Earthworm (b) Lower invertebrates
(c) Scorpion (d) Snake

96. In Hydra, waste material of food digestion and nitrogenous waste material are removed respectively from ***(2001)***
(a) mouth and mouth
(b) body wall and body wall
(c) mouth and body wall
(d) mouth and tentacles.

97. Similarity in Ascaris lumbricoides and Anopheles stephensi is ***(2000)***
(a) sexual dimorphism
(b) metamerism
(c) anaerobic respiration
(d) endoparasitism.

98. Which of the following characters is absent in all chordates? ***(2000)***
(a) Diaphragm
(b) Coelom
(c) Pharyngeal gill clefts
(d) Dorsal nerve cord

99. What is true for mammalia? ***(2000)***
(a) Platypus is oviparous.
(b) Bats have feather.
(c) Elephant is ovoviviparous.
(d) Diaphragm is absent in them.

100. Aquatic reptiles are ***(1999)***
(a) ureotelic (b) ureotelic in water
(c) ammonotelic (d) ureotelic over land.

101. Temperature changes, in the environment, affect most of the animals which are ***(1999)***
(a) poikilothermic (b) homoiothermic
(c) aquatic (d) desert living.

102. The canal system is a characteristic feature of ***(1999)***
(a) echinoderms (b) sponges
(c) helminthes (d) coelenterates.

103. Which of the following is not found in birds? ***(1999)***
(a) Pelvic girdle (b) Pectoral girdle
(c) Hindlimb (d) Forelimb

104. The long bones are hollow and connected by air passages. They are the characteristics of ***(1998)***
(a) reptilia (b) land vertebrates
(c) aves (d) mammals.

105. Solenocytes are the main excretory structures in ***(1998)***
(a) echinodermates (b) platyhelminthes
(c) annelids (d) molluscs.

106. Most appropriate term to describe the life cycle of Obelia is ***(1998)***
(a) metamorphosis (b) neoteny
(c) metagenesis (d) all of these.

107 . Sound box of birds is called ***(1992)***
(a) pygostyle (b) larynx
(c) syrinx (d) synsacrum.

108. The excretory structures of flatworms/ Taenia are ***(1991)***
(a) flame cells (b) protonephridia
(c) Malpighian tubules (d) green glands.

109. What is common among silverfish, scorpion, crab and honey bee? ***(1997)***
(a) Jointed legs (b) Metamorphosis
(c) Compound eyes (d) Poison glands

110. Which of the following statements is without exception for sponges? ***(1996)***
(a) They all have calcareous spicules.
(b) They have high regenerative power.
(c) They are found only in marine water.
(d) They are all radially symmetrical.

111. Pneumatic bone is found in ***(1996)***
(a) shark (b) Rana
(c) pigeon (d) whale.

112. The nephridia in earthworm are analogous to **(1996)**
(a) nematoblasts of Hydra
(b) flame cells of Planaria
(c) gills of prawn
(d) trachea of insects.

113. Which of the following is common among mammals? ***(1996)***
(a) They undergo no moulting.
(b) They have seven cervical vertebrae.
(c) They are carnivores.
(d) They have ventral nerve cord.

114. The organisms attached to the substratum, generally, possess ***(1995)***
(a) one single opening of the digestive canal
(b) cilia on the surface to create water current
(c) radial symmetry
(d) asymmetrical body.

115. A common characteristic of all vertebrates without exception is ***(1994)***
(a) the division of body into head, neck, trunk and tail
(b) their body covered with an exoskeleton
(c) the possession of two pairs of functional appendages
(d) the presence of well-developed skull.

116. One of the special characters of coelenterata only is the occurrence of ***(1994)***
(a) polymorphism (b) flame cells
(c) hermaphroditism (d) nematocysts.

117. Radial symmetry is, usually, exhibited in animals which ***(1994)***
(a) are attached to the substratum
(b) have one opening of alimentary canal
(c) live in water
(d) have ciliary mode of feeding.

118. Which of the following is an example of platyhelminthes? ***(1994)***
(a) Plasmodium (b) Schistosoma
(c) Trypanosoma (d) Wuchereria

119. Among the following organisms point out a completely non-parasitic form ***(1994)***
(a) Tapeworm (b) Mosquito
(c) Sea anemone (d) Leech.

120. Tube feet are the characteristic structures of ***(1994)***
(a) starfish (b) jellyfish
(c) crayfish (d) cuttlefish.

121. Which of the following does not have an open circulatory system? ***(1994)***
(a) Frog's tadpole (b) Prawn
(c) Chelifer (d) Cockroach

122. Which is common between ostrich, penguin and kiwi? ***(1993)***
(a) Running birds (b) Migratory birds
(c) Flightless birds (d) Four toed birds

123. Budding is a normal mode of asexual reproduction in ***(1993)***
(a) starfish and Hydra
(b) Hydra and sponges
(c) tapeworm and Hydra
(d) sponge and starfish.

124. A larval stage occurs in the life history of all members of the group ***(1993)***
(a) frog, lizard and cockroach
(b) Ascaris, housefly and frog
(c) housefly, earthworm and mosquito
(d) butterfly, frog and mosquito.

125. Gorilla, chimpanzee, monkeys and humans belong to the same ***(1993)***
(a) species (b) genus
(c) family (d) order.

126. What is common in whale, bat and rat? (1993)
(a) Absence of neck
(b) Muscular diaphragm between thorax and abdomen
(c) Extra-abdominal testes to avoid high temperature of body
(d) Presence of external ears

ANSWER KEY

1.	(d)	2.	(b)	3.	(d)	4.	(a)	5.	(a)	6.	(a)	7.	(d)
8.	(d)	9.	(b)	10.	(c)	11.	(d)	12.	(d)	13.	(d)	14.	(c)
15.	(d)	16.	(a)	17.	(d)	18.	(b)	19.	(a)	20.	(d)	21.	(b)
22.	(a)	23.	(d)	24.	(b)	25.	(c)	26.	(b)	27.	(a)	28.	(c)
29.	(b)	30.	(b)	31.	(b)	32.	(a)	33.	(b)	34.	(b)	35.	(a)
36.	(c)	37.	(a)	38.	(d)	39.	(d)	40.	(b)	41.	(a)	42.	(*)
43.	(a)	44.	(a)	45.	(d)	46.	(b)	47.	(b)	48.	(a)	49.	(a)
50.	(c)	51.	(d)	52.	(d)	53.	(d)	54.	(d)	55.	(d)	56.	(a)
57.	(d)	58.	(b)	59.	(d)	60.	(c)	61.	(*)	62.	(c)	63.	(d)
64.	(d)	65.	(c)	66.	(b)	67.	(d)	68.	(b)	69.	(c)	70.	(d)
71.	(a)	72.	(c)	73.	(a)	74.	(d)	75.	(a)	76.	(d)	77.	(a)
78.	(c)	79.	(c)	80.	(a)	81.	(d)	82.	(b)	83.	(a)	84.	(a)
85.	(c)	86.	(a)	87.	(d)	88.	(b)	89.	(b)	90.	(b)	91.	(b)
92.	(d)	93.	(a)	94.	(d)	95.	(d)	96.	(c)	97.	(a)	98.	(a)
99.	(a)	100.	(b)	101.	(a)	102.	(b)	103.	(d)	104.	(c)	105.	(b)
106.	(c)	107.	(c)	108.	(a)	109.	(a)	110.	(b)	111.	(c)	112.	(b)
113.	(a)	114.	(c)	115.	(d)	116.	(d)	117.	(a)	118.	(b)	119.	(c)
120.	(a)	121.	(a)	122.	(c)	123.	(b)	124.	(d)	125.	(d)	126.	(b)

HINTS & EXPLANATIONS

1. (d) Adults of hemichordates have bilateral symmetry.

2. (b) : Mollusca shows organ system level of organisation with unsegmented body (except Neopilina which is a segmented mollusc) having distinct head, muscular foot and visceral hump. They usually show bilateral symmetry but some molluscs (example Pila) become asymmetrical due to torsion.

3. (d)

4. (a) : Triploblastic is a condition which describes an animal having a body composed of three embryonic germ layers : the ectoderm, mesoderm and endoderm. Most multicellular animals belonging to Phylum Platyhelminthes to Phylum Chordata are triploblastic. Ctenophores, sponges and corals are diploblastic.

5. (a): Acoelomates are animals having no body cavity or coelom. Examples are poriferans, coelenterates, ctenophora, platyhelminthes. In pseudocoelomates, body space is pseudocoelom or false coelom. Examples are aschelminthes. In coelomates, body space is a true coelom enclosed by mesoderm on both sides. Remaining phyla from annelida to arthropoda are coelomates. Molluscs and insects are coelomates while flatworms are acoelomates.

6. (a) :Aschelminthes is a phylum consisting of pseudocoelomates. These are mostly aquatic, free living or parasitic. Their body is slender, bilaterally symmetrical and triploblastic.

7. **(d)** The term metamerism refers to a linear repetition of parts in an animal body. It occurs in three highly organized phyla : Annelida, Arthropoda and Chordata. Each segment is called a metamere, or somite. Segmentation often affects both external and internal structures. Such a condition is called metameric segmentation. In chordates, the segmentation is apparent only in the embryonic stage. In the adult chordates, segmentation is visible in the internal structures, such as vertebrae, ribs, nerves and blood vessels.

8. **(d)**: Echinoderms are triploblastic animals with organ system level of organisation. Larval forms possess bilateral symmetry while adults have radial symmetry.

9. **(b)**: Hydra, has tissue level of organization. Its body is multicellular and the cells occur in 2 distinct layers or tissues of specialized cells. Sponges have cellular level of organization. Liver fluke and Ascaris have organ-system level of organization.

10. **(c)**: Coelom is a fluid-filled cavity that forms the main body cavity of vertebrate and most invertebrate animals. It is found between mesoderm and body wall (endoderm).

11. **(d)**

12. **(d)**: The unique mammalian characters are mammary glands (milk producing glands), presence of hair and external ears or pinnae.

13. **(d)**: Chordates possess dorsal, hollow, single nerve cord, closed circulatory system, paired pharyngeal gill slits, ventral muscular heart, triploblastic and coelomate animals.

14. **(c)**: The body of arthropods is covered by chitinous exoskeleton.

15. **(d)** : The alimentary canal of birds have additional chambers, the crop and gizzard. Crop stores and softens the food however the gizzard helps in crushing and chewing the food, e.g., Pavo, Psittacula, Corvus.

16. **(a)**: Phylum chorodata possesses three sub-phylum (Urochordata, Cephalochordata, Vertebrata) which possess notochord at some stage of their life. The members of subphylum Vertebrata possess notochord during the embryonic period. The notochord is replaced by a cartilaginous or bony vertebral column in the adult. Thus, all vertebrates are chordates but all chordates are not vertebrates.

17. **(d)**: Physalia - Portuguese man of war
Limulus - Living fossil
Ancylostoma - Hookworm
Pinctada - Pearl oyster

18. **(b)**

19. **(a)** : Metagenesis is observed in Obelia which belongs to the Phylum Coelenterata. Comb plates present in ctenophores help in locomotion.

20. **(d)**

21. **(b)**: Platyhelminthes are bilaterally symmetrical, triploblastic and acoelomate animals with organ level of organisation.

22. **(a)**

23. **(d)**: In Urochordata, notochord is present only in larval tail. Phylum Chordata is divided into three subphyla : Urochordata or Tunicata, Cephalochordata and Vertebrata.

24. **(b)**

25. **(c)**: The buccal cavity of Pila (apple snail) possess rasping organ, radula, with transverse row of teeth for cutting grass. Bombyx (silk moth), an insect has Malpighian tubules, as excretory organ. Pleurobrachia is a ctenophore having

eight ciliary plates called comb plates. Taenia is a platyhelminth having flame cells for excretion and osmoregulation.

26. **(b)**

27. **(a)**: Metamorphosis is the process of transformation of an immature larva into an adult form in two or more distinct stages. Animals that undergo metamorphosis are said to have indirect development, e.g., tunicates, moth, starfish, etc. In case of earthworm, development is direct which means no larval stage is present and hence, there is no metamorphosis.

28. **(c)**: The alimentary canal of birds have additional chambers, the crop and gizzard. Crop stores and softens the food however the gizzard helps in crushing and chewing the food, e.g., Pavo, Psittacula, Corvus.

29. **(b)**: Homeotherms are the animals that maintain constant body temperature, irrespective of surrounding temperature by metabolic activity, e.g., birds and mammals. Turtle (Chelone) belongs to Class Reptilia and is poikilotherm or cold blooded.

30. **(b)**: An important characteristics that hemichordates and chordates share is presence of pharyngeal gill slits. Gill slits are dorsal in position in hemichordates whereas they are lateral in chordates.

31. **(b)** : Whales, dolphins and seals are examples of aquatic mammals. Trygon and sharks are cartilaginous fishes.

32. **(a)**: Perissodactyla represents the order of horse. Equidae is the family, caballus is the subspecies whereas E. ferus is the species of horse.

33. **(b)**: Spongocoel is the central body cavity of the sponges. It is lined by highly specialised flagellated cells called choanocytes.

34. **(b)**: Ornithorhynchus and Tachyglossus are oviparous mammals. Crocodile is a reptile which possesses four chambered heart. In cartilaginous fish (except Chimaera) gills are not covered by an operculum.

35. **(a)**: All birds are oviparous while all mammals except Ornithorhynchus (duck billed platypus) and Echidna or Tachyglossus (spiny anteater) are viviparous.

36. **(c)**: Phylum Chordata includes both jawless vertebrates (Agnatha) and jawed vertebrates (Gnathostomata), Crocodile of Class Reptilia has four chambered heart with two auricles and two ventricles. Duck billed platypus and spiny anteater are oviparous mammals.

37. **(a)**: Parapodia are flattened, fleshy, vertical flap-like outgrowths of body wall found in annelids on lateral sides of trunk segments. These are hollow structures enclosing coelom which is continuous with that of trunk segments. These serve the dual purpose of locomotion and respiration.

38. **(d)**: Phylum Porifera (the sponges) has cellular level of body organisation, with inner cellular layer consisting of highly specialised flagellated cells called choanocytes (or collar cells). The development in this phylum is indirect as it includes a free swimming larva called amphiblastula or parenchymula for dispersal of the species.

39. **(d)**: An alternation of generation between asexual and sexual phases of an organism is referred to as metagenesis. E.g., in Obelia (a coelenterate), polyps reproduce asexually and medusae reproduce sexually.

40. **(b)**: Petromyzon (Lamprey) belongs to the Class Cyclostomata of Phylum Chordata. It is a jawless fish which lays eggs in fresh water.

The eggs hatch in about 3 weeks into minute transparent larvae called ammocoetes. After metamorphosis, the young lampreys swim down to the sea where they remain for 3 or 4 years before reaching maturity, when they once again migrate to streams or rivers to spawn and die. Gonads become mature at that time when adults return to rivers for spawning.

41. **(a)**: Trichinella spiralis is a minute nematode parasite that shows viviparity i.e., produces live youngs (larvae) not eggs. The adults of T. spiralis live in the human small intestine, where the females release large numbers of larvae. These larvae bore through the intestine and can cause trichinosis or trichiniasis which has symptoms like diarrohea, nausea, vertigo, pain in limbs and fever etc.

Humans get infected after eating imperfectly cooked meat infected with the parasite's larval cysts.

42. **(*)** : None of the options is correct.

Cyclostomes do not have paired appendages. Skin in Aves is neither moist nor glandular. Only preen gland is present at the base of tail. Chondrichthyes members have gills without operculum, except Chimaera. Prototherian mammals do not have ear pinnae and aquatic mammals lack hindlimbs (like whales and dolphins).

43. **(a)**: Duck-billed platypus is an egg laying mammal. It is found in the rivers in Eastern Australia and Tasmania. It is a beaver like monotreme about $50-60 cm$ long and well adapted to live in water. Usually, two eggs are laid at a time. The female curls around them for incubation and remains inactive for about two weeks. Newly hatched young ones are very immature, naked, blind and each is 2.5 cm long.

44. **(a)**: Exoskeleton made of cuticle has enabled insects to live on land and to diversify to almost all the possible habitats. It gives them protection, support and also helps to prevent desiccation.

45. **(d)**: Cnidarians are the sac-like animals which are aquatic, mostly marine except a few like Hydra, are fresh water forms. They are the simplest organisms that have attained a tissue level of organization. Members of Ctenophora, Cephalochordata and Echinodermata are exclusively marine.

46. **(b)**: Planaria possesses high degree of regeneration. Both epimorphosis, in which the missing parts are formed and morphallaxis, in which the whole body can be regenerated from a fragment of the body.

47. **(b)**: Torpedo is a bottom-living marine fish, discharging electricity which is sufficient to stun preys such as small fishes, etc. A pair of electric organs are situated on the dorsal side of the trunk region. Infact the electric organs are the modified lateral muscle-plates innervated by the cranial nerves.

48. **(a)**: Spiny anteater (Echidna) is a prototherian mammal whereas, sea urchins and sea cucumber are echinoderms. Silver fish (Lepisma) is an insect, Cuttle fish (Sepia) is a mollusc and flying fish (Exocoetus) is a bony fish. Centipede is Class Chilopoda, Millipede is Class Diplopoda and Scorpion and Spider are Class Arachnida of Phylum Arthropoda.

49. **(a)**: Prawn, Scorpion and Locusta belong to the Phylum Arthropoda. All other animal categories are given below:
Sponge $\rightarrow$ Porifera
Sea anemone $\rightarrow$ Coelenterata
Starfish $\rightarrow$ Echinodermata
Malarial parasite, Amoeba $\rightarrow$ Protozoa

Mosquito → Arthropoda
Earthworm → Annelida
Pinworm → Aschelminthes
Tapeworm → Platyhelminthes

50. **(c)**

51. **(d)**: Phylum Arthropoda is the largest phylum of Animalia which includes insects. Examples include Apis, silkworm, Laccifer, silver fish (Lepisma), locust, etc. Puffer fish and flying fish (Exocoetus) are examples of Superclass Pisces, while cuttle fish (Sepia) belongs to Phylum Mollusca.

52. **(d)**: Reptiles represent the first class of vertebrates fully adapted for life in dry places on land. The characters of reptiles are in fact a combination of characters that are found in fish and amphibians on one hand and birds and mammals on the other. Their exoskeleton is of horny epidermal scales, shields, plates and scutes. The skin is dry, cornified and devoid of glands. Reptiles lack external ears.

53. **(d)** : In ctenophores, asexual reproduction is absent. They are monoecious and fertilization is generally external. In cnidaria, asexual reproduction (budding) is found in the polyps and sexual reproduction is found in the medusa form. Both asexual and sexual reproduction occur in porifera (sponges). Asexual reproduction occurs by budding and gemmules. In protozoa, asexual reproduction takes place by binary fission, budding, etc., and sexual reproduction takes place by syngamy and conjugation.

54. **(d)**: Duckbilled platypus is oviparous and belongs to Class Mammalia. Millipede belongs to Class Diplopoda. Sea anemone has two germ layers, i.e., diploblastic. Silver fish (Lepisma) belongs to nonchordata. It is an insect.

55. **(d)**: Sharks and dogfishes have cylindrical body while skates and rays have both of their pectoral fins fused. It gives a wing-like appearance and are not distinct from body.

56. **(a)** Pila belongs to Phylum Mollusca. The body of molluscs (soft bodied animals) is unsegmented, with a distinct head, muscular foot and visceral hump. Radula is found in mouth of Pila.

57. **(d)**: Sea horse (Hippocampus) and flying fish (Exocoetus) belong to Class Osteichthyes of super class pisces. They have two chambered heart (one auricle and one ventricle) and are cold blooded animals.

58. **(b)**: Heart is generally 3-chambered in reptiles but in crocodile, it is 4-chambered. Sponges are generally marine and have collared cells but few fresh water forms can also be seen like Spongilla. All mammals are viviparous (giving birth to young ones) with an exception, Ornithorhynchus (platypus), which is oviparous (egg laying).

59. **(d)**: Tail end is straight in female Ascaris, while tail end is curved ventrally in male Ascaris. Anal cerci is present in both male and female cockroach, while anal style is present only in the male cockroach. The forelimbs in both frogs (male and female) bear small articular pads dorsally at the joints of digit, but the males possess a special nuptial, copulatory pad on ventral side of the first finger of each forelimb. Copulatory pad appears merely as rough patches, but during breeding season, these become thick and sticky. In copulation, the male strongly grips a female under her armpits by means of these pads. Claspers are modified inner edges of pelvic fins in male sharks.

60. **(c)**

61. **(*)**: None of the options is correct.

Ascaris is member of Phylum Nematoda, which are round worms. They do not have segmented body. In Ascaris female is longer than male.

Salamandra is member of amphibia. Salamanders do not have tympanum, although they have greatly reduced middle ears and fertilization is usually internal in them.

Pteropus is member of Class Mammalia. They are viviparous. A mantle of golden hair covers the head, neck and shoulders in Pteropus.

Aurelia is member of coelenterata, which has tissue level of organization. Its epidermis contain cnidoblasts (stinging cells) for defence and offence purpose.

62. **(c)**: Humans are mammals which are chordates. Phylum Chordata includes animals which possess a notochord either throughout or during early embryonic life. In Ascidia (urochordata), notochord is present only in larval tail while in Amphioxus (cephalochordata), it extends from head to tail region and is persistent throughout their life. It is replaced by a vertebral column in adult frog.

63. **(d)** :The animals which possess true coelom are called eucoelomates or coelomates. The true coelom is a body cavity which arises as a cavity in embryonic mesoderm. True coelom is of two types; schizocoelom (schizocoel) and enterocoelom (enterocoel). Schizocoelom develops as a split in the mesoderm sheet. It is found in annelids, arthropods, molluscs. In enterocoelom, mesoderm arises from the wall of the embryonic cut of enteron as hollow outgrowths. It occurs in echinoderms and chordates.

64. **(d)**: In Fasciola (flatworms) the body has a single cavity with one opening to the outside. The single opening functions as both mouth for ingestion (intake of food) and anus for egestion (undigested food is passed out). It is called blind sac plan. Other examples are coelenterates.

65. **(c)**: Spongilla is a common, widely distributed fresh water sponge belonging to Phylum Porifera. Canal system in Spongilla is with choanocytes restricted to small rounded chambers. It is not found in leech, dolphin and penguin.

66. **(b)**: Nephridia is the excretory organ of the earthworm. Earthworms have three types of nephridial structures called as septal, integumentary and pharyngeal nephridia. These three nephridial structures are present on different positions in the body and also vary in structures. Septal and pharyngeal nephridia are both enteronephric i.e., nitrogen products are expelled in gut. Integumentary nephridia is exonephric i.e., nitrogen waste products are directly discharged outside.

67. **(d)**: Animals belonging to Phylum Chordata are fundamentally characterised by the presence of a notochord, a dorsal hollow nerve cord and paired pharyngeal gill slits. Crocodile, penguin, whale and dogfish are all chordates. All of them have gill slits or have had it during embryonic development. Thus, paired gill slits are present in these animals at some stage of life.

68. **(b)**: Agnatha is subphylum or superclass of marine and fresh water vertebrates that lack jaws. They are fish-like animals with cartilaginous skeletons and well-developed sucking mouth parts with horny teeth. The only living agnathans are lampreys and hagfishes (Class Cyclostomata), which are parasites or scavengers.

69. **(c)**: Birds have originated from some ancestral reptilian stalk. These two classes have so many features in common that link the two groups.

The evidence of reptilian ancestry of birds is furnished by their comparative anatomy, embryology and palaeontology. One of the features is that all birds have horny epidermal scales confined to the lower parts of their legs and feet, which are exactly like the epidermal scales of the reptiles.

70. **(d)**: Ascaris belongs to the Phylum Nematoda of Superphylum Aschelminthes. They have a cylindrical body without showing any metamerism, a pseudocoel (false coelom) and a complete digestive tract lined by endodermal epithelium. The cuticle covering the body surface bears minute transverse striations giving a pseudosegmented appearance to the worm.

71. **(a)** : Scorpion, spider and cockroach belong to Phylum Arthropoda and are invertebrates. They possess ventral solid central nervous system which consists of a dorsal brain connected with a nerve ring to a double ventral nerve cord.

72. **(c)** : Arthropods are the largest phylum of Kingdom Animalia that characteristically possesses an outer body layer - the cuticle. The body is composed of segments usually forming distinct specialized body regions, i.e., head, thorax and abdomen. In them the trachea or windpipe or book lungs are the respiratory organs found in terrestrial forms, which help in respiration.

73. **(a)**: Phylum Annelida comprises invertebrates, which are segmented worms having cylindrical soft bodies showing metameric segmentation. These are triploblastic animals showing bilateral symmetry. A true coelom is present which is filled with coelomic fluid containing cells. Annelids are perhaps the first animals to have a true schizocoelic coelom.

74. **(d)**: Reptiles have two auricles and a partly divided ventricle except crocodiles which have four-chambered heart. Obelia shows metagenesis i.e., alternation of generations which may be defined as a phenomenon in which diploid asexual phase alternates with haploid sexual phase. Lemur has a thecodent teeth i.e., the teeth are embedded in the sockets of the jaw bone.

75. **(a)**

76. **(d)**: Homoiothermy is the maintenance by an animal in which body temperature remains constant and does not change with the change of environmental temperature. Homoiothermy occurs in birds and mammals, which are described as endotherms. The heat produced by their tissue metabolism and the heat lost to the environment are balanced by various means to keep body temperature constant: 36–38°C in mammals and 38–40°C in birds. The hypothalamus in the brain monitors blood temperature and controls thermoregulation by both nervous and hormonal means. Thus, parrot (bird), platypus and kangaroo (mammals) are homoiothermic animals.

77. **(a)** :Nereis, scorpion, cockroach and silver fish are all invertebrates and thus possess dorsal heart. Nereis is a marine animal while other animals mentioned in the question are terrestrial. Nereis belongs to Phylum Annelida while rest of the animals belong to Phylum Arthropoda. Jointed appendages are present in scorpion, cockroach and silver fish.

78. **(c)**: Ctenophora is a small phylum of exclusively marine, invertebrate animals. Ctenoplana and Beroe are examples of ctenophora. They have biradial symmetry (a combination of radial and bilateral symmetries). They lack the specialized stinging cells (nematocysts) found in coelenterates, but one species (Haeckelia rubra) incorporates those of its jellyfish prey for its own defense.

79. (c) : Centipede, cockroach and crab all belong to Phylum Arthropoda which are characterized by jointed legs and chitinous exoskeleton. Arthropods have bilaterally symmetrical and metamerically segmented body with haemocoel and open blood vascular system.

80. (a): Kangaroo, hedgehog, dolphin and Loris are mammals and thus give brith to young ones. Ostrich and kiwi are birds that lay eggs. Platypus is a most primitive living mammal that lays eggs. Other animals in the options are mammals and give birth to young ones.

81. (d): Mollusca includes those animals which have soft bodies, usually furnished with a shell. The body is often divided into a head, with eyes or tentacles, a muscular foot and a visceral mass housing the organs. Loligo (squid or sea arrow), Teredo (shipworm), Octopus are some of their examples. In option (a) Spongilia and Euplectella belong to porifera but Pennatula (the sea pen or sea feather) belongs to coelenterata. In option (b) Physalia and Aurelia belong to cnidaria but Bonellia belongs to Phylum Annelida. In option (c) Planaria and Schistosoma belong to platyhelminthes but Enterobius (Pinworm) belongs to aschelminthes.

82. (b) : Protista is the kingdom of unicellular eukaryotes. The protists include heterotrophs, autotrophs and some organisms that can vary their nutritional mode depending upon environmental conditions. Protists occur in freshwater, saltwater, soil, and as symbionts within other organisms. Trypanosoma, Noctiluca, Monocystis and Giardia are all unicellular protists.

83. (a) : Platyhelminthes do not have body cavity so they are acoelomates. In annelids, the body cavity is true and schizocoelous. Both annelids and platyhelminthes have bilateral symmetry.

84. (a) : Prawn has one pair of antennae, one on either side, just below the antennules. They are sensory, excretory and balancing in function. Antennules are attached on either side, below the bases of eye stalks. They are tactile in function. Nematocysts are present in cnidoblasts that act as organs of offence and defence. Millipedes belong to Class Myriapoda. They are called thousand leggers because of possession of numerous walking legs. Body is made up of small head and 40 trunk segments, each with two pairs of jointed legs. Animals belonging to Phylum Porifera are mostly marine and a few are freshwater.

85. (c): Mammals have twelve pair of cranial nerves. Ten pairs of cranial nerves are present in fish and amphibians. Reptiles and birds also have 12 pairs of cranial nerves.

86. (a) : Body in arthropoda is segmented. Segments are grouped into 3 forms - head, thorax and abdomen. When head and thorax are fused then they are referred to as cephalothorax. Class Insecta of Phylum Arthropoda have body divided into head, thorax and abdomen.

87. (d): It is universally accepted that amphibians (frogs) have originated from fishes. Resemblance of amphibia to fish is seen in most systems of the body. Both are cold blooded. Fish respire by gills and also tadpole of frog respires by gills. To prevent dessication in air, both usually lay eggs in water.

88. (b):The unique feature of mammals is the presence of diaphragm. It is a membrane that separates thoracic cavity from abdominal cavity. The cavity of other animals is not divided into thoracic and abdominal cavities. Homeothermy, four chambered heart and rib cage are the characters of mammals as well as some other animals also.

89. (b): Sycon, belonging to the Phylum Porifera, are multicellular organisms with cellular level of body organisation. The constituent cells perform their functions more or less independently. No distinct tissue or organs are present in it.

90. (b): In Musca, development is indirect with complete metamorphosis (holometaboly) including four stages as follows

- egg, larva, pupa and adult. In complete metamorphosis, larva after hatching, moults several times to become a fully grown one. It later becomes a pupa within a secreted case, called the puparium. Pupa differentiates into the young adult that breaks the puparium open and emerges outside. Then it grows to a mature form.

91. (b) : Silver fish is an insect in which respiration occurs by tracheae. These communicate with the exterior by paired apertures, called spiracles. Respiratory system of scorpion consists of 4 pairs of book lungs that communicate with the outer air through stigma. In sea squirt, respiration occurs through pharyngeal slits. In dolphin, respiration occurs by lungs

92. (d): Hydra which belongs to the Phylum Coelenterata has nerve cells but no brain. Its nervous system consists of nerve cells and their processes. Sensory cells are also present. Sponges do not have nerve cells, they lack nervous system. Earthworm (annelida) has nervous system consisting of a circumenteric nerve ring and a solid, double, midventral nerve cord with ganglia. Cockroach (arthropoda) has the nervous system as that of earthworm.

93. (a): Chordates are the animals that have notochord, a skeletal rod present at some stage in life cycle. In lower vertebrates, notochord persists throughout life while in higher vertebrates it is replaced by vertebral column in adults. Nonchordates never develop notochord, not even in embryonic stage.

94. (d): In molluscs, blood often has a copper-containing, blue respiratory pigment called haemocyanin. In insects, the blood called haemolymph is colourless. In echinodermates, blood is colourless as it has no respiratory pigment. In annelids, the blood is red with haemoglobin dissolved in plasma.

95. (d): Snakes are limbless reptiles with elongated cylindrical body, covered with overlapping scales differentiated into shields and plates and have post anal tail which is long.

96. (c): In Hydra indigestible residues are egested through mouth, for there is no anus. Egestion occurs by a sudden squirt due to muscular contraction of body, so that the debris is thrown at a distance. Hydra has neither blood, blood vessels, nor organs of excretion. Due to thinness of body wall and circulation of water in gastrovascular cavity, most cells of body remain freely exposed to the surrounding water. Therefore, excretion of waste nitrogenous matter (chiefly ammonia) occurs directly by diffusion through cell membranes in the outside world.

97. (a) : Sexual dimorphism is the difference in the form of individuals of different sexes but of same species. Sexes in Ascaris are separate and sexual dimorphism is well defined. Males are smaller than females. They possess a recurved tail with pre and post anal papillae, a cloaca and a pair of spicules or penial setae. In Anopheles, the ends of maxillary palps in males are club-shaped while in females they are not.

98. **(a)**: Diaphragm is a membrane that separates thoracic cavity from abdominal cavity. It is present only in mammals. All other chordates do not have diaphragm as their body cavity is not divided into thoracic and abdominal cavities.

99. **(a)**: Mammals are viviparous i.e., they give birth to young ones. Protherians (e.g., Platypus) are primitive mammals and lay eggs, so they are oviparous.

100. **(b)**: The waste material of aquatic reptiles chiefly consists of urea, so they are ureotelic. Land forms are uricotelic i.e., their waste material consists of uric acid.

101. **(a)**: Poikilothermic animals are those whose body temperature varies with the temperature of the environment. All animals except birds and mammals are poikilothermic.

102. **(b)**

103. **(d)**: Forelimbs are absent in birds as they are modified into wings for flight. They are attached high on the back to the anterior or thoracic region of the trunk and are very powerful when compared with the size and strength of the bird. Each wing is elongated, flattened and distally pointed with its longitudinal axis at right angles to that of the trunk.

104. **(c)** :Aves are the animals that fly so their body weight should be less and for this their bones are hollow and connected by air passages.

105. **(b)**: Solenocytes are also called flame cells. It is a cup shaped cell which contains group of cilia and this is the main excretory organ of platyhelminthes.

106. **(c)**:Obelia belongs to the Phylum Coelenterata. In Obelia, life-cycle includes two clearly defined phases: a fixed polypoid phase (hydroid colony) and a pelagic medusoid phase. Hydroid colony has no gonads and reproduces by asexual budding to give rise to medusae. On the other hand, medusae reproduce exclusively by sexual method (ova and sperms) to give rise to new hydroid colonies. This fact apparently seems to have given rise to the idea of alternation of generations, also called metagenesis.

107. **(c)**: At the posterior end or base of the trachea, at its junction with the bronchi, is found a special structure, the syrinx or voice box, concerned with sound production. It is characteristic of birds as it does not occur in other vertebrates.

108. **(a)**: Flame cells are scattered throughout parenchyma from which they remove metabolic wastes. A flame cell is of irregular shape, with granular cytoplasm and a nucleus. Bundle of cilia, or flame, arises from basal granules near nucleus. Cilia are enclosed into a funnel-shaped lumen formed by the terminal blind end of a capillary. Protonephridia are found in flatworms, Malpighian tubules in insects and green glands in crustaceans.

109. **(a)**

110. **(b)**: Sponges may have calcareous or siliceous spicules. All sponges are not marine, some are freshwater living also. Sponges may be asymmetrical or bilaterally symmetrical, besides being radially symmetrical. So, these characters are with exception. The character without exception is the regenerative power of sponges.

All sponges have a good power of regeneration. They can regrow any part of the body lost or cut off. Small fragments can grow into a complete sponge.

111. **(c)**: Pneumatic bone is present in pigeon to keep it light weight because it has to fly. Pneumatic bone has a hollow cavity, which makes it light.

112. (b): Analogous organs are organs of very disparate organisms and are superficially similar but have evolved from vastly different origins. They have same function but different structure. The nephridia in earthworm are analogous to flame cells of Planaria since both of them have excretory functions. Nematoblasts of Hydra are organs of locomotion, food capture and anchorage. Gills and trachea are organs of respiration in prawn and insects respectively.

113.(a) : Mammals do not undergo moulting. Moulting is usually exhibited by invertebrates. In many vertebrate species, cervical vertebrae are variable in number, however almost all mammals have seven cervical vertebrae including those with short neck such as elephants or whales and those with very long necks, such as giraffes. But there are a few exceptional cases in which there are nine cervical vertebrae in mammals. All the mammals are not carnivorous, they may be herbivorous, carnivorous and omnivorous also. Mammals have dorsal nerve cord.

114. (c): The organisms attached to the substratum possess radial symmetry in all vertical planes. All the animals belonging to cnidaria (e.g., jellyfish) and echinodermata (e.g., starfish) are radially symmetrical and typically sessile in their adult form. In radial symmetry the parts in an organ or organism when cut through the centre in any direction produces two halves that are mirror images of each other.

115. (d): The sub-phylum vertebrata or craniata have a well developed central nervous system that is differentiated into brain and spinal cord. Brain is protected by a brain box called cranium, so they are also called as craniata.

116. (d): The cells characteristic of the coelenterates include stinging cells (cnidocytes or cnidoblasts or nematoblasts) for offence and defence. The stinging cells, when discharged, give out from a sac, the cnide or cnidocyst or nematocyst, a long thread-tube that may coil around the prey, or attach to it, or inject a toxin, called hypnotoxin, into it to paralyse it.

117. (a)

118. (b) : Platyhelminthes have soft and dorsoventrally flattened body with bilateral symmetry. Plasmodium and Trypanosoma belong to Phylum Protozoa while Wuchereria belongs to Phylum Aschelminthes.

119. (c): Sea anemone is completely non-parasitic form. It shows the example of mutualism. Sea-anemone attaches itself to shell used by a hermit crab. The anemone obtains nourishment from the scraps of food left by the crab and is transported from place to place when the crab moves. The crab is protected by the stinging cells in the tentacles of sea anemone.

120. (a) : Starfish belongs to the Phylum Echinodermata who have developed tube feet for locomotion. The tube feet generally protrude out through special radial areas called ambulacra. They are extended and retracted by variations in hydraulic pressure of fluid in them and by contractions of their muscles.

121. (a): In the open circulatory system, the blood is not confined to the blood vessels, but it flows in the open spaces. Prawn, Chelifer and cockroach have open circulatory system. Frog's tadpole has closed circulatory system, that is the blood flows in the blood vessels.

122. (c): Ostrich, penguin and kiwi are flightless birds

123. (b): Budding is an asexual mode of reproduction in Hydra and sponges. Bud is formed as an outgrowth on the body surface, then detached to form new animal.

124. (d): In butterfly, the larval stage is known as caterpillar, in frog is known as tadpole and in mosquito is known as wriggler.

125. (d): Gorilla, chimpanzee, monkeys and humans belong to the same Order i.e., Primates. They have well developed brain, flat nails on fingers and toes. First digit is usually opposable, an adaptation for grasping. Eyes are typically large and turned forward.

126. (b): Whale, bat and rat are mammals. Diaphragm is present in mammals. The diaphragm separates the thoracic cavity (with lung and heart) from the abdominal cavity (with digestive system and urogenital system).

Chapter : 05 MORPHOLOGY OF FLOWERING PLANTS

THE ROOT

1. The roots that originate from the base of the stem are *(2020)*
(a) fibrous roots (b) primary roots
(c) prop roots (d) lateral roots.

2. Sweet potato is a modified *(2018)*
(a) stem (b) adventitious root
(c) tap root (d) rhizome.

3. Roots play insignificant role in absorption of water in *(2015)*
(a) pea (b) wheat
(c) sunflower (d) Pistia.

4. Pneumatophores are found in *(2000)*
(a) the vegetation which is found in marshy and saline lake
(b) the vegetation which found in acidic soil
(c) xerophytes
(d) epiphytes.

5. The plant, which bears clinging roots, is(1999)
(a) screw pine (b) Podostemon
(c) Trapa (d) orchid.

6. Velamen is found in *(1991)*
(a) roots of screwpine
(b) aerial and terrestrial roots of orchids
(c) leaves of Ficus elastic
(d) aerial roots of orchids.

THE STEM

7. Identify the correct set of statements : *(2022)*
(A) The leaflets are modified into pointed hard thorns in Citrus and Bougainvillea
(B) Axillary buds form slender and spirally coiled tendrils in cucumber and pumpkin
(C) Stem is flattened and fleshy in Opuntia and modified to perform the function of leaves
(D) Rhizophora shows vertically upward growing roots that help to get oxygen for respiration
(E) Subaerially growing stems in grasses and strawberry help in vegetative propagation.

Choose the correct answer from the options given below:
(a) (B) and (C) only
(b) (A) and (D) only
(c) (B), (C), (D) and (E) only
(d) (A), (B), (D) and (E) only

8. In Bougainvillea, thorns are the modifications of *(2017)*
(a) adventitious root (b) stem
(c) leaf (d) stipules.

9. Which of the following is not a stem modification? *(NEET-I 2016)*
(a) Tendrils of cucumber
(b) Flattened structures of Opuntia
(c) Pitcher of Nepenthes
(d) Thorns of citrus

10. Stems modified into flat green organs performing the functions of leaves are known as *(NEET-I 2016)*
(a) phylloclades (b) scales
(c) cladodes (d) phyllodes.

11. An example of edible underground stem is *(2014)*
(a) carrot (b) groundnut
(c) sweet potato (d) potato.

12. Sweet potato is homologous to *(Mains 2011)*
(a) potato (b) Colocasia
(c) ginger (d) turnip.

13. Which one of the following is a xerophytic plant in which the stem is modified into the flat green and succulent structure? *(Mains 2010)*
(a) Opuntia (b) Casuarina
(c) Hydrilla (d) Acacia

14. What is the eye of potato? ***(2001)***
(a) Axillary bud (b) Accessory bud
(c) Adventitious bud (d) Apical bud

15. New banana plants develop from ***(1990)***
(a) rhizome (b) sucker
(c) stolon (d) seed.

THE LEAF

16. Leaves become modified into spines in ***(2015 Cancelled)***
(a) onion (b) silk cotton
(c) Opuntia (d) pea.

17. How many plants among China rose, Ocimum, sunflower, mustard, Alstonia, guava, Calotropis and Nerium (oleander) have opposite phyllotaxy? ***(Karnataka NEET 2013)***
(a) Three (b) Four
(c) Five (d) Two

18. Phyllode is present in ***(2012)***
(a) Asparagus (b) Euphorbia
(c) Australian Acacia (d) Opuntia.

19. Whorled, simple leaves with reticulate venation are present in ***(Mains 2011)***
(a) Calotropis (b) neem
(c) China rose (d) Alstonia.

THE INFLORESCENCE

20. Given below are two statements : One is labelled as Assertion (A) and the other is labelled as Reason (R):

Assertion (A) : A flower is defined as modified shoot wherein the shoot apical meristem changes to floral meristem.

Reason (R) : Internode of the shoot gets condensed to produce different floral appendages laterally at successive nodes instead of leaves.

In the light of the above statements, choose the correct answer from the options given below :

(a) (A) is true but (R) is false.
(b) (A) is false but (R) is true.
(c) Both (A) and (R) are true and (R) is the correct explanation of (A).
(d) Both (A) and (R) are true but (R) is not the correct explanation of (A).

21. Inflorescence is racemose in ***(Karnataka NEET 2013)***
(a) brinjal (b) tulip
(c) Aloe (d) soybean.

22. In a cymose inflorescence the main axis ***(Karnataka NEET 2013)***
(a) has unlimited growth
(b) bears a solitary flower
(c) has unlimited growth but lateral branches end in flowers
(d) terminates in a flower.

23. Cymose inflorescence is present in ***(2012)***
(a) Solanum (b) Sesbania
(c) Trifolium (d) Brassica.

24. Long filamentous threads protruding at the end of a young cob of maize are ***(2006)***
(a) hairs (b) anthers
(c) styles (d) ovaries.

25. Hair found in the inflorescence of Zea mays are the modification of ***(2000)***
(a) style (b) stigma
(c) spathe (d) filaments.

26. Hypanthodium is a specialised type of (1994)
(a) fruit (b) inflorescence
(c) thalamus (d) ovary.

THE FLOWER

27. Axile placentation is observed in
(a) tomato, Dianthus and pea
(b) China rose, Petunia and lemon
(c) mustard, cucumber and primrose
(d) China rose, beans and lupin.

28. The flowers are zygomorphic in ***(2022)***
(A) Mustard (B) Gulmohar
(C) Cassia (D) Datura

(E) Chilly

Choose the correct answer from the options given below :

(a) (A), (B), (C) only (b) (B), (C) only
(c) (D), (E) only (d) (C), (D), (E) only

29. Which one of the following plants shows vexillary aestivation and diadelphous stamens? ***(2022)***

(a) Colchicum autumnale
(b) Pisum sativum
(c) Allium cepa
(d) Solanum nigrum

30. Diadelphous stamens are found in ***(2021)***
(a) China rose and citrus
(b) China rose
(c) citrus
(d) pea.

31. Ray florets have ***(2020)***
(a) inferior ovary (b) superior ovary
(c) hypogynous ovary (d) half inferior ovary.

32. The ovary is half inferior in ***(2020)***
(a) brinjal (b) mustard
(c) sunflower (d) plum.

33. Placentation in which ovules develop on the inner wall of the ovary or in peripheral part, is ***(2019)***

(a) free central (b) basal
(c) axile (d) parietal.

34. Match the placental types (column-I) with their examples (column-II). ***(Odisha NEET 2019)***

Column-I	Column-II
(A) Basal	(i) Mustard
(B) Axile	(ii) China rose
(C) Parietal	(iii) Dianthus
(D) Free central	(iv) Sunflower

Choose the correct answer from the following options.

(a) (A)-(ii), (B)-(iii), (C)-(iv), (D)-(i)
(b) (A)-(i), (B)-(ii), (C)-(iii), (D)-(iv)
(c) (A)-(iv), (B)-(ii), (C)-(i), (D)-(iii)
(d) (A)-(iii), (B)-(iv), (C)-(i), (D)-(ii)

35. The term 'polyadelphous' is related to ***(NEET-II 2016)***

(a) gynoecium (b) androecium
(c) corolla (d) calyx.

36. How many plants among Indigofera, Sesbania, Salvia, Allium, Aloe, mustard, groundnut, radish, gram and turnip have stamens with different lengths in their flowers? ***(NEET-II 2016)***
(a) Three (b) Four
(c) Five (d) Six

37. Radial symmetry is found in the flowers of ***(NEET-II 2016)***

(a) Brassica (b) Trifolium
(c) Pisum (d) Cassia.

38. Free central placentation is found in ***(NEET-II 2016)***

(a) Dianthus (b) Argemone
(c) Brassica (d) Citrus.

39. The standard petal of a papilionaceous corolla is also called ***(NEET-I 2016)***
(a) vexillum (b) corona
(c) carina (d) pappus.

40. Among China rose, mustard, brinjal, potato, guava, cucumber, onion and tulip, how many plants have superior ovary? ***(2015)***
(a) Three (b) Four
(c) Five (d) Six

41. Axile placentation is present in ***(2015)***
(a) pea (b) Argemone
(c) Dianthus (d) lemon.

42. Keel is the characteristic feature of flower of ***(2015 Cancelled)***

(a) Aloe (b) tomato
(c) tulip (d) Indigofera.

43. When the margins of sepals or petals overlap one another without any particular direction, the condition is termed as ***(2014)***
(a) vexillary (b) imbricate
(c) twisted (d) valvate.

44. Among bitter gourd, mustard, brinjal, pumpkin, china rose, lupin, cucumber, sunhemp, gram, guava, bean, chilli, plum, Petunia, tomato, rose, Withania, potato, onion, Aloe and tulip how many plants have hypogynous flower? ***(2013)***
(a) Fifteen (b) Eighteen
(c) Six (d) Ten

45. In China rose, the flowers are ***(2013)***
(a) zygomorphic, hypogynous with imbricate aestivation
(b) zygomorphic, epigynous with twisted aestivation
(c) actinomorphic, hypogynous with twisted aestivation
(d) actinomorphic, epigynous with valvate aestivation.

46. Among flowers of Calotropis, tulip, Sesbania, Asparagus, Colchicum, sweet pea, Petunia, Indigofera, mustard, soybean, tobacco and groundnut, how many plants have corolla with valvate aestivation? ***(Karnataka NEET 2013)***
(a) Six (b) Seven
(c) Eight (d) Five

47. Placentation in tomato and lemon is ***(2012)***
(a) parietal (b) free central
(c) marginal (d) axile.

48. The gynoecium consists of many free pistils in flowers of ***(2012)***
(a) Aloe (b) tomato
(c) Papaver (d) Michelia.

49. How many plants in the list given below have marginal placentation? ***(Mains 2012)***

Mustard, Gram, Tulip, Asparagus, Arhar, Sun-hemp, Chilli, Colchicum, Onion, Moong, Pea, Tobacco, Lupin
(a) Four (b) Five
(c) Six (d) Three

50. Flowers are zygomorphic in ***(2011)***
(a) mustard (b) gulmohar
(c) tomato (d) Datura.

51. The ovary is half inferior in flowers of ***(2011)***
(a) peach (b) cucumber
(c) cotton (d) guava.

52. Which one of the following figures represents the placentation in Dianthus? ***(Mains 2011)***

(a) 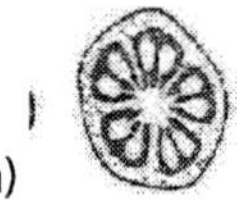 (b) 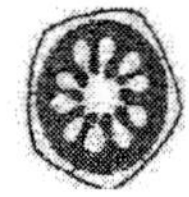

(c) 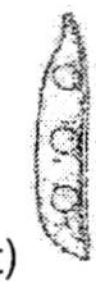 (d) 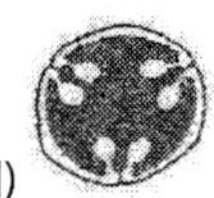

53. In unilocular ovary with a single ovule, the placentation is ***(2010)***
(a) marginal (b) basal
(c) free central (d) axile.

54. Keel is characteristic of the flowers of ***2010)***
(a) gulmohur (b) Cassia
(c) Calotropis (d) bean.

55. Ovary is half inferior in the flowers of ***(2010)***
(a) guava (b) plum
(c) brinjal (d) cucumber.

56. The technical term used for the androecium in flower of China rose (Hibiscus rosa sinensis) is ***(2010)***
(a) monadelphous (b) diadelphous
(c) polyandrous (d) polyadelphous.

57. Aestivation of petals in the flower of cotton is correctly shown in (Mains 2010)

(a) 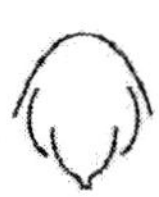 (b) 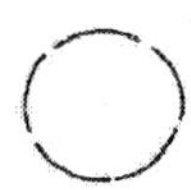

(c) 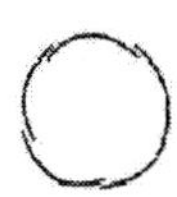 (d) 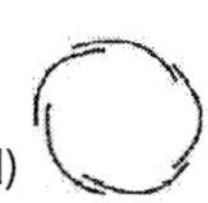

58. An example of axile placentation is (2009)
(a) Dianthus (b) lemon
(c) marigold (d) Argemone.

59. Replum is present in the ovary of flower of *(2008)*
(a) sunflower (b) pea
(c) lemon (d) mustard.

60. Angiosperm, to which the largest flowers belong, is *(1999)*
(a) total root parasite
(b) partial root parasite
(c) total stem parasite
(d) partial stem parasite.

THE FRUIT

61. Coconut fruit is a *(2017)*
(a) berry (b) nut
(c) capsule (d) drupe.

62. Placenta and pericarp are both edible portions in *(2014)*
(a) apple (b) banana
(c) tomato (d) potato.

63. An aggregate fruit is one which develops from *(2014)*
(a) multicarpellary syncarpous gynoecium
(b) multicarpellary apocarpous gynoecium
(c) complete inflorescence
(d) multicarpellary superior ovary.

64. How many plants in the list given below have composite fruits that develop from an inflorescence? *(2012)*
Walnut, poppy, radish, fig, pineapple, apple, tomato, mulberry
(a) Four (b) Five
(c) Two (d) Three

65. A drupe develops in *(2011)*
(a) mango (b) wheat
(c) pea (d) tomato.

66. A fruit developed from hypanthodium inflorescence is called *(2009)*
(a) sorosis (b) syconus
(c) caryopsis (d) hesperidium.

67. The fleshy receptacle of syconus of fig encloses a number of *(2008)*
(a) berries (b) mericarps
(c) achenes (d) samaras.

68. The fruit is chambered, developed from inferior ovary and has seeds with succulent testa in *(2008)*
(a) guava (b) cucumber
(c) pomegranate (d) orange.

69. In which of the following fruits, the edible part is the aril? *(2006)*
(a) Litchi (b) Custard apple
(c) Pomegranate (d) Orange

70. Which of the following represents the edible part of the fruit of litchi? *(2005)*
(a) Mesocarp (b) Endocarp
(c) Pericarp (d) Juicy aril

71. Edible part of mango is *(2004)*
(a) endocarp (b) receptacle
(c) epicarp (d) mesocarp.

72. Juicy hair-like structures observed in the lemon fruit develop from *(2003)*
(a) exocarp
(b) mesocarp
(c) endocarp
(d) mesocarp and endocarp.

73. Geocarpic fruit is *(2002)*
(a) potato (b) peanut
(c) onion (d) garlic.

74. Edible part in mango is *(2002)*
(a) mesocarp (b) epicarp
(c) endocarp (d) epidermis.

75. Geocarpic fruit is *(2000)*
(a) carrot (b) radish
(c) groundnut (d) turnip.

76. Which plant will lose its economic value, if its fruits are produced by induced parthenocarpy? ***(1997)***
(a) Orange (b) Banana
(c) Grape (d) Pomegranate

77. Which of the following is a 'true fruit'? ***(1996)***
(a) Banana (b) Fig
(c) Apple (d) Pear

78. Fruit of Mangifera indica is ***(1991)***
(a) berry (b) drupe
(c) capsule (d) siliqua.

79. Mango juice is obtained from ***(1989)***
(a) epicarp
(b) mesocarp
(c) endocarp
(d) pericarp and thalamus.

80. Fruit of groundnut is ***(1988)***
(a) legume (b) caryopsis
(c) berry (d) nut.

THE SEED

81. The body of the ovule is fused within the funicle at ***(2020)***
(a) hilum (b) micropyle
(c) nucellus (d) chalaza.

82. The morphological nature of the edible part of coconut is ***(2017)***
(a) cotyledon (b) endosperm
(c) pericarp (d) perisperm.

83. Cotyledon of maize grain is called ***(NEET-I 2016)***
(a) coleoptile (b) scutellum
(c) plumule (d) coleorhiza.

84. The wheat grain has an embryo with one large, shield shaped cotyledon known as ***(2015)***
(a) scutellum (b) coleoptile
(c) epiblast (d) coleorhiza.

85. Which one of the following statements is correct? ***(2014)***
(a) The seed in grasses is not endospermic.
(b) Mango is a parthenocarpic fruit.
(c) A proteinaceous aleurone layer is present in maize grain.
(d) A sterile pistil is called a staminode.

86. The coconut water and the edible part of coconut are equivalent to ***(2012)***
(a) endosperm (b) endocarp
(c) mesocarp (d) embryo.

87. Which one of the following statements is correct? ***(2011)***
(a) In tomato, fruit is a capsule.
(b) Seeds of orchids have oil-rich endosperm.
(c) Placentation in primose is basal.
(d) Flower of tulip is a modified shoot.

88. The scutellum observed in a grain of wheat or maize is comparable to which part of the seed in other monocotyledons? ***(2010)***
(a) Cotyledon (b) Endosperm
(c) Aleurone layer (d) Plumule

89. Cotyledons and testa respectively are edible parts in ***(2009)***
(a) walnut and tamarind
(b) french bean and coconut
(c) cashew nut and litchi
(d) groundnut and pomegranate.

90. An example of a seed with endosperm, perisperm, and caruncle is ***(2009)***
(a) coffee (b) lily
(c) castor (d) cotton.

91. Endosperm is consumed by developing embryo in the seed of ***(2008)***
(a) pea (b) maize
(c) coconut (d) castor.

92. The aleurone layer in maize grain is specially rich in ***(2003)***
(a) proteins (b) starch
(c) lipids (d) auxins.

93. In groundnut the food/oil reserve is present in ***(1990)***
(a) epicarp (b) mesocarp
(c) endosperm (d) cotyledons.

SEMI-TECHNICAL DESCRIPTION OF A TYPICAL FLOWERING PLANT

94. Floral features are chiefly used in angiosperm identification because ***(1998)***
(a) flowers can be safely pressed
(b) reproductive parts are more stable and conservative than vegetative parts
(c) flowers are nice to work with
(d) flowers are of various colours.

DESCRIPTION OF SOME IMPORTANT FAMILIES

95. Family Fabaceae differs from Solanaceae and Liliaceae. With respect to the stamens, pick out the characteristics specific to family Fabaceae but not found in Solanaceae or Liliaceae. ***(2023)***
(a) Monoadelphous and monothecous anthers
(b) Epiphyllous and dithecous anthers
(c) Diadelphous and dithecous anthers
(d) Polyadelphous and epipetalous stamens

96. Match Column - I with Column - II.

List-I	List-II
(p) $\%\ ⚥\ K_{(5)}\ C_{1+2+(2)}A_{(9)+1}\underline{G}_1$	(i) Brassicaceae
(q) $\oplus\ ⚥\ K_{(5)}\ \widehat{C_{(5)}A_5}\underline{G}_{(2)}$	(ii) Liliaceae
(r) $Br\ \oplus\ ⚥\ \widehat{P_{(3+3)}A_{3+3}}\underline{G}_{(3)}$	(iii) Fabaceae
(s) $\oplus\ ⚥\ K_{2+2}C_4A_{2+4}\underline{G}_{(2)}$	(iv) Solanaceae

Select the correct answer from the options given below.

	(p)	(q)	(r)	(s)
(a)	(iv)	(ii)	(i)	(iii)
(b)	(iii)	(iv)	(ii)	(i)
(c)	(i)	(ii)	(iii)	(iv)
(d)	(ii)	(iii)	(iv)	(i)

97. Tricarpellary, syncarpous gynoecium is found in flowers of ***(NEET-I 2016)***
(a) Fabaceae (b) Poaceae
(c) Liliaceae (d) Solanaceae

98. $\oplus\ ⚥\ K_{(5)}\ \widehat{C_{(5)}}\ A_5\ \underline{G}_{(2)}$ is the floral formula of ***(2015 Cancelled)***
(a) Petunia (b) Brassica
(c) Allium (d) Sesbania.

99. Vexillary aestivation is characteristic of the Family ***(2012)***
(a) Fabaceae (b) Asteraceae
(c) Solanaceae (d) Brassicaceae.

100. The correct floral formula of chilli is ***(Mains 2010)***

(a) $\oplus\ ⚥\ K_{(5)}\ C_5\ A_5\ \underline{G}_{(2)}$

(b) $\oplus\ ⚥\ K_{(5)}\ \widehat{C_{(5)}}\ A_5\ \underline{G}_{(2)}$

(c) $\oplus\ ⚥\ K_{(5)}\ C_{(5)}\ A_{(5)}\ \underline{G}_2$

(d) $\oplus\ ⚥\ K_5\ \widehat{C_5\ A_{(5)}}\ \underline{G}_2$..

101. The correct floral formula of soybean is ***(Mains 2010)***

(a) $\%\ ⚥\ K_{(5)}\ C_{1+(2)+2}\ A_{(9)+1}\underline{G}_1$

(b) $\%\ ⚥\ K_5\ C_{1+(2)+2}\ A_{(9)+1}\underline{G}_1$

(c) $\%\ ⚥\ K_{(5)}\ C_{1+2+(2)}\ A_{(9)+1}\underline{G}_1$

(d) $\%\ ⚥\ K_{(5)}\ C_{1+2+(2)}\ A_{1+(9)}\underline{G}_1$

102. Consider the following four statements (i), (ii), (iii) and (iv) and select the right option for two correct statements. ***(Mains 2010)***

Statements :

(i) In vexillary aestivation, the large posterior petal is called-standard, two lateral ones are wings and two small anterior petals are termed keel.

(ii) The floral formula for Liliaceae is $Br\ \oplus\ ⚥\ \widehat{P_{(3+3)}A_{3+3}}\underline{G}_{(3)}$.

(iii) In pea flower the stamens are monodelphous.

(iv) The floral formula for Solanaceae is $\oplus ⚥ K_{(3)} C_{(3)} A_{(4)} \underline{G}_{(2)}$.

The correct statements are

(a) (i) and (iii) (b) (i) and (ii)
(c) (ii) and (iii) (d) (iii) and (iv).

103. The floral formula $\oplus ⚥ K_{(5)} \widehat{C_{(5)} A_5} \underline{G}_{(2)}$ is that of *(2009)*

(a) soybean (b) sunhemp
(c) tobacco (d) tulip.

104. Pentamerous actinomorphic flowers, bicarpellary ovary with oblique septa, and fruit capsule or berry, are characteristic features of *(2006)*

(a) Liliaceae (b) Asteraceae
(c) Brassicaceae (d) Solanaceae.

105. Bicarpellary gynoecium and oblique ovary occurs in *(2001)*

(a) mustard (b) banana
(c) Pisum (d) brinjal

106. Tetradynamous conditions occur in *(2001)*

(a) Cruciferae (b) Malvaceae
(c) Solanaceae (d) Liliaceae

107. Which is expressing right appropriate pairing? *(2000)*

(a) Brassicaceae - sunflower
(b) Malvaceae - cotton
(c) Papilionaceae - Catechu
(d) Liliaceae - wheat

108. Pulses are obtained from *(1993)*

(a) Fabaceae (b) Asteraceae
(c) Poaceae (d) Solanaceae.

109. Epipetalous stamens with free filaments and fused anthers occur in *(1992)*

(a) Asteraceae (b) Solanaceae
(c) Liliaceae (d) Poaceae.

110. Floral formula of tomato/tobacco is **(1992, 1989)**

(a) $\oplus ⚥ K_{4-5}A_{10}G_{(2)}$ (b) $\oplus ⚥ K_{2+2}C_4A_{2+4}G_1$

(c) $\oplus ⚥ P_2A_3G_1$ (d) $\oplus ⚥ K_{(5)}\widehat{C_{(5)}A_5}\underline{G}_{(2)}$.

111. $\oplus ⚥ K_{(5)}\widehat{C_{(5)}A_5}\underline{G}_{(2)}$ is floral formula of *(1991)*

(a) Liliaccae (b) Solanaceae
(c) Asteraceae (d) Fabaceae.

112. Epipetalous and syngenesious stamens occur in *(1991)*

(a) Solanaceae (b) Brassicaceae
(c) Fabaceae (d) Asteraceae.

113. A family delimited by type of inflorescence is *(1991)*

(a) Fabaceae (b) Asteraceae
(c) Solanaceae (d) Liliaceae.

114. Syngenesious condition is found in *(1991)*

(a) Asteraceae (b) Labiatae
(c) Solanaceae (d) Fabaceae.

ANSWER KEY

1.	(a)	2.	(b)	3.	(d)	4.	(a)	5.	(d)	6.	(d)	7.	(c)
8.	(b)	9.	(c)	10.	(a)	11.	(d)	12.	(d)	13.	(a)	14.	(a)
15.	(b)	16.	(c)	17.	(a)	18.	(c)	19.	(d)	20.	(c)	21.	(d)
22.	(d)	23.	(a)	24.	(c)	25.	(a)	26.	(b)	27.	(b)	28.	(b)
29.	(b)	30.	(d)	31.	(a)	32.	(d)	33.	(d)	34.	(c)	35.	(b)
36.	(b)	37.	(a)	38.	(a)	39.	(a)	40.	(d)	41.	(d)	42.	(d)
43.	(b)	44.	(a)	45.	(c)	46.	(b)	47.	(d)	48.	(d)	49.	(c)
50.	(b)	51.	(a)	52.	(b)	53.	(b)	54.	(d)	55.	(b)	56.	(a)
57.	(d)	58.	(b)	59.	(d)	60.	(a)	61.	(d)	62.	(c)	63.	(b)
64.	(d)	65.	(a)	66.	(b)	67.	(c)	68.	(c)	69.	(a)	70.	(d)
71.	(d)	72.	(c)	73.	(b)	74.	(a)	75.	(c)	76.	(d)	77.	(a)
78.	(b)	79.	(b)	80.	(a)	81.	(a)	82.	(b)	83.	(b)	84.	(a)
85.	(c)	86.	(a)	87.	(d)	88.	(a)	89.	(d)	90.	(c)	91.	(a)
92.	(a)	93.	(d)	94.	(b)	95.	(c)	96.	(b)	97.	(c)	98.	(a)
99.	(a)	100.	(b)	101.	(c)	102.	(b)	103.	(c)	104.	(d)	105.	(d)
106.	(a)	107.	(b)	108.	(a)	109.	(a)	110.	(d)	111.	(b)	112.	(d)
113.	(b)	114.	(a)										

HINTS & EXPLANATIONS

1. (a): In monocotyledonous plants, the primary root is short lived and is replaced by a large number of roots. These roots originate from the base of the stem and constitute the fibrous root system, e.g., wheat plant.

2. (b): Sweet potato (Ipomoea batatas) is swollen single root tuber that does not assume a definite shape. It is a modified adventitious root for storage of food.

3. (d): Pistia (water lettuce) is a floating aquatic plant. In aquatic plants, roots are generally poorly developed and do not take part in absorption of water. Water is absorbed by the general body surface in these plants.

4. (a): These special roots, called pneumatophores or knees, develop in mangrove plants, i.e., plants growing in saline marshes. These roots grow vertically upward and are negatively geotropic. Air enters these roots through minute breathing pores called pneumathodes, present on the tips of vertical roots. These plants include Rhizophora, Heritiera, Avicennia, etc.

5. (d): Clinging roots arise from the nodes of stem and penetrate the stem of the host plant. It helps in fixing the plant to the host. It is found in orchids. Orchids bear three types of roots - clinging roots for fixation, absorbing roots for absorbing mineral salts and water and epiphytic roots for absorbing moisture from air.

6. (d): Velamen is found in aerial roots of orchids. In many epiphytic orchids, the aerial roots are covered by a hygroscopic velamen tissue. They absorb water from the atmosphere.

7. **(c)**: The axillary buds of stem are modified into pointed hard thorns in Citrus and Bougainvillea.

8. **(b)**

9. **(c)**: Pitcher of Nepenthes is a modification of leaf. In Nepenthes, the pitchers are meant for catching and digesting insects. The lamina is modified into pitcher. The leaf apex gives rise to a coloured lid for attracting the insects.

10. **(a)**: Phylloclades are flattened green stems which have taken over the function of photosynthesis while cladodes are only the branches of stem that are modified to take over the function of leaves.

11. **(d)**: Carrot and sweet potato are root modifications while edible part of groundnut is seed. Potato is an edible underground stem.

12. **(d)**: Sweet potato is homologous to turnip as both are having same origin, i.e,, both are root but modified for different functions. Sweet potato is a modified root for storage and vegetative propagation while turnip is modified for storage only.

13. **(a)**: Opuntia is a xerophytic plant which lives in dry habitat. The plant has fleshy organs where water and mucilage are stored. The stem is modified into flat green structure, called as phylloclade.

14. **(a)**: A tuber is the swollen tip of the underground branch. Tubers are round or oval in shape. Each tuber has many notches on the surface called 'eyes'. These are in fact axillary buds which grow into new plants during favourable conditions.

15. **(b)**: Suckers are the sub-aerial modification of stem. They grow obliquely upward from the main stem producing roots from the underground nodes. The sucker like structures in banana are also called sword suckers, which give rise to new leafy trunk.

16. **(c)**: In xerophytic plants, the leaves modify into sharp, pointed spines, e.g., Solanum surattense, Opuntia, Asparagus, etc. This modification is either for protection of plant or to lessen transpiration, or for both.

17. **(a)**: In opposite phyllotaxy, two leaves are borne on the opposite sides of a single node. It is of two types; (i) opposite and superposed, (ii) opposite and decussate. Ocimum, guava and Calotropis have opposite decussate phyllotaxy.

18. **(c)**: In several species of Acacia found in the deserts of Australia the bipinnate lamina is absent. Instead petiole and part of the rachis become flattened into sickle-shaped structure for performing the function of food synthesis. Such a flattened petiole which carries out the functions of the lamina is called phyllode. Formation of phyllode is a mechanism to reduce transpiration because (i) it is vertically placed and (ii) has fewer stomata.

19. **(d)**: In Alstonia, five or more leaves arises from each node, so it shows whorled phyllotaxy. The leaves are leathery, sessile, simple which are elliptical or ovate or wedge shaped at the base. It is used in traditional medicines.

20. **(c)**: A flower is a modified shoot wherein the shoot apical meristem changes to floral meristem. Internodes do not elongate and the axis gets condensed. When these axis gets condensed, the apex produces different floral appendages laterally at successive nodes instead of leaves.

21. **(d)**: Racemose inflorescence is also called indefinite and indeterminate type. Growth of the peduncle is indefinite. Here the terminal bud will not modify into a flower. Flowers develop in acropetal succession, i.e., mature flowers are towards the base and the younger ones towards the tip of the peduncle. Flowers open

in centripetal succession, i.e,, opening of flowers proceeds from the periphery to the centre of the inflorescence. Peduncle may be unbranched or branched. Soybean belongs to Family Fabaceae which has racemose inflorescence.

22. (d): Cymose inflorescence is also called definite or determinate inflorescence. Growth of the peduncle is definite. Here, the terminal bud is modified into a flower. Flowers develop in basipetal succession, i.e., mature flowers are towards the apex and young flower buds are towards the base. Flowers open in centrifugal sequence, i.e., flowers open from centre to the periphery of the inflorescence, e.g., Solanum, Ranunculus, Datura, Gossypium, etc.

23. (a)

24. (c): In maize the male inflorescence occupies the terminal position on the main axis, whereas the female inflorescence (ear or cob) is borne on modified lateral branches in the axils of leaves. The ear producing branch has short internodes and bears a female spike at its apex. Each spikelet has a pair of small membranous glumes and two florets. The feathery styles of the female florets are long and emerge out of the cobs to expose stigma for wind pollination.

25. (a)

26. (b): Inflorescence is the cluster of flowers or arrangement of flowers on the floral axis. Hypanthodium is the characterstic inflorescence of Ficus (Family Moraceae). Here a cup-shaped cavity with an apical opening or ostiole is formed by a fleshy receptacle, which is guarded by inwardly projecting hairs and bear flowers on the inner wall of the cavity, i.e., female (♀) flowers at the base and male (♂) flowers above.

27. (b): When placenta is axial and the ovules are attached to it in a multilocular ovary, the placentation is said to be axile, as in china rose, tomato, Petunia, lemon. Dianthus and Primrose have free central placentation. Pea, beans and lupin have marginal placentation, while mustard and cucumber have parietal placentation.

28. (b): Zygomorphic flower can be divided into two similar halves only in one particular vertical plane, e.g., gulmohar, Cassia. Flowers of mustard, Datura and chilly are actinomorphic. Actinomorphic flowers can be divided into two equal radial halves in any radial plane passing through the centre.

29. (b): Colchicum autumnale, Allium cepa and Solanum nigrum show valvate aestivation.

30. (d): Pea (Pisum sativum) belongs to Family Fabaceae in which all stamens are united and form two bundles.

31. (a): The ovary is inferior in ray florets of sunflower. It possess epigynous flower i.e., the margin of thalamus grows upward enclosing the ovary completely and getting fused with it, the other parts of flower arise above the ovary.

32. (d): The ovary is superior in brinjal and mustard while it is inferior in sunflower.

33. (d): Parietal placentation is found in compound or syncarpous ovary. There are two or more longitudinal placentae or files of ovules attached to the ovary wall. The ovary is usually unilocular but becomes falsely two or more locular due to ingrowth of placentae or formation of false septa.

34. (c)

35. (b): Polyadelphous condition represents cohesion of stamens. In this condition stamens of a flower are fused by their filaments only to form many groups, e.g., Citrus.

36. (b)

37. (a): The flowers of Brassica are radially symmetrical whereas flowers of Trifolium, Pisum and Cassia are zygomorphic.

38. (a): Free central placentation is found in Dianthus. Parietal placentation is present in Argemone and Brassica whereas Citrus has axile placentation in ovary.

39. (a): The posterior large bilobed petal of a papilionaceous corolla is called standard or vexillum. It overlaps the two smaller lateral petals known as wings or alae.

40. (d): China rose, mustard, brinjal, potato, onion and tulip are the plants that have superior ovary whereas in guava and cucumber, ovary is inferior.

41. (d): Axile placentation occurs in syncarpous pistils. The ovary is partitioned into two or more chambers. Placentae occur in the central region where the septa meet so that, an axile column bearing ovules is formed, e.g., shoe flower (pentalocular), lcmon (multilocular), etc.

42. (d) : The flowers of Family Papilionaceae have butterfly shaped corolla (papilionaceous corolla). Posterior or outermost petal is the largest and is called standard or vexillum, two lateral petals are similar and generally clawed, are called wings or alae and the two anterior petals called keel are fused enclosing stamens and carpels. This type of petal arrangement is found in bean, gram, pea, Indigofera, etc.

43. (b): Aestivation is the arrangements of accessory floral organs (sepals or petals) in relation to one another in floral bud. It may be of open, valvate, twisted or imbricate type. In imbricate aestivation there is an irregular overlapping of petals or sepals by one another. Cassia, gulmohar, etc., show imbricate aestivation.

44. (a): In the hypogynous flower the gynoecium occupies the highest position while the other parts are situated below it. The ovary in such flowers is said to be superior, e.g., mustard, China rose and brinjal. All the given plants except bitter gourd, pumpkin, cucumber, guava, plum and rose have hypogynous flower.

45. (c): In China rose the flowers are actinomorphic, i.e., it can be divided into two equal radial halves in any radial plane passing through the centre; they are hypogynous, i.e., the gynoecium occupies the highest position, while the other parts are situated below it; they have twisted aestivation, i.e., one margin of petal overlaps that of the next one and so on.

46. (b): The mode of arrangement of the sepals or petals with respect to one another in the floral bud is termed as aestivation. In valvate aestivation, sepals or petals or tepals just touch each other without any overlapping. Calotropis, tulip, Asparagus, Colchicum, Petunia, mustard and tobacco have valvate aestivation.

47. (d)

48. (d): Gynoecium is the female reproductive organ of a flower. It may be apocarpous (pistils separated), e.g., Michelia or syncarpous (fused), e.g., tomato.

49. (c): Gram, arhar, sunhemp, moong, pea and lupin belong to Family Fabaceae which is characterised by marginal placentation.

50. (b): Flowers of gulmohar have bilateral symmetry. So, they are called zygomorphic. Datura, mustard and tomato have actinomorphic flowers.

51. (a): If gynoecium is situated in the centre and other parts of the flower are located on the rim of the thalamus almost at the same level, it is called perigynous. The ovary here is said to be half inferior, e.g., plum, rose, peach.

52. (b): The given figure in option (b) represents the free central placentation. In free central placentation, ovary is unilocular and ovules are borne on the axis in the center of the ovary and septa are absent. It is seen in Dianthus and Primrose.

53. (b): In basal type of placentation the ovary is unilocular and ovules and generally reduced to one borne at the base of the ovary.

54. (d)

55. (b): If gynoecium is situated in the centre and other parts of the flower are located on the rim of the thalamus almost at the same level, it is called perigynous. The ovary here is said to be half inferior, e.g., plum, rose, peach.

56. (a): China rose of Family Malvaceae possess numerous stamens. The filaments of stamens are united in one group thus forming a staminal tube around the style. Such stamens are called monadelphous.

57. (d): In cotton, China rose and lady's finger margins of sepals or petals overlap that of the next one this mode of arrangement (aestivation) is called twisted.

58. (b)

59. (d): Replum is a false septum formed due to the ingrowth of parietal placenta. This makes the ovary bilocular. It is mainly seen in the ovary of flowers of Brassicaceae (Cruciferae) Family, e.g., mustard, candytuft, etc.

60. (a): Rafflesia is a specialised total root parasite as the vegetative parts of its body are reduced and the whole body is within the host root and only structure which is visible outside, is the biggest flower. The diameter of the flower is one meter and its weight is about 10 kg. Its pollination is done by elephant. The flowers are fleshy white and they emit smell, which resembles the smell of decaying meat.

61. (d): Coconut fruit is fibrous drupe with a fibrous mesocarp.

62. (c): A true fruit consists of a pericarp (fruit wall) formed from ovary wall and seeds formed from ovules. Pericarp is divisible into epicarp, mesocarp and endocarp. Tomato is a berry fruit derived from bicarpellary, syncarpous, bi- to tetralocular ovary with swollen placenta. Berry consists of a membranous skin represented by epicarp. Mesocarp is the middle fleshy part. Endocarp, septa and placenta are pulpy and edible.

63. (b): An aggregate fruit or etaerio is a group of simple fruitlets that develop from free ovaries (apocarpous condition) of a single flower (single gynoecium).

64. (d): A composite or multiple fruit is a group of fruitlets which develop from the different flowers of an inflorescence. It is of two main types, sorosis (e.g., mulberry, pineapple, jackfruit) and syconus (e.g., peepal, banyan, fig, etc.)

65. (a): Drupe is a fleshy fruit that develops from either one or several fused carpels and contains one or many seeds. The seeds are enclosed by the hard protective endocarp (pericarp) of the fruit, e.g., mango. In mango the pericarp is well differentiated into an outer thin epicarp, a middle fleshy edible mesocarp and an inner stony hard endocarp.

66. (b): Syconus fruit develops from a hypanthodium inflorescence, e.g., Ficus. Hypanthodium is a box like inflorescence where the box is formed by the fleshly receptacle. It opens to exterior by a single pore called ostiole. The hollow pear shaped fleshy receptacle encloses a number of minute male and female flowers, it becomes fleshy and forms the fruit.

67. (c): Syconus develop from hypanthodium type of inflorescence. The flask shaped fleshy receptacle encloses female flower which produces small achene like fruitlets and has a small pore protected by scale leaves, e.g., syconus of fig (Ficus carica).

68. (c): In pomegranate, the whole fruit is covered by a hard rind made up of exocarp and a part of mesocarp. It develops from multilocular syncarpous inferior ovary. Mesocarp forms plate like infolding (i.e., chambered) and the seeds are covered by endocarp and contain hright red succulent testa.

69. (a): In litchi, aril forms the edtble part in fruit. It is a collar like outgrowth from the base of the ovule forming a kind of third integument. Litchi is a nut. In litchi, the epicarp and mesocarp (layers of pericarp) together become leathery and the endocarp is membranous.

70. (d)

71. (d): Mango (Mangifera indica) of Family Anacardiaceae is a drupe. The edible part in mango is mesocarp.

72. (c): Lemon is a hesperidium type of fruit. It is many chambered fleshy fruit developing from a multicarpellary, syncarpous, multilocular, superior ovary bearing seeds on axile placentation. The leathery epicarp of hesperidium has many glands of aromatic oil. The mesocarp, represented by white fibres, is fused to the epicarp. The epicarp and mesocarp together form the rind. The endocarp is thin and papery. It projects inwards and forms many compartments. The inner wall of endocarp gives out many juicy succulent hairs which form the edible part of the fruit. Hesperidium is a characteristic fruit of the Rutaceae, e.g., Citrus aurantifolia (lemon), Citrus reticulata (orange), etc.

73. (b)

74. (a): Mango (Mangifera indica) of Family Anacardiaceae is a drupe. The edible part in mango is mesocarp.

75. (c)

76. (d): Development of fruits without fertilisation is called parthenocarpy and such fruits are called parthenocarpic fruits. Since in pomegranate juicy testa is the edible part and parthenocarpy will make the fruit seedless and hence they will be useless.

77. (a) : A fruit is a ripened ovary. On the basis of the formation of fruits, they are classified into two types - true fruits and false fruits. True fruits are developed from the ovary only. Banana is a fleshy fruit - berry. It develops from multicarpellary syncarpous superior or inferior ovary. The pericarp of berries is differentiated into epicarp, mesocarp and endocarp (like drupes) but the endocarp is not stony as in drupes. Apple and pear are pome. Pome is a false fruit in which the edible part is thalamus where the true fruit remains embedded. Fig is a composite fruit. These fruits are the products of the whole inflorescence together with its component parts.

78. (b)

79. (b)

80. (a): Fruit of groundnut is legume. It is developed from monocarpellary ovary but dehisces by both sutures from apex downward.

81. (a) The hilum is a scar on the seed coat where funicle and body of ovule is attached.

82. (b)

83. (b): The seeds of monocotyledonous plants have only one cotyledon. In Family Poaceae (e.g., wheat, maize, etc.), this cotyledon is called scutellum, situated towards lateral side of embryonal axis. It provides nourishment to the developing embryo.

84. (a)

85. (c): Grass seeds are endospermic. Mango is a seeded fruit. A sterile pistil is called pistillode and a sterile stamen is called staminode. Maize grains consist of fruit wall, seed coat, endosperm and embryo. The endosperm occupies most of the grains interior and consists of two parts, horny aleurone layer and mainly storage layers. The aleurone layer lies immediately below the grain covering and is 1-3 cell thick. Aleurone cells are thick walled with cytoplasm filled with aleurone grains which produce enzymes during seed germination to mobilise stored nutrients.

86. (a): Coconut fruit is a drupe. It has a membranous epicarp, fibrous mesocarp and stony endocarp. The endocarp encloses a single seed with brown testa that contains a small embryo and a white oily endosperm (edible part) with watery fluid called coconut water.

87. (d)

88. (a): Scutellum is the tissue in a grass or wheat or maize seed that lies between the embryo and the endosperm. It is the modified cotyledon, being specialised for the digestion and absorption of the endosperm.

89. (d): Groundnut is dry, one chambered, one seeded fruit developing from a superior bi or polycarpellary ovary. The edible part is cotyledons and embryo lobe. Pomegranate is balausta type of fruit. The fruits develop from multilocular syncarpous inferior ovary. Testa is fleshy and edible.

90. (c): In castor seed, testa and tegmen are united together. Seed coat is tough and bright due to scleroprotein. Over narrower end a brownish pad is found which is called caruncle. Caruncle is carbohydrate in nature. This protects micropyle and develops as an integumental outgrowth after fertilisation. Below seed coat a very thin membrane is found over kernel and called perisperm (the persistant nucellus). Below perisperm there is a large, white, swollen and oily mass called endsoperm.

91. (a): During the process of the development of the embryo, the food stored up in the endosperm is continuously drawn up by the developing embryo and thus completely exhausted. Such seeds are known as exalbuminous or nonendospermic. The common examples of exalbuminous are gram, pea, bean, tamarind, orchid, etc.

92. (a): In monocotyledons the seeds are generally endospermous. The internal structure of grain can be studied in a longitudinal section. It shows two distinct regions upper large region, the endosperm and lower smaller region, the embryo. The endosperm is surrounded by a special one cell thick layer, called aleurone layer. It is filled with aleurone grains which are proteinaceous in nature.

93. (d): In groundnut the food/oil reserve is present in cotyledons. It is very important commercial crop of Leguminosae.

94. (b) Floral features are used to identify angiosperms because reproductive parts are more stable and conservative than vegetative parts.

95. (c): Fabaceae stamens are united in two bundles i.e., diadelphous. Anther is dithecous i.e., each lobe of anther having two theca. Monoadelphous and epipetalous stamen is found in Solanaceae family. Epiphyllous stamen is found in Liliaceae family.

96. (b)

97. (c): Members of Liliaceae possess tricarpellary, syncarpous gynoecium with superior ovary. The ovary is trilocular with two to many ovules in each loculus.

98. (a): The given floral formula is of Family Solanaceae. Among the given options, only Petunia belongs to Family Solanaceae. Allium is a member of Family Liliaceae, Sesbania is of Family Leguminosae and Brassica is a member of Family Brassicaceae or Cruciferae.

99. (a): Vexillary aestivation is a characteristic of Family Fabaceae. In it, the posterior largest petal (standard) overlaps two lateral petals (wings) which in turn overlap two anterior petals (keel). It is also called papilionaceous corolla.

100.(b): Chilli is the member of Solanaceae, in which flowers are bisexual (⚥), actinomorphic (⊕); calyx -5 and gamosepalous, corolla - 5 and gamopetalous; androecium - 5, free, epipetalous basifixed, inferior; gynoecium - bicarpellary, syncarpous and ovary superior. So, floral formula of chilli is ⊕ ⚥ $K_{(5)}\widehat{C_{(5)}A_5}\underline{G}_{(2)}$.

101. (c): The plants belonging to the Family Fabaceae such as soybean, pea, sem, moong, gram, etc. have the floral formula % ⚥ $K_{(5)}\ C_{1+2+(2)}\ A_{(9)+1}\ \underline{G}_1$.

102. (b): Flowers in pea have diadelphous stamens. The floral formula for Solanaceae is ⊕ ⚥ $K_{(5)}\ \widehat{C_{(5)}\ A_5}\ \underline{G}_{(2)}$.

103.(c): The floral formula of tobacco is ⊕ ⚥ $K_{(5)}\ \widehat{C_{(5)}\ A_5}\ \underline{G}_{(2)}$. It belongs to the Family Solanaceae. The flower is actinomorphic, bisexual, 5 sepals gamosepalous, 5 gamopetalous corolla, 5 epipetalous stamens and 2 carpels syncarpous having superior ovary.

104.(d): A pentamerous actinomorphic flower is one where the floral parts are in multiples of five and the flower can be divided into two equal halves in more than one plane. Gynoecium is bicarpellary, syncarpous, forming a superior bilocular ovary. Each locule has many ovule on axile placentation. Members of Solanaceae are characterised by the presence of an obliquely placed septum in the ovary and highly swollen placentae.

105.(d): Brinjal or Solanum melongena belongs to Family Solanaceae. The fruits are rich in iodine. They are used in the form of vegetable. Gynoecium is bicarpellary, syncarpous, forming a superior bilocular ovary. Each locule has many ovules on axile placentation. Members of Solanaceae are characterised by the presence of an obliquely placed septum in the ovary and highly swollen placentae. The oblique septum is probably due to shifting in the position of the ovary.

106. (a): In tetradynamous condition there are six stamens, 4 are long and 2 are short, i.e., 4 + 2 arrangement of stamens. It is characterstic feature of Cruciferae members. In Liliaceae 6 stamens are arranged in whorls of 3 each (3+3). In Solanaceae there are 5 stamens they are epipetalous and polyandrous. In Malvaceae there are numerous stamens that are monadelphous.

107. (b): Malvaceae is also known as cotton family or mallow family. The plants of this family are cosmopolitan in distribution, although more common in tropical (warm) regions. Gossypium (cotton) is an important genera of this family. Sunflower belongs to Family Compositae. Wheat belong to Family Poaceae. Catechu belongs to Family Mimosaceae.

108. (a): Pulses are obtained from Fabaceae.

109. **(a)**: Epipetalous stamens with free filaments and fused anthers occur in Asteraceae. Asteraceae possess five stamens with free filaments. This family shows syngenesious condition in which anthers are united forming a tube around the style.

110. **(d)**

111. **(b)**

112. **(d)**: Syngenesious condition is found in Asteraceae. It is the condition when stamens are united by their anthers (filaments free). Epipetalous condition is also seen here.

113. **(b)**: A family delimited by type of inflorescence is Asteraceae. Asteraceae possess head or capitulum inflorescence, which is racemose and is surrounded by an involucre of bracts.

114. **(a)**: Syngenesious condition is found in Asteraceae. It is the condition when stamens are united by their anthers (filaments free). Epipetalous condition is also seen here.

Chapter : 06

ANATOMY OF FLOWERING PLANTS

THE TISSUES

1. Given below are two statements. ***(2023)***

Statement I : Endarch and exarch are the terms often used for describing the position of secondary xylem in the plant body.

Statement II: Exarch condition is the most common feature of the root system..

In the light of the above statements, choose the correct answer from the options given below:
(a) Statement I is correct but statement II is false.
(b) Statement I is incorrect but statement II is true
(c) Both statement I and statement II are true.
(d) Both statement I and statement II are false.

2. Phloem in gymnosperms lacks ***(2019)***
(a) both sieve tubes and companion cells
(b) albuminous cells and sieve cells
(c) sieve tubes only
(d) companion cells only.

3. Regeneration of damaged growing grass following grazing is largely due to ***(Odisha NEET 2019)***
(a) lateral meristem (b) apical meristem
(c) intercalary meristem (d) secondary meristem

4. Tracheids differ from other tracheary elements in ***(2014)***
(a) having Casparian strips
(b) being imperforate
(c) lacking nucleus
(d) being lignified.

5. Meristematic tissue responsible for increase in girth of tree trunk is ***(Karnataka NEET 2013)***
(a) intercalary meristem
(b) lateral meristem
(c) phellogen
(d) apical meristem.

6. Gymnosperms are also called soft wood spermatophytes because they lack ***(2012)***
(a) cambium
(b) phloem fibres
(c) thick-walled tracheids
(d) xylem fibres.

7. Companion cells are closely associated with ***(2012)***
(a) sieve elements (b) vessel elements
(c) trichomes (d) guard cells.

8. Function of companion cells is ***(Mains 2011)***
(a) providing energy to sieve elements for active transport
(b) providing water to phloem
(c) loading of sucrose into sieve elements by passive transport
(d) loading of sucrose into sieve elements.

9. Which one of the following is not a lateral meristem? ***(2010)***
(a) Intrafascicular cambium
(b) Interfascicular cambium
(c) Phellogen
(d) Intercalary meristem

10. The chief water conducting elements of xylem in gymnosperms are ***(2010)***
(a) vessels (b) fibres
(c) transfusion tissue (d) tracheids.

11. Transport of food material in higher plants takes place through ***(Mains 2010)***
(a) companion cells (b) transfusion tissue
(c) tracheids (d) sieve elements.

12. The length of different internodes in a culm of sugarcane is variable because of ***(2008)***
(a) size of leaf lamina at the node below each internode
(b) intercalary meristem
(c) shoot apical meristem
(d) position of axillary buds.

13. A common structural feature of vessel elements and sieve tube elements is ***(2006)***

(a) enucleate condition

(b) thick secondary walls

(c) pores on lateral walls

(d) presence of P-protein.

14. The apical meristem of the root is present ***(2003)***

(a) only in radicals

(b) only in tap roots

(c) only in adventitious roots

(d) in all the roots.

15. The cells of the quiescent centre are characterised by ***(2003)***

(a) having dense cytoplasm and prominent nuclei

(b) having light cytoplasm and small nuclei

(c) dividing regularly to add to the corpus

(d) dividing regularly to add to tunica.

16. Which of the following statements is true? ***(2002)***

(a) Vessels are multicellular with wide lumen.

(b) Tracheids are multicellular with narrow lumen.

(c) Vessels are unicellular with narrow lumen.

(d) Tracheids are unicellular with wide lumen.

17. Axillary bud and terminal bud derived from the activity of ***(2002)***

(a) lateral meristem

(b) intercalary meristem

(c) apical meristem

(d) parenchyma.

18. Vessels are found in ***(2002)***

(a) all angiosperms and some gymnosperm

(b) most of angiosperms and few gymnosperms

(c) all angiosperms, all gymnosperms and some pteridophyta

(d) all pteridophyta.

19. At maturity, which of the following is non-nucleated? ***(1997)***

(a) Palisade cell (b) Cortical cell

(c) Sieve cell (d) Companion cell

20. Which of the following is not true about 'sclereids'? ***(1996)***

(a) These are groups of living cells.

(b) These are found in nut shells, guava pulp, pear.

(c) These are also called stone cells.

(d) These are form of sclerenchyma with fibres.

21. Which of the following plant cells will show totipotency? ***(1993)***

(a) Sieve tubes (b) Xylem vessels

(c) Meristem (d) Cork cells

22. An organised and differentiated cellular structure having cytoplasm but no nucleus is ***(1991)***

(a) vessels

(b) xylem parenchyma

(c) sieve tubes

(d) tracheids.

23. Sieve tubes are suited for translocation of food because they possess ***(1989)***

(a) bordered pits(b) no end walls

(c) broader lumen and perforated cross walls

(d) no protoplasm.

24. Death of protoplasm is a pre-requisite for a vital function like ***(1989)***

(a) transport of sap (b) transport of food

(c) absorption of water(d) gaseous exchange.

25. Which meristem helps in increasing girth? ***(1988)***

(a) Lateral meristem

(b) Intercalary meristem

(c) Primary meristem

(d) Apical meristem

THE TISSUE SYSTEM

26. Read the following statements about the vascular bundles. ***(2022)***

(A) In roots, xylem and phloem in a vascular bundle are arranged in an alternate manner along the different radii.

(B) Conjoint closed vascular bundles do not possess cambium.

(C) In open vascular bundles, cambium is present in between xylem and phloem.

(D) The vascular bundles of dicotyledonous stem possess endarch protoxylem.

(E) In monocotyledonous root, usually there are more than six xylem bundles present.

Choose the correct answer from the options given below.

(a) (A), (B) and (D) only
(b) (B), (C), (D) and (E) only
(c) (A), (B), (C) and (D) only
(d) (A), (C), (D) and (E) only

27. Match List-I with List-II. ***(2021)***

List-I	**List-II**
(p) Cells with active cell division capacity	(i) Vascular tissues
(q) Tissue having all cells similar in structure and function	(ii) Meristematic tissue
(r) Tissue having different types of cells	(iii) Sclereids
(s) Dead cells with highly thickened walls and narrow lumen	(iv) Simple tissue

Select the correct answer from the options given below.

	p	q	r	s
(a)	(iii)	(ii)	(iv)	(i)
(b)	(ii)	(iv)	(i)	(iii)
(c)	(iv)	(iii)	(ii)	(i)
(d)	(i)	(ii)	(iii)	(iv)

28. Stomata in grass leaf are ***(2018)***

(a) dumb-bell shaped (b) kidney-shaped
(c) rectangular (d) barrel-shaped.

29. Specialised epidermal cells surrounding the guard cells are called ***(NEET-I 2016)***

(a) bulliform cells (b) lenticels
(c) complementary cells (d) subsidiary cells.

30. Vascular bundles in monocotyledons are considered closed because ***(2015 Cancelled)***

(a) there are no vessels with perforations
(b) xylem is surrounded all around by phloem
(c) a bundle sheath surrounds each bundle
(d) cambium is absent.

31. Which of the following statements is not true for stomatal apparatus? ***(Karnataka NEET 2013)***

(a) Guard cells invariably possess chloroplasts and mitochondria.
(b) Guard cells are always surrounded by subsidiary cells.
(c) Stomata are involved in gaseous exchange.
(d) Inner wall of guard cells are thick.

32. Closed vascular bundles lack ***(2012)***

(a) ground tissue (b) conjunctive tissue
(c) cambium (d) pith.

33. Ground tissue includes ***(2011)***

(a) all tissues external to endodermis
(b) all tissues except epidermis and vascular bundles
(c) epidermis and cortex
(d) all tissues internal to endodermis.

34. Some vascular bundles are described as open because these ***(Mains 2011)***

(a) are surrounded by pericycle but no endodermis
(b) are capable of producing secondary xylem and phloem
(c) possess conjunctive tissue between xylem and phloem
(d) are not surrounded by pericycle.

35. Given below is the diagram of a stomatal apparatus. In which of the following all the four parts labelled as A, B, C and D are correctly identified? ***(Mains 2010)***

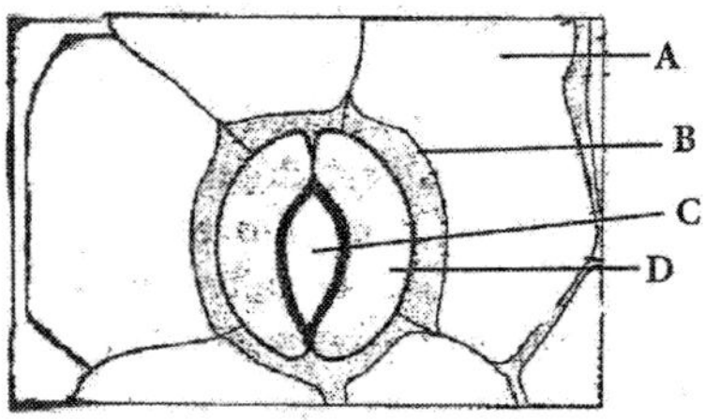

	A	B	C	D
(a)	Subsidiary cell	Epidermal cell	Guard cell	Stomatal aperture
(b)	Guard cell	Stomatal aperture	Subsidiary cell	Epidermal cell
(c)	Epidermal cell	Guard cell	Stomatal cell	Subsidiary aperture
(d)	Epidermal cell	Subsidiary cell	Stomatal aperture	Guard cell

36. In barley stem vascular bundles are ***(2009)***
(a) closed and scattered
(b) open and in a ring
(c) closed and radial
(d) open and scattered.

ANATOMY OF DICOTYLEDONOUS AND MONOCOTYLEDONOUS PLANTS

37. The transverse section of a plant shows following anatomical features : ***(2020)***
(i) Large number of scattered vascular bundles surrounded by bundle sheath
(ii) Large conspicuous parenchymatous ground tissue
(iii) vascular bundles conjoint and closed
(iv) phloem parenchyma absent
Identify the category of plant and its part.
(a) Monocotyledonous stem.
(b) Monocotyledonous root
(c) Dicotyledonous stem
(d) Dicotyledonous root

38. Grass leaves curl inwards during very dry weather. Select the most appropriate reason from the following. ***(2019)***
(a) Tyloses in vessels
(b) Closure of stomata
(c) Flaccidity of bulliform cells
(d) Shrinkage of air spaces in spongy mesophyll

39. In the dicot root the vascular cambium originates from ***(Odisha NEET 2019)***
(a) tissue located below the phloem bundles and a portion of pericycle tissue above protoxylem
(b) cortical region
(c) parenchyma between endodermis and pericycle
(d) intrafascicular and interfascicular tissue in a ring.

40. Casparian strips occur in ***(2018)***
(a) epidermis (b) pericycle
(c) cortex (d) endodermis.

41. Root hair develop from the region of ***(2017)***
(a) elongation
(b) root cap
(c) meristematic activity
(d) maturation.

42. Cortex is the region found between ***(NEET-II 2016)***
(a) epidermis and stele
(b) pericycle and endodermis
(c) endodermis and pith
(d) endodermis and vascular bundle.

43. A major characteristic of monocot root is the presence of ***(2015 Cancelled)***
(a) vasculature without cambium
(b) cambium sandwiched between phloem and xylem along the radius
(c) open vascular bundles
(d) scattered vascular bundles

44. You are given a fairly old piece of dicot stem and a dicot root. Which of the following anatomical structures will you use to distinguish between the two? ***(2014)***
(a) Secondary xylem
(b) Secondary phloem
(c) Protoxylem
(d) Cortical cells

45. Water containing cavities in vascular bundles are found in ***(2012)***
(a) sunflower (b) maize
(c) Cycas (d) Pinus.

46. As compared to a dicot root, a monocot root has ***(Mains 2012)***
(a) more abundant secondary xylem
(b) many xylem bundles
(c) inconspicuous annual rings
(d) relatively thicker periderm.

47. Palisade parenchyma is absent in leaves of ***(2009)***
(a) mustard (b) soybean
(c) gram (d) Sorghum.

48. Anatomically fairly old dicotyledonous root is distinguished from the dicotyledonous stem by ***(2009)***
(a) absence of secondary phloem
(b) presence of cortex
(c) position of protoxylem
(d) absence of secondary xylem.

49. Passage cells are thin walled cells found in ***(2007)***
(a) phloem elements that serve as entry points for substance for transport to other plant parts
(b) testa of seeds to enable emergence of growing embryonic axis during seed germination
(c) central region of style through which the pollen tube grows towards the ovary
(d) endodermis of roots facilitating rapid transport of water from cortex to pericycle.

50. In a woody dicotyledonous tree, which of the following parts will mainly consist of primary tissues? ***(2005)***
(a) All parts
(b) Stem and root
(c) Flowers, fruits and leaves
(d) Shoot tips and root tips

51. Four radial vascular bundle are found in ***(2002)***
(a) dicot root (b) monocot root
(c) dicot stem (d) monocot stem.

52. Casparian strips are found in ***(1999)***
(a) epidermis (b) hypodermis
(c) periderm (d) endodermis.

53. A plant bears fruit, has a column of vascular tissue and a tap root system. This plant is a ***(1994)***
(a) angiosperm and dicot
(b) gymnosperm and dicot
(c) angiosperm and monocot
(d) gymnosperm and monocot.

54. What is true about a monocot leaf? ***(1992, 1990)***
(a) Reticulate venation
(b) Absence of bulliform cells from epidermis
(c) Mesophyll not differentiated into palisade and spongy tissues
(d) Well differentiated mesophyll

55. Pericycle of roots produces ***(1990)***
(a) mechanical support
(b) lateral roots
(c) vascular bundles
(d) adventitious buds.

ANSWER KEY

1.	(b)	2.	(a)	3.	(c)	4.	(b)	5.	(b)	6.	(d)	7.	(a)
8.	(d)	9.	(d)	10.	(d)	11.	(d)	12.	(b)	13.	(a)	14.	(d)
15.	(b)	16.	(a)	17.	(c)	18.	(b)	19.	(c)	20.	(a)	21.	(c)
22.	(c)	23.	(c)	24.	(a)	25.	(a)	26.	(*)	27.	(b)	28.	(a)
29.	(d)	30.	(d)	31.	(b)	32.	(c)	33.	(b)	34.	(b)	35.	(d)
36.	(a)	37.	(a)	38.	(c)	39.	(a)	40.	(d)	41.	(d)	42.	(a)
43.	(a)	44.	(c)	45.	(b)	46.	(b)	47.	(d)	48.	(c)	49.	(d)
50.	(d)	51.	(a)	52.	(d)	53.	(a)	54.	(c)	55.	(b)		

HINTS & EXPLANATIONS

1. (b) : Endarch and exarch are the terms often used for describing the position of primary xylem in the plant body. Primary xylem is of two types - protoxylem and metaxylem. In roots, protoxylem lies towards the centre. This arrangement of primary xylem is called exarch.

2. (a) : In gymnosperms phloem is without companion cells and sieve tubes.

3. (c)

4. (b) : Tracheids are elongated, dead cells with hard lignified walls, wide lumens and narrow walls with spiral, annular, reticulate, scalariform and pitted thickening but without perforated end walls of septa. That is, they have intact end walls unlike vessels. Vessels are long cylindrical tube like structures made of many cells, called vessel members, each with lignified walls and a large central cavity. Vessel members are interconnected through perforation in their common walls.

5. (b) :Lateral meristems are the meristems which are present along the lateral sides of stem and roots. They divide only in radial direction. Intrastelar or vascular cambium ring formed by intra-fascicular (also called fascicular) and inter-fascicular cambium; and cork cambium (phellogen) are examples of this type of meristem. These meristems are responsible for increase in girth of stem and roots.

6. (d)

7. (a) :Companion cell is a type of cell found within the phloem of flowering plants. Each companion cell is usually closely associated with a sieve element. They remain connected with sieve cells by plasmodesmata. They help in loading of phloem sieve cells with sugars through active transport.

8. (d) :Companion cells move sugar and amino acids into and out of the sieve elements. In "source" tissue such as leaf companion cells use transmembrane proteins to take up sugar and amino acids by active transport. Movement of sugars in the phloem begins at the source, where sugars are loaded (actively transported) into a sieve tube. Loading sets up a water potential gradient that facilitates movement of sugar.

9. (d) :Meristem is classified on the basis of position in plant bodies into lateral meristem, apical meristem and intercalary meristem. Lateral meristem is present on the lateral sides, e.g., vascular cambium (fascicular and interfascicular cambium) and cork cambium (phellogen).

10. (d) :The chief water conducting elements of xylem in gymnosperms are tracheids. These are elongated cells with tapering ends and are dead because of deposition of lignin. These show scalariform, annular, reticulate or bordered pitted thickening. These are the only water conducting xylem elements in both gymnosperms and pteridophytes. Generally vessels are absent in gymnosperms with exceptions like Gnetum, Welwitschia, Ephedra.

11. (d)

12. (b) :Internode is the part of a plant stem, that occurs between two adjacent nodes. Intercalary meristem is internodal in position and is found in the stem of grasses and other monocotyledonous plants. In early stages the internode is wholly or partially meristematic but later on some of its parts become matured more rapidly than the rest so a definite continuous sequence of development is maintained i.e., mature tissue left behind whereas new ones grow which later shows variable length.

13. (a) :Xylem vessels are hollow, elongated cells with open ends and pitted walls. Cells wall are lignified. At maturity nucleus is absent in vessels. Sieve tube members are long, slender, tube-like cells joined end to end, to form long tubular channels - the sieve tubes. Sieve tube members possess specialized sieve areas on the end walls called sieve plate. Young sieve tube members have abundant cytoplasm but there is no nucleus. The nucleus disintegrates during their development.

14. (d) :Parts of typical root : root cap, meristematic growing region, zone of elongation, root hair zone, zone of meristematic cells.

Apical meristem is terminal in position and responsible for terminal growth of the plant. Apical meristem is present at all root tips and shoot tips.

15. (b) :In the apices of some roots, there is a central region of cells which normally does not divide. This central inactive region was called quiescent centre by Clowes. The cells of this region have lesser amount of RNA and DNA so they have small nuclei. These cells also have a lower rate of protein synthesis. Mitochondria and endoplasmic reticulum are less developed. The cells of the quiescent centre are usually inactive. However, if already existing meristematic cells are injured or become inactive due to any other reason, the cells of quiescent centre become active.

16. (a) :Xylem is the principal water conducting tissue of the plant. It consists of four types of cells-tracheids, vessels, xylem fibres and xylem parenchyma. The tracheids and vessels together are known as tracheary elements. Tracheids are characteristic of all vascular plant. Tracheids originate from single cells. These are single elongated cells with tapering ends. The end walls are without perforations. Their length varies from 1 to 3 mm. Tracheids are devoid of protoplast, hence dead; fairly large cavity of these cells is without any contents. The wall of tracheids is moderately thick and usually lignified.

17. (c) :Apical meristems are situated at the tips of the root and shoot. They take part in initial growth. Plants elongate and increase in height as a result of divisions in this meristem. Promeristem and primary meristem (root and shoot apices) are included in this type of meristem.

18. (b): Vessels are found in the wood of almost all the angiosperms except certain primitive members of the order Ranales (vesseless dicots), e.g., *Trochodendron, Tetracentron, Drimys, Pseudowintera*, etc. Vessels also occur in some pteridophytes, such as Selaginella and in the members of order Gnetales of gymnosperms (e.g., *Gnetum, Ephedra* and *Welwitschia*)

19. (c) :In pteridophytes and gymnosperms, sieve tubes are not arranged in linear rows and hence called sieve cells. Sieve tube elements are the conducting elements of phloem. These are arranged end to end in linear rows with sieve plate between two sieve tube elements. In the sieve plate, there are present sieve pores. Sieve tube elements are living and have thin cellulosic walls in young cells but they become thick walled and are without nuclei at maturity.

20. (a) : Sclereids are a type of sclerenchyma cells. They are short or irregular, their walls are very thick, irrergular and the lumen is very narrow. These are dead cells and do not perform any metabolic functions. They show different types of lignin depositions and also have pits.

21. (c) : Meristems show the totipotency whereas xylem vessels and cork cells are dead cells while sieve tube cells do not possess nuclei.

22. (c) : An organised and differentiated cellular structure having cytoplasm but no nucleus are sieve tubes. The sieve tubes are living cells. Their walls are thicker than surrounding parenchyma cells. Sometimes they have a special, shining nacreous thickening. Cytoplasm occurs in the form of thin lining enclosing a big central vacuole.

23.(c) : Sieve tubes are suited for translocation of food because they possess broader lumen and perforated cross walls. Sieve tubes are elongated tubular conducting channels of phloem. The end wall possess many small pores and have thin cellulosic wall.

24 (a) : Death of protoplasm is a pre-requisite for a vital function like transport of sap. Xylem is a dead tissue (except xylem parenchyma) and do not have protoplasm, xylem performs the function of transport of water or sap inside the plant from roots to leaves.

25.(a) :The meristem that helps in increasing girth is lateral meristem. The lateral meristem is responsible for lateral growth of the plant i.e., growth in thickness e.g., cambium and cork cambium. It divides only periclinally or radially and is responsible for increase in girth or diameter.

26. (*) None of the options is correct.

All statements are correct.

27. (b)

28. (a): Grass being a monocot, has dumb-bell shaped guard cells. Guard cells are generally bean shaped or kidney shaped in dicots.

29.(d) :The leaf and stem epidermis of plant is covered with pores called stomata. Each stomata is surrounded by a pair of specialised epidermal cells known as guard cells which are in some cases further surrounded by another category of less modified epidermal cells known as subsidiary cells which provide support to the guard cells.

30. (d)

31.(b) :The epidermal surface of the leaf exhibits 1,000 to 60,000 minute openings called stomata. The stomata are bordered by two specialised epidermal cells - the guard cells which in some cases are accompanied by subsidiary cells. The walls of guard cells are unevenly thickened. Each guard cell has thick, inelastic inner wall and thin, elastic outer wall. Stomatal aperture is present in between the guard cells. Guard cells are not always surrounded by accessory cells or subsidiary cells.

32.(c) : Vascular bundle consists of complex tissues, the phloem and xylem. In dicots, between xylem and phloem, cambium is present which helps in secondary growth. This type of vascular bundle is called open. While in monocots cambium is absent, so these are called closed vascular bundles.

33.(b) : Ground tissue can be defined as all the tissues except epidermis and vascular bundles. Ground tissue constitutes the interior of organs except vascular system. It consists of simple tissues such as parenchyma, collenchyma and sclerenchyma.

34. (b) : In dicot stem, cambium is present between xylem and phloem, such vascular bundles are called open. Cambium constitutes meristematic cells which produce secondary xylem and phloem.

35.(d) A - Epidermal cell

B - Subsidiary cell

C - Stomatal aperture

D - Guard cell

36 (a) : Barley is a monocotyledonous plant. The vascular bundle of stem is conjoint, collateral,exarch and closed (because cambium is absent). It is also scattered throughout the ground tissue.

37. (a)

38.(c) : In grasses, certain adaxial epidermal cells along the veins modify themselves into large, empty, colourless cells. These are called bulliform cells. When the bulliform cells in the leaves have absorbed water and are turgid, the leaf surface is exposed. When they are flaccid due to water stress, they make the leaves curl inwards to minimise water loss.

39. (a)

40.(d) : Casparian strip is a band of thickening present on the radial and tangential walls of the endodermis. It is made up of both suberin and lignin.

41.(d) : Root hair are lateral tubular outgrowths that develop from the outer cells of zone of maturation or root hair zone.

42. (a)

43.(a) : In monocot root, a large number of vascular bundles are arranged in the form of a ring around the central pith. Vascular bundles are closed because there is no cambium present between the xylem and phloem.

44.(c) :In stems, the protoxylem lies towards the centre (pith) and the metaxylem lies towards the periphery. This type of primary xylem is called endarch. In root, the protoxylem lies towards periphery and metaxylem lies towards the centre, such arrangement is called exarch.

45. (b)

46.(b) :In monocot root, secondary growth is absent and vascular cylinder is in the form of several alternate and radial xylem and phloem bundles. The vascular bundles are arranged in the form of ring around central pith. Their number in maize ranges between 20 - 30 whereas in Pandanus and palms, they may be upto 100 . Because of the presence of numerous xylem bundles and exarch condition, xylem of monocot root is polyarch. On the other hand, in dicot root, xylem and phloem are equal in number (2-6) and alternately arranged i.e., they lie on different radii hence called radial bundles. According to number of ray (equivalent to number of xylem or phloem bundles) the roots may be diarch, triarch, tetrarch, pentarch or hexarch.

47. (d) : Palisade parenchyma is absent in leaves of Sorghum. It is a monocot plant where the parenchyma tissues of the leaves are not differentiated into palisade and spongy.

48.(c) : In dicot root the protoxylem is located near the periphery of the vascular cylinder, the metaxylem farther inward. In roots xylem is exarch or centripetal. In dicot stem the protoxylem is located near the centre of vascular bundle and metaxylem is located near the periphery i.e., the xylem is endarch or centrifugal.

49.(d) : Endodermis is a single layered structure which separates cortex from stele. There are both thick walled and thin walled cells in the endodermis. The thin walled cells are known as passage cells or transfusion cells which are opposite the protoxylem groups. These cells help in rapid transport of water from cortex to pericycle.

50 (d) : Primary tissues are those meristematic tissues that are derived directly from embryonal tissues, e.g., shoot apex and root apex.

51.(a) : The vascular tissue of the root is characterised by radial arrangement of vascular bundles i.e., xylem and phloem occur in separate patches on alternate radii. The number of xylem and phloem groups vary from two to six. But tetrarch condition (four vascular bundles) is more common. Monocot root generally has more than six vascular bundles (polyarch). Vascular bundles in dicot stems are conjoint, collateral or bicollateral, endarch and open. They are arranged in a ring.

In monocot stems the vascular bundles are conjoint, collateral, endarch and closed. They are scattered in the ground tissue.

52.(d) : Endodermis is single layered structure which separates cortex from stele. The cells of endodermis are barrelshaped without intercellular spaces, living and containing starch. The radial and tangential walls of endodermal cells possess thickenings of lignin, suberin and cutin in the form of strips or bands, which are known as casparian bands or Casparian strips.

53.(a) : In angiosperms, seeds are produced inside the ripened ovary called fruit. However in gymnosperms the seeds are not produced inside a fruit. In angiosperms vascular tissue includes both tracheids and vessels and in gymnosperms the vascular tissue contains only tracheids and not vessels. Tap root is the primary root that develops from the radicle.

It forms lateral branches which are further branched to form tertiary roots. These are generally found in dicotyledons. In monocotyledons, primary root is short lived, tap root is absent and adventitious roots are found.

54.(c) : In monocot leaf, mesophyll cells are not differentiated into palisade and spongy tissues. But there is well differentiated mesophyll cells in dicot stem. Also in the upper epidermis, there are some large cells found in groups which are called bulliform cells. The venation pattern in monocot is parallel.

55.(b) : Pericycle of root produces lateral roots. Endodermis is followed by pericycle. Usually it is a continuous layer but in some monocots it is interrupted by xylem and phloem. It is the site of origin of lateral roots and cork cambium. The root branches are, therefore described as endogenous in origin.

ANIMAL TISSUES

1. Given below are two statements: **(2023)**

Statement I: Ligaments are dense irregular tissue.

Statement II: Cartilage is dense regular tissue.

In the light of the above statements, choose the correct answer from the options given below:
(a) Statement I is true but statement II is false.
(b) Statement I is false but statement II is true.
(c) Both statement I and statement II are true.
(d) Both statement I and statement II are false.

2. Match List I with List II. **(2023)**

List I	List II
A. Mast cells	I. Ciliated epithelium
B. Inner surface of bronchiole	II. Areolar connective tissue
C. Blood	III. Cuboidal epithelium
D. Tubular parts of nephron	IV. Specialised connective tissue

Choose the correct answer from the options give below:
(a) A-II, B-I, C-IV, D-III (b) A-III, B-IV, C-II, D-I
(c) A-I, B-II, C-IV, D-III (d) A-II, B-III, C-I, D-IV

3. Which of the following is not a connective tissue? **(2022)**
(a) Blood (b) Adipose tissue
(c) Cartilage (d) Neuroglia

4. Which of the following is present between the adjacent bones of the vertebral column ? **(2022)**
(a) Intercalated discs (b) Cartilage
(c) Areolar tissue (d) Smooth muscle

5. Match list-I with list-II. **(2022)**

List-I	List-II
(A) Bronchioles	(i) Dense regular connective tissue
(B) Goblet cell	(ii) Loose connective tissue
(C) Tendons	(iii) Glandular tissue
(D) Adipose Tissue	(iv) Ciliated epithelium

Choose the correct answer from the option given below :
(a) (A)-(iv), (B)-(iii), (C)-(i), (D)-(ii)
(b) (A)-(i), (B)-(ii), (C)-(iii), (D)-(iv)
(c) (A)-(ii), (B)-(i), (C)-(iv), (D)-(iii)
(d) (A)-(iii), (B)-(iv), (C)-(ii), (D)-(i)

6. Which of the following statements wrongly represents the nature of smooth muscle? **(2021)**
(a) These muscles are present in the wall of blood vessels.
(b) These muscle have no striations.
(c) They are involuntary muscles.
(d) Communication among the cells is performed by intercalated discs.

7. Identify the types of cell junctions that help to stop the leakage of the substances across a tissue and facilitation of communication with neighbouring cells via rapid transfer of ions and molecules. **(2021)**
(a) Adhering junctions and gap junctions, respectively.
(b) Gap junctions and adhering junctions, respectively.
(c) Tight junctions and gap junctions, respectively.
(d) Adhering junctions and tight junctions, respectively.

8. Cuboidal epithelium with brush border of microvilli is found in **(2020)**
(a) lining of intestine
(b) ducts of salivary glands
(c) proximal convoluted tubule of nephron
(d) Eustachian tube.

9. Goblet cells of alimentary canal are modified from ***(2020)***
(a) squamous epithelial cells
(b) columnar epithelial cells
(c) chondrocytes
(d) compound epithelial cells.

10. The ciliated epithelial cells are required to move particles or mucus in a specific direction. In humans, these cells are mainly present in ***(2019)***
(a) bronchioles and Fallopian tubes
(b) bile duct and bronchioles
(c) Fallopian tubes and pancreatic duct
(d) Eustachian tube and salivary duct.

11. Match the following cell structure with its characteristic feature. ***(Odisha NEET 2019)***

(A) Tight	(i) Cement neighbouring junctions
(B) Adhering junctions cells together to form sheet	(ii) Transmit information through chemical to another cells
(C) Gap junctions	(iii) Establish a barrier to prevent leakage of fluid across epithelial cells
(D) Synaptic junctions	(iv) Cytoplasmic channels to facilitate communication between adjacent cells

Select correct option from the following

	(A)	(B)	(C)	(D)
(a)	(ii)	(iv)	(i)	(iii)
(b)	(iv)	(ii)	(i)	(iii)
(c)	(iii)	(i)	(iv)	(ii)
(d)	(iv)	(iii)	(i)	(ii)

12. Smooth muscles are ***(NEET-II 2016)***
(a) involuntary, fusiform, non-striated
(b) voluntary, multinucleate, cylindrical
(c) involuntary, cylindrical, striated
(d) voluntary, spindle-shaped, uninucleate.

13. Which type of tissue correctly matches with its location? ***(NEET-I 2016)***

	Tissue	Location
(a)	Transitional epithelium	Tip of nose
(b)	Cuboidal epithelium	Lining of stomach
(c)	Smooth muscle	Wall of intestine
(d)	Areolar tissue	Tendons

14. The function of the gap junction is to (2015)
(a) separate two cells from each other
(b) stop substance from leaking across a tissue
(c) performing cementing to keep neighbouring cells together
(d) facilitate communication between adjoining cells by connecting the cytoplasm for rapid transfer of ions, small molecules and some large molecules.

15. Choose the correctly matched pair. ***(2014)***
(a) Tendon - Specialized connective tissue
(b) Adipose tissue - Dense connective tissue
(c) Areolar tissue - Loose connective tissue
(d) Cartilage - Loose connective tissue

16. Choose the correctly matched pair. ***(2014)***
(a) Inner lining of - Ciliated epithelium salivary ducts
(b) Moist surface - Glandular epithelium of buccal cavity
(c) Tubular parts of -Cuboidal epithelium nephrons
(d) Inner surface of - Squamous epithelium bronchioles

17. Identify the tissue shown in the diagram and match with its characteristics and its location. ***(Karnataka NEET 2013)***

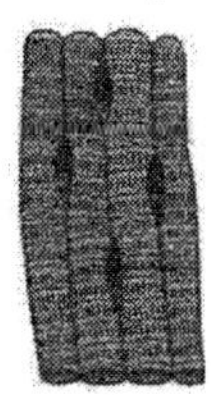

(a) Smooth muscles, show branching, found in the wall of the heart
(b) Cardiac muscles, unbranched muscles,

found in the walls of the heart

(c) Striated muscles, tapering at both ends, attached with the bones of the ribs

(d) Skeletal muscles show striations and are closely attached with the bones of the limbs

18. Given below is the diagrammatic sketch of a certain type of connective tissue. Identify the parts labelled A, B, C and D and select the right option about them. ***(Mains 2012)***

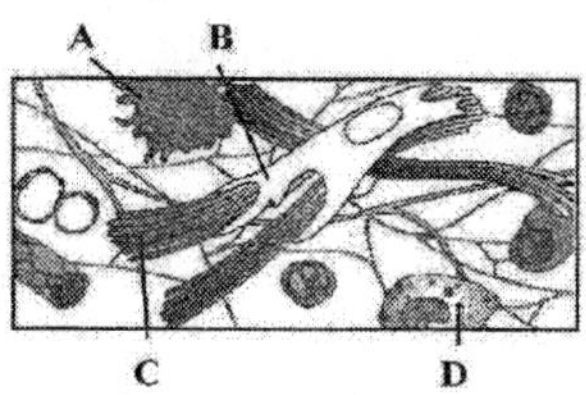

A B C D

	A	B	C	D
(a)	Macrophage	Fibroblast	Collagen fibres	Mast cell
(b)	Mast cell	Macrophage	Fibroblast	Collagen fibres
(c)	Macrophage	Collagen fibres	Fibroblast	Mast cell
(d)	Mast cell	Collagen fibres	Fibroblast	Macro-phage

19. The supportive skeletal structures in the human external ears and in the nose tip are examples of ***(Mains 2012)***

(a) ligament (b) areolar tissue

(c) bone (d) cartilage.

20. The four sketches (A, B, C and D) given below, represent four different types of animal tissues. Which one of these is correctly identified in the options given, along with its correct location and function? ***(Mains 2012)***

(A)

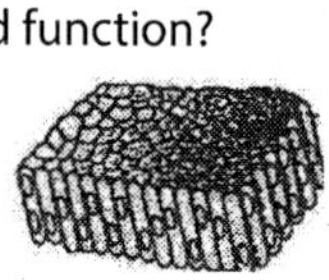

(B)

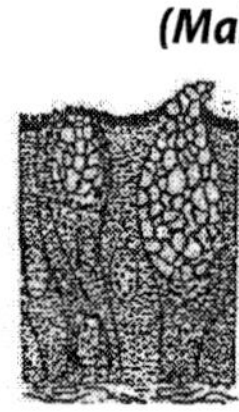

(C)

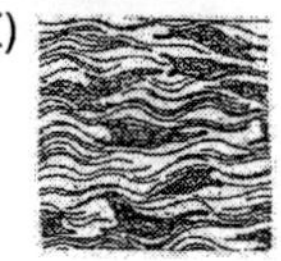

(D)

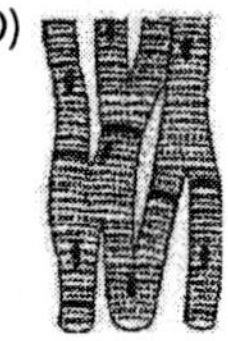

	Tissue	Location	Function
(a)	(B) Glandular epithelium	Intestine	Secretion
(b)	(C) Collagen fibres	Cartilage	Attach skeletal muscles to bones
(c)	(D) Smooth muscle tissue	Heart	Heart contraction
(d)	(A) Columnar epithelium	Nephron	Secretion and absorption

21. The ciliated columnar epithelial cells in humans are known to occur in ***(2011)***

(a) Eustachian tube and stomach lining

(b) bronchioles and Fallopian tube

(c) bile duct and oesophagus

(d) Fallopian tube and urethra.

22. The cells lining the blood vessels belong to the category of ***(Mains 2011, 2010)***

(a) smooth muscle tissue

(b) squamous epithelium

(c) columnar epithelium

(d) connective tissue.

23. Which one of the following is correct pairing of a body part and the kind of muscle tissue that moves it? ***(2009)***

(a) Biceps of upper arm - Smooth muscle fibres

(b) Abdominal wall - Smooth muscle

(c) Iris – Involuntary smooth muscle

(d) Heart wall – Involuntary unstriated muscle

24. The epithelial tissue present on the inner surface of bronchioles and Fallopian tubes is ***(2009)***

(a) glandular

(b) ciliated

(c) squamous

(d) cuboidal.

25. The cell junctions called tight, adhering and gap junctions are found in ***(2009)***
(a) connective tissue
(b) epithelial tissue
(c) neural tissue
(d) muscular tissue.

26. The kind of tissue that forms the supportive structure in our pinna (external ears) is also found in ***(2009)***
(a) nails (b) ear ossicles
(c) tip of the nose (d) vertebrae.

27. Which one of the following pairs of structures distinguishes a nerve cell from other types of cell? ***(2007)***
(a) Vacuoles and fibres
(b) Flagellum and medullary sheath
(c) Nucleus and mitochondria
(d) Perikaryon and dendrites

28. In which one of the following preparations are you likely to come across cell junctions most frequently? ***(2007)***
(a) Thrombocytes (b) Tendon
(c) Hyaline cartilage (d) Ciliated epithelium

29. Areolar connective tissue joins ***(2006)***
(a) bones with bones
(b) fat body with muscles
(c) integument with muscles
(d) bones with muscles.

30. Mast cells secrete ***(2006)***
(a) haemoglobin (b) hippurin
(c) myoglobin (d) histamine.

31. Four healthy people in their twenties got involved in injuries resulting in damage and death of few cells of the following. Which of the cells are least likely to be replaced by new cells? ***(2005)***
(a) Liver cells (b) Neurons
(c) Malpighian layer of the skin
(d) Osteocytes

32. Mast cells of connective tissue contain ***(2004)***
(a) vasopressin and relaxin
(b) heparin and histamine
(c) heparin and calcitonin
(d) serotonin and melanin.

33. Which one of the following contains the largest quantity of extracellular material? ***(2003)***
(a) Striated muscle(b) Areolar tissue
(c) Stratified epithelium
(d) Myelinated nerve fibres

34. Collagen is ***(2002)***
(a) fibrous protein (b) globular protein
(c) lipid (d) carbohydrate.

35. During an injury nasal septum gets damaged and for its recovery which cartilage is preferred? ***(2001)***
(a) Elastic cartilage (b) Hyaline cartilage
(c) Calcified cartilage (d) Fibrous cartilage

36. Which cells do not form layer and remains structurally separate? ***(2001)***
(a) Epithelial cells (b) Muscle cells
(c) Nerve cells (d) Gland cells

37. Proteoglycan in cartilages which is a part of polysaccharide is ***(2000)***
(a) chondroitin (b) ossein
(c) casein (d) cartilagin.

38. Characteristic of simple epithelium is that they ***(2000)***
(a) are arranged indiscriminately
(b) make a definite layer
(c) continue to divide and help in organ function
(d) none of the above.

39. Ligament is a/an ***(1999)***
(a) inelastic white fibrous tissue
(b) modified white fibrous tissue
(c) modified yellow elastic fibrous tissue
(d) none of the above.

40. Tendon is made up of ***(1999)***
(a) yellow fibrous connective tissue
(b) modified white fibrous tissue
(c) areolar tissue
(d) adipose tissue.

41. In mammals, histamine is secreted by **(1998)**
(a) lymphocytes (b) mast cells
(c) fibroblasts (d) histiocytes.

42. Protein present in cartilage is **(1997)**
(a) cartilagin (b) ossein
(c) chondrin (d) none of these.

43. Basement membrane is made up of **(1997)**
(a) no cell product of epithelial cell
(b) endodermal cell
(c) Mesodermal cells
(d) both (b) and (c).

44. Stratum germinativum is an example of which kind of epithelium? **(1997)**
(a) Columnar (b) Squamous
(c) Cuboidal (d) Ciliated

45. An epithelial tissue which has thin flat cells, arranged edge to edge so as to appear like closely packed tiles, is found to be present at **(1994)**
(a) outer surface of ovary
(b) inner lining of Fallopian tube
(c) inner lining of stomach
(d) inner lining of cheeks.

46. Hair present in the skin are **(1993)**
(a) epidermal in origin and made of dead cells
(b) epidermal in origin and made of living cells
(c) dermal in origin and made of living cells
(d) dermal in origin and made of dead cells.

47. The layer of actively dividing cells of skin is termed as **1993)**
(a) stratum compactum
(b) stratum corneum
(c) stratum malpighii/stratum germinativum
(d) stratum lucidum.

48. Formation of cartilage bones involves **(1993)**
(a) deposition of bony matter by osteoblasts and resorption by chondroclasts
(b) deposition of bony matter by osteoclasts
(c) deposition of bony matter by osteoclasts only
(d) deposition of bony matter by osteoblasts only.

49. Characteristics of smooth muscle fibres are **(1992)**
(a) spindle-shaped, unbranched, nonstriated, uninucleate and involuntary
(b) spindle-shaped, unbranched, unstriped, multinucleate and involuntary
(c) cylindrical, unbranched, unstriped, multinucleate and involuntary
(d) cylindrical, unbranched, striated, multinucleate and voluntary.

50. Haversian canals occur in **(1989)**
(a) humerus (b) pubis
(c) scapula (d) clavicle.

51. Histamine secreting cells are found in **(1989)**
(a) connective tissues (b) lungs
(c) muscular tissue (d) nervous tissue.

52. Mineral found in red pigment of vertebrate blood is **(1989)**
(a) magnesium (b) iron
(c) calcium (d) copper.

COCKROACH

53. Match List I with List II. **(2023)**

List I	List II
A. Taenia	I. Nephridia
B. Paramecium	II. Contractile vacuole
C. Periplaneta	III. Flame cells
D. Pheretima	IV. Urecose gland

Choose the correct answer from the options give below:
(a) A-III, B-II, C-IV, D-I (b) A-II, B-I, C-IV, D-III
(c) A-I, B-II, C-III, D-IV (d) A-I, B-II, C-IV, D-III

54. Which of the following is characteristic feature of cockroach regarding sexual dimorphism? **(2023)**
(a) Presence of sclerites
(b) Presence of anal cerci
(c) Dark brown body colour and anal cerci
(d) Presence of anal styles

55. In cockroach, excretion is brought about by ***(2023)***

A. Phallic gland

B. Urecose gland

C. Nephrocytes

D. Fat body

E. Collaterial glands.

Choose the correct answer from the options given below:

(a) B, C and D only (b) B and D only
(c) A and E only (d) A, B and E only

56. Tegmina in cockroach, arises from ***(2022)***
(a) prothorax
(b) mesothorax
(c) metathorax
(d) prothorax and mesothorax.

57. Which of the following characteristics is incorrect with respect to cockroach? ***(2021)***
(a) 10th abdominal segment in both sexes, bears a pair of anal cerci.
(b) A ring of gastric caeca is present at the junction of midgut and hind gut.
(c) Hypopharynx lies within the cavity enclosed by the mouth parts.
(d) In females, 7th -9th sterna together form a genital pouch.

58. If the head of cockroach is removed, it may live for few days because ***(2020)***
(a) the supra-oesophageal ganglia of the cockroach are situated in ventral part of abdomen
(b) the cockroach does not have nervous system
(c) the head holds a small proportion of a nervous system while the rest is situated along the ventral part of its body
(d) the head holds a $1/3^{rd}$ of a nervous system while the rest is situated along the dorsal part of its body.

59. Select the correct sequence of organs in the alimentary canal of cockroach starting from mouth. ***(2019)***
(a) Pharynx → Oesophagus → Ileum → Crop → Gizzard → Colon → Rectum
(b) Pharynx → Oesophagus → Crop → Gizzard → Ileum → Colon → Rectum
(c) Pharynx → Oesophagus → Gizzard → Crop → Ileum → Colon → Rectum
(d) Pharynx → Oesophagus → Gizzard → Ileum→ Crop → Colon → Rectum

60. Which of the following features is used to identify a male cockroach from a female cockroach? ***(2018)***
(a) Presence of a boat-shaped sternum on the 9th abdominal segment
(b) Presence of caudal styles
(c) Forewings with darker tegmina
(d) Presence of anal cerci

61. In male cockroaches, sperms are stored in which part of the reproductive system? ***(NEET-II 2016)***
(a) Seminal vesicles (b) Mushroom glands
(c) Testes (d) Vas deferens

62. Which of the following features is not present in *Periplaneta americana*? ***(NEET-I 2016)***
(a) Exoskeleton composed of N-acetylglucosamine
(b) Metamerically segmented body
(c) Schizocoelom as body cavity
(d) Indeterminate and radial cleavage during embryonic development

63. The body cells in cockroach discharge their nitrogenous waste in the haemolymph mainly in the form of ***(2015)***
(a) urea (b) calcium carbonate
(c) ammonia (d) potassium urate.

64. The terga, sterna and pleura of cockroach body are joined by ***(2015 Cancelled)***
(a) arthrodial membrane
(b) cartilage
(c) cementing glue
(d) muscular tissue.

65. What external changes are visible after the last moult of a cockroach nymph? ***(2013)***
(a) Both forewings and hindwings develop
(b) Labium develops
(c) Mandibles become harder
(d) Anal cerci develop

66. Select the correct option with respect to cockroaches. ***(Karnataka NEET 2013)***
(a) Malpighian tubules convert nitrogenous wastes into urea.
(b) Males bear short anal styles not present in females.
(c) Nervous system comprises of a dorsal nerve cord and ten pairs of ganglia.
(d) The forewings are tegmina which are used in flight.

67. Which one of the following is one of the paths followed by air or O2 during respiration in the adult male Periplaneta americana as it enters the animal body? ***(Karnataka NEET 2013)***
(a) Spiracle in metathorax, trachea, tracheoles, oxygen diffuses into cells
(b) Mouth, bronchial tube, trachea, oxygen enters cells
(c) Spiracles in prothorax, tracheoles, trachea, oxygen diffuses into cells
(d) Hypopharynx, mouth, pharynx, trachea tissues

68. Select the correct statement from the ones given below with respect to Periplaneta americana. ***(2012)***
(a) Nervous system located dorsally, consists of segmentally arranged ganglia joined by a pair of longitudinal connectives.
(b) Males bear a pair of short thread like anal styles.
(c) There are 16 very long Malpighian tubules present at the junctions of midgut and hindgut.
(d) Grinding of food is carried out only by the mouth parts.

69. Which of the following happens in the common cockroach? ***(2011)***
(a) Malpighian tubules are excretory organs projecting out from the colon.
(b) Oxygen is transported by haemoglobin in blood.
(c) Nitrogenous excretory product is urea.
(d) The food is ground by mandibles and gizzard.

70. Assertion (A) : Periplaneta americana is nocturnal, omnivorous, household pest. ***(1992)***

Reason (R): It is because it acts as scavenger.
(a) A is true but R is false.
(b) A is false but R is true.
(c) Both A and R are true and R is correct explanation of A.
(d) Both A and R are true but R is not correct explanation of A.

71. Male and female cockroaches can be distinguished externally through ***(1991)***
(a) anal styles in male
(b) anal cerci in female
(c) anal style and antennae in females
(d) both (b) and (c).

FROG

72. Select the correct route for the passage of sperms in male frogs. ***(2017)***
(a) Testes - Vasa efferentia - Kidney - Seminal vesicle - Urinogenital duct - Cloaca
(b) Testes - Vasa efferentia - Bidder's canal -Ureter - Cloaca
(c) Testes - Vasa efferentia - Kidney - Bidder's canal - Urinogenital duct - Cloaca
(d) Testes - Bidder's canal - Kidney - Vasa efferentia - Urinogenital duct - Cloaca

73. Frog's heart when taken out of the body continues to beat for sometime.

Select the best option from the following statements. ***(2017)***
(1) Frog is a poikilotherm.
(2) Frog does not have any coronary circulation.

(3) Heart is "myogenic" in nature.

(4) Heart is autoexcitable.

(a) Only (4) (b) (1) and (2)

(c) (3) and (4) (d) Only (3)

74. Compared to those of humans, the erythrocytes in frog are ***(2012)***

(a) without nucleus but with haemoglobin

(b) nucleated and with haemoglobin

(c) very much smaller and fewer

(d) nucleated and without haemoglobin.

75. Frogs differ from humans in possessing ***(Mains 2011)***

(a) paired cerebral hemispheres

(b) hepatic portal system

(c) nucleated red blood cells

(d) thyroid as well as parathyroid.

76. Ureters act as urinogenital ducts in ***(Mains 2011)***

(a) human males

(b) human females

(c) both male and female frogs

(d) male frogs.

77. Consider the following four statements (A-D) related to the common frog Rana tigrina, and select the correct option stating which ones are true (T) and which ones are false (F). ***(Mains 2011)***

Statements:

A. On dry land it would die due to lack of O2 if its mouth is forcibly kept closed for a few days.

B. It has four-chambered heart.

C. On dry land it turns uricotelic from ureotelic.

D. Its life-history is carried out in pond water.

	A	B	C	D
(a)	T	F	F	T
(b)	T	T	F	F
(c)	F	F	T	T
(d)	F	T	T	F

78. Which one of the following is the true description about an animal concerned? ***(2008)***

(a) Rat - Left kidney is slightly higher in position than the right one

(b) Cockroach - 10 pairs of spiracles (2 pairs on thorax and 8 pairs on abdomen)

(c) Earthworm - The alimentary canal consists of a sequence of pharynx, oesophagus, stomach, gizzard and intestine

(d) Frog - Body divisible into three regions head, neck and trunk

79. What happens if bone of frog is kept in dilute hydrochloric acid? ***(2000)***

(a) Will become flexible

(b) Will turn black

(c) Will break into pieces

(d) Will shrink

80. The roof of the cranium of frog is formed by ***(1997)***

(a) frontoparietal

(b) orbitosphenoid

(c) parasphenoid

(d) alisphenoid.

81. In frog, the surface of attachment of tongue is ***(1997)***

(a) pterygoid (b) hyoid apparatus

(c) parasphenoid (d) palatine.

82. In frog, "fenestra ovalis" is ***(1997)***

(a) the communication between the pharynx and the tympanic cavity

(b) the external opening of the tympanic cavity which is covered by the tympanic membrane

(c) the air filled cavity of the middle ear

(d) the opening in the auditory capsule which separates the middle ear from the internal ear.

83. The kidney of an adult frog is ***(1997)***

(a) metanephros (b) opisthonephros

(c) pronephros (d) mesonephros.

84. Mucus helps frog in forming ***(1993)***
(a) thick skin (b) dry skin
(c) smooth skin (d) moist skin.

85. Bullfrog of India is ***(1992)***
(a) Rana tigrina (b) R. sylvatica
(c) R. catesbeiana (d) R. esculenta.

86. Addition of a trace of thyroxine or iodine in water containing tadpoles will ***(1990)***
(a) keep them in larval stage
(b) hasten their metamorphosis
(c) slow down their metamorphosis
(d) kill the tadpoles.

ANSWER KEY

1.	(d)	2.	(a)	3.	(d)	4.	(b)	5.	(a)	6.	(d)	7.	(c)
8.	(c)	9.	(b)	10.	(a)	11.	(c)	12.	(a)	13.	(c)	14.	(d)
15.	(c)	16.	(c)	17.	(d)	18.	(a)	19.	(d)	20.	(a)	21.	(b)
22.	(b)	23.	(b, c)	24.	(b)	25.	(b)	26.	(c)	27.	(d)	28.	(d)
29.	(c)	30.	(d)	31.	(b)	32.	(b)	33.	(b)	34.	(a)	35.	(b)
36.	(c)	37.	(a)	38.	(b)	39.	(c)	40.	(b)	41.	(b)	42.	(c)
43.	(a)	44.	(a)	45.	(d)	46.	(a)	47.	(c)	48.	(a)	49.	(a)
50.	(a)	51.	(a)	52.	(b)	53.	(a)	54.	(d)	55.	(a)	56.	(b)
57.	(b)	58.	(c)	59.	(b)	60.	(b)	61.	(a)	62.	(d)	63.	(d)
64.	(a)	65.	(a)	66.	(b)	67.	(a)	68.	(b)	69.	(d)	70.	(d)
71.	(a)	72.	(c)	73.	(c)	74.	(b)	75.	(c)	76.	(d)	77.	(*)
78.	(b)	79.	(a)	80.	(a)	81.	(b)	82.	(c)	83.	(d)	84.	(d)
85.	(a)	86.	(b)										

HINTS & EXPLANATIONS

1. (d) :Ligaments are dense regular connective tissue. Cartilage, bones and blood are types of specialised connective tissue.

2. (a) : Mast cells → Areolar connective tissue

Inner surface of bronchiole → Ciliated epithelium

Blood → Specialised connective tissue

Tubular parts of nephron ® Cuboidal epithelium

3. (d) : Neuroglia, also called glial cells which constitute the rest of neural system protect and support neurons.

4. (b) : Cartilage is present in the tip of nose, outer ear joints, between adjacent bones of the vertebral column, limbs and hands in adults.

5. (a) : Bronchioles - Ciliated epithelium

Goblet cell - Glandular tissue

Tendons - Dense regular connective tissue

Adipose Tissue - Loose connective tissue

6. (d) : Intercalated discs are present in cardiac muscle that communicate at some fusion points and allow the cells to contract as a unit.

7. (c) : Tight junctions help to stop substances from leaking across a tissue. Gap junctions facilitate the cells to communicate with each other by connecting the cytoplasm of adjoning cells, for rapid transfer of ions, small molecules and certain big molecules.

8. (c) : The cuboidal epithelium is composed of a single layer of cube-like cells which is commonly found in ducts of glands and tubular parts of nephrons in kidneys and its main functions are secretion and absorption. The epithelium of proximal convoluted tubule (PCT) of nephron in the kidney has microvilli.

9. (b) : Certain cells of columnar epithelial cells contain muscles and are called goblet cells as they look like goblet. Such cells are present in alimentary canal.

10. (a)

11. (c)

12. (a) : Smooth muscle fibres are elongated and spindle-shaped (fusiform). Each fibre contains a single oval nucleus surrounded by cytoplasm (sarcoplasm). In cytoplasm, myofibrils are arranged longitudinally. These fibres lack striations and sarcolemma. However, are enclosed by plasma membrane.

13. (c) : Tip of nose has elastic cartilage. Simple columnar epithelium lines the stomach. Tendon is white fibrous connective tissue. Posterior part of intestine has single unit smooth muscle in which all fibres of muscle contract simultaneously as single unit.

14. (d) : Most cells in animal tissues (with the exception of a few terminally differentiated cells such as skeletal muscle cells and blood cells) are in communication with their adjoining cells via gap junctions. At the place where gap junction is present, membranes of two adjacent cells are separated by a uniform narrow gap of about 2-4 nm. The gap is spanned by channel forming proteins called connexins, which allow inorganic ions and other small water soluble molecules to pass directly from cytoplasm of one cell to cytoplasm of other cell.

15. (c) : Areolar tissue is the most widely distributed loose connective tissue in the body. Tendon is a type of dense connective tissue, adipose tissue is a fat-storing loose connective tissue and cartilage is a specialised connective tissue.

16. (c) : Inner lining of salivary ducts - Simple cuboidal epithelium

Moist surface of buccal cavity- Non-keratinized stratified squamous

Inner surface of bronchioles - Ciliated columnar epithelium

17. (d) : Locomotion (performed by limbs) in humans depends on the movements of muscle fibres. Skeletal muscles are attached to the bones by tendons and help in the movement of the parts of skeleton. These muscles are under the control of conscious mind and are called voluntary muscles. Under the microscope, these muscles show transverse stripes and hence are designated as striated muscles.

18. (a)

19. (d) : Cartilage is a semi-rigid supportive or skeletal connective tissue in which matrix is solid and made of mucoprotein or proteoglycan called chondrin. It is of four types - hyaline, fibrous, calcified and elastic. Yellow elastic fibrocartilage is found in pinna and external auditory canal of the ear, Eustachian tube, epiglottis and tip of the nose. Its matrix contains numerous yellow fibres which form a network by uniting with one another. Due to the presence of yellow fibres, the cartilage becomes more flexible. Hence, it provides flexibility to these organs.

20. (a) : Intestine is lined by glandular epithelium which is secretory in function. The glands found in intestine are exocrine and may be unicellular or multicellular. When unicellular glands secrete mucus, they are called mucous cells or goblet cells and are common in the columnar epithelium of intestine. When unicellular glands secrete a clear watery fluid, they are called serous cells which are also present in intestinal glands. On the other hand, multicellular glands consist of a duct and secretory portion, both formed of epithelial cells. They are further of two types: tubular and saccular. In tubular glands secretory portion is tube like, for example, Crypts of Lieberkuhn (a type of simple straight tubular glands found in intestine) and Brunner's gland (a type of simple branched tubular glands found in intestine).

21. (b) : The ciliated columnar epithelial cells in humans are present in the nasal passages, oviducts (Fallopian tubes), terminal bronchioles, ventricles of the brain and central canal of the spinal cord of the embryo. Columnar ciliated epithelium consists of columnar cells, which bear cilia on the free surface.

22. (b) : Simple squamous epithelium is composed of large flat cells whose edges fit closely together like the tiles in a floor, hence it is also called pavement epithelium. The nuclei of the cells are flattened and often lie at the centre of the cells and cause bulgings of cells surface. The epithelium lines the blood vessels, lymph vessels, heart, terminal bronchioles, alveoli of the lungs, walls of the Bowman's capsules, descending limbs of loop of Henle. In the blood vessels and heart it is called endothelium.

23. (b, c) : Smooth muscles are called involuntary muscles as action of these muscles is controlled by autonomic nervous system i.e., not under the control of animal's will. Iris of eyes consist of smooth involuntary muscles. Abdominal wall also have smooth muscles. Biceps of upper arm is made of skeletal muscles while heart wall consists of cardiac muscles.

24. (b) : The ciliated columnar epithelial cells in humans are present in the nasal passages, oviducts (Fallopian tubes) terminal bronchioles, ventricles of the brain and central canal of the spinal cord of the embryo. Columnar ciliated epithelium consists of columnar cells, which bear cilia on the free surface.

25. (b) : Epithelial tissues consist of variously shaped cells closely arranged in one or more layers. The cells are held together by intercellular junctions like tight, adhering and gap junctions.

26. (c) : Yellow elastic fibrocartilage, a type of skeletal tissue, is found in the pinna, Eustachian tubes, epiglottis and tip of the nose. It is a type of cartilage and due to presence of yellow fibres, it becomes more flexible.

27. (d) : Neuron (nerve cell) is one of the basic functional units of the nervous system. Neuron is a cell specialized to transmit electrical nerve impulse and so carry information from one part of the body to another. Each neuron has an enlarged portion, the cell body (perikaryon), containing the nucleus; from the body extend several processes (dendrites) through which impulses enter from their branches. A longer process, the nerve fibre, extends outward and carries impulses away from the cell body. This is normally unbranched except at the nerve ending. The point of contact of one neuron with another is known as a synapse.

28. (d) : Cell junctions come across most frequently in the preparation of ciliated epithelium. A cell junction is a structure within a tissue of a multicellular organism. They consist of protein complexes and provide contact between neighbouring cells, between a cell and the extracellular matrix, or they built up the paracellular barrier of epithelia and control the paracellular transport.

29. (c) : Areolar tissue is a loose connective tissue comprised of a semifluid ground substance containing several kinds of loosely arranged fibres. Its function is to attach the skin to the underlying tissues, to fill the spaces between various organs and thus holds them in place, and surrounds and supports the blood vessels.

30. (d) : Mast cells are granulated wandering cells that are found in connective tissue. Their granules contain histamine which is a vasodilator. It causes running nose, sneezing and itching; and narrows the airways in the lungs. Their granules also contain heparin which is an anticoagulant and serotonin which acts as a mediator of inflammation and allergic reactions.

31. (b) : Neurons are least likely to be replaced by new cells as they have least regeneration power.

32. (b)

33. (b) : In areolar tissue, there is more intercellular space, so largest quantity of extracellular material is present in this tissue. It contains all cell types and fibres of connective tissue. There is a thin layer of extracellular fluid in stratified epithelium whereas striated muscle is attached with tendons and there is very less amount of extracellular fluid in myelinated nerve fibre.

34. (a) : Collagen is an insoluble fibrous protein found extensively in the connective tissue of skin, tendons and bone. Collagen accounts for over 30% of the total body protein of mammals. Globular proteins have compact rounded molecules and are usually water soluble. Lipid is a diverse group of organic compounds, that are insoluble in water but soluble in organic solvents. Carbohydrates are compounds of carbon, hydrogen and oxygen.

35. (b) : Nasal septum consists of hyaline cartilage. It is bluish-green and translucent in appearance. It has fewer very fine white fibres in the matrix. This type of cartilage gives flexibility and support at the joints. Elastic, calcified and fibrous cartilages occur in other parts of body.

36. (c) : Nerve cells are the highly excitable cells, specialized for impulse conduction. They originate from neural plate of embryonic ectoderm and serve as structural and functional units of nervous tissue.

37. (a) : Proteoglycans consist of polysaccharide attached with a protein chondroitin. It is present in cartilage as well as in extracellular material. Ossein is a protein present in matrix of bone. Casein is a milk protein.

38. (b) : Simple epithelium consists of a single layer of cells resting on a basement membrane. This makes a definite layer.

39. (c) : Ligament occurs in the form of cords in a modified yellow elastic fibrous tissue and connects bone with a bone. Modified white fibrous tissue is present in the tendons.

40. (b) : White fibrous tissue has two forms : cords and sheets. The white fibres run parallel to form cords, called tendons. Tendon attaches a muscle to a bone. It consists of collagen fibres and are therefore inelastic. They ensure that the force exerted by muscular contraction is transmitted to the relevant part of the body to be moved.

41. (b)

42. (c) : Chondrin is a protein present in the matrix of cartilage. It forms a constituent of a compound called chondrin sulphate. Chondrin sulphate consists of proteoglycans, that is protein chains bonded to long chains of disaccharide hyaluronic acid.

43. (a) : Basement membrane (basal lamina) is a thin sheet of fibrous proteins that underlies and supports the cells of an epithelium, separating this from underlying tissue. Basement membranes are components of the extracellular matrix (= the viscous watery fluid that surrounds cells in animal tissue) and help to regulate passage of materials between epithelial cells and adjacent blood vessels. Each consists of a framework of collagen fibrils within which are glycosaminoglycans (mucopolysaccharides) and laminins, which are proteins that bind the basement membrane to neighbouring cells via cell adhesion molecules.

44. (a) : Stratum germinativum (also stratum basale or basal cell layer) is the layer of keratinocytes that lies at the base of the epidermis immediately above the dermis. It consists of a single layer of tall, simple columnar epithelial cells lying on a basement membrane. These cells undergo rapid cell division, mitosis to replenish the regular loss of skin by shedding from the surface. About 25% of the cells are melanocytes, which produce melanin which provides pigmentation for skin and hair.

45. (d) : An epithelial tissue which has thin flat cells, arranged edge to edge so as to appear like closely packed tiles is known as pseudostratified epithelium. It covers moist surfaces where there is little wear and tear by friction such as inner lining of cheeks.

46. (a) : Each hair is present in a tubular pit called hair follicle which is made up by sinking of epidermis. Living cells are present only at the base of hair i.e. in hair papilla, rest of the hair is dead and is divisible into outer cuticle, middle cortex and inner medulla.

47. (c) : Stratum malpighii/stratum germinativum is the innermost layer of the skin consisting of one celled thick columnar epithelial cells. It lies on the basement layer. Its cells are active and continuously produce new cells by mitotic division that is why called germinative layer.

48. (a) : Bone is an unusual tissue in that it is continually being reconstructed. The osteoblasts secrete bone matrix, whereas the large, much branched, motile, lysosome-rich, multinucleate cells, called osteoclasts, destroy bone matrix. The twin process of resorption and resconstruction enables a particular bone to remodel its structure to meet any change in the mechanical requirements of the animal during its development.

49. (a)

50. (a) : Long bones, such as the humerus and femur, have a cavity, the marrow cavity, at the centre. The substance of the bone is distinguishable into 3 regions : periosteum, matrix and endosteum. The matrix of bone along with the bone forming cells (osteoblasts) is arranged in concentric layers (lamellae) round the small canals which run parallel to the long axis (shaft) of the bone. These canals, called Haversian canals, are interconnected with one another via Volkmann's canals and contain a blood vessel, a nerve and a lymph vessel.

51. (a) : Mast cells are found in the matrix of areolar connective tissue and secrete histamine (vasodilator), serotonin (vasoconstrictor) and heparin (anticoagulant). These take part in allergic reactions and also help in a body defence.

52. (b) : Red pigment of vertebrate blood is haemoglobin. Haemoglobin is a conjugated protein. It consists of a basic protein globin joined to a nonprotein group heme, hence the name haemoglobin. Heme is an iron-porphyrin ring. A mammalian haemoglobin molecule is a complex of 4 heme molecules joined with 4 globin molecules.

53.(a) Taenia → Flame cells

Paramecium → Contractile vacuole

Periplaneta → Urecose gland

Pheretima → Nephridia

54.(d) : Cockroach shows sexual dimorphism, i.e., the sex can be distinguished from the other externally. Male cockroach bears a pair of short, thread like anal styles which are absent in females. Dark brown body colour, anal cerci and sclerites are present in both male and female cockroaches.

55.(a) : In cockroach, excretion is performed by Malpighian tubules. Alongwith this, fat body, nephrocytes and urecose glands also help in excretion.

56.(b) : In cockroach, the first pair of wings called tegmina (forewings) comes out from the mesothorax.

57.(b) : In cockroach, a ring of 6-8 blind tubules called hepatic or gastric caeca is present at the junction of foregut and midgut.

58.(c) : The head holds a bit of a nervous system of cockroach while the rest is situated along the ventral (bellyside) part of its body. So, if the head of a cockroach is cut off, it will still live for as long as one week.

59. (b)

60.(b) : Male cockroach bears a pair of short thread-like anal/caudal styles which are absent in females. They project backwardly from the sides of 9th abdominal segment in male cockroach.

61.(a) : Seminal vesicles are numerous small sacs present on ventral surface of anterior part of the ejaculatory duct which store sperms.

62.(d) : In insect, cleavage is superficial.

63.(d) : In cockroach, Malpighian tubules extract metabolic wastes like potassium and sodium urate, water and carbon dioxide from the blood. In the Malpighian tubules bicarbonates of potassium and sodium, water and uric acid are formed. A large amount of water and bicarbonates of potassium and sodium are reabsorbed by the cells of Malpighian tubules and then transferred to the blood (haemolymph). Uric acid is carried to the alimentary canal of the insect and is finally passed out through anus.

64.(a) : Arthrodial membrane is a tough, flexible cuticle that joins the skeletal elements of cockroach and other arthropods. It connects terga, pleura and sterna of cockroach body.

65.(a) : Cockroach undergoes paurometabolous development. The nymph moults about 6-7 times to reach the adult form. The next to last nymphal stage has wing pads but only adult cockroaches have wings.

66.(b) : Malpighian tubules are the main excretory structures in cockroach. They extract nitrogenous wastes and water from haemolymph and reabsorb certain salts resulting in precipitation of uric acid. So, cockroach is uricotelic. Males have paired anal styles on 9th abdominal sternite which are absent in females.

67. (a) : The respiratory system is well developed in a cockroach in order to compensate the poorly developed circulatory system. It consists of tracheae, tracheoles and spiracles. The main tracheal trunks open to the exterior on body surface through 10 pairs of segmentally arranged apertures termed spiracles or stigmata. Two pairs of spiracles are thoracic, one between pro and mesothorax and the other between meso and metathorax. Haemocoel contains a network of elastic, closed and branching air tubes or tracheae. The ultimate finer branches of tracheae are called tracheoles which come in contact with the individual body cells. The elaborate tracheal system carries oxygen directly to all the body cells.

68.(b) : The posterior segment of cockroaches bear appendages named as anal cerci. These are found in both male and female. But male cockroach can be distinguished by female ones by the presence of an extra pair of accessory appendages named as anal styles. It assists during copulation.

69.(d) : Mouth part of cockroach contains two mandibles, which bear teeth. When both the mandibles work simultaneously in a horizontal plane, the food matter is cut and masticated into fine and smaller pieces. Gizzard is a part of alimentary canal. It bears six muscular folds which are covered by chitinous conical plates, the teeth, used for grinding the food.

70.(d) : Cockroaches are found in places where there is warmth, dampness and plenty of organic food to devour. Indoors, they are a common pest in kitchens, latrines, hotels, restaurants, godowns, storerooms, board ships, etc. Cockroaches are nocturnal creatures. During daytime, they remain inactive and hiding. During night, they show much activity and run here and there in search of food. Being omnivorous and scavengerous in diet, they devour any animal or vegetable substance etc., causing great loss.

71.(a) : In male cockroach, 9th sternum bears a pair of short, unjointed thread-like anal styles which are absent in female. Anal cerci and antennae are present in both male and female cockroaches.

72. (c) The correct route for transport of sperms in male frog is

Testes$\rightarrow$ Vasa efferentia $\rightarrow$ Kidney $\rightarrow$ Bidder's canal $\rightarrow$ Urinogenital duct $\rightarrow$ Cloaca.

73. (c) : Frog's heart is myogenic, i.e., heartbeat originates from muscles of heart. Hence, it is autorhythmic. Wave of contraction originates from sinus venosus and spreads to wall of sinus venosus and both auricles. This compels the heart to beat. Due to this reason, frog's heart will continue to beat as long as it gets supply of ATP.

74. (b) : Human erythrocytes are enucleated, discoidal while in frogs erythrocytes are large, oval and biconvex nucleated cells. Erythrocytes are the carriers of haemoglobin.

75. (c)

76. (d) : In male frogs, two ureters act as urinogenital duct which open into the cloaca. They run backwards from the kidneys and open into the cloaca. In female ureters carry urine alone, while in male both sperms and urine are carried. Hence, are called urinogenital ducts.

77. (*) : None of the options is correct.

Frog respires in three different manners; cutaneous or skin respiration; buccopharyngeal respiration; pulmonary or lung respiration. Lungs are poorly developed in frog, the inadequate supply of O_2 obtained through lungs is supplemented through moist skin and buccal cavity. Hence, first statement is false. Heart of frog has three chambers, two atria and one ventricle. Hence, second statement is false. The frog excretes urea and thus is a ureotelic animal. The elimination of nitrogenous wastes is carried out by a well developed excretory system. The excretory system consists of a pair of kidneys, ureters, cloaca and urinary bladder. Frog do not change into uricotelic animal in any condition. Hence, third statement is false. In frog, fertilization is external and takes place in water. Within two weeks, fertilized eggs or zygotes develop into free-swimming aquatic larvae, called tadpoles, which undergo metamorphosis to become adult terrestrial frogs.

78.(b) : There are 10 pairs of spiracles in cockroach. Two pairs are thoracic in which first pair is known as mesothoracic, lying infront of the mesothorax between the bases of first and second pair of legs and are the largest. The second pair is called metathoracic. Abdominal spiracles are eight pairs. The first pair is dorsal in position and lies on the lateral margins of the first abdominal tergum. The remaining are situated on the sides of their corresponding segments on the pleura between the terga and sterna.

79. (a) : Main component of bone is collagen which is a complex combination of amino acids. When frog's bone is treated with HCl , these compounds are broken down and the bone becomes flexible.

80. (a) : Fronto-parietals are a pair of long, broad, flattened and membranous bones. They are united along the mid-dorsal line and form the whole roof of cranium. In larval frog, each fronto-parietal occurs into separate frontal and parietal parts, but in adult frog, they become fused to form a single frontoparietal. The entire floor of cranium is covered and strengthened by a large parasphenoid bone.

81. (b) : In adult frog, gills disappear and their skeletal framework is also reduced to form hyoid apparatus. It lies below tongue in the floor of mouth and provides surface of attachment to the tongue.

82. (c) : The bony partition between tympanic cavity (cavity of middle ear) and auditory capsule (internal ear) is perforated by a small window-like oval aperture, the fenestra ovalis, which remains closed by a membrane and a cartilaginous nodule, the stapedial plate.

83. (d) : Mesonephros kidney is present in both adult as well as embryo of frog. A mesonephros develops from the middle part of intermediate mesoderm, posterior to each pronephros soon after its degeneration.

84. (d) : Mucus helps frog in forming moist skin as skin is its respiratory organ.

85. (a) :The common Indian bull frog Rana tigrina lives in or near permanent freshwater lakes, ponds and streams. It lives in the water most of the time. It lives near water mainly for two reasons : (i) To keep skin moist to carry on cutaneous respiration and (ii) To immediately jump or slip into water to escape from enemies.

86. (b) : In 1912, Gudernatsch discovered that metamorphosis in frog's tadpole is increased by the thyroxine hormone which has the iodine as the main constituent. If thyroxine or iodine is added in water having tadpoles in it, then it increases the rate of metamorphosis in tadpole.

Chapter : 08

CELL-THE UNIT OF LIFE

CELL THEORY

1. The concept of *"Omnis cellula-e-cellula"* regarding cell division was first proposed by **(2019)**
(a) Aristotle (b) Rudolf Virchow
(c) Theodore Schwann (d) Schleiden.

2. Which is correct about cell theory in view of current status of our knowledge about cell structure? **(1993)**
(a) It needs modification due to discovery of subcellular structures like chloroplasts and mitochondria.
(b) Modified cell theory means that all living being are composed of cells capable of reproducing.
(c) Cell theory does not hold good because all living beings (e.g., viruses) do not have cellular organisation.
(d) Cell theory means that all living objects consists of cells whether or not capable of reproducing.

3. Names of Schleiden and Schwann are associated with **(1993)**
(a) protoplasm as the physical basis of life
(b) cell theory
(c) theory of cell lineage
(d) nucleus functions as control centre of cell.

AN OVERVIEW OF CELL

4. Angstrom (Å) is equal to **(1992)**
(a) 0.01 mm (b) 0.001 mm
(c) 0.0001 mm (d) 0.00001 mm

5. Organelles can be separated from cell homogenate through **(1989)**
(a) chromatography
(b) X-rays diffraction
(c) differential centrifugation
(d) auto-radiography.

PROKARYOTIC CELLS

6. Which of the following statements about inclusion bodies is incorrect? **(2020)**
(a) They are not bound by any membrane.
(b) These are involved in ingestion of food particles.
(c) They lie free in the cytoplasm.
(d) These represent reserve material in cytoplasm.

7. Select the wrong statement. **(NEET-II 2016)**
(a) Bacterial cell wall is made up of peptidoglycan.
(b) Pili and fimbriae are mainly involved in motility of bacterial cells.
(c) Cyanobacteria lack flagellated cells.
(d) Mycoplasma is a wall-less microorganism.

8. Which of the following structures is not found in a prokaryotic cell? **(2015)**
(a) Mesosome (b) Plasma membrane
(c) Nuclear envelope (d) Ribosome

9. The structures that help some bacteria to attach to rocks and/or host tissues are **(2015)**
(a) mesosomes (b) holdfast
(c) rhizoids (d) fimbriae.

10. Which one of the following is not an inclusion body found in prokaryotes? **(2015 Cancelled)**
(a) Glycogen granule
(b) Polysome
(c) Phosphate granule
(d) Cyanophycean granule

11. Which structures perform the function of mitochondria in bacteria? **(2014)**
(a) Nucleoid (b) Ribosomes
(c) Cell wall (d) Mesosomes

12. The motile bacteria are able to move by ***(2014)***
(a) fimbriae (b) flagella
(c) cilia (d) pili.

13. Why is a capsule advantageous to a bacterium? ***(Karnataka NEET 2013)***
(a) It protects the bacterium from desiccation.
(b) It provides means of locomotion.
(c) It allows bacterium to "hide" from host's immune system.
(d) It allows the bacterium to attach to the surface.

14. The term 'glycocalyx' is used for ***(Karnataka NEET 2013)***
(a) a layer present between cell wall and membrane of bacteria
(b) cell wall of bacteria
(c) bacterial cell glyco-engineered to possess N-glycosylated proteins
(d) a layer surrounding the cell wall of bacteria.

15. Chromosomes in a bacterial cell can be 1–3 in number and ***(2003)***
(a) are always circular
(b) are always linear
(c) can be either circular or linear, but never both within the same cell
(d) can be circular as well as linear within the same cell.

16. Photosynthetic bacteria have pigments in ***(1999)***
(a) chromoplasts (b) chromatophores
(c) leucoplasts (d) chloroplasts.

17. The site of respiration in bacteria is ***(1997)***
(a) ribosome (b) microsome
(c) episome (d) mesosome.

EUKARYOTIC CELLS

18. Which of the following functions is carried out by cytoskeleton in a cell? ***(2023)***
(a) Motility (b) Transportation
(c) Nuclear division (d) Protein synthesis

19. Which of the following are not considered as the part of endomembrane system? ***(2023)***

A. Mitochondria

B. Endoplasmic Reticulum

C. Chloroplasts

D. Golgi complex

E. Peroxisomes

Choose the most appropriate answer from the options given below.
(a) A and D only (b) A, D and E only
(c) B and D only (d) A, C and E only

20. How many different proteins does the ribosome consist of? ***(2023)***
(a) 40 (b) 20
(c) 80 (d) 60

21. Match list-I with list-II. ***(2022)***

List-I	List-II
(a) Metacentric chromosome	(i) Centromere situated close to the end forming one extremely short and one very long arm
(b) Acrocentric chromosome	(ii) Centromere at the terminal end
(c) Sub-metacentric	(iii) Centromere in the middle forming two equal arms of chromosomes
(d) chromosome	(iv) Centromere slightly away from the middle forming longer arm one shorter arm and one

Choose the correct answer from the options given below:
(a) (A)-(iii),(B)-(i),(C)-(iv),(D)-(ii)
(b) (A)-(i),(B)-(iii),(C)-(ii),(D)-(iv)
(c) (A)-(ii), (B)-(iii), (C)-(iv), (D)-(i)
(d) (A)-(I), (B)-(ii), (C)-(iii), (D)-(iv)

22. Which of the following statements with respect to endoplasmic reticulum is incorrect? ***(2022)***
(a) RER has ribosomes attached to ER
(b) SER is devoid of ribosomes
(c) In prokaryotes only RER are present
(d) SER are the sites for lipid synthesis

23. Which of the following is an incorrect statement? ***(2021)***

(a) Nuclear pores act as passages for proteins and RNA molecules in both directions between nucleus and cytoplasm.

(b) Mature sieve tube elements possess a conspicuous nucleus and usual cytoplasmic organelles.

(c) Microbodies are present both in plant and animal cells.

(d) The perinuclear space forms a barrier between the materials present inside the nucleus and that of the cytoplasm.

24. Match List-I with List-II. ***(2021)***

List-I	List-II
(p) Cristae	(i) Primary constriction in chromosome
(q) Thylakoids	(ii) Disc-shaped sacs in Golgi apparatus
(r) Centromere	(iii) Infoldings in mitochondria
(s) Cisternae	(iv) Flattened membranous sacs in stroma of plastids

Choose the correct answer from the options given below.

	(p)	(q)	(r)	(s)
(a)	(ii)	(iii)	(iv)	(i)
(b)	(iv)	(iii)	(ii)	(i)
(c)	(i)	(iv)	(iii)	(ii)
(d)	(iii)	(iv)	(i)	(ii)

25. When the centromere is situated in the middle of two equal arms of chromosomes, the chromosome is referred as ***(2021)***

(a) acrocentric (b) metacentric

(c) telocentric (d) sub-metacentric.

26. The organelles that are included in the endomembrane system are ***(2021)***

(a) Golgi complex, endoplasmic reticulum, mitochondria and lysosomes

(b) Endoplasmic reticulum, mitochondria, ribosomes and lysosomes

(c) Endoplasmic reticulum, Golgi complex, lysosomes and vacuoles

(d) Golgi complex, mitochondria, ribosomes and lysosomes.

27. Which is the important site of formation of glycoproteins and glycolipids in eukaryotic cells? ***(2020)***

(a) Endoplasmic reticulum

(b) Peroxisomes

(c) Golgi bodies (d) Polysomes

28. Which of the following statements is not correct? ***(2019)***

(a) Lysosomes are formed by the process of packaging in the endoplasmic reticulum.

(b) Lysosomes have numerous hydrolytic enzymes.

(c) The hydrolytic enzymes of lysosomes are active under acidic pH.

(d) Lysosomes are membrane-bound structures.

29. Which of the following statements regarding mitochondria is incorrect? ***(2019)***

(a) Mitochondrial matrix contains single circular DNA molecule and ribosomes.

(b) Outer membrane is permeable to monomers of carbohydrates, fats and proteins.

(c) Enzymes of electron transport are embedded in outer membrane.

(d) Inner membrane is convoluted with infoldings.

30. The shorter and longer arms of a sub-metacentric chromosome are referred to as ***(2019)***

(a) m-arm and n-arm respectively

(b) s-arm and l-arm respectively

(c) p-arm and q-arm respectively

(d) q-arm and p-arm respectively.

31. Which of the following pairs of organelles does not contain DNA? ***(2019)***

(a) Nuclear envelope and Mitochondria

(b) Mitochondria and Lysosome

(c) Chloroplast and Vacuoles

(d) Lysosomes and Vacuoles

32. Match the column I with column II. ***(Odisha NEET 2019)***

Column-I	Column-II
A. Golgi apparatus	(i) Synthesis of protein
B. Lysosomes	(ii) Trap waste and excretory products
C. Vacuoles	(iii) Formation of glycoproteins and glycolipids
D. Ribosomes	(iv) Digesting biomolecules

Choose the right match from options given below.

(a) A-(iii), B-(iv), C-(ii), D-(i)
(b) A-(iv), B-(iii), C-(i), D-(ii)
(c) A-(iii), B-(ii), C-(iv), D-(i)
(d) A-(i), B-(ii), C-(iv), D-(iii)

33. Which of the following is true for nucleolus? ***(2018)***

(a) Larger nucleoli are present in dividing cells.
(b) It is a membrane-bound structure.
(c) It takes part in spindle formation.
(d) It is a site for active ribosomal RNA synthesis.

34. The Golgi complex participates in ***(2018)***

(a) fatty acid breakdown
(b) formation of secretory vesicles
(c) respiration in bacteria
(d) activation of amino acid.

35. Which of the following events does not occur in rough endoplasmic reticulum? ***(2018)***

(a) Protein folding
(b) Protein glycosylation
(c) Cleavage of signal peptide
(d) Phospholipid synthesis

36. Select the incorrect match. ***(2018)***

(a) Lampbrush - Diplotene bivalents chromosomes
(b) Allosomes - Sex chromosomes
(c) Sub-metacentric - L-shaped chromosomes
(d) Polytene - Oocytes of chromosomes amphibians

37. Which of the following cell organelles is responsible for extracting energy from carbohydrates to form ATP? ***(2017)***

(a) Ribosome (b) Chloroplast
(c) Mitochondrion (d) Lysosome

38. Select the mismatch. ***(NEET-II 2016)***

(a) Gas vacuoles - Green bacteria
(b) Large central vacuoles - Animal cells
(c) Protists - Eukaryotes
(d) Methanogens - Prokaryotes

39. A cell organelle containing hydrolytic enzymes is ***(NEET-II 2016)***

(a) lysosome (b) microsome
(c) ribosome (d) mesosome.

40. Mitochondria and chloroplast are (NEET-I 2016)

(A) semi-autonomous organelles
(B) formed by division of pre-existing organelles and they contain DNA but lack protein synthesising machinery.

Which one of the following options is correct?

(a) (A) is true but (B) is false.
(b) Both (A) and (B) are false.
(c) Both (A) and (B) are correct.
(d) (B) is true but (A) is false.

41. Microtubules are the constituents of ***(NEET-I 2016)***

(a) centrioles, spindle fibres and chromatin
(b) centrosome, nucleosome and centrioles
(c) cilia, flagella and peroxisomes
(d) spindle fibres, centrioles and cilia.

42. Which one of the following cell organelles is enclosed by a single membrane? ***(NEET I 2016)***

(a) Lysosomes (b) Nuclei
(c) Mitochondria (d) Chloroplasts

43. Water soluble pigments found in plant cell vacuoles are ***(NEET-I 2016)***

(a) carotenoids (b) anthocyanins
(c) xanthophylls (d) chlorophylls.

44. Match the columns and identify the correct option. ***(2015)***

Column I	Column II
A. Thylakoids	(i) Disc-shaped sacs in Golgi apparatus
B. Cristae	(ii) Condensed structure of DNA
C. Cisternae	(iii) Flat membranous sacs in stroma
D. Chromatin	(iv) Infoldings in mitochondria

(a) A-(iii), B-(i), C-(iv), D-(ii)
(b) A-(iii), B-(iv), C-(ii), D-(i)
(c) A-(iv), B-(iii), C-(i), D-(ii)
(d) A-(iii), B-(iv), C-(i), D-(ii)

45. Cellular organelles with membranes are ***(2015)***
(a) endoplasmic reticulum, ribosomes and nuclei
(b) lysosomes, Golgi apparatus and mitochondria
(c) nuclei, ribosomes and mitochondria
(d) chromosomes, ribosomes and endoplasmic reticulum.

46. Which of the following are not membrane bound? ***(2015)***
(a) Lysosomes (b) Mesosomes
(c) Vacuoles (d) Ribosomes

47. DNA is not present in ***(2015 Cancelled)***
(a) nucleus (b) mitochondria
(c) chloroplast (d) ribosomes.

48. Nuclear envelope is a derivative of ***(2015 Cancelled)***
(a) microtubules
(b) rough endoplasmic reticulum
(c) smooth endoplasmic reticulum
(d) membrane of Golgi complex.

49. The structures that are formed by stacking of organised flattened membranous sacs in the chloroplasts are ***(2015 Cancelled)***
(a) stroma lamellae (b) stroma
(c) cristae (d) grana.

50. Select the correct matching in the following pai rs. ***(2015 Cancelled)***
(a) Rough ER - Synthesis of glycogen
(b) Rough ER - Oxidation of fatty acids
(c) Smooth ER - Oxidation of phospholipids
(d) Smooth ER - Synthesis of lipids

51. The chromosomes in which centromere is situated close to one end are ***(2015 Cancelled)***
(a) telocentric (b) sub-metacentric
(c) metacentric (d) acrocentric.

52. The solid linear cytoskeletal elements having a diameter of 6 nm and made up of a single type of monomer are known as ***(2014)***
(a) microtubules
(b) microfilaments
(c) intermediate filaments
(d) lamins.

53. The osmotic expansion of a cell kept in water is chiefly regulated by ***(2014)***
(a) mitochondria (b) vacuoles
(c) plastids (d) ribosomes.

54. Match the following and select the correct answer. ***(2014)***

(A) Centriole	(i) Infoldings in mitochondria
(B) Chlorophyll	(ii) Thylakoids
(C) Cristae	(iii) Nucleic acids
(D) Ribozymes	(iv) Basal body of cilia or flagella

	A	B	C	D
(a)	(iv)	(ii)	(i)	(iii)
(b)	(i)	(ii)	(iv)	(iii)
(c)	(i)	(iii)	(ii)	(iv)
(d)	(iv)	(iii)	(i)	(ii)

55. The Golgi complex plays a major role ***(2013)***
(a) as energy transferring organelles
(b) in post translational modification of proteins and glycosylation of lipids
(c) in trapping the light and transforming it into chemical energy
(d) in digesting proteins and carbohydrates.

56. Which one of the following organelle in the figure correctly matches with its function? ***(2013)***

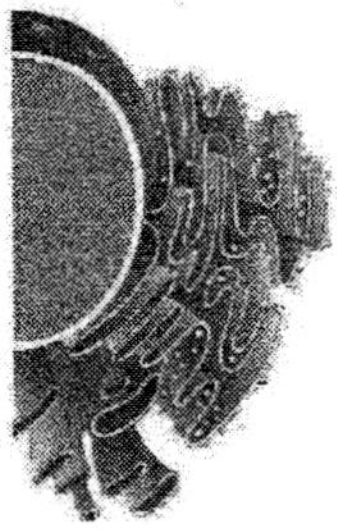

(a) Golgi apparatus, formation of glycolipids
(b) Rough endoplasmic reticulum, protein synthesis
(c) Rough endoplasmic reticulum, formation of glycoproteins
(d) Golgi apparatus, protein synthesis

57. A major site for synthesis of lipids is ***(2013)***
(a) symplast (b) nucleoplasm
(c) RER (d) SER

58. Which of the following types of plastid does not contain stored food material? ***(Karnataka NEET 2013)***
(a) Chromoplasts (b) Elaioplasts
(c) Aleuroplasts (d) Amyloplasts

59. Select the alternative giving correct identification and function of the organelle 'A' in the diagram. ***(Karnataka NEET 2013)***

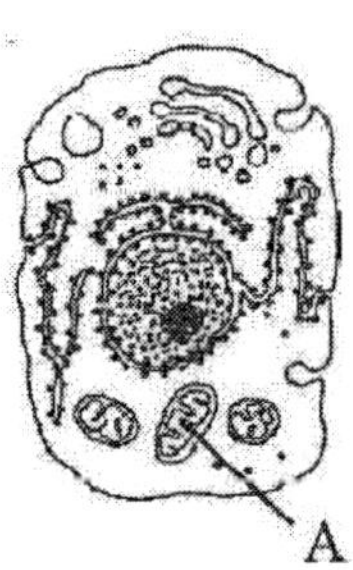

(a) Mitochondria - Produce cellular energy in the form of ATP
(b) Golgi body - Provides packaging material
(c) Lysosomes - Secrete hydrolytic enzymes
(d) Endoplasmic reticulum - Synthesis of lipids

60. Select the correct statement from the following regarding cell membrane. ***(2012)***
(a) Na+ and K+ ions move across cell membrane by passive transport.
(b) Proteins make up 60 to 70% of the cell membrane.
(c) Lipids are arranged in a bilayer with polar heads towards the inner part.
(d) Fluid mosaic model of cell membrane was proposed by Singer and Nicolson.

61. What is true about ribosomes? ***(2012)***
(a) The prokaryotic ribosomes are 80 S, where "S" stands for sedimentation coefficient.
(b) These are composed of ribonucleic acid and proteins.
(c) These are found only in eukaryotic cells.
(d) These are self-splicing introns of some RNAs.

62. Which one of the following does not differ in E.coli and Chlamydomonas? ***(2012)***
(a) Ribosomes
(b) Chromosomal organization
(c) Cell wall
(d) Cell membrane

63. Which one of the following cellular parts is correctly described? ***(Mains 2012)***
(a) Thylakoids - flattened membranous sacs forming the grana of chloroplasts
(b) Centrioles - sites for active RNA synthesis
(c) Ribosomes - those on chloroplasts are larger (80S) while those in the cytoplasm are smaller (70S)
(d) Lysosomes - optimally active at a pH of about 8.5

64. Which one of the following structures is an organelle within an organelle? ***(Mains 2012)***
(a) Ribosome (b) Peroxisome
(c) ER (d) Mesosome

65. Peptide synthesis inside a cell takes place in ***(2011)***
(a) chloroplast (b) mitochondria
(c) chromoplast (d) ribosomes.

66. Important site for formation of glycoproteins and glycolipids is ***(2011)***

(a) vacuole (b) Golgi apparatus
(c) plastid (d) lysosome.

67. Which one of the following is not considered as a part of the endomembrane system? ***(Mains 2011)***

(a) Golgi complex (b) Peroxisome
(c) Vacuole (d) Lysosome

68. The figure below shows the structure of a mitochondrion with its four parts labelled A, B, C and D. Select the part correctly matched with its function. ***(Mains 2011)***

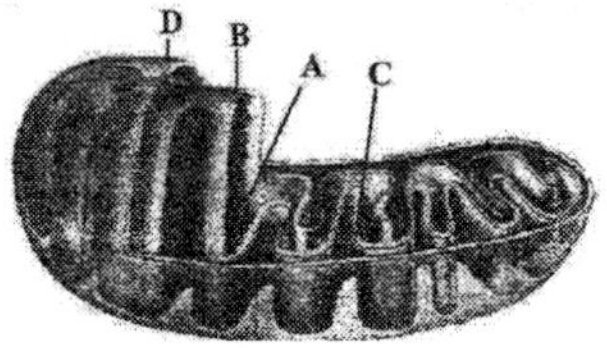

(a) D (outer membrane) - gives rise to inner membrane by splitting
(b) B (inner membrane) - forms infoldings called cristae
(c) C (crista) - possesses single circular DNA molecule and ribosomes
(d) A (matrix) - major site for respiratory chain enzymes

69. The plasma membrane consists mainly of ***(2010)***

(a) phospholipids embedded in a protein bilayer
(b) proteins embedded in a phospholipid bilayer
(c) proteins embedded in a polymer of glucose molecules
(d) proteins embedded in a carbohydrate bilayer.

70. The main area of various types of activities of a cell is ***(2010)***

(a) plasma membrane (b) mitochondrion
(c) cytoplasm (d) nucleus.

71. Which one of the following has its own DNA? ***(2010)***

(a) Mitochondria (b) Dictyosome
(c) Lysosome (d) Peroxisome

72. Which one of the following structures between two adjacent cells is an effective transport pathway? ***(2010)***

(a) Plasmodesmata
(b) Plastoquinones
(c) Endoplasmic reticulum
(d) Plasmalemma

73. An elaborate network of filamentous proteinaceous structures present in the cytoplasm which helps in the maintenance of cell shape is called ***(Mains 2010)***

(a) thylakoid
(b) endoplasmic reticulum
(c) plasmalemma
(d) cytoskeleton.

74. Identify the components labelled A, B, C, and D in the diagram below from the list (i) to (viii) given along with Components : (Mains 2010)

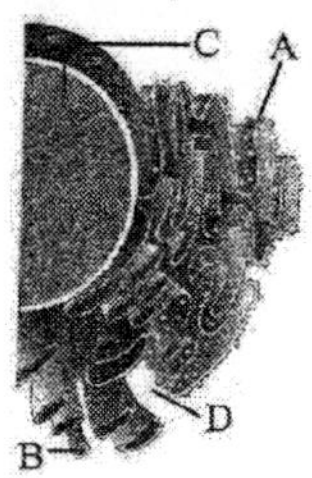

(i) Cristae of mitochondria
(ii) Inner membrane of mitochondria
(iii) Cytoplasm
(iv) Smooth endoplasmic reticulum
(v) Rough endoplasmic reticulum
(vi) Mitochondrial matrix
(vii) Cell vacuole
(viii) Nucleus

The correct components are:

	A	B	C	D
(a)	(v)	(iv)	(viii)	(iii)
(b)	(i)	(iv)	(viii)	(vi)
(c)	(vi)	(v)	(iv)	(vii)
(d)	(v)	(i)	(iii)	(ii)

75. Middle lamella is composed mainly of **(2009)**
(a) muramic acid (b) calcium pectate
(c) phosphoglycerides (d) hemicellulose.

76. Cytoskeleton is made up of **(2009)**
(a) callose deposits
(b) cellulosic microfibrils
(c) proteinaceous filaments
(d) calcium carbonate granules.

77. Plasmodesmata are **(2009)**
(a) locomotory structures
(b) membranes connecting the nucleus with plasmalemma
(c) connections between adjacent cells
(d) lignified cemented layers between cells.

78. In germinating seeds, fatty acids are degraded exclusively in the **(2008)**
(a) peroxisomes (b) mitochondria
(c) proplastids (d) glyoxysomes.

79. Vacuole in a plant cell **(2008)**
(a) lacks membrane and contains air
(b) lacks membrane and contains water and excretory substances
(c) is membrane-bound and contains storage proteins and lipids
(d) is membrane-bound and contains water and excretory substances.

80. Keeping in view the 'fluid mosaic model' for the structure of cell membrane, which one of the following statement is correct with respect to the movements of lipids and proteins from one lipid monolayer to the other (described as flip-flop movement)? **(2008)**
(a) While proteins can flip-flop, lipids can not
(b) Neither lipids, nor proteins can flip-flop
(c) Both lipids and proteins can flip-flop
(d) While lipids can rarely flip-flop, proteins cannot.

81. Which one of the following is not a constituent of cell membrane? **(2007)**
(a) Glycolipids (b) Proline
(c) Phospholipids (d) Cholesterol

82. Select the wrong statement from the following. **(2007)**
(a) Both chloroplasts and mitochondria have an internal compartment, the thylakoid space bounded by the thylakoid membrane.
(b) Both chloroplasts and mitochondria contain DNA.
(c) The chloroplasts are generally much larger than mitochondria.
(d) Both chloroplasts and mitochondria contain an inner and an outer membrane.

83. Which of the following statements regarding mitochondrial membrane is not correct? **(2006)**
(a) The outer membrane resembles a sieve.
(b) The outer membrane is permeable to all kinds of molecules.
(c) The enzymes of the electron transfer chain are embedded in the outer membrane.
(d) The inner membrane is highly convoluted forming a series of infoldings.

84. Which of the following statements regarding cilia is not correct? **(2006)**
(a) Cilia contain an outer ring of nine doublet microtubules surrounding two singlet microtubules.
(b) The organised beating of cilia is controlled by fluxes of Ca^{2+} across the membrane.
(c) Cilia are hair-like cellular appendages.
(d) Microtubules of cilia are composed of tubulin.

85. Chlorophyll in chloroplasts is located in **(2005)**
(a) grana (b) pyrenoid
(c) stroma (d) both grana and stroma.

86. According to widely accepted "fluid mosaic model" cell membranes are semi-fluid, where lipids and integral proteins can diffuse randomly. In recent years, this model has been modified in several respects. In this regard, which of the following statements is incorrect? **(2005)**
(a) Proteins in cell membranes can travel within the lipid bilayer.

(b) Proteins can also undergo flip-flop movements in the lipid bilayer.
(c) Proteins can remain confined within certain domains of the membrane.
(d) Many proteins remain completely embedded within the lipid bilayer.

87. Centromere is required for ***(2005)***
(a) movement of chromosomes towards poles
(b) cytoplasmic cleavage
(c) crossing over
(d) transcription.

88. The main organelle involved in modification and outing of newly synthesized proteins to their destinations is ***(2005)***
(a) chloroplast
(b) mitochondria
(c) lysosome
(d) endoplasmic reticulum.

89. In chloroplasts, chlorophyll is present in the ***(2004)***
(a) outer membrane (b) inner membrane
(c) thylakoids (d) stroma.

90. Ribosomes are produced in ***(2002)***
(a) nucleolus (b) cytoplasm
(c) mitochondria (d) Golgi body.

91. In fluid mosaic model of plasma membrane, ***(2002)***
(a) upper layer is non-polar and hydrophilic
(b) upper layer is polar and hydrophobic
(c) phospholipids form a bimolecular layer in middle part
(d) proteins form a middle layer.

92. Element necessary for the middle lamella is ***(2001)***
(a) Ca (b) Zn (c) K (d) Cu.

93. Microtubules are absent in ***(2001)***
(a) mitochondria (b) flagella
(c) spindle fibres (d) centrioles.

94. Lysosome contains ***(2000)***
(a) oxidative enzymes (b) hydrolytic enzymes
(c) reductive enzymes (d) anabolic enzymes.

95. Which of the following ribosomes are engaged in protein synthesis in animal cell? ***(2000)***
(a) Ribosomes which occur on nuclear membrane and ER
(b) Ribosomes of only cytosol
(c) Ribosomes of only nucleolus and cytosol
(d) Ribosomes of only mitochondria and cytosol

96. Function of telomeres in nucleus is ***(2000)***
(a) poleward movement
(b) to initiate the RNA synthesis
(c) to seal the ends of chromosome
(d) to recognise the homologous chromosome.

97. The proteins are synthesised at ***(1999)***
(a) centrosomes (b) Golgi bodies
(c) ribosomes (d) mitochondria.

98. Lysosomes are rich in ***(1996)***
(a) nucleic acids
(b) hydrolytic enzymes
(c) carbohydrates
(d) hormones.

99. Which of the following organelles contain enzymes that have digestive action? ***(1994)***
(a) Ribosomes (b) Polysomes
(c) Plastids (d) Lysosomes

100. In mitochondria, cristae act as sites for ***(1994)***
(a) protein synthesis
(b) phosphorylation of flavoproteins
(c) breakdown of macromolecules
(d) oxidation-reduction reaction.

101. Centromere is required for ***(1994)***
(a) replication of DNA
(b) chromosome segregation
(c) pole ward movement of chromosomes
(d) cytoplasmic cleavage.

102. Which one of the following organelles is located near the nucleus and contains a collection of flattened membrane bound cisternae? ***(1994)***
(a) Nucleolus (b) Mitochondrion
(c) Centriole (d) Golgi apparatus

103. The inner membrane of the mitochondria is usually, highly convoluted forming a series of infoldings known as ***(1994)***
(a) thylakoids (b) lamellae
(c) cristae (d) grana.

104. Besides giving out secretory vesicles, the Golgi apparatus is also concerned with the formation of ***(1994)***
(a) lysosomes
(b) plastids
(c) grana of chloroplasts
(d) cell plates after cell division in plants.

105. Active and passive transports across cell membrane differ in ***(1993)***
(a) passive transport is non selective
(b) passive transport is along the concentration gradient while active transport is due to metabolic energy
(c) active transport is more rapid
(d) passive transport is confined to anions while active transport is confined to cations.

106. In plant cells, peroxisomes are associated with ***(1993)***
(a) photorespiration (b) phototropism
(c) photoperiodism (d) photosynthesis.

107. Membranous bag with hydrolytic enzymes which is used for controlling intracellular digestion of macromolecules is ***(1993)***
(a) endoplasmic reticulum
(b) nucleosome
(c) lysosome
(d) phagosome.

108. Golgi apparatus is absent in ***(1993)***
(a) higher plants
(b) yeast
(c) bacteria and blue-green algae
(d) none.

109. Cell recognition and adhesion occur due to biochemicals of cell membranes named ***(1993)***
(a) proteins
(b) lipids
(c) proteins and lipids
(d) glycoproteins and glycolipids.

110. In salivary gland chromosomes/polytene chromosomes, pairing is ***(1993)***
(a) absent
(b) occasional
(c) formed between non-homologous chromosomes
(d) formed between homologous chromosomes.

111. All types of plastids possess essentially the same structure because they ***(1993)***
(a) perform the same function
(b) store food materials like starch, fat and protein
(c) occur in aerial parts
(d) can transform from one form to another.

112. An outer covering membrane is absent over ***(1992)***
(a) nucleolus (b) lysosome
(c) mitochondrion (d) plastid.

113. Oxysomes or F0 – F1 particles occur on ***(1992)***
(a) thylakoids
(b) mitochondrial surface
(c) inner mitochondrial membrane
(d) chloroplast surface.

114. Ribosomes are the centre for ***(1992)***
(a) respiration (b) photosynthesis
(c) protein synthesis (d) fat synthesis.

115. Cell wall shows ***(1991)***
(a) complete permeability
(b) semipermeability
(c) differential permeability
(d) impermeability.

116. Ribosomes were discovered by ***(1991)***
(a) Golgi (b) Porter
(c) de Robertis (d) Palade.

117. Fluid mosaic model of cell membrane was put forward by ***(1991)***
(a) Danielli and Davson
(b) Singer and Nicolson
(c) Garner and Allard
(d) Watson and Crick.

118. The latest model for plasma membrane is ***(1990)***
(a) lamellar model
(b) unit membrane model
(c) fluid mosaic model
(d) molecular lipid model.

119. Polyribosomes are aggregates of ***(1989)***
(a) ribosomes and rRNA
(b) only rRNA
(c) peroxisomes
(d) several ribosomes held together by string of mRNA.

120. Plasma membrane is made of ***(1989)***
(a) proteins and carbohydrates
(b) proteins and lipids
(c) proteins, lipids and carbohydrates
(d) proteins, some nucleic acid and lipids.

121. According to fluid mosaic model, plasma membrane is composed of ***(1988)***
(a) phospholipids and oligosaccharides
(b) phospholipids and hemicellulose
(c) phospholipids and integral proteins
(d) phospholipids, extrinsic proteins and intrinsic proteins.

ANSWER KEY

1.	(b)	2.	(c)	3.	(b)	4.	(c)	5.	(c)	6.	(b)	7.	(b)
8.	(c)	9.	(d)	10.	(b)	11.	(d)	12.	(b)	13.	(a)	14.	(d)
15.	(a)	16.	(b)	17.	(d)	18.	(a)	19.	(d)	20.	(c)	21.	(a)
22.	(c)	23.	(b)	24.	(d)	25.	(b)	26.	(c)	27.	(c)	28.	(a)
29.	(c)	30.	(c)	31.	(d)	32.	(a)	33.	(d)	34.	(b)	35.	(d)
36.	(d)	37.	(c)	38.	(b)	39.	(a)	40.	(a)	41.	(d)	42.	(a)
43.	(b)	44.	(d)	45.	(b)	46.	(d)	47.	(d)	48.	(b)	49.	(d)
50.	(d)	51.	(d)	52.	(b)	53.	(b)	54.	(a)	55.	(b)	56.	(b)
57.	(d)	58.	(a)	59.	(a)	60.	(d)	61.	(b)	62.	(d)	63.	(a)
64.	(a)	65.	(d)	66.	(b)	67.	(b)	68.	(b)	69.	(b)	70.	(c)
71.	(a)	72.	(a)	73.	(d)	74.	(a)	75.	(b)	76.	(c)	77.	(c)
78.	(d)	79.	(d)	80.	(d)	81.	(b)	82.	(a)	83.	(c)	84.	(b)
85.	(a)	86.	(b)	87.	(a)	88.	(d)	89.	(c)	90.	(a)	91.	(c)
92.	(a)	93.	(a)	94.	(b)	95.	(a)	96.	(c)	97.	(c)	98.	(b)
99.	(d)	100.	(d)	101.	(c)	102.	(d)	103.	(c)	104.	(a)	105.	(b)
106.	(a)	107.	(c)	108.	(c)	109.	(d)	110.	(d)	111.	(d)	112.	(a)
113.	(c)	114.	(c)	115.	(a)	116.	(d)	117.	(b)	118.	(c)	119.	(d)
120.	(c)	121.	(d)										

HINTS & EXPLANATIONS

1.(b) Rudolf Virchow (1855) observed that new cells develop by division of the pre-existing cells- "Omnis cellula- e-cellula" (theory of cell lineage or common ancestry). The finding gave cell theory its final shape.

2. (c) Viruses are an exceptions to the cell theory as they are obligate parasites (subcellular in nature).

3.(b) Names of Schleiden and Schwann were associated with cell theory in 1839. The concept that "All living organisms are composed of cell" is known as cell theory.

4.(c) An angstrom (symbol "Å") is a non-SI unit of length that is internationally recognised, equal to 0.1 nanometer (nm). It can be written in scientific notations as 1×10^{-10} m. It is used in expressing the size of atoms, length of chemical bonds, etc. It is named after Anders Jonas Angstrom.

Angstrom =0.0001μm

5.(c) Organelles can be separated from cell homogenate through differential centrifugation. The basic principle involved here is sedimentation of particles in a suspension by centrifugal force. In a centrifuge, the particles sediment at different rates when an accelerating force is subjected. The rate of sedimentation depends upon the size of the particles, its shape and density.

6. (b) Reserve material in prokaryotic cells are stored in the cytoplasm in the form of inclusion bodies. These are not bound by any membrane system and lie free in the cytoplasm, e.g., phosphate granules, cyanophycean granules and glycogen granules.

7. (b) Pili and fimbriae are bacterial appendages which are not involved in locomotion. Actually, pili are long, fewer and thick tubular outgrowths which develop in response to F+ or fertility factor in Gram negative bacteria. Being long they are helpful in attaching to recipient cell and forming conjugation tube. Fimbriae are small bristle-like fibres sprouting from cell surface in large number. There are 300–400 of them per cell. They are involved in attaching bacteria to solid surfaces.

8. (c) A prokaryotic cell is characterised by absence of an organised nucleus and membrane bound cell organelles. DNA is naked i.e., without a nuclear envelope and lies variously coiled in the cytoplasm. It is commonly called nucleoid or genophore. Mesosomes, plasma membrane and 70S ribosomes are present in a prokaryotic cell.

9. (d)

10. (b) Polysome is not an inclusion body. It is an aggregation of ribosomes formed under conditions of high concentration of magnesium. An inclusion body is any of various particulate structures, usually proteins, formed after viral infections in a prokaryotic or eukaryotic cell.

11. (d) Mesosome is characteristic circular to villiform specialisation of bacterial cell membrane that develops as an ingrowth. It consists of vesicles, tubules and lamellae. Mesosomes may be septal or lateral. Septal mesosome connects nucleoid with plasma membrane and assists in replication and septum formation during cells division. Lateral mesosome is not connected with nucleoid and contains respiratory enzymes and performs functions similar to eukarytoic mitochondria and hence is also called chondrioid. They also increase the surface area of plasma membrane and enzymatic contact.

12. (b) Flagellum is the organ of motility in bacteria. Bacterial flagella are unistranded, equivalent to a single microtubular fibre and formed of protein called flagellin. They perform rotatory movements.

13. (a) S-type bacteria or virulent bacteria are capsulated. The capsule is made up of polysaccharides and amino acids. It is a tough and thick mucilage covering. It gives protection to bacteria against host's immune system. The capsule is considered a virulence factor because it enhances the ability of bacteria to cause disease. Capsule contains water and mucilage, thus protects bacteria against desiccation. Capsule also helps the bacterium to adhere (attach) to the surface.

14. (d) Glycocalyx is a sticky, gelatinous material that collects outside the cell wall of bacteria to form an additional surface layer. When this layer is firmly attached to the surface of the cell, it is called a capsule. If it is loosely distributed around the cell, the glycocalyx is called a slime layer.

15. (a) Bacterial cells do not have nucleus, characteristic of eukaryotic cells. Nuclear material of bacteria lies free in the cell in the form of an irregular, thin, fibrillar and circular single molecule of DNA, called nucleoid or chromatin body. This DNA, sometimes attached at one or more points to a mesosome, frequently runs parallel to the axis of the cell. Bacterial DNA is not associated with histone protein and does not coil to form welldefined chromosomes during the multiplication. In addition to circular DNA, a small amount of subsidiary extrachromosomal DNA is also present as plasmids or episomes.

16. (b) Photosynthetic bacteria have chromatophores which are membrane bound vesicular structures which are extensions of cytoplasmic membrane. They contain photosynthetic pigments along with enzymes and electron carriers for photosynthetic phosphorylation. These pigments are bacteriochlorophyll and bacteriophaeophytin. Leucoplasts, chloroplasts and chromoplasts are different types of plastids which occur in plants and some protistans.

17. (d) Mesosomes are complex, intracellular, membranous structures within the cytoplasm, that are formed by the infoldings of the cytoplasmic membrane. Surface of mesosomes have many enzymes which take part in respiration, e.g., oxidases and dehydrogenases. Mesosomes are also known to help in the separation of two daughter molecules of DNA during cell division. They are also called mitochondria of bacterial cell.

18. (a) Cytoskeleton is an elaborate network of filamentous proteinaceous structures consisting of microtubules, microfilaments and intermediate filaments present in the cytoplasm. It is involved in many functions such as motility, mechanical support and maintenance of the shape of the cell.

19. (d) The endomembrane system include endoplasmic reticulum (ER) (B), Golgi complex (D), lysosomes and vacuoles because functions of these organelles are coordinated. But the functions of the mitochondria (A), chloroplast (C) and peroxisomes (E) are not coordinated, with above components so, these are not considered as part of the endomembrane system.

20. (c)

21. (a)

22. (c) The rough endoplasmic reticulum, peroxisomes and mitochondria are bound by their own membranes and are only found in eukaryotic cells. So, SER and RER are not found in prokaryotic cells as they are exclusive to eukaryotic cells.

23. (b) Sieve tube elements lack nucleus at maturity and they are associated with companion cells for support.

24. (d)

25. (b) Depending upon the position of centromere, chromosomes are of four types:

(i) Acrocentric-Centromere is situated inner to telomere.

(ii) Metacentric - Centromere present in the middle of chromosome.

(iii)Telocentric - Centromere terminal in the area of telomere.

(iv)Sub-metacentric - Centromere occurs slightly away from the middle of chromosome.

26. (c) The endomembrane system include endoplasmic reticulum (ER), Golgi complex, lysosomes and vacuoles.

27. (c) Golgi apparatus is the important site of formation of glycoproteins and glycolipids. Protein synthesised by the rough endoplasmic reticulum and lipids synthesised by smooth endoplasmic reticulum reach the cisternae of the Golgi apparatus. Here, they combine with carbohydrates to form glycoproteins and glycolipids.

28. (a) Lysosomes are single membrane bound vesicles which contain hydrolytic enzymes. Lysosomes are believed to be formed by the joint activity of ER and Golgi complex. Precursors of hydrolytic enzymes are synthesised at RER and are transferred to the forming face of Golgi complex. These precursors are then changed to enzymes. Enzymes are then packed in larger vesicles and are pinched off at maturing face.

These vesicles combine with endosomes to produce lysosomes. Lysosomal enzymes function in acidic medium or pH 4.5. This pH is lower than that of cytoplasm.

29. (c) Enzymes of electron transport are embedded in the inner membrane of mitochondria.

30. (c) The short arm of chromosome is termed as the p (petit) arm and longer arm is referred as q arm.

31. (d)

33. (d) Nucleolus is naked (devoid of membrane), round or slightly irregular structure which is attached to the chromatin at a specific region called nucleolar organiser region (NOR). Nucleolus is a site for rRNA synthesis. Nucleolus disappears when the cell undergoes division and reappears after its completion.

34. (b) Golgi complex is a complex cytoplasmic structure made up of smooth membrane saccules or cisternae, a network of tubules with vesicles and vacuoles, which takes part in membrane transformation, secretion and production of complex biochemicals. One face of Golgi apparatus in convex (forming, cis) face while the other is concave (maturing, trans) face. Cis face receives contents from endoplasmic reticulum which then reaches trans face and bud off as secretory vesicles.

35. (d) Smooth endoplasmic reticulum is involved in the production of lipids and sterols. Complexing of lipids and proteins to form lipoproteins occurs in SER. RER is involved in protein folding, glycosyation of protein and cleavage of signal peptide.

36. (d) Polytene chromosomes are giant chromosomes formed by somatic pairing between homologous chromosomes and repeated replication (endomitosis) of their chromonemata. They are quite common in salivary glands of insects and are therefore, popularly known as salivary chromosomes.

37. (c) Mitochondria are miniature biochemical factories where food stuffs or respiratory substrates are completely oxidised to carbon dioxide and water. The energy liberated in the process is initially stored in the form of reduced coenzymes and reduced prosthetic groups. The latter soon undergo oxidation and form energy rich ATP. ATP comes out of mitochondria and helps perform various energy requiring processes of the cell like muscle contraction, nerve impulse conduction, biosynthesis, membrane transport, cell division, movement, etc. Because of the formation of ATP, the mitochondria are called power houses of the cell.

38. (b) Large central vacuoles are the characteristic of plant cell, not animal cell which may have many small scattered vacuoles.

39. (a) Lysosomes are small vesicles which are bounded by a single membrane and contain hydrolytic enzymes in the form of minute crystalline or semicrystalline granules of 5-8 nm. About 50 enzymes have been recorded to occur in them. All the enzymes do not occur in the same lysosome but there are different sets of enzymes in different types of lysosomes. The important enzymes are acid phosphatases, sulphatases, proteases, peptidases, nucleases, lipases and carbohydrases. They are also called acid hydrolases because these digestive enzymes usually function in acidic medium or pH of 4-5.

40. (a) Both mitochondria and chloroplast are semi-autonomous organelles. They have their own DNA which produces its own mRNA, tRNA and rRNA. These organelles also possess their own ribosomes and hence are able to synthesise some of their proteins.

41. (d) Microtubules are unbranched hollow submicroscopic tubules of protein tubulin which develop on specific nucleating regions. It can undergo quick growth or dissolution at their ends by assembly or disassembly of monomers. They are present in the cytoplasm as well as in specialised structures like centrioles, basal bodies, cilia or flagella, sensory hair, equatorial ring of thrombocytes, spindle apparatus, chromosome fibres, nerve processes, sperm tails, axostyle of parasitic flagellates, fibre system of Stentor, cytopharyngeal basket of Nassula, etc.

42. (a) Lysosomes are small vesicles bounded by a single membrane and contain hydrolytic enzymes. Nucleus, mitochondria and chloroplasts are double membrane bound cell organelles.

43. (b) Anthocyanins are water soluble pigments, which commonly occur in membrane enclosed vacuoles. They are responsible for colour of fruits, flowers and petals.

44. (d)

45. (b)

46. (d)

47. (d) Ribosome is a small spherical body within a living cell that is the site of protein synthesis. Ribosomes consist of two subunits, one large and one small, each of which comprises some RNA (called ribosomal RNA) and proteins. They do not have any DNA.

48. (b) Recent developments have shown that nuclear membrane is derived from rough endoplasmic reticulum. During cell division, nuclear membrane is disintegrated. The nuclear envelope transmembrane proteins are absorbed in the RER. Once the division is completed, RER reassembles the nuclear envelope.

49. (d) A chloroplast is a vesicle, bound by an

envelope of two unit membranes and filled with a fluid matrix called stroma. The lamellae, after separation from the inner membrane, usually take the form of closed, flattened, ovoid sacs, the thylakoids, which lie closely packed in piles, the grana.

50. (d) Smooth endoplasmic reticulum (SER) is a system of smooth membranes (i.e., membranes not having ribosomes) within the cytoplasm of plant and animal cells. It forms a link between the cell and nuclear membranes. It is the site of important metabolic reactions, including phospholipids and fatty acid synthesis. In animal cells, lipid-like steroidal hormones are also synthesised.

51. (d) Centromere is a part of a chromosome that attaches to the spindle during cell division. A chromosome with the centromere close to one end is acrocentric.

52. (b) Microfilaments are ultramicroscopic long, cylindrical rods that occur in eukaryotic plants and animals. They are 6-8 nm in thickness. Microtubules are hollow microscopic tubular structures with an external diameter of 24 nm and of variable length. They are composed of tubulin. Intermediate filaments are the numerous microscopic protein fibres of about 10 nm thickness that form part of the cytoskeleton. They are made up of a variety of proteins, e.g., keratin in nails.

53. (b) Vacuoles are non-cytoplasmic areas present inside cytoplasm and separated from latter by tonoplast. They are believed to be formed by expansion and pinching off from ER. There occurs a large central vacuole and many small vacuoles in plant cells. They play a major role in osmotic expansion of a cell.

54. (a)

55. (b) Post-translational modification is a step in protein biosynthesis. Proteins are created on ribosomes translating mRNA into polypeptide chains. These polypeptide chains undergo post-translational modification, such as folding, cutting and other processes, before becoming the mature protein product. Proteins synthesised by the rough endoplasmic reticulum and lipids synthesised by smooth endoplasmic reticulum reach the cisternae of the Golgi apparatus. Here, they combine with carbohydrates to form glycoproteins and glycolipids. This process is called glycosylation.

56. (b) The given figure shows endoplasmic reticulum bearing ribosomes on its surface. It is called rough endoplasmic reticulum or RER. RER is actively involved in protein synthesis and secretion.

57.(d) Smooth endoplasmic reticulum (SER) is a system of smooth membranes (i.e., membranes not having ribosomes) within the cytoplasm of plant and animal cells. It forms a link between the cell and nuclear membranes. It is the site of important metabolic reactions, including phospholipid and fatty acid synthesis. In animal cells, lipid-like steroidal hormones are also synthesised.

58.(a) Chromoplasts are coloured plastids. They do not contain stored food material. Chromoplasts are formed either from leucoplasts or chloroplasts. Chromoplasts provide colour to many flowers for attracting pollinating insects. They also provide colour to fruits for attracting animals for dispersal.

59.(a) Mitochondria are miniature biochemical factories where food stuffs or respiratory substrates are completely oxidised to carbon dioxide and water. The energy liberated in the process is initially stored in the form of reduced coenzymes and reduced prosthetic groups. The latter soon undergo oxidation and form energy rich ATP. ATP comes out of mitochondria and helps perform various energy requiring processes of the cell like muscle contraction, nerve impulse conduction, biosynthesis, membrane transport, cell division, movement, etc. Because of the formation of ATP, the mitochondria are called power houses of the cell.

60.(d) According to the fluid mosaic model of cell membrane structure proposed by Singer and Nicolson (1972). Plasma membrane contains about 50-60% proteins and 50-40% lipids. Lipids form a bilayer with hydrophilic heads pointing outwards. Cell membrane allows transport of some molecules by passive transport, e.g., water, neutral solutes while some are transported actively, e.g., Na+/K+ pump.

61.(b) Ribosome is a small spherical body within a living cell that is the site of protein synthesis. Ribosomes consist of two subunits, one large and one small, each of which comprises some RNA (called ribosomal RNA) and protein. They do not have any DNA.

62.(d) E.coli (bacteria) is prokaryote while Chlamydomonas (algae) is eukaryote. Ribosomes of both groups differ being 70S in prokaryotes and 80S in eukaryotes. Prokaryotic chromosomes lack histone protein unlike eukaryotic ones. Cell wall organisation also differs as bacterial cell wall is rich in muramic acid while algal cell wall is cellulosic. It is the cell membrane which has similar organisation in both the groups.

63.(a) Thylakoids are the flattened sac-like membranous structures that are stacked on top of one another to form the grana of plant chloroplast. Chlorophyll and other photosynthetic pigments are situated in the thylakoid membranes, which are the site for the light-dependent reactions of photosynthesis.

64.(a) Ribosomes occur in all living cells except mammalian erythrocytes or red blood corpuscles. Depending upon the place of their occurrence, ribosomes are of two types-cytoplasmic ribosomes and organelle ribosomes. The cytoplasmic ribosomes (cytoribosomes) may remain free in the cytoplasmic matrix or attached to the cytosolic surface of endoplasmic reticulum with the help of special ribophorin or SRP protein. The organelle ribosomes are found in plastids (plastiribosomes) and mitochondria (mitoribosomes) Cytoplasmic ribosome are of 80S type in eukaryotic cell whereas organelle ribosomes are of 70S type.

65.(d) Peptide synthesis inside a cell takes place in ribosome. Ribosomes are found in all cells and are involved in protein synthesis. The major constituents of ribosomes are RNA and proteins present in approximately equal amounts.

66.(b) Golgi apparatus principally performs the function of packaging materials. The newly synthesized proteins are handed over to the Golgi apparatus which are catalysed by the addition of carbohydrates, lipid or sulphates moieties to the proteins. Golgi apparatus is the important site of formation of glycoproteins and glycolipids.

67.(b) While each of the membranous organelles is distinct in terms of its structure and function, many of these are considered together as an endomembrane system because their functions are coordinated. The endomembrane system includes endoplasmic reticulum (ER), Golgi complex, lysosomes and vacuoles. Since the functions of the mitochondria, chloroplast and peroxisomes are not coordinated with the above components, these are not considered as part of the endomembrane system.

68. (b)

69.(b) Plasma membrane consists of lipids (20-79%), proteins (20-70%), carbohydrates (1-5%) and water (20%) Lipid molecules possess both hydrophobic and hydrophilic ends and are thus arranged in the form of lipid bilayer. Most common lipid of the bilayer is phospholipid. Protein molecules occur at places both inside (intrinsic proteins) and on the outer side (extrinsic proteins) of the phospholipid bilayer.

70.(c) Cytoplasm is granular, crystallo-colloidal complex that forms the living protoplasm of a cell excluding its nucleus. It consists of proteins, nucleic acids, fats, carbohydrates, vitamins, minerals, waste metabolites and all the organelles. It is the main area for various types of activities of a cell like respiration, nutrition, storage, etc.

71.(a) Both mitochondria and chloroplast are semi-autonomous organelles. They have their own DNA which produces its own mRNA, tRNA and rRNA. These organelles also possess their own ribosomes and hence are able to synthesise some of their proteins.

72.(a) Plasmodesmata are fine cytoplasmic strands that connect the protoplasts of adjacent plant cells by passing through their cell walls. Plasmodesmata are cylindrical in shape (about 20-40 nm in diameter) and are lined by the plasma membrane of the two adjacent cells. They permit the passage of substances including ions, sugars, amino acids and macromolecules between cells.

73. (d)

74.(a) A - Rough endoplasmic reticulum

B - Smooth endoplasmic reticulum

C - Nucleus

D - Cytoplasm

75.(b) Middle lamella of cell wall is composed of calcium and magnesium pectate. It joins the adjoining cells together and thus acts as a cementing layer.

76.(c) The ability of eukaryotic cells to adopt a variety of shapes and to carry out coordinated and directed movements depends on the cytoskeleton. The main proteins that are present in the cytoskeleton are tubulin (in the microtubules), actin, myosin, tropomyosin (in the microfilaments) and keratins, vimentin, desmin, lamin, etc, (in intermediate filaments).

77. (c) Plasmodesmata are fine cytoplasmic strands that connect the protoplasts of adjacent plant cells by passing through their cell walls. Plasmodesmata are cylindrical in shape (about 20-40 nm in diameter) and are lined by the plasma membrane of the two adjacent cells. They permit the passage of substances including ions, sugars, amino acids and macromolecules between cells.

78.(d) Glyoxysomes are small, spherical vesicles enclosed by a single unit membrane. Glyoxysomes are generally found in cells of yeast, Neurospora and in germinating fatty seeds where fat is being converted into carbohydrates, i.e., glyoxylate cycle (gluconeogenesis).

79.(d) In a plant cell, vacuole may be defined as a non-living reservoir, bounded by a differentially or selectively permeable membrane, the tonoplast. It is filled with a highly concentrated solution called vascular sap or cell sap which contains many dissolved solutes such as organic acids, soluble carbohydrates, soluble nitrogenous compounds as nitrates, enzyme, tannins, chlorides, phosphates, amino acids alkaloids and anthocyanin pigments.

80.(d) According to fluid mosaic model, there is rapid internal motion involving flexing, within each lipid molecule a rapid lateral diffusion of the lipids is possible and a slow 'flip-flop' motion, i.e., a transfer of lipid molecules from one side of the bilayer to the other, is also possible. The lipid molecules might also rotate about their axes. The proteins of the membrane are concerned with the enzymatic activity of the membrane, with transport of molecules, and with a receptor function whereas, the lipid bilayer provides the permeability barrier.

81.(b) Chemically, a biomembrane consists of lipids (20-70%), proteins (20-70%), carbohydrates (1-5%) and water (20%). The important lipids of the membrane are phospholipids (some hundred types), sterols, (e.g. cholesterol), glycolipids, sphingolipid (e.g., sphingomyelin, cerebrosides). Proteins can be fibrous or globular structural carrier, receptor or enzymatic.

82.(a) The outer membrane of mitochondrion is smooth, freely permeable to most small molecules, contains fewer enzymes and is poor in proteins. It has porin proteins which form channels for the passage of molecules through it. It allows uptake of substrates and release of ATP. The inner membrane is semipermeable and regulates the passage of materials into and out of the mitochondrion. It is rich in enzymes and carrier proteins (permeases). It is usually produced into numerous infolds called cristae (singular crista). It bears minute regularly spaced lollipop-shaped particles known as oxysomes. The rest of the inner membrane contains the electron carrier molecules of the electron transport chain.

83. (c)

84. (b)

85.(a) Thylakoids are the flattened sac-like membranous structures that are stacked on top of one another to form the grana of plant chloroplast. Chlorophyll and other photosynthetic pigments are situated in the thylakoid membranes, which are the site for the light-dependent reactions of photosynthesis.

86.(b) According to fluid mosaic model, there is rapid internal motion involving flexing, within each lipid molecule a rapid lateral diffusion of the lipids is possible and a slow 'flip-flop' motion, i.e., a transfer of lipid molecules from one side of the bilayer to the other, is also possible. The lipid molecules might also rotate about their axes. The proteins of the membrane are concerned with the enzymatic activity of the membrane, with transport of molecules, and with a receptor function whereas, the lipid bilayer provides the permeability barrier.

87.(a) Centromere is the point at which the two chromatids of a chromosome are held together. During movement of chromosomes, the spindle fibres (on which the chromatids move) are attached to the centromere.

88.(d) The proteins formed on ribosomes pass into the ER lumen where they are modified. Then the modified proteins move on into the transitional area, where the ER buds off membranous sacs, the transport vesicles, carrying the proteins to the Golgi apparatus.

89.(c) Thylakoids are the flattened sac-like membranous structures that are stacked on top of one another to form the grana of plant chloroplast. Chlorophyll and other photosynthetic pigments are situated in the thylakoid membranes, which are the site for the light-dependent reactions of photosynthesis.

90.(a) Nucleolus synthesises and stores RNA. The ribosomal proteins are synthesized in the cytoplasm and shift to the nucleolus for the formation of ribosomal subunits by complexing with rRNA.

91. (c)

92.(a) Middle lamella is the first formed layer, present in between the two adjacent cells. It is situated outside the primary cell wall. It is made up of calcium and magnesium pectate.

93. (a)

94.(b) A lysosome is a tiny sac bounded by a single unit membrane of lipoprotein. It contains a dense, finely granular fluid. The latter consists of glycoprotein hydrolytic (digestive) enzymes called acid hydrolases. These include proteases, lipases, nucleases, glycosidases, sulphatases, acid phosphatases, etc.

95.(a) Ribosomes present in nuclear membrane and endoplasmic reticulum take part in protein synthesis. Two or more ribosomes simultaneously engaged in protein synthesis on the same m RNA strand forming polyribosomes. The ribosome functions as a template, bringing together different components required for protein synthesis.

96. (c)

97.(c) The ribosomes provide space for the synthesis of proteins in the cell. Hence, they are known as the "protein factories" of the cell. The ribosomes bound to the membranes generally synthesise proteins for export as secretions by exocytosis or for incorporation into membranes or for inclusion into lysosomes. The free ribosomes generally produce enzymic proteins for use in the cell itself.

98.(b) A lysosome is a tiny sac bounded by a single unit membrane of lipoprotein. It contains a dense, finely granular fluid. The latter consists of glycoprotein hydrolytic (digestive) enzymes called acid hydrolases. These include proteases, lipases, nucleases, glycosidases, sulphatases, acid phosphatases, etc.

99.(d) A lysosome is a tiny sac bounded by a single unit membrane of lipoprotein. It contains a dense, finely granular fluid. The latter consists of glycoprotein hydrolytic (digestive) enzymes called acid hydrolases. These include proteases, lipases, nucleases, glycosidases, sulphatases, acid phosphatases, etc.

100.(d) Respiratory chain is located in the inner membrane (cristae) of mitochondria. It consists of a series of proteins containing oxidation-reduction groups. Chemical treatment of the mitochondrial membrane results in the isolation of five complexes which have been designated as complexes I, II, III, IV and V.

101. (c)

102. (d)

103. (c)

104.(a) The two poles of a Golgi apparatus are called cis face and trans face, which act respectively as the receiving and shipping departments.

The vesicles lie near the ends and concave surface of the Golgi complex. They are pinched off from the tubules of the cisternae. The Golgi complex gives rise to primary lysosomes by budding from the *trans* face of cisternae.

105.(b) Passive transport takes place along the concentration gradient whereas active transport takes place against the concentration gradient and require energy.

106.(a) In plant cells, peroxisomes are associated with photorespiration. Peroxisomes are found only in C3 plants where a wasteful phenomenon of photorespiration occurs. The other organelles associated with this process are chloroplast and mitochondria. Peroxisomes are also reported in animal cells, i.e., liver and kidney cells. The peroxisome contains several enzyme such as amino transferase, glycolate oxidase, glyoxylate reductase, peroxidase and catalase, etc.

107. (c) A lysosome is a tiny sac bounded by a single unit membrane of lipoprotein. It contains a dense, finely granular fluid. The latter consists of glycoprotein hydrolytic (digestive) enzymes called acid hydrolases. These include proteases, lipases, nucleases, glycosidases, sulphatases, acid phosphatases, etc.

108.(c) Golgi apparatus is absent in bacteria and blue green algae. Golgi bodies are absent in prokaryotic cells and present in eukaryotic cells except in male gametes of bryophytes and pteridophytes, mammalian RBCs, sieve tubes of plants, etc.

109.(d) Cell recognition and adhesion occur due to biochemicals of cell membranes named glycoproteins and glycolipids. These are formed due to small carbohydrate molecules present on lipids and extrinsic proteins.

110.(d) In salivary gland chromosomes/polytene chromosomes, pairing is formed between homologous chromosomes. A characteristic feature of these chromosomes is that somatic pairing occurs in them and hence their number appears half of normal somatic cells.

111. (d) All the plastids have a common origin and one type of plastid can change into another. Plastids are of 2 main types : leucoplasts and chromoplasts. The leucoplasts are colourless and occur in the cells not exposed to sunlight. The chromoplasts are coloured occur in the cells exposed to sunlight.

112.(a) An outer covering membrane is absent over nucleolus. Nucleolus is a dense, spherical, colloidal body which remains attached with nucleolar organizing chromosomes. It was discovered by Fontana (1781) and termed as nucleolus by Bowman (1840). The main function of nucleolus is the synthesis of ribosomal RNA and it is called store house of RNA. It plays an important role in cell division also.

113.(c) Oxysomes or F0 – F1 particles occurs on inner mitochondrial membrane. Each particle is made up of base, stalk and head and is about 10 mm in length. The number of oxysomes per mitochondrion varies from 104–105. Chemically, these are made up of phospholipid core and protein cortex. Oxysomes have ATP as enzyme molecules and therefore, responsible for ATP synthesis. These elementary particles are also called F0–F1 particles by some workers. The base of these is called F0 subunit and head is called F1 subunit.

114.(c) The ribosomes provide space for the synthesis of proteins in the cell. Hence, they are known as the "protein factories" of the cell. The ribosomes bound to the membranes generally synthesise proteins for export as secretions by exocytosis or for incorporation into membranes or for inclusion into lysosomes. The free ribosomes generally produce enzymic proteins for use in the cell itself.

115.(a) Cell wall shows complete permeability because it helps in the transport of substances into and out of the cell. The main function of cell wall is to provide mechanical support.

116.(d) In plant cells ribosomes were first of all observed by Robinson and Brown (1953) in bean roots. In animal cells, these were discovered by Palade (1955), hence are called Palade particles.

117. (b)

118. (c)

119.(d) Polyribosomes are aggregates of several ribosomes held together by string of mRNA Polyribosomes consists of 4–8 ribosomes which are attached to a single strand of messenger RNA or mRNA. This mechanism helps in synthesis of several copies of the same protein.

120.(c) Plasma membrane consists of lipids (20-79%), proteins (20-70%), carbohydrates (1-5%) and water (20%) Lipid molecules possess both hydrophobic and hydrophilic ends and are thus arranged in the form of lipid bilayer. Most common lipid of the bilayer is phospholipid. Protein molecules occur at places both inside (intrinsic proteins) and on the outer side (extrinsic proteins) of the phospholipid bilayer.

121.(d) Plasma membrane consists of lipids (20-79%), proteins (20-70%), carbohydrates (1-5%) and water (20%) Lipid molecules possess both hydrophobic and hydrophilic ends and are thus arranged in the form of lipid bilayer. Most common lipid of the bilayer is phospholipid. Protein molecules occur at places both inside (intrinsic proteins) and on the outer side (extrinsic proteins) of the phospholipid bilayer.

Chapter : 09

BIOMOLECULES

HOW TO ANALYSE CHEMICAL COMPOSITION?

1. Read the following statements on lipids and find out correct set of statement. ***(2022)***

(A) Lecithin found in the plasma membrane is a glycolipid

(B) Saturated fatty acids possess one or more C = C bonds

(C) Gingely oil has lower melting point, hence remains as oil in winter

(D) Lipids are generally insoluble in water but soluble in some organic solvents

(E) When fatty acid is esterified with glycerol, monoglycerides are formed

Choose the correct answer from the options given below.

(a) (A), (B) and (C) only (b) (A), (D) and (E) only
(c) (C), (D) and (E) only (d) (A), (B) and (D) only

2. A dehydration reaction links two glucose molecules to produce maltose. If the formula for glucose is $C_6H_{12}O_6$ then what is the formula for maltose?
(2022)

(a) $C_{12}H_{20}O_{10}$ (b) $C_{12}H_{24}O_{12}$
(c) $C_{12}H_{22}O_{11}$ (d) $C_{12}H_{24}O_{11}$

3. Following are the statements with reference to lipids. ***(2021)***

(A) Lipids having only single bonds are called unsaturated fatty acids.

(B) Lecithin is a phospholipid.

(C) Trihydroxy propane is glycerol.

(D) Palmitic acid has 20 carbon atoms including carboxyl carbon.

(E) Arachidonic acid has 16 carbon atoms.

Choose the correct answer from the options given below.

(a) (B) and (E) only (b) (A) and (B) only
(c) (C) and (D) only (d) (B) and (C) only

4. Identify the basic amino acid from the following. ***(2020)***

(a) Tyrosine (b) Glutamic Acid
(c) Lysine (d) Valine

5. The two functional groups characteristic of sugars are ***(2018)***

(a) hydroxyl and methyl
(b) carbonyl and methyl
(c) carbonyl and phosphate
(d) carbonyl and hydroxyl.

6. A typical fat molecule is made up of ***(NEET-I 2016)***

(a) one glycerol and one fatty acid molecule
(b) three glycerol and three fatty acid molecules
(c) three glycerol molecules and one fatty acid molecule
(d) one glycerol and three fatty acid molecules.

7. A phosphoglyceride is always made up of (2013)

(a) a saturated or unsaturated fatty acid esterified to a glycerol molecule to which a phosphate group is also attached
(b) a saturated or unsaturated fatty acid esterified to a phosphate group which is also attached to a glycerol molecule
(c) only a saturated fatty acid esterified to a glycerol molecule to which a phosphate group is also attached
(d) only an unsaturated fatty acid esterified to a glycerol molecule to which a phosphate group is also attached.

8. Uridine, present only in RNA is a ***(Karnataka NEET 2013)***

(a) nucleoside (b) nucleotide
(c) purine (d) pyrimidine

9. Which one out of A - D given below correctly represents the structural formula of the basic amino acid? ***(2012)***

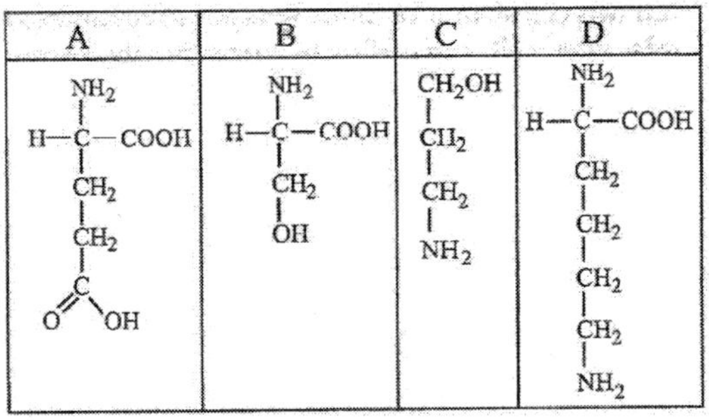

(a) C (b) D (c) A (d) B

10. The given diagrammatic representation shows one of the categories of small molecular weight organic compounds in the living tissues. Identify the category shown and the one blank ***(2012)***

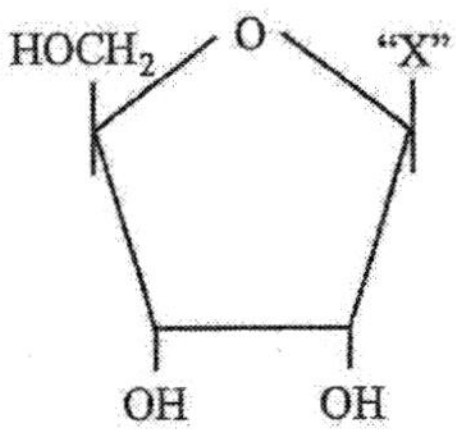

component " X" in it.

Category	Component
(a) Cholesterol	Guanine
(b) Amino acid	NH_2
(c) Nucleotide	Adenine
(d) Nucleoside	Uracil

11. Which one of the following biomolecules is correctly characterized? ***(Mains 2012)***

(a) Lecithin-a phosphorylated glyceride found in cell membrane.

(b) Palmitic acid - an unsaturated fatty acid with 18 carbon atoms.

(c) Adenylic acid - adenosine with a glucose phosphate molecule.

(d) Alanine amino acid - contains an amino group and an acidic group anywhere in the molecule.

12. Which one of the following structural formulae of two organic compounds is correctly identified along with its related function? ***(2011)***

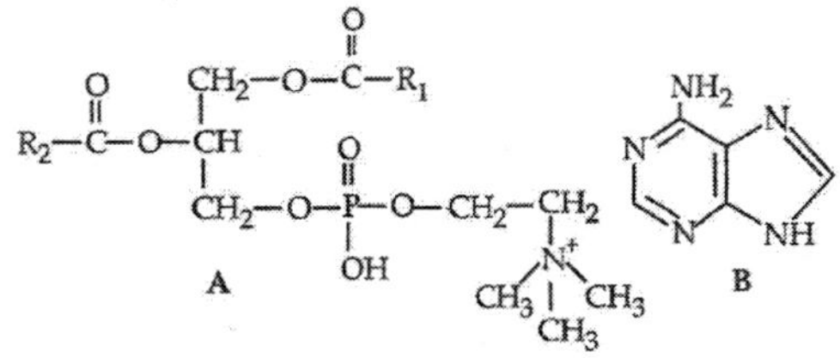

(a) B : Adenine – A nucleotide that makes up nucleic acids

(b) A : Triglyceride - Major source of energy

(c) B : Uracil - A component of DNA

(d) A: Lecithin - A component of cell membrane

13. About 98 percent of the mass of every living organism is composed of just six elements including carbon, hydrogen, nitrogen, oxygen and ***(2007)***

(a) sulphur and magnesium

(b) magnesium and sodium

(c) calcium and phosphorus

(d) phosphorus and sulphur.

14. Which of the following is the simplest amino acid? ***(2005)***

(a) Alanine (b) Asparagine

(c) Glycine (d) Tyrosine

15. The major role of minor elements inside living organisms is to act as ***(2003)***

(a) co-factors of enzymes

(b) building blocks of important amino acids

(c) constituent of hormones

(d) binder of cell structure.

16. Lipids are insoluble in water because lipid molecules are ***(2002)***

(a) hydrophilic (b) hydrophobic

(c) neutral (d) zwitter ions.

17. Essential amino acid is ***(2000)***

(a) phenylalanine (b) glycine

(c) aspartic acid (d) serine.

18. What are the most diverse molecules in the cell? ***(1996)***
(a) Lipids (b) Mineral salts
(c) Proteins (d) Carbohydrates

19. The four elements that make up 99% of all elements found in a living system are ***(1994)***
(a) C, H, O and P (b) C, N, O and P
(c) H, O, C and N (d) C, H, O and S

20. Amino acids are mostly synthesised from ***(1992)***
(a) mineral salts (b) fatty acids
(c) volatile acids (d) a-ketoglutaric acid.

21. Living cell contains 60–95% water. Water present in human body is ***(1992)***
(a) 60–65% (b) 50 –55%
(c) 75 – 80% (d) 65 – 70%

PRIMARY AND SECONDARY METABOLITES

22. Which of the following are not secondary metabolites in plants? ***(2021)***
(a) Rubber, gums
(b) Morphine, codeine
(c) Amino acids, glucose
(d) Vinblastin, curcumin

23. Identify the incorrect pair. ***(2021)***
(a) Drugs - Ricin
(b) Alkaloids - Codeine
(c) Toxin - Abrin
(d) Lectins - Concanavalin A

24. Secondary metabolites such as nicotine, strychnine and caffeine are produced by plants for their ***(2020)***
(a) nutritive value
(b) growth response
(c) defence action
(d) effect on reproduction.

25. Concanavalin A is ***(2019)***
(a) a pigment (b) an alkaloid
(c) an essential oil (d) a lectin

Proteins

26. Which one of the following is the most abundant protein in the animals? ***(2020)***
(a) Haemoglobin (b) Collagen
(c) Lectin (d) Insulin

27. Which of the following glucose transporters is insulin-dependent? ***(2019)***
(a) GLUT IV (b) GLUT I
(c) GLUT II (d) GLUT III

28. Which one is the most abundant protein in the animal world? ***(2012)***
(a) Trypsin (b) Haemoglobin
(c) Collagen (d) Insulin

29. Which of the following have carbohydrate as prosthetic group? ***(2000)***
(a) Glycoprotein (b) Chromoprotein
(c) Lipoprotein (d) Nucleoprotein

POLYSACCHARIDES

30. Cellulose does not form blue colour with iodine because ***(2023)***
(a) It does not contain complex helices and hence cannot hold iodine molecules.
(b) It breaks down when iodine reacts with it.
(c) It is a disaccharide.
(d) It is a helical molecule.

31. Match list-I with list-II.

List-I (Biological molecules)	List-II (Biological functions)
(A) Glycogen	(i) Hormone
(B) Globulin	(ii) Biocatalyst
(C) Steroids	(iii) Antibody
(D) Thrombin	(iv) Storage product

Choose the correct answer from the options given below : ***(2022)***
(a) (A)-(iii), (B)-(ii), (C)-(iv), (D)-(i)
(b) (A)-(iv), (B)-(ii), (C)-(i), (D)-(iii)
(c) (A)-(ii), (B)-(iv), (C)-(iii), (D)-(i)
(d) (A)-(iv), (B)-(iii), (C)-(i), (D)-(ii)

32. Which one of the following statements is wrong? ***(NEET-I 2016)***

(a) Uracil is a pyrimidine.

(b) Glycine is a sulphur containing amino acid.

(c) Sucrose is a disaccharide.

(d) Cellulose is a polysaccharide.

33. The chitinous exoskeleton of arthropods is formed by the polymerisation of ***(2015)***

(a) N - acetyl glucosamine

(b) lipoglycans

(c) keratin sulphate and chondroitin sulphate

(d) D - glucosamine.

34. Which one of the following is a non - reducing carbohydrate? ***(2014)***

(a) Maltose (b) Sucrose

(c) Lactose (d) Ribose 5-phosphate

35. Macromolecule chitin is ***(2013)***

(a) sulphur containing polysaccharide

(b) simple polysaccharide

(c) nitrogen containing polysaccharide

(d) phosphorus containing polysaccharide.

36. Carbohydrates are commonly found as starch in plants storage organs. Which of the following five properties of starch (1-5) make it useful as a storage material? ***(2008)***

(1) Easily translocated

(2) Chemically non-reactive

(3) Easily digested by animals

(4) Osmotically inactive

(5) Synthesized during photosynthesis

The useful properties are

(a) (1), (3) and (5) (b) (1) and (5)

(c) (2) and (3) (d) (2) and (4).

37. Cellulose is the major component of cell walls of ***(2008)***

(a) Pseudomonas (b) Saccharomyces

(c) Pythium (d) Xanthomonas.

38. Carbohydrates, the most abundant biomolecule on earth, are produced by ***(2005)***

(a) some bacteria, algae and green plant cells

(b) fungi, algae and green plant cells

(c) all bacteria, fungi and algae

(d) viruses, fungi and bacteria.

39. Which of the following is a reducing sugar? ***(2002)***

(a) Galactose

(b) Gluconic acid

(c) b-methyl galactoside

(d) Sucrose

40. Cellulose, the most important constituent of plant cell wall is made up of ***(1998)***

(a) branched chain of glucose molecules linked by β–1, 4 glycosidic bond in straight chain and α–1, 6 glycosidic bond at the site of branching

(b) unbranched chain of glucose molecules linked by β–1, 4 glycosidic bond

(c) branched chain of glucose molecules linked by α–1, 6 glycosidic bond at the site of branching

(d) unbranched chain of glucose molecules linked by α–1, 4 glycosidic bond.

41. Lactose is composed of ***(1998)***

(a) glucose + galactose

(b) fructose + galactose

(c) glucose + fructose

(d) glucose + glucose.

42. In which of the following groups are all polysaccharides? ***(1996)***

(a) Sucrose, glucose and fructose

(b) Maltose, lactose and fructose

(c) Glycogen, sucrose and maltose

(d) Glycogen, cellulose and starch

43. Glycogen is a polymer of ***(1993)***

(a) galactose (b) glucose

(c) fructose (d) sucrose.

NUCLEIC ACIDS

44. Which of the following are not polymeric? ***(2017)***
(a) Proteins (b) Polysaccharides
(c) Lipids (d) Nucleic acids

45. Nucleotides are building blocks of nucleic acids. Each nucleotide is a composite molecule formed by ***(2005)***
(a) base-sugar-phosphate
(b) base-sugar-OH
(c) (base-sugar-phosphate)
(d) sugar-phosphate

46. Which purine base is found in RNA? ***(1996)***
(a) Thymine (b) Uracil
(c) Cytosine (d) Guanine

47. In RNA, thymine is replaced by ***(1992)***
(a) adenine (b) guanine
(c) cytosine (d) uracil.

48. Adenine is ***(1992)***
(a) purine (b) pyrimidine
(c) nucleoside (d) nucleotide.

49. A nucleotide is formed of ***(1991)***
(a) purine, pyrimidine and phosphate
(b) purine, sugar and phosphate
(c) nitrogen base, sugar and phosphate
(d) pyrimidine, sugar and phosphate.

50. DNA is composed of repeating units of ***(1991)***
(a) ribonucleosides
(b) deoxyribonucleosides
(c) ribonucleotides
(d) deoxyribonucleotides.

51. The basic unit of nucleic acid is ***(1991)***
(a) pentose sugar (b) nucleoid
(c) nucleoside (d) nucleotide.

52. RNA does not possess ***(1988)***
(a) uracil (b) thymine
(c) adenine (d) cytosine.

STRUCTURE OF PROTEINS

53. Given below are two statements: ***(2023)***
Statement I : A protein is imagined as a line, the left end represented by first amino acid (C-terminal) and the right end represented by last amino acid (N-terminal)
Statement II : Adult human haemoglobin, consists of 4 subunits (two subunits of α type and two subunits of β type.)
In the light of the above statements, choose the correct answer from the options given below:
(a) Statement I is true but Statement II is false.
(b) Statement I is false but Statement II is true
(c) Both Statement I and Statement II are true.
(d) Both Statement I and Statement II are false.

54. "Ramachandran plot" is used to confirm the structure of ***(Odisha NEET 2019)***
(a) RNA (b) proteins
(c) triacylglycerides (d) DNA.

55. Which of the following is the least likely to be involved in stabilising the three-dimensional folding of most proteins? ***(NEET-II 2016)***
(a) Hydrogen bonds
(b) Electrostatic interaction
(c) Hydrophobic interaction
(d) Ester bonds

56. The figure shows a hypothetical tetrapeptide portion of a protein with parts labelled A-D. Which one of the following options is correct?
(Karnataka NEET 2013)

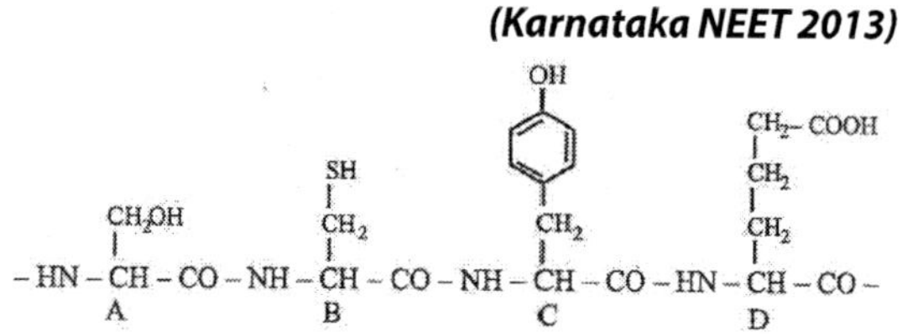

(a) D is the acidic amino acid-glutamic acid.
(b) C is an aromatic amino acid-tryptophan.
(c) A is the C-terminal amino acid and D is N -terminal amino acid
(d) A is a sulphur containing amino acid methionine.

NATURE OF BOND LINKING MONOMERS IN A POLYMER

57. Match List-I with List-II. ***(2021)***

List-I	List-II
(p) Protein	(i) C = C double bonds
(q) Unsaturated fatty acid	(ii) Phosphodiester bonds
(r) Nucleic acid	(iii) Glycosidic bonds
(s) Polysaccharide	(iv) Peptide bonds

Select the correct answer from the options given below.

	(p)	(q)	(r)	(s)
(a)	(iv)	(iii)	(i)	(ii)
(b)	(iv)	(i)	(ii)	(iii)
(c)	(i)	(iv)	(iii)	(ii)
(d)	(ii)	(i)	(iv)	(iii)

58. Identify the substances having glycosidic bond and peptide bond, respectively in their structure. ***(2020)***
(a) Chitin, cholesterol (b) Glycerol, trypsin
(c) Cellulose, lecithin (d) Inulin, insulin

59. Which of the following biomolecules does have a phosphodiester bond? ***(2015)***
(a) Amino acids in a polypeptide
(b) Nucleic acids in a nucleotide
(c) Fatty acids in a diglyceride
(d) Monosaccharides in a polysaccharide

METABOLIC BASIS FOR LIVING

60. ATP is ***(2000)***
(a) nucleotide (b) nucleoside
(c) nucleic acid (d) vitamin.

ENZYMES

61. Melonate inhibits the growth of pathogenic bacteria by inhibiting the activity of ***(2023)***
(a) Lipase
(b) Dinitrogenase
(c) Succinic dehydrogenase
(d) Amylase

62. Given below are two statements: ***(2023)***

Statement I: Low temperature preserves the enzyme in a temporarily inactive state whereas high temperature destroys enzymatic activity because proteins are denatured by heat.

Statement II: When the inhibitor closely resembles the substrate in its molecular structure and inhibits the activity of the enzyme, it is known as competitive inhibitor.

In the light of the above statements, choose the correct answer from the options given below:
(a) Statement I is true but Statement II is false.
(b) Statement I is false but Statement II is true.
(c) Both Statement I and Statement II are true.
(d) Both Statement I and Statement II are false.

63. Match the following. ***(2020)***

(A) Inhibitor of catalytic activity	(i) Ricin
(B) Possess peptide	(ii) Malonate
(C) Cell wall material in fungi	(iii) Chitin
(D) Secondary metabolite	(iv) Collagen

Choose the correct option from the following:

	(p)	(q)	(r)	(s)
(a)	(ii)	(iv)	(iii)	(i)
(b)	(iii)	(i)	(iv)	(ii)
(c)	(iii)	(iv)	(i)	(ii)
(d)	(ii)	(iii)	(i)	(iv)

64. Consider the following statements. ***(2019)***
(A) Coenzyme or metal ion that is tightly bound to enzyme protein is called prosthetic group.
(B) A complete catalytic active enzyme with its bound prosthetic group is called apoenzyme.

Select the correct option.
(a) (A) is false but (B) is true.
(b) Both (A) and (B) are true.
(c) (A) is true but (B) is false.
(d) Both (A) and (B) are false.

65. Prosthetic groups differ from co-enzymes in tha t ***(Odisha NEET 2019)***
(a) they require metal ions for their activity
(b) they (prosthetic groups) are tightly bound to apoenzymes
(c) their association with apoenzymes is transient
(d) they can serve as co-factors in a number of enzyme-catalyzed reactions.

66. Which of the following statements is correct with reference to enzymes? ***(2017)***
(a) Holoenzyme = Apoenzyme + Coenzyme
(b) Coenzyme = Apoenzyme + Holoenzyme
(c) Holoenzyme = Coenzyme + Co-factor
(d) Apoenzyme = Holoenzyme + Coenzyme

67. A non-proteinaceous enzyme is ***(NEET-II 2016)***
(a) lysozyme (b) ribozyme
(c) ligase (d) deoxyribonuclease.

68. Which of the following describes the given graph correctly? ***(NEET-II 2016)***

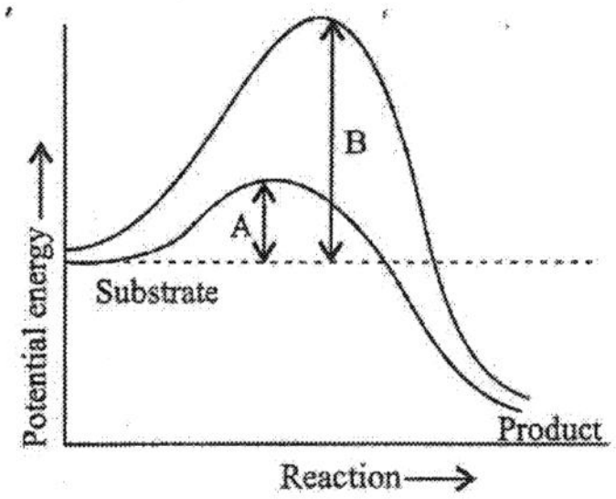

(a) Endothermic reaction with energy A in presence of enzyme and B in absence of enzyme.
(b) Exothermic reaction with energy A in presence of enzyme and B in absence of enzyme.
(c) Endothermic reaction with energy A in absence of enzyme and B in presence of enzyme.
(d) Exothermic reaction with energy A in absence of enzyme and B in presence of enzyme.

69. Which one of the following statements is incorrect? ***(2015 Cancelled)***
(a) The competitive inhibitor does not affect the rate of breakdown of the enzyme-substrate complex.
(b) The presence of the competitive inhibitor decreases the Km of the enzyme for the substrate.
(c) A competitive inhibitor reacts reversibly with the enzyme to form an enzyme-inhibitor complex.
(d) In competitive inhibition, the inhibitor molecule is not chemically changed by the enzyme.

70. Select the option which is not correct with respect to enzyme action. ***(2014)***
(a) Substrate binds with enzyme at its active site.
(b) Addition of lot of succinate does not reverse the inhibition of succinic dehydrogenase by malonate.
(c) A non-competitive inhibitor binds the enzyme at a site distinct from that which binds the substrate.
(d) Malonate is a competitive inhibitor of succinic dehydrogenase.

71. Transition state structure of the substrate formed during an enzymatic reaction is ***(2013)***
(a) transient and unstable
(b) permanent and stable
(c) transient but stable
(d) permanent but unstable.

72. The essential chemical components of many coenzymes are ***(2013)***
(a) carbohydrates (b) vitamins
(c) proteins (d) nucleic acids.

73. Which of the following statements about enzymes is wrong? ***(Karnataka NEET 2013)***
(a) Enzymes are denatured at high temperatures.
(b) Enzymes are mostly proteins but some are lipids also.
(c) Enzymes are highly specific.
(d) Enzymes require optimum pH and temperature for maximum activity.

74. The curve given below shows enzymatic activity in relation to three conditions (pH, temperature and substrate concentration). ***(2011)***

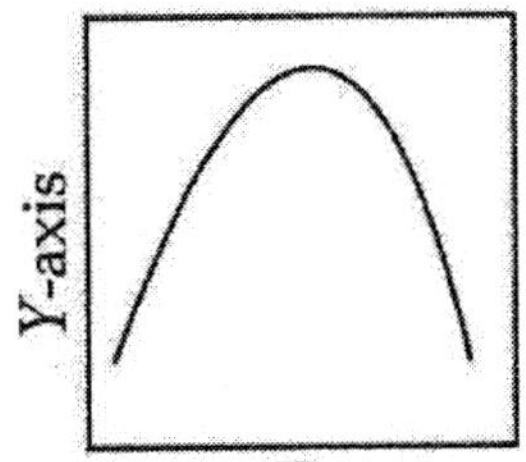

What do the two axes (X and Y) represent?

	X-axis	Y-axis
(a)	Enzymatic activity	pH
(b)	Temperature	Enzyme activity
(c)	Substrate concentration	Enzymatic activity
(d)	Enzymatic activity	Temperature

75. Three of the following statements about enzymes are correct and one is wrong. Which one is wrong? ***(Mains 2010)***

(a) Enzymes require optimum pH for maximal activity.

(b) Enzymes are denatured at high temperature but in certain exceptional organisms they are effective even at temperatures 80° – 90°C.

(c) Enzymes are highly specific.

(d) Most enzymes are proteins but some are lipids.

76. The figure given below shows the conversion of a substrate into product by an enzyme. In which one of the four options (A-D) the components of

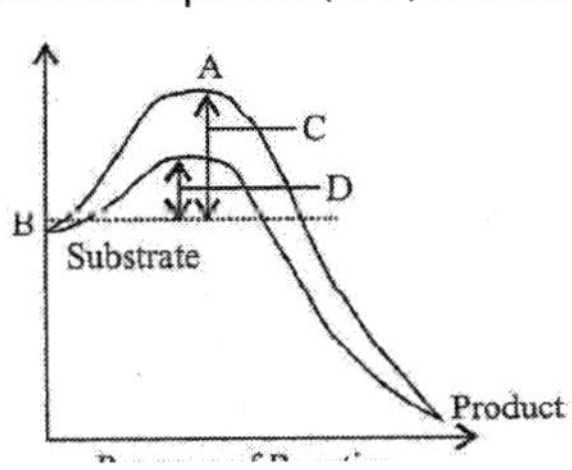

Progress of Reaction reaction labelled as A, B, C and D are identified correctly? ***(Mains 2010)***

	A	B	C	D
(a)	Potential energy	Transition state	Activation energy with enzyme	Activation energy without enzyme
(b)	Transition state	Potential energy	Activation energy without enzyme	Activation energy with enzyme
(c)	Potential	Transition energy	Activation state with enzyme	Activation energyenergy without enzyme
(d)	Activation energy with enzyme	Transition state	Activation energy without enzyme	Potential energy

77. A competitive inhibitor of succinic dehydrogenase is ***(2008)***

(a) a-ketoglutarate (b) malate

(c) malonate (d) oxaloacetate.

78. An organic substance bound to an enzyme and essential for its activity is called ***(2006)***

(a) isoenzyme (b) coenzyme

(c) holoenzyme (d) apoenzyme.

79. The catalytic efficiency of two different enzymes can be compared by the ***(2005)***

(a) formation of the product

(b) pH of optimum value

(c) Km value

(d) molecular size of the enzyme.

80. Which one of the following statements regarding enzyme inhibition is correct? ***(2005)***

(a) Competitive inhibition is seen when a substrate competes with an enzyme for binding to an inhibitor protein.

(b) Competitive inhibition is seen when the substrate and the inhibitor compete for the active site on the enzyme.

(c) Non-competitive inhibition of an enzyme can be overcome by adding large amount of substrate.

(d) Non-competitive inhibitors often bind to the enzyme irreversibly.

81. Enzymes, vitamins and hormones can be classified into a single category of biological chemicals, because all of these ***(2005)***
(a) help in regulating metabolism
(b) are exclusively synthesized in the body of a living organism as at present
(c) are conjugated proteins
(d) enhance oxidative metabolism.

82. Role of an enzyme in reactions is to/as ***(2000)***
(a) decrease activation energy
(b) increase activation energy
(c) inorganic catalyst
(d) none of the above.

83. Which factor is responsible for inhibition of enzymatic process during feedback? ***(2000)***
(a) Substrate (b) Enzymes
(c) End product (d) Temperature

84. Enzymes are not found in ***(2000)***
(a) fungi (b) algae
(c) virus (d) cyanobacteria.

85. Co-factor (prosthetic group) is a part of holoenzyme. It is ***(1997)***
(a) loosely attached organic part
(b) loosely attached inorganic part
(c) accessory non-protein substance attached firmly
(d) none of these.

ANSWER KEY

1.	(c)	2	(c)	3.	(d)	4.	(c)	5.	(d)	6.	(d)	7.	(a)
8.	(a)	9.	(b)	10.	(d)	11.	(a)	12.	(d)	13.	(d)	14.	(c)
15.	(a)	16.	(b)	17.	(a)	18.	(c)	19.	(c)	20.	(d)	21.	(d)
22.	(c)	23.	(a)	24.	(c)	25.	(d)	26.	(b)	27.	(a)	28.	(c)
29.	(a)	30.	(a)	31.	(d)	32.	(b)	33.	(a)	34.	(b)	35.	(c)
36.	(d)	37.	(c)	38.	(a)	39.	(a)	40.	(b)	41.	(a)	42.	(d)
43.	(b)	44.	(c)	45.	(a)	46.	(d)	47.	(d)	48.	(a)	49.	(c)
50.	(d)	51.	(d)	52.	(b)	53.	(b)	54.	(b)	55.	(d)	56.	(*)
57.	(b)	58.	(d)	59.	(b)	60.	(a)	61.	(c)	62.	(c)	63.	(a)
64.	(d)	65.	(b)	66.	(a)	67.	(b)	68.	(b)	69.	(b)	70.	(b)
71.	(a)	72.	(b)	73.	(b)	74.	(b)	75.	(d)	76.	(b)	77.	(c,d)
78.	(b)	79.	(c)	80.	(b)	81.	(a)	82.	(a)	83.	(c)	84.	(c)
85.	(c)												

HINTS & EXPLANATIONS

1. **(c)**:Lecithin is a phospholipid. Saturated fatty acids do not possess double bond.

2. **(c)** : Maltose is a disaccharide made up two units of glucose with a chemical formula $C_{12}H_{22}O_{11}$

3. **(d)**: Unsaturated fatty acids contain one or more double C = C bonds. Palmitic acids and arachidonic acid has 16 and 20 carbons respectively including carboxyl carbon.

4. **(c)**: Glutamic acid, valine and tyrosine are acidic, neutral and aromatic acid respectively.

5. **(d)**: Carbohydrates (commonly called sugars) are chemically defined as polyhydroxy aldehyde or ketones. All sugar molecules have one carbonyl group (-CO-) in addition to hydroxyl group (OH) on other carbon atoms.

6. **(d)**: Neutral or true fats are triglycerides which are formed by esterification of three molecules of fatty acids with one molecule of trihydric alcohol, glycerol (glycerine or trihydroxy propane).

7. **(a)**: Phosphoglycerides are the triesters of fatty acids (either saturated or unsaturated) and glycerol to which a phosphate group is also attached.

8. **(a)**: A nucleoside is pentose sugar and base together, without the phosphate group. Uracil is present as uridine in RNA only.

   Uracil + Ribose $\rightarrow$ Uridine

9. **(b)**: Basic amino acids have an additional amino group without forming amides, thus they are diamino monocarboxylic acids e.g., arginine, lysine, etc.

10. **(d)**: The given structure corresponds with the structure of ribose sugar. As it lacks a phosphoric acid hence it can be a nucleoside not a nucleotide.

11. **(a)**: Lecithin is a triglyceride lipid where one fatty acid is replaced by phosphoric acid which is linked to additional nitrogenous group called choline. It is a common membrane lipid. It is an amphipathic phospholipid having both hydrophilic polar and hydrophobic non-polar groups. The hydrocarbon chains of two fatty acids function as hydrophobic non-polar tails whereas the phosphate and choline behave as hydrophilic polar head group of the molecule.

    Palmitic acid is a saturated fatty acid (as it does not possess double bonds in its carbon chain) and contains 16 carbon atoms with formula $C_{16}H_{22}O_2$

    Adenylic acid or adenosine monophosphate is a nucleotide formed by union of adenine (nitrogenous base), ribose (pentose sugar) and phosphate. It is formed through phosphorylation of nucleoside as phosphate combines with sugar molecule at its 5′ carbon atom. Amino acids are organic acids with carboxylic group (–COOH) having amino group (–NH_2) generally attached to α–carbon or carbon next to carboxylic group. Alanine is a nonpolar and neutral amino acid having one methyl group and having amino group attached to carbon next to carboxylic group.

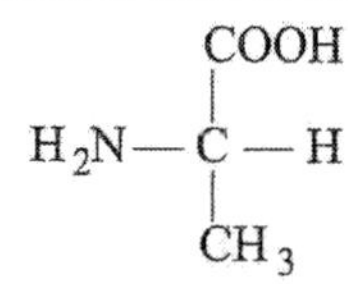

Alanine

12. **(d)** : 'A' is a structural formula of lecithin.

    Alanine It is probably the most common phospholipid. Phospholipids are major components in the lipid bilayers of cell membrane.

13. **(d)**: Living organisms requires 6 elements in relatively large amounts. C, H, O, N, P, S.

These elements contribute to the structural organization of living organisms

14. **(c)**: Glycine is considered as the simplest amino acid as it has one amino group, one carboxylic group and no substituent functional group.

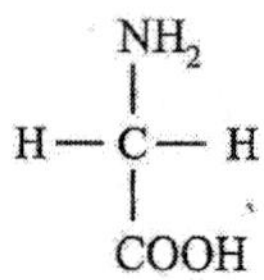

15. **(a)**: Minor elements are those which are required in quantity of less than milligram/gram of dry matter but they are essential for proper growth and development of an organism e.g., Cl, Mn, B, Zn, Cu, Mo, etc. These elements work as nonprotein cofactor in enzymes e.g., Zn, Cu etc. They also take part in oxidation reduction reactions e.g., Cu, with variable valency. Chloride ion enhances activity of salivary amylase. Zinc is required for activity of carbonic anhydrase and alcohol dehydrogenase, etc.

16. **(b)**: Lipid molecules are insoluble or sparingly soluble in water but are freely soluble in organic solvents like ether, alcohol and benzene. Insolubility of lipids in water is due to the fact that the polar groups they contain are much smaller than their nonpolar portions. The nonpolar chains are long complex hydrophobic hydrocarbon chains. If shaken in water lipids often form small droplets or micelles. The complex formed is called emulsions. These non polar proteins give them water repellent or hydrophobic property.

17. **(a)**: Essential amino acids are those amino acids that must be ingested in food for survival as they are not synthesised in the body. There are 7 essential amino acids. Glycine, aspartic acid and serine are non-essential amino acids as they can be synthesized in the body.

18. **(c)**: Proteins show enormous diversity because of different proportions and sequences of twenty amino acid within the protein molecule. A large number of permutations and combinations of these amino acids are responsible for the unlimited variety of proteins. Proteins are the most abundant and most varied of the macromolecules having one or more polypeptides (chains of amino acids). The proteins constitute almost 50% of the total dry weight of the cell. Proteins may be simple or conjugated. Among conjugated, proteins may be phosphoprotein, glycoprotein, nucleoprotein, chromoprotein, lipoprotein, flavoprotein, metalloprotein, etc. Functionally, proteins may be structural protein, enzymes, hormones, respiratory pigment, etc.

19. **(c)**:Carbon, hydrogen, oxygen and nitrogen are called four big elements of living body. They make up about 99% of the mass of most cells. As C, H, O and N are lightest elements so the bonds they form are the strongest covalent bonds. So that the compounds formed are stable, varied in size and shapes. Carbon constitutes more than 50% of the dry matter. It has been observed that human body contains 0.5% hydrogen, 18.5% carbon, 65% oxygen and 3.3% nitrogen. Other elements are present in very lesser amount.

20. **(d)**: Amino acids are mostly synthesised from α-ketoglutaric acid. These are the precursors of amino acids. A five carbon compound formed during Krebs' cycle is α–ketoglutaric acid which is the first dicarboxylic acid formed. Pyruvic acid converted into alanine, α–ketoglutaric acid into glutamic acid, OAA into aspartic acid, polymerization of such amino acids results into formation of proteins.

21. **(d)**: Water is the most abundant substance of

living beings. The water content of actively living cells varies between 60 – 95%. In human beings, maximum water content found in the embryo is 90–95%. Water content decreases thereafter in adult and the aged where it is 65 – 70%.

22. (c): Amino acid and glucose are required for basic metabolic processes and are directly involved in normal growth and development, so these are categorised under primary metabolites.

23. (a): Ricin is a toxin.

24. (c): Nicotine, strychnine and caffeine are the examples of alkaloids. These are produced by plants and are used by them in their defense against herbivores and pathogens.

25. (d): Concanavalin A, a lectin is a secondary metabolite, which has no direct function in growth and development of plants, rather are found at particular stages of development.

26. (b): Collagen is the most abundant protein in animal world. RuBisCO is the most abundant protein in the world of the bisphere.

27. (a): GLUT stands for glucose transport protein channel. They are of different types. Glucose transporter type 4 (GLUTIV) is a protein encoded in humans by the SLC2A4 gene. It is insulin regulated glucose transporter found primarily in adipose tissues and striated muscles.

28. (c): Collagen is an insoluble fibrous protein found extensively in the connective tissue of skin, tendons and bone. Collagen accounts for over 30% of the total body proteins of mammals and it is the most abundant animal protein.

29. (a): Glycoproteins are proteins that contain sugars like carbohydrates as prosthetic group. In most glycoproteins, the linkage is between asparagine and N-acetyl-D-glucosamine. Some glycoproteins are immunoglobulins, membrane proteins and muscle proteins. Lipoproteins are protein complexed with lipids like triglycerides, phospholipids etc. Nucleoproteins are proteins associated with nucleic acids and chromoproteins are proteins associated with pigments e.g., cytochrome, phytochrome.

30. (a)

31. (d)

32. (b): Glycine is a neutral amino acid. Cysteine and methionine are sulphur containing amino acid.

33. (a): Chitin is a structural polysaccharide that constitutes the exoskeleton of arthropods. It is a complex carbohydrate in which N-acetyl glucosamine monomers are joined together by (1, 4)β-linkages. Chitinous exoskeleton provides strength and elasticity to arthropods.

34. (b): In non-reducing sugars, a free aldehyde or ketonic group is absent. Sucrose is a non-reducing sugar formed by condensation of one molecule each of glucose and fructose with release of a water molecule. A glycosidic bond is established between carbon atom 1 of glucose and carbon atom 2 of fructose.

35. (c)

36. (d): Starch is the major storage carbohydrate of plants. In most plant species, it is accumulated in the chloroplast of leaves, whereas in storage organ it accumulates in amyloplast as reserve starch. It is the osmotically inactive form of photosynthetic product and is a hexosan polysaccharide made of large number of glucose unit so, chemically non-reactive.

37. (c): The cell wall of most fungi consist of chitin or cellulose. In Pythium, the hyphal wall contains cellulose whereas, in yeast the cell wall is thin and is composed of chitin in combination with other compounds (carbohydrates, glucan and mannan). The bacterial cell wall contains N-acetyl glucosamine and N-acetyl muramic acid.

38. (a): Carbohydrates are organic compounds synthesized in the chlorophyll containing cells of some bacteria, algae and green plant cells, during photosynthesis. Certain photoautotrophic bacteria e.g., Green sulphur bacteria and purple sulphur bacteria contain pigments like chlorobium chlorophyll and bacteriochlorophyll respectively that helps them in photosynthesis.

39. (a): All those sugars which have free aldehyde or ketone group are called reducing sugars. These are able to reduce cupric ions (Cu^{+2}) into cuprous ions (Cu^{+}). Sucrose, starch are non-reducing sugars.

40. (b): Cellulose is the most abundant carbohydrate Cellulose molecule is composed of 1600 to 6000 glucose molecules joined together. Those polymers form long twisting macromolecules of cellulose. The chains are unbranched and linear. The successive glucose residues are joined together by β–1–4, linkages.

41. (a): Lactose is popularly known as milk sugar. It is a disaccharide composed of one molecule of glucose and one molecule of galactose. The covalent bond that joins these two monosaccharide units is called glycosidic bond or glycosidic linkage. It is a reducing sugar.

42. (d): Polysaccharides are complex long chain carbohydrates which are formed by dehydrate synthesis or polymerisation of more than 10 but generally very large number of units called monosaccharides. Starch, glycogen and cellulose are all polysaccharides. Starch is a glucosan homopolysaccharide which is the main reserve food of plants. Glycogen is also a glucosan homopoly-saccharide which is the major reserve food of fungi, animals and some bacteria. It is also called animal starch. Cellulose is the structural polysaccharide of plant cell walls, some fungi, protists. It is a fibrous glucosan homopolysaccharide of high tensile strength.

43. (b): Glycogen (animal starch) is a polysaccharide consisting of a highly branched polymer of glucose occurring in animal tissues, especially in liver and muscle cells. It is the major store of carbohydrate energy in animal cells.

44. (c): Lipids are fatty acids esters of alcohols and related substances. Polysaccharides are polymers of monosaccharides. Proteins are polymers of amino acids and nucleic acids are polymer of nucleotides.

45. (a): Each nucleotide consists of three distinct units - a phosphate group derived from phosphoric acid, a pentose sugar and a ring shaped nitrogenous base.

Nucleoside + Phosphoric acid → Nucleotide + H_2O

46. (d): The bases are of two types-purines and pyrimidines. The purine derivatives adenine (A) and guanine (G) are double ring structures whereas pyrimidine derivatives thymine, cytosine and uracil are single ring structures. Thymine (T) and cytosine (C) are found in DNA and cytosine (C) and uracil (U) are found in RNA.

47. (d)

48. (a)

49. (c): Nucleotide is an organic compound consisting of a nitrogen-containing purine or pyrimidine base linked to a sugar (ribose or deoxyribose) and a phosphate group.

50. (d): DNA is the largest macromolecule in the organisms. It is a long, double chain of deoxy-ribonucleotide or deoxyribotide units. The two deoxyribonucleotide chains are twisted around a common axis to form a right-handed double helix (spiral) that encloses a cylindrical space in it. Each deoxyribonucleotide unit, in turn, consists of three different molecules : phosphate, (PO_4^{3-}), a 5-carbon deoxyribose sugar ($C_5H_{10}O_4$) and a nitrogenous base.

51. (d): The nucleic acids (DNA and RNA) are the molecules having complex structure and very high molecular weights. The nucleic acid is composed of a large number of nucleotide molecules joined into a linear, unbranched chain. Nucleotide is an organic compound consisting of a nitrogen-containing purine or pyrimidine base linked to a sugar (ribose or deoxyribose) and a phosphate group.

52. (b)

53. (b): A protein is imagined as line, the left end represents first amino acid (N-terminal amino acid) and right end represents the last amino acid (C-terminal amino acid).

54. (b)

55. (d):Tertiary structure or three dimensional structure of protein is stabilised by several types of bonds-hydrogen bonds, ionic bonds, van der Waal's interactions, covalent bonds and hydrophobic bonds.

56. (*) : None of the options is correct.

A – Serine (Neutral – Polar)

B – Cysteine (Neutral – Polar)

C – Tyrosine (Neutral – Polar)

S – Not an amino acid

57. (b)

58. (d)

59. (b)

60. (a): ATP is a nucleotide as it is composed of adenine, ribose sugar and phosphoric acid. There are two additional phosphate groups attached to the phosphate group of AMP. The last two phosphate molecules are connected by high energy bonds.

61.(c) : In competitive inhibition, the inhibitor closely resembles the real substrate in its molecular structure and inhibits the activity of the enzyme. Due to its close structural similarity with the substrate, the inhibitor competes with substrate for the substrate binding site of enzymes. Consequently, the substrate cannot bind and as a result, the enzyme action declines. Inhibition of succinic dehydrogenase by malonate is one of the example of competitive inhibition. Malonate closely resembles the substrate succinate in structure. Such competitive inhibitors are often used to inhibit the growth of pathogenic bacteria.

62. (c)

63. (a)

64. (d): Enzymes could be simple or conjugated (holoenzyme). Conjugated enzymes are formed of two parts - a protein part called apoenzyme and a non-protein part named co-factor. Co-factors are bound to the enzyme to make it catalytically active. There are three types of cofactors : prosthetic groups, co-enzymes and metal ions. Prosthetic groups are organic compounds and are distinguished from other cofactors in which they are tightly bound to the apoenzyme. Co-enzymes are organic compounds but their association with the apoenzyme is only transient, occurring during the course of catalysis. A number of enzymes require metal ions for their activity which form coordination one or more coordination bonds with the substrate.

65. (b)

66. (a): Holoenzyme is the complete conjugate enzyme consisting of an apoenzyme and a cofactor. Cofactor may be organic or inorganic in nature. Organic cofactors are of two types- coenzyme and prosthetic group.

67. (b): A ribozyme is a ribonucleic acid (RNA) enzyme that catalyses a chemical reaction in a similar way to that of a protein enzyme. These are found in ribosomes and are also called catalytic RNAs.

68. (b)

69. (b): Competitive inhibition is a reversible inhibition where inhibitor competes with the normal substrate for the active site of enzyme. A competitive inhibitor is usually chemically similar to the normal substrate and therefore, fits into the active site of an enzyme and binds with it. The inhibition is thus due to substrate analogue. The enzyme, now cannot act upon the substrate and reaction products are not formed. E.g., the activity of succinate dehydrogenase is inhibited by malonate. Km value or Michaelis constant is defined as the substrate concentration at which half of the enzyme molecules are forming enzyme substrate (ES) complex or concentration of the substrate when the velocity of the enzyme reaction is half the maximal possible. A smaller Km value indicates greater affinity of the enzyme for its substrate, hence, shows a quicker reaction. The competitive inhibitor decreases the affinity of enzyme for substrate, thus increases the Km value.

70. (b):The reduction of activity of succinate dehydrogenase by malonate is an example of competitive inhibition.Competitive inhibition is a reversible inhibition where inhibitor competes with the normal substrate for the active site of enzyme. A competitive inhibitor is usually similar to the normal substrate and therefore, fits into the active site of an enzyme and binds with it. The enzyme, now cannot act upon the substrate and reaction products are not formed. Hence, action of an enzyme may be reduced or inhibited. Since a competitive inhibitor occupies the site only temporarily, the enzyme action is not permanently affected. Thus, addition of a lot of succinate can reverse the inhibition of succinate dehydrogenase by malonate.

71. (a): Transition state is formation of unstable intermediate structural state. During this, substrate bonds are broken and new bonds are established that transform the substrate molecules into products. This state is transient and highly unstable.

72. (b): Coenzyme is the non protein organic group which gets attached to the apoenzyme to form holoenzyme or conjugate enzyme. It helps in removing a product of chemical reaction besides bringing contact between the substrate and the enzyme. Most of the coenzymes are made of water soluble vitamins B and C, e.g., thiamine, riboflavin, nicotinamide, pyridoxine.

73. (b): Enzymes are mostly proteins but some are RNA (ribozymes). No lipid working as enzymes are known.

74. (b): Enzymes generally function in a narrow range of temperature and pH. Each enzyme shows its highest activity at a particular temperature and pH called the optimum temperature and optimum pH. Activity declines both below and above the optimum values. X-axis always represents temperature or pH and Y axis represents enzyme activity.

75. (d)

76. (b)

77. (c,d): Malonate or oxaloacetate, which resemble succinate in structure and inhibit the activity of succinate dehydrogenase. Such competitive inhibitors are often used in control of bacterial pathogen.

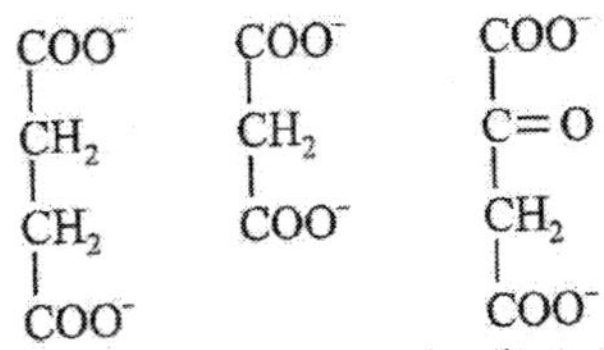

Succinate Malonate Oxaloacetate

78. (b): Enzymes are simple if they are made of only proteins (e.g., pepsin, amylase, etc.) while conjugate enzymes have an additional non-protein cofactor which may be organic or inorganic. Loosely attached organic cofactor is coenzyme. It plays an accessory role in enzyme catalysed processes often by acting as a donor or acceptor of a substance involved in the reaction. ATP and NAD are common coenzymes.

79. (c): Km value or Michaelis constant is defined as the substrate concentration at which half of the enzyme molecules are forming (ES) complex or concentration of the substrate when the velocity of the enzyme reaction is half the maximal possible. The Km varies from enzyme to enzyme and is used in characterizing the different enzymes. A smaller Km value indicates greater affinity of the enzyme for its substrate, hence, shows a quicker reaction. Km value is a constant characteristic of an enzyme for its conversion of a substrate.

80. (b)

81. (a): Enzymes control all the life processes. They increase the rate of a biological reaction. The magnitude of increase may be greater than those affected by other catalysts.

Vitamins are accessory indispensable food factor, organic in nature (organic acid, amino acid, esters, alcohols, steroids, etc.) required by an organism in small amounts to maintain normal growth and regulate the metabolic processes.

Hormones are biologically active organic substance that are produced in minute quantities by some specialised organs and exert physiological effects at sites far from their origin.

82. (a): All molecules require certain amount of energy for activation (to overcome energy barrier) before they can react. This energy is called activation energy. This energy is recovered when products are formed. The essence of an enzyme is its ability to speed up (catalyze) a reaction by making or breaking specific covalent bonds (bonds in which atoms are held together by sharing of electrons). Enzymes act by somehow lowering the temperature at which a given bond is unstable i.e., they speed up a reaction by lowering the activation energy. It is the magnitude of the activation energy which determines how fast the reaction will proceed.

83. (c): Feedback inhibition or end product inhibition is the inhibition of the activity of an enzyme catalysing some early reactions of the series by the end product of the metabolic pathway. For example, a substrate A is converted into a product F through B, C, D and E intermediate products. As the concentration of end product F increases, it diffuses to allosteric enzyme (E1) causing a reduced synthesis of the product B which in turn lowers the rate of enzymatic reactions in rest of the pathway.

84. (c) : Viruses do not have enzymes so they cannot synthesize proteins. They multiply only inside the living host cell and for multiplication and metabolism they take over the machinery of the host cell. They lack their own cellular machinery and enzymes.

85. (c)

Chapter : 10 CELL CYCLE AND CELL DIVISION

CELL CYCLE

1. Match List I with List II : ***(2023)***

List I	List II
A. M Phase	I. Proteins are synthesized
B. G_2 Phase	II. Inactive phase
C.Quiescent stage	III. Interval between mitosis and initiation of DNA replication
D. G_1 Phase	IV. Equational division

Choose the correct answer from the options given below:

(a) A-IV, B-I, C-II, D-III
(b) A-II, B-IV, C-I, D-III
(c) A-III, B-II, C-IV, D-I
(d) A-IV, B-II, C-I, D-III

2. Among eukaryotes, replication of DNA takes place in - ***(2023)***

(a) G1 phase (b) G2 phase
(c) M phase (d) S phase

3. Given below are two statements: ***(2023)***

Statement I : During G_0 phase of cell cycle, the cell is metabolically inactive.

Statement II : The centrosome undergoes duplication during S phase of interphase.

In the light of the above statements, choose the most appropriate answer from the options given below:

(a) Statement I is correct but Statement II is incorrect.
(b) Statement I is incorrect but Statement II is correct.
(c) Both Statement I and Statement II are correct.
(d) Both Statement I and Statement II are incorrect.

4. Match List-I with List-II. ***(2021)***

List-I	List-II
(p) S phase	(i) Proteins are synthesised
(q) G_2 phase	(ii) Inactive phase
(r) Quiescent stage	(iii) Interval between mitosis and initiation of DNA replication
(s) G_1 phase	(iv) DNA replication

Select the correct answer from the options given below.

	(p)	(q)	(r)	(s)
(a)	(ii)	(iv)	(iii)	(i)
(b)	(iii)	(ii)	(i)	(iv)
(c)	(iv)	(ii)	(iii)	(i)
(d)	(iv)	(i)	(ii)	(iii)

5. The fruit fly has 8 chromosomes (2n) in each cell. During interphase of mitosis if the number of chromosomes at G1 phase is 8 , what would be the number of chromosomes after S phase? ***(2021)***

(a) 32 (b) 8 (c) 16 (d) 4

6. The centriole undergoes duplication during ***(2021)***

(a) G2 phase (b) S-phase
(c) prophase (d) metaphase

7. Identify the correct statement with regard to G1 phase (Gap 1) of interphase. ***(2020)***

(a) DNA synthesis or replication takes place.
(b) Reorganisation of all cell components takes place.
(c) Cell is metabolically active, grows but does not replicate its DNA.
(d) Nuclear division takes place.

8. Some dividing cells exit the cell cycle and enter vegetative inactive stage. This is called quiescent stage (G0). This process occurs at the end of ***(2020)***
(a) M phase (b) G1 phase
(c) S phase (d) G2 phase.

9. Cells in G0 phase ***(2019)***
(a) terminate the cell cycle
(b) exit the cell cycle
(c) enter the cell cycle
(d) suspend the cell cycle.

10. The correct sequence of phases of cell cycle is ***(2019)***
(a) G1→S→G2→M (b) M→G1→G2→S
(c) G1→G2→S→M (d) S→G1→G2→M.

11. During cell growth, DNA synthesis takes place on ***(NEET-II 2016)***
(a) S-phase (b) G1-phase
(c) G2-phase (d) M phase.

12. When cell has stalled DNA replication fork, which checkpoint should be predominantly activated? ***(NEET-II 2016)***
(a) G1/S (b) G2/M
(c) M (d) Both G2/M and M

13. A somatic cell that has just completed the S phase of its cell cycle, as compared to gamete of the same species, has ***(2015 Cancelled)***
(a) twice the number of chromosomes and four times the amount of DNA
(b) four times the number of chromosomes and twice the amount of DNA
(c) twice the number of chromosomes and twice the amount of DNA
(d) same number of chromosomes but twice the amount of DNA.

14. During which phase(s) of cell cycle, amount of DNA in a cell remains at 4C level if the initial amount is denoted as 2C? ***(2014)***
(a) G0 and G1 (b) G1 and S
(c) Only G2 (d) G2 and M

15. In 'S' phase of the cell cycle ***(2014)***
(a) amount of DNA doubles in each cell
(b) amount of DNA remains same in each cell
(c) chromosome number is increased
(d) amount of DNA is reduced to half in each cell.

16. Given below is a schematic break-up of the phases/ stages of cell cycle. Which one of the following is the correct indication of the stage/ phase in the cell cycle? ***(2009)***

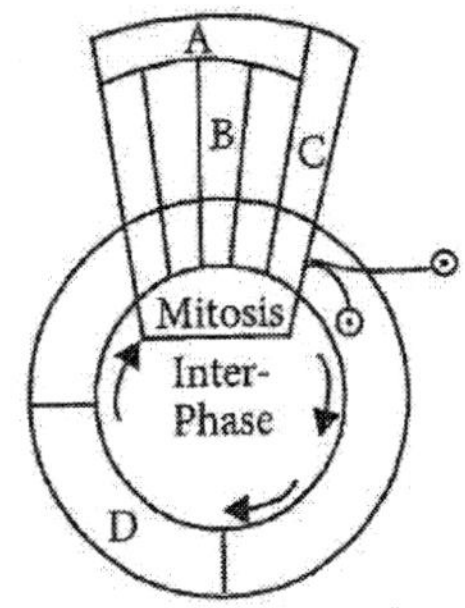

(a) C - karyokinesis
(b) D - synthetic phase
(c) A - cytokinesis
(d) B - metaphase

17. At what stage of the cell cycle are histone proteins synthesized in a eukaryotic cell? ***(2005)***
(a) During G2 stage of prophase
(b) During S-phase
(c) During entire prophase
(d) During telophase

18. In the somatic cell cycle ***(2004)***
(a) in G1 phase DNA content is double the amount of DNA present in the original cell
(b) DNA replication takes place in S phase
(c) a short interphase is followed by a long mitotic phase
(d) G2 phase follows mitotic phase.

19. In which stage of cell cycle, DNA replication occurs? ***(2000)***
(a) G1-phase (b) S-phase
(c) G2-phase (d) M-phase

20. Which typical stage is known for DNA replication? ***(1996)***
(a) S-phase (b) G2-phase
(c) metaphase (d) G1-phase

21. In a somatic cell cycle, DNA synthesis takes place in ***(1994)***
(a) G1 phase (b) prophase of mitosis
(c) S-phase (d) G2 phase.

M PHASE AND SIGNIFICANCE OF MITOSIS

22. Which one of the following never occurs during mitotic cell division? ***(2022)***
(a) Spindle fibres attach to kinetochores of chromosomes
(b) Movement of centrioles towards opposite poles
(c) Pairing of homologous chromosomes
(d) Coiling and condensation of the chromatids

23. Select the incorrect statement with reference to mitosis. ***(2022)***
(a) All the chromosomes lie at the equator at metaphase.
(b) Spindle fibres attach to centromere of chromosomes.
(c) Chromosomes decondense at telophase.
(d) Splitting of centromere occurs at anaphase.

24. Which of the following options gives the correct sequence of events during mitosis? ***(2017)***
(a) Condensation → Nuclear membrane disassembly → Arrangement at equator → Centromere division → Segregation → Telophase
(b) Condensation → Crossing over → Nuclear membrane disassembly → Segregation → Telophase
(c) Condensation → Arrangement at equator → Centromere division → Segregation → Telophase
(d) Condensation → Nuclear membrane disassembly → Crossing over → Segregation → Telophase

25. Anaphase Promoting Complex (APC) is a protein degradation machinery necessary for proper mitosis of animal cell. If APC is defective in a human cell, which of the following is expected to occur? ***(2017)***
(a) Chromosomes will be fragmented.
(b) Chromosomes will not segregate.
(c) Recombination of chromosome arms will occur.
(d) Chromosomes will not condense.

26. Spindle fibres attach on to ***(NEET-I 2016)***
(a) centromere of the chromosome
(b) kinetosome of the chromosome
(c) telomere of the chromosome
(d) kinetochore of the chromosome.

27. Which of the following is not a characteristic feature during mitosis in somatic cells? ***(NEET-I 2016)***
(a) Chromosome movement
(b) Synapsis
(c) Spindle fibres
(d) Disappearance of nucleolus

28. A stage in cell division is shown in the figure. ***(2013)***

Select the answer which gives correct identification of the stage with its characteristics.

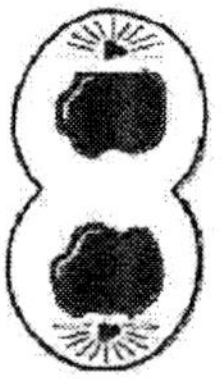

(a)	Cytokinesis	Cell plate formed, mitochondria distributed between two daughter cells.
(b)	Telophase	Endoplasmic reticulum and nucleolus not reformed yet.
(c)	Telophase	Nuclear envelope reforms, Golgi complex reforms.
(d)	Late anaphase	Chromosomes move away from equatorial plate, Golgi complex not present.

29. During the metaphase stage of mitosis, spindle fibres attach to chromosomes at ***(Karnataka NEET 2013)***

(a) kinetochore
(b) both centromere and kinetochore
(c) centromere, kinetochore and areas adjoining centromere
(d) centromere.

30. A stage of mitosis is shown in the diagram. Which stage is it and what are its characteristics? ***(Karnataka NEET 2013)***

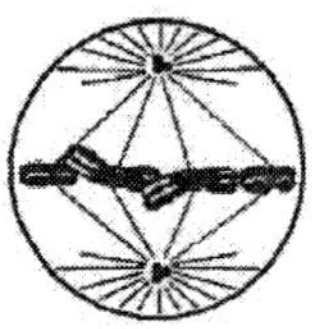

(a) Metaphase-Spindle fibers attached to kinetochores, centromeres split and chromatids separate.
(b) Metaphase - Chromosomes moved to spindle equator, chromosomes made up of two sister chromatids.
(c) Anaphase - Centromeres split and chromatids separate and start moving away.
(d) Late prophase - Chromosomes move to spindle equator.

31. Select the correct option with respect to mitosis. ***(2011)***

(a) Chromatids separate but remain in the centre of the cell in anaphase.
(b) Chromatids start moving towards opposite poles in telophase.
(c) Golgi complex and endoplasmic reticulum are still visible at the end of prophase.
(d) Chromosomes move to the spindle equator and get aligned along equatorial plate in metaphase.

32. At metaphase, chromosomes are attached to the spindle fibres by their ***(Mains 2011)***

(a) satellites (b) secondary constrictions
(c) kinetochores (d) centromeres.

33. During mitosis, ER and nucleolus begin to disappear at ***(2010)***

(a) late prophase (b) early metaphase
(c) late metaphase (d) early prophase.

34. Which stages of cell division do the following figures A and B represent respectively? (2010)

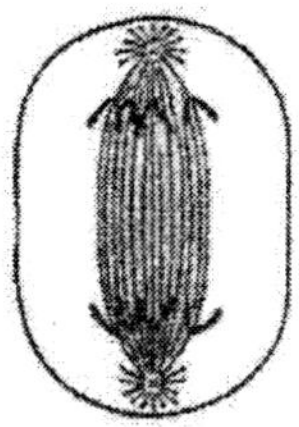

Fig. A

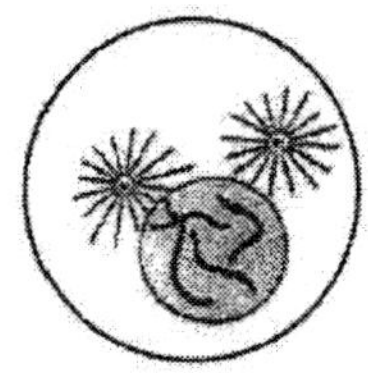

Fig. B

	A	B
(a)	Metaphase	Telophase
(b)	Telophase	Metaphase
(c)	Late anaphase	Prophase
(d)	Prophase	Anaphase

35. If you are provided with root-tips of onion in your class and are asked to count the chromosomes, which of the following stages can you most conveniently look into? ***(2004)***

(a) Metaphase (b) Telophase
(c) Anaphase (d) Prophase

36. Which one of the following precedes reformation of the nuclear envelope during M phase of the cell cycle? ***(2004)***

(a) Decondensation from chromosomes and reassembly of the nuclear lamina
(b) Transcription from chromosomes and reassembly of the nuclear lamina
(c) Formation of the contractile ring and formation of the phragmoplast
(d) Formation of the contractile ring and transcription from chromosome

37. Mitotic spindle is mainly composed of which protein? ***(2002)***

(a) Actin (b) Tubulin
(c) Actomyosin (d) Myoglobin

38. Best material for the study of mitosis in laboratory is ***(2002)***
(a) anther (b) root tip
(c) leaf tip (d) ovary.

39. Spindle fibre unite with which structure of chromosomes? ***(2000)***
(a) Chromocentre (b) Chromomere
(c) Kinetochore (d) Centriole

40. Microtubule is involved in the ***(1998)***
(a) muscle contraction
(b) membrane architecture
(c) cell division
(d) DNA recognition.

41. How many mitotic divisions are needed for a single cell to make 128 cells? ***(1997)***
(a) 28 (b) 32 (c) 7 (d) 14

42. During cell division in apical meristem, the nuclear membrane appears in ***(1997)***
(a) telophase (b) cytokinesis
(c) metaphase (d) anaphase.

43. Which of the following structures will not be common to mitotic cell of a higher plant? ***(1997)***
(a) Centriole (b) Spindle fibre
(c) Cell plate (d) Centromere

44. Colchicine is an inhibitory chemical, which ***(1996)***
(a) stops the functioning of centriole
(b) prevents attaching of centromeres with rays
(c) prevents the spindle formation in mitosis
(d) prevents the formation of equatorial plane.

45. Which of the following represents the best stage to view the shape, size and number of chromosomes? ***(1994)***
(a) Prophase (b) Metaphase
(c) Interphase (d) Telophase

46. Mitotic anaphase differs from metaphase in possessing ***(1991)***
(a) same number of chromosomes and same number of chromatids
(b) half number of chromosomes and half number of chromatids
(c) half number of chromosomes and same number of chromatids
(d) same number of chromosomes and half number of chromatids.

MEIOSIS AND SIGNIFICANCE OF MEIOSIS

47. The process of appearance of recombination nodules occurs at which sub stage of prophase I in meiosis? ***(2023)***
(a) Diplotene (b) Diakinesis
(c) Zygotene (d) Pachytene

48. Which of the following stages of meiosis involves division of centromere? ***(2023)***
(a) Anaphase II (b) Telophase
(c) Metaphase I (d) Metaphase II

49. Select the correct statements. ***(2023)***

A. Tetrad formation is seen during Leptotene.

B. During Anaphase, the centromeres split and chromatids separate.

C. Terminalization takes place during Pachytene.

D. Nucleolus, Golgi complex and ER are reformed during Telophase.

E. Crossing over takes place between sister chromatids of homologous chromosome.

Choose the correct answer from the options given below:
(a) A, C and E only (b) B and E only
(c) A and C only (d) B and D only

50. The appearance of recombination nodules on homologous chromosomes during meiosis characterises ***(2022)***
(a) synaptonemal complex
(b) bivalent
(c) sites at which crossing over occurs
(d) terminalisation.

51. Regarding meiosis, which of the statements is incorrect? ***(2022)***

(a) There are two stages in meiosis, meiosis-I and II.

(b) DNA replication occurs in S phase of meiosis-II.

(c) Pairing of homologous chromosomes and recombination occurs in meiosis-I.

(d) Four haploid cells are formed at the end of meiosis-II.

52. Which of the following stages of meiosis involves division of centromere? ***(2021)***

(a) Telophase II (b) Metaphase I

(c) Metaphase II (d) Anaphase II

53. Which stage of meiotic prophase shows terminalisation of chiasmata as its distinctive feature? ***(2021)***

(a) Pachytene (b) Leptotene

(c) Zygotene (d) Diakinesis

54. Dissolution of the synaptonemal complex occurs during ***(2020)***

(a) pachytene (b) zygotene

(c) diplotene (d) leptotene.

55. Match the following with respect to meiosis. ***(2020)***

(A) Zygotene (i) Terminalization

(B) Pachytene (ii) Chiasmata

(C) Diplotene (iii) Crossing over

(D) Diakinesis (iv) Synapsis

Select the correct option from the following

	(A)	(B)	(C)	(D)
(a)	(iii)	(iv)	(i)	(ii)
(b)	(iv)	(iii)	(ii)	(i)
(c)	(i)	(ii)	(iv)	(iii)
(d)	(II)	(iv)	(iii)	(i)

56. Crossing over takes place between which chromatids and in which stage of the cell cycle ? ***(Odisha NEET 2019)***

(a) Non-sister chromatids of non-homologous chromosomes at Zygotene stage of prophase I.

(b) Non-sister chromatids of homologous chromosomes at Pachytene stage of prophase I.

(c) Non-sister chromatids of homologous chromosomes at Zygotene stage of prophase I.

(d) Non-sister chromatids of non-homologous chromosomes at Pachytene stage of prophase I.

57. The stage during which separation of the paired homologous chromosomes begins is ***(2018)***

(a) pachytene (b) diplotene

(c) diakinesis (d) zygotene.

58. Match the stages of meiosis in column I to their characteristic features in column II and select the correct option using the codes given below. ***(NEET-II 2016)***

Column I	Column II
A. Pachytene	(i) Pairing of homologous chromosomes
B. Metaphase I	(ii) Terminalisation of chiasmata
C. Diakinesis	(iii) Crossing-over takes place
D. Zygotene	(iv) Chromosomes align at equatorial plate

(a) A-(iii), B-(iv), C-(ii), D-(i)

(b) A-(i), B-(iv), C-(ii), D-(iii)

(c) A-(ii), B-(iv), C-(iii), D-(i)

(d) A-(iv), B-(iii), C-(ii), D-(i)

59. In meiosis crossing over is initiated at ***(NEET-I 2016)***

(a) zygotene (b) diplotene

(c) pachytene (d) leptotene.

60. Arrange the following events of meiosis in correct sequence ***(2015)***

(i) Crossing over

(ii) Synapsis

(iii) Terminalisation of chiasmata

(iv) Disappearance of nucleolus

(a) (i), (ii), (iii), (iv) (b) (ii), (iii), (iv), (i)

(c) (ii), (i), (iv), (iii) (d) (ii), (i), (iii), (iv)

61. Select the correct option. ***(2015 Cancelled)***

Column I	Column II
A Synapsis aligns homologous chromosomes	(i) Anaphase II
B Synthesis of RNA and protein	(ii) Zygotene
C Action of enzyme recombinase	(iii) G2-phase
D Centromeres do not separate but chromatids move towards opposite poles	(iv) Anaphase I
	(v) Pachytene

(a) A-(i), B-(ii), C-(v), D-(iv)
(b) A-(ii), B-(iii), C-(iv), D-(v)
(c) A-(ii), B-(i), C-(iii), D-(iv)
(d) A-(ii), B-(iii), C-(v), D-(iv)

62. The enzyme recombinase is required at which stage of meiosis? ***(2014)***
(a) Pachytene (b) Zygotene
(c) Diplotene (d) Diakinesis

63. The complex formed by a pair of synapsed homologous chromosomes is called ***(2013)***
(a) bivalent (b) axoneme
(c) equatorial plate (d) kinetochore.

64. During meiosis I, the chromosomes start pairing at ***(Karnataka NEET 2013)***
(a) zygotene (b) pachytene
(c) diplotene (d) leptotene.

65. During gamete formation, the enzyme recombinase participates during ***(2012)***
(a) metaphase I (b) anaphase II
(c) prophase I (d) prophase II.

66. The given figure is the representation of a certain event at a particular stage of a type of cell division. Which is this stage? ***(2012)***

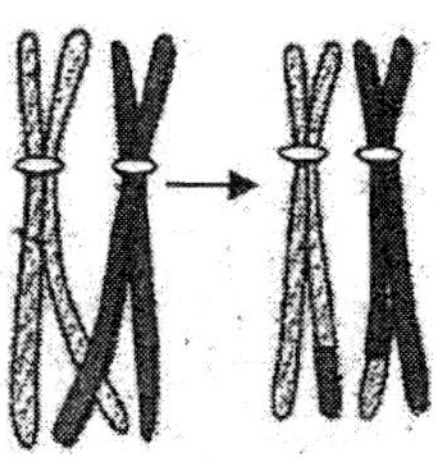

(a) Prophase I during meiosis
(b) Prophase II during meiosis
(c) Prophase of mitosis
(d) Both prophase and metaphase of mitosis

67. Identify the meiotic stage in which the homologous chromosomes separate while the sister chromatids remain associated at their centromeres. ***(Mains 2012)***
(a) Metaphase I (b) Metaphase II
(c) Anaphase I (d) Anaphase II

68. Synapsis occurs between ***(2009)***
(a) mRNA and ribosomes
(b) spindle fibres and centromere
(c) two homologous chromosomes
(d) a male and a female gamete.

69. When paternal and maternal chromosomes change their materials with each other in cell division this event is called ***(1996)***
(a) bivalent-forming (b) dyad-forming
(c) synapsis (d) crossing-over.

70. Which statement best explains the evolutionary advantage of meiosis? ***(1994)***
(a) Meiosis is necessary for sexual reproduction.
(b) Genetic recombinations are possible from generation to generation.
(c) Meiosis alternates with mitosis from generation to generation.
(d) The same genetic system is passed on from generation to generation.

71. Meiosis II performs ***(1993)***
(a) separation of sex chromosomes
(b) synthesis of DNA and centromere
(c) separation of homologous chromosomes
(d) separation of chromatids.

72. Number of chromatids at metaphase is **(1992)**
(a) two each in mitosis and meiosis
(b) two in mitosis and one in meiosis
(c) two in mitosis and four in meiosis
(d) one in mitosis and two in meiosis.

73. In meiosis, the daughter cells differ from parent cell as well as amongst themselves due to ***(1991)***
(a) segregation, independent assortment and crossing over
(b) segregation and crossing over
(c) independent assortment and crossing over
(d) segregation and independent assortment.

74. Meiosis I is reductional division. Meiosis II is equational division due to ***(1988)***
(a) pairing of homologous chromosomes
(b) crossing over
(c) separation of chromatids
(d) disjunction of homologous chromosomes.

ANSWER KEY

1.	(a)	2.	(d)	3.	(b)	4.	(d)	5.	(b)	6.	(b)	7.	(c)
8.	(b)	9.	(b)	10.	(a)	11.	(a)	12.	(a)	13.	(a)	14.	(d)
15.	(a)	16.	(b)	17.	(b)	18.	(b)	19.	(b)	20.	(a)	21.	(c)
22.	(c)	23.	(b)	24.	(a)	25.	(b)	26.	(d)	27.	(b)	28.	(c)
29.	(a)	30.	(b)	31.	(d)	32.	(c)	33.	(d)	34.	(c)	35.	(a)
36.	(c)	37.	(b)	38.	(b)	39.	(c)	40.	(c)	41.	(c)	42.	(a)
43.	(a)	44.	(c)	45.	(b)	46.	(d)	47.	(d)	48.	(a)	49.	(d)
50.	(c)	51.	(b)	52.	(d)	53.	(d)	54.	(c)	55.	(b)	56.	(b)
57.	(b)	58.	(a)	59.	(c)	60.	(d)	61.	(d)	62.	(a)	63.	(a)
64.	(a)	65.	(c)	66.	(a)	67.	(c)	68.	(c)	69.	(d)	70.	(b)
71.	(d)	72.	(a)	73.	(a)	74.	(c)						

HINTS & EXPLANATIONS

1. **(a)**

2. **(d)**: S or synthesis phase marks the period during which DNA synthesis or replication takes place. During this phase, the amount of DNA per cell doubles. If the initial amount of DNA is denoted as 2C, then it increases to 4C.

3. **(b)**: The cells in G_0 phase (quiescent stage) of cell cycle are metabolically active but no longer proliferate unless called on to do so depending on the requirements of the organisms. During S-phase of interphase, the centrosome begins to divide in centriole containing cells to form two centrosomes or centriole pair.

4. **(d)**

5. **(b)**: In S-phase, the amount of DNA per cell doubles. However, there is no change in the chromosome number. So, in fruit fly the number of chromosomes will remain same i.e. 8.

6. **(b)**: The centriole undergoes duplication during S-phase which plays role in formation of the spindle fibres required to separate chromosomes during mitosis.

7. **(c)**: S or synthesis phase marks the period during which DNA synthesis takes place. Reorganisation of all cellular components takes place in M-phase. This phase also start with nuclear division (Karyokinesis).

8. **(b)**

9. **(b)**: Some cells in the adult animals do not appear to exhibit division (e.g., heart cells) and many other cells divide only occasionally, as needed to replace cells that have been lost because of injury or cell death. These cells that do not divide further exit G1 phase to enter an inactive stage called quiescent stage(G_0) of the cell cycle. Cells in this stage remain metabolically active but no longer proliferate unless called on to do so depending on the requirement of the organism.

10. **(a)**

11. **(a)**: In S-phase (synthetic phase) of cell cycle, the chromosomes replicate. For this their DNA molecules function as templates and form carbon copies. The DNA content doubles i.e., 1C to 2C for haploid cells and 2C to 4C for diploid cells. As a result duplicate sets of genes are formed. Along with replication of DNA new chromatin fibres are formed which, however, remain attached in pairs and the number of chromosomes does not increase. As chromatin fibres are elongated chromosomes, each chromosome comes to have two chromatin threads or sister chromatids which remain attached at a common point called centromere.

12. **(a)**: If cell has stalled DNA replication fork, it implies that it has entered S-phase and G1/S check point is still activated to check the machinery of replication.

13. **(a)**: In diploid cells (somatic cells) during G1 phase, DNA content is 2C and chromosome number is 2n whereas in haploid cells (gamete) during G1 phase, DNA content is 1C and chromosome number is n. S phase is marked by replication of DNA and the amount of DNA per cell is doubled i.e., it becomes 4C in somatic cells, whereas chromosome number remains same i.e., 2n. Thus, a somatic cell which has just completed S phase, will have 4CDNA content but 2n chromosome number, while the gamete cell has 1 C DNA content and n chromosome number.

14. **(d)**: In the G2 and M phase of the cell cycle, the amount of DNA in a cell remains at 4C level when the initial amount is denoted as 2C. In M-phase, both 4C and 2C of DNA are present in different stages. S phase marks the period during which the amount of DNA in the cell doubles.

15. **(a)**

16. **(b)**

17. **(b)**: During S phase or synthetic phase the replication of DNA takes place. For replication of DNA, histone proteins are required so they are also synthesized during this phase. It takes about 30% – 50% of the total cell cycle.

18. **(b)**

19. **(b)**

20. **(a)**

21. **(c)**

22. **(c)** : Pairing of homologous chromosomes characteristic of meiotic cell division.

23. **(b)**

24. **(a)**: Mitosis is divided into four phases : prophase, metaphase, anaphase and telophase. During prophase the indistinct and interwined DNA molecules condenses to form elongated chromosomes. The nuclear membrane disintegrates during prometaphase. During metaphase, the chromosomes align themselves at the equatorial plate. During anaphase, centromere of each chromosome divides into two so that each chromosome comes to have its own centromere. Chromatids move towards opposite poles along the path of their chromosome fibres. Finally during telophase, two chromosome groups reorganise to form two nuclei. Nuclear envelope reappears, Golgi complex and endoplasmic reticulum are reformed.

Option (c) also gives the correct sequence of events but it misses step II (nuclear membrane disassembly). Hence, is ruled out as best appropriate answer is option (a).

25. (b): During anaphase in mitosis, sister chromatids segregate at opposite poles. Therefore, a defective APC will affect chromosome segregation.

26. (d): Small disc-shaped structures at the surface of the centromeres are called kinetochores. These structures serve as the sites of attachment of spindle fibres to the chromosomes that are moved into position at the centre of the cell.

27. (b): Synapsis is the process of association of homologous chromosomes. It takes place during zygotene stage of prophase I of meiosis. This stage is not seen during mitosis.

28. (c): The figure given in the question shows a stage of mitotic cell division called as telophase stage. The individual chromosomes are no longer seen and chromatin material tends to collect in a mass at the two poles. This is the stage which shows the following key events:

Chromosomes cluster at opposite spindle poles and their identity is lost as discrete elements.

Nuclear envelope assembles around the chromosome clusters.

Nucleolus, Golgi complex and ER reform.

29. (a): In metaphase, chromosomes consisting of two sister chromatids get arranged at equator. Discontinuous fibres radiate out from two spindle poles and get connected to the disc shaped structure at the surface of the centromere called kinetochores. These are known as chromosome fibres or tractile fibrils. A kinetochore is a complex protein structure that is analogous to a ring for the microtubule hook; it is the point where microtubules attach themselves to the chromosome.

30. (b)

31.(d) : The plane of alignment of the chromosomes at metaphase is referred to as the metaphase plate. The key features of metaphase are, (1) Spindle fibres attach to kinetochores of chromosomes (2) Chromosomes are moved to spindle equator and get aligned along metaphase plate through spindle fibres to both poles.

32. (c): The key feature of metaphase is the attachment of spindle fibres to kinetochores of chromosomes. Kinetochores are disc-shaped structures at the surface of the centromeres. These structures serve as the sites of attachment of spindle fibres to the chromosomes that are moved into position.

33. (d): During early prophase of mitosis, nucleus and cell become spheroid. Viscosity and refractivity of cytoplasm increases. DNA molecules condense to form shortened chromosome. Endoplasmic reticulum and nucleolus starts disappearing.

34. (c)

35. (a): Metaphase is the best time to count and study the number and morphology of chromosomes. The distinctly visible chromosome arrange themselves at the equatorial or metaphasic plate. The centromeres lie at the equatorial plate while the limbs are placed variously according to their size and spiral arrangement. At prophase the chromosomes appear thin and filamentous, forming a network. So they are not very clearly visible. At telophase the chromosomes uncoil and lengthen and therefore are not clearly seen.

Anaphase also shows chromosomes distinctly and they can be counted. But during anaphase chromatids separate and start moving towards opposite pole. So for counting chromosomes metaphase is the best stage.

36. **(c)**: M phase or mitotic phase is the actual division phase and formation of contractile ring and formation of phragmoplast precedes reformation of nuclear envelope. Contractile ring is belt-like bundle of actin and myosin that appears during cell division immediately below the plasma membrane. Contraction of this ring leads to the separation of the two daughter cells.

Phragmoplast is the region of plant cell cytoplasm that becomes evident in the latter stages of mitosis. It forms from the residual microtubules of the polar mitotic spindle and appears to function in transporting materials to the new cell plate forming between the daughter cells. Once the cell plate is complete, the phragmoplast is divided and gradually disappears, the cell plate finally becoming transformed into the middle lamella lying between the new cell walls.

37. **(b)**: A spindle of fine fibres begins to develop during prophase. It consists of microtubules which are made of protein called tubulin and certain other associated proteins. These delicate fibres radiate from the centriole and constitute aster.

As actin is involved as contractile machinery in many non muscle cells. Myoglobin is present in muscles which can bind to oxygen.

38. **(b)**: Mitosis occurs both in somatic cells as well as in germ cells of the gonads. In plants mitosis occurs in the meristematic cells of root tip or shoot tip. These cells divide at a faster rate. So the root tip shows active cell division and are used in the laboratory to study mitosis.

39. **(c)**

40. **(c)**: Microtubules are unbranched hollow submicroscopic tubules of protein tubulin which develop on specific nucleating regions and can undergo quick growth or dissolution at their ends by assembly or disassembly of monomers. Microtubules form spindle during cell division. Centrioles help in cell division by forming spindle poles or microtubules. In animal cells, microfilament collect in the middle region of the cell below the cell membrane. They induce the cell membrane to invaginate.

In plant cells, cell plate is formed to separate the two daughter cells. Some of the spindle fibres called interzonal microtubules are deposited around phragmoplast. Vesicles from Golgi apparatus are deposited and coalesce on the phragmoplast to form a cell plate.

41. **(c)**: Mitosis is an equational division where after division each cell produces two daughter cells, therefore after 7 divisions one cell will give 128 cells in case of mitosis.

$$1 \xrightarrow{1} 2 \xrightarrow{2} 4 \xrightarrow{3} 8 \xrightarrow{4} 16 \xrightarrow{5} 32 \xrightarrow{6} 64 \xrightarrow{7} 128$$

42. **(a)**: In apical meristems mitotic divisions occur at a rapid rate. In late telophase of mitosis, a nuclear membrane appears on the outside from either pieces of nuclear envelope or endoplasmic reticulum. The telophase may last as long as the prophase.

43. **(a)**: The centrioles occur in nearly all animal cells and in motile plant cells, such as zoospores of algae, sperm cells of ferns, and motile algae. They are absent in amoebae, prokaryotic cells, higher gymnosperms and all angiosperms.

44. **(c):** Colchicine is an alkaloid derived from the autumn crocus, Colchicum autumnale. It inhibits spindle formation in cells during mitosis so that chromosomes cannot separate during anaphase, thus inducing multiple sets of chromosomes. Colchicine is used in genetics, cytology, and plant breeding research and also in cancer therapy to inhibit cell division.

45. **(b)**

46. **(d):** Mitotic anaphase differs from metaphase in possessing same number of chromosomes and half number of chromatids. During anaphase of mitosis, chromosomes divide at the point of centromere or kinetochore and thus two sister chromatids are formed which are called as chromosomes. While during metaphase, chromosomes become maximally distinct due to further contraction and thus size of chromosomes is measured at mitotic metaphase.

47. **(d)**: During pachytene stage of prophase I of meiosis, the four chromatids of each bivalent chromosomes become distinct and clearly appear as tetrad. This stage is characterised by the appearance of recombination nodules, the sites at which crossing over occurs between non-sister chromatids of the homologous chromosomes.

48. **(a)**: Anaphase II begins with the simultaneous splitting of the centromere of each chromosome allowing them to move toward opposite poles of the cell.

49. **(d)**: Bivalent is formed during zygotene stage of prophase I. The four chromatids of each bivalent chromosomes become distinct and clearly visible as tetrad during pachytene of prophase I. Terminalisation of chiasmata occur during diakinesis of prophase I. Crossing over is the exchange of genetic material between non-sister chromatids of the homologous chromosomes.

50. **(c):** Pachytene stage of prophase I of meiosis I is characterised by the appearance of recombination nodules, the sites at which crossing over occurs between non sister chromatids of the homologous chromosomes.

51. **(b):** Meiosis II is similar to mitosis . However, there is no "S' phase in meiosis II. DNA replication occurs during S-phase of interphase.

52. **(d):** Anaphase II begins with the simultaneous splitting of the centromere of each chromosome allowing them to move toward opposite poles of the cell by shortening of microtubules attached to kinetochores.

53. **(d)**

54. **(c):** During diplotene in prophase I of meiosis I dissolution of the nucleoprotein synaptonemal complex occurs.

55. **(b)**

56. **(b)**

57. **(b):** During diplotene, the nucleoprotein fusion complex of synapsed chromosomes dissolves partially therefore homologous chromosomes separate except in the region of crossing over.

58. **(a)**

59. **(c):** Crossing over is a process of exchange of genetic material or chromatid segments between two homologous chromosomes. It is initiated during pachytene stage of meiosis.

60. **(d):** Prophase-I of meiosis has been divided into five substages which occur in the sequence as : Leptotene $\rightarrow$ Zygotene $\rightarrow$ Pachytene $\rightarrow$Diplotene $\rightarrow$ Diakinesis.

Synapsis i.e. pairing of homologous chromosomes occurs during zygotene Crossing over i.e., exchange of chromatid segments occurs during pachytene. Terminalisation of chiasmata i.e., shifting of chiasmata towards the ends of chromosomes and complete disappearance of nucleolus take place during diakinesis.

61. **(d)**

Synapsis aligns homologous chromosomes	–	Zygotene
Synthesis of RNA and protein	–	G_2 phase
Action of enzyme recombinase	–	Pachytene
Centromeres do not separate but chromatids move towards opposite poles	–	Anaphase I

62. **(a)**: Pachytene stage is characterized by the appearance of recombination nodules, the sites at which crossing over occurs between non-sister chromatids of the homologous chromosomes. Nodules contain multi enzyme complex called recombinase. Recombinase is made of endonuclease, exonuclease, unwindase, R-protein, etc.

63. **(a):** During zygotene stage chromosomes start pairing together and this process of association is called synapsis. Such paired chromosomes are called homologous chromosomes. Electron micrographs of this stage indicate that chromosome synapsis is accompanied by the formation of complex structure called synaptonemal complex. The complex formed by a pair of synapsed homologous chromosomes is called a bivalent or a tetrad.

64. **(a)**

65. **(c):** During gamete formation, the enzyme recombinase participates during pachytene stage of prophase I. This stage is characterized by the appearance of recombination nodules, the sites at which crossing over occurs between non-sister chromatids of the homologous chromosomes. Crossing over is the exchange of genetic material between two homologous chromosomes. Crossing over is also an enzyme-mediated process and the enzyme involved is called recombinase.

66. **(a):** The given figure shows crossing over i.e., exchange of segments between two homologous chromosomes. Crossing over is characteristic of meiosis and occurs during pachytene stage of prophase I.

67. **(c):** During anaphase I, from each tetrad two chromatids of a chromosome move as a unit (dyad) to one pole of a spindle and the remaining two chromatids of its homologue migrate to the opposite pole. Thus, the homologous chromosomes of each pair, rather than the chromatids of a chromosome, are separated. As a result, half of the chromosomes, which appear in early prophase, go to each pole. Thus the paternal and maternal chromosomes of each homologous pair segregate during anaphase I independently of the other chromosomes.

68. **(c):** During zygotene or zygonema of meiotic prophase I the chromosomes become shorter and thicker. The homologous chromosomes come to lie side-by-side in pairs. This pairing of homologous chromosomes is known as synapsis. A pair of homologous chromosomes lying together is called a bivalent.

69. **(d):** Crossing over is responsible for inducing variability. It involves an exchange of equal segments of non-sister chromatids belonging to two different but homologous chromosomes. Crossing over takes place at four stranded stage. Only two of the four chromatids take part in crossing over. The other two are called non crossovers. Zygotene is characterized by pairing of homologous chromosomes which is called synapsis.

70. **(b)**: Meiosis involves exchange of genes between homologous chromosomes. So the gametes produced are genetically different from each other. Offsprings produced by the fusion of gametes therefore also show recombinations or genetic variations. These variations in the offsprings make organisms more adaptable to the environment and these have a definite role in evolution.

71. **(d)**: Meiosis II is shorter than the typical mitotic division because of the shortening of prophase of this division. The division maintains the number of chromosomes produce at the end of reduction division. Hence, it is called homotypic or equational division, though it is similar to mitosis. The main function of homotypic division or meiosis II is to separate the chromatids of univalent chromosomes which differ from each other in their linkage groups due to crossing over.

72. **(a)**: Number of chromatids at metaphase is two each in mitosis and meiosis. Chromatid is a half chromosome during duplication in early prophase and metaphase of mitosis and between diplotene and the second metaphase of meiosis. After these stages chromatids are called a daughter chromosomes.

73. **(a)**: In meiosis, the daughter cells differ from parent cell as well as amongst themselves due to segregation, independent assortment and crossing over. Daughter cells inhibit variations. Meiosis leads to recombinations or new combinations of genes or characters as a result of crossing over. Due to these recombinations, variations are created, which have role in process of evolution.

74. **(c)**: The two divisions of meiosis are called the first and the second meiotic divisions. In meiosis I, the number of chromosomes are reduced from diploid to haploid condition, whereas in meiosis II, the two chromatids of each chromosomes separate from each other and go to separate daughter cells, as a result the number of chromosomes remains the same as produced by meiosis I.

Chapter : 11 PHOTOSYNTHESIS IN HIGHER PLANTS

EARLY EXPERIMENTS

1. One scientist cultured Cladophora in a suspension of Azotobacter and illuminated the culture by splitting light through a prism. He observed that bacteria accumulated mainly in the region of ***(Odisha NEET 2019)***
(a) violet and green light
(b) indigo and green light
(c) orange and yellow light
(d) blue and red light.

2. Oxygen is not produced during photosynthesis by ***(2018)***
(a) Green sulphur bacteria
(b) Nostoc
(c) Cycas
(d) Chara.

3. Anoxygenic photosynthesis is characteristic of ***(2014)***
(a) Rhodospirillum (b) Spirogyra
(c) Chlamydomonas (d) Ulva.

4. Oxygenic photosynthesis occurs in ***(2009)***
(a) Oscillatoria (c) Chlorobium
(b) Rhodospirillum (d) Chromatium.

WHERE DOES PHOTOSYNTHESIS TAKE PLACE?

5. Stroma in the chloroplasts of higher plant contains ***(2009)***
(a) light-dependent reaction enzymes
(b) ribosomes
(c) chlorophyll
(d) light-independent reaction enzymes.

HOW MANY TYPES OF PIGMENTS ARE INVOLVED IN PHOTOSYNTHESIS?

6. Emerson's enhancement effect and Red drop have been instrumental in the discovery of ***(NEET-I 2016)***
(a) photophosphorylation and cyclic electron transport
(b) oxidative phosphorylation
(c) photophosphorylation and non-cyclic electron transport
(d) two photosystems operating simultaneously.

7. Chromatophores take part in ***(2015)***
(a) movement (b) respiration
(c) photosynthesis (d) growth.

8. Which fractions of the visible spectrum of solar radiations are primarily absorbed by carotenoids of the higher plants? ***(2003)***
(a) Blue and green (b) Green and red
(c) Red and violet (d) Violet and blue

9. Which element is located at the centre of the porphyrin ring in chlorophyll? ***(2003)***
(a) Calcium (b) Magnesium
(c) Potassium (d) Manganese

10. Chlorophyll a molecule at its carbon atom 3 of the pyrrole ring II has one of the following ***(1997)***
(a) carboxylic group (b) magnesium
(c) aldehyde group (d) methyl group

11. The core metal of chlorophyll is ***(1997)***
(a) Ni (b) Cu (c) Fe (d) Mg.

12. Chlorophyll a occurs in ***(1992)***
(a) all photosynthetic autotrophs
(b) in all higher plants
(c) all oxygen liberating autotrophs
(d) all plants except fungi.

13. Photosynthetic pigments found in the chloroplasts occur in ***(1991)***
(a) thylakoid membranes (b) plastoglobules
(c) matrix (d) chloroplast envelope.

WHAT IS LIGHT REACTION?

14. The reaction centre in PS II has an absorption maxima at ***(2023)***
(a) 660 nm (b) 780 nm
(c) 680 nm (d) 700 nm.

15. Which of the following is not a product of light reaction of photosynthesis? ***(2018)***
(a) ATP (b) NADH
(c) NADPH (d) Oxygen

16. Which of the following absorb light energy for photosynthesis? ***(2002)***
(a) Chlorophyll (b) Water molecule
(c) O_2 (d) RuBP

17. The first step for initiation of photosynthesis will be ***(2000)***
(a) photolysis of water
(b) excitement of chlorophyll molecules due to absorption of light
(c) ATP formation
(d) glucose formation.

18. NADPH2 is generated through ***(1997)***
(a) photosystem II (b) anaerobic respiration
(c) glycolysis (d) photosystem I.

19. Which of the following pigments acts as a reactioncentre during photosynthesis? ***(1994)***
(a) Carotene (b) Phytochrome
(c) P_{700} (d) Cytochrome

THE ELECTRON TRANSPORT

20. Which of the following combinations is required for chemiosmosis? ***(2023)***
(a) Proton pump, electron gradient, ATP synthase
(b) Proton pump, electron gradient, NADP synthase
(c) Membrane, proton pump, proton gradient, ATP synthase
(d) Membrane, proton pump, proton gradient, NADP synthase

21. Which one of the following is not true regarding the release of energy during ATP synthesis through chemiosmosis? It involves ***(2022)***
(a) breakdown of proton gradient
(b) breakdown of electron gradient
(c) movement of protons across the membrane to the stroma
(d) reduction of NADP to $NADPH_2$ on the stroma side of the membrane.

22. In light reaction, plastoquinone facilitates the transfer of electrons from ***(2020)***
(a) PS-II to $Cytb_6f$ complex
(b) $Cytb_6f$ complex to PS-I
(c) PS-I to $NADP^+$
(d) PS-I to ATP synthase.

23. In a chloroplast the highest number of protons are found in ***(NEET-I 2016)***
(a) intermembrane space
(b) antennae complex
(c) stroma
(d) lumen of thylakoids.

24. Read the following four statements (A - D). ***(Mains 2012)***

(A) Both photophosphorylation and oxidative phosphorylation involve uphill transport of protons across the membrane.

(B) In dicot stems, a new cambium originates from cells of pericycle at the time of secondary growth.

(C) Stamens in flowers of Gloriosa and Petunia are polyandrous.

(D) Symbiotic nitrogen fixers occur in free-living state also in soil.

How many of the above statements are right?
(a) Two (b) Three
(c) Four (d) One

25. Which one of the following is essential for photolysis of water? ***(Mains 2011)***
(a) Manganese (b) Zinc
(c) Copper (d) Boron

26. Read the following four statements, (i), (ii), (iii) and (iv) and select the right option having both correct statements. ***(Mains 2010)***

Statements :

(i) Z scheme of light reaction takes place in presence of PSI only.

(ii) Only PSI is functional in cyclic photophosphorylation.

(iii) Cyclic photophosphorylation results into synthesis of ATP and $NADPH_2$.

(iv) Stroma lamellae lack PSII as well as NADP.

(a) (ii) and (iv) (b) (i) and (ii)
(c) (ii) and (iii) (d) (iii) and (iv)

27. Cyclic photophosphorylation results in the formation of ***(2009)***

(a) ATP and NADPH (b) ATP, NADPH and O_2
(c) ATP (d) NADPH.

28. Electrons from excited chlorophyll molecule of photosystem II are accepted first by ***(2008)***

(a) quinone (b) ferredoxin
(c) cytochrome-b (d) cytochrome-f.

29. The first acceptor of electrons from an excited chlorophyll molecule of photosystem II is ***(2007)***

(a) iron-sulphur protein
(b) ferredoxin
(c) quinone
(d) cytochrome.

30. In photosystem I, the first electron acceptor is ***(2006)***

(a) an iron-sulphur protein
(b) ferredoxin
(c) cytochrome
(d) plastocyanin.

31. Which one of the following concerns photophosphorylation? ***(2003)***

(a) $ADP + AMP \xrightarrow{\text{Light energy}} ATP$
(b) $ADP + \text{Inorganic } PO_4 \xrightarrow{\text{Light energy}} ATP$
(c) $ADP + \text{Inorganic } PO_4 \longrightarrow ATP$
(d) $AMP + \text{Inorganic } PO_4 \xrightarrow{\text{Light energy}} ATP$

32. In photosynthesis energy from light reaction to dark reaction is transferred in the form of ***(2002)***

(a) ADP (b) ATP
(c) RuDP (d) chlorophyll.

33. Which pigment system is inactivated in red drop? ***(2001)***

(a) PS-I and PS-II (b) PS-I
(c) PS-II (d) None of these

34. During light reaction of photosynthesis, which of the following phenomenon is observed during cyclic phosphorylation as well as non-cyclic phosphorylation? ***(1994)***

(a) Release of O_2
(b) Formation of ATP
(c) Formation of NADPH
(d) Involvement of PS I and PS II pigment systems

35. A photosynthesising plant is releasing ^{18}O more than the normal. The plant must have been supplied with ***(1993)***

(a) O_3 (b) H_2O with ^{18}O
(c) CO_2 with ^{18}O (d) $C_6H_{12}O_6$ with ^{18}O

36. Photosystem II occurs in ***(1992)***

(a) stroma (b) cytochrome
(c) grana (d) mitochondrial surface.

37. $NADP^+$ is reduced to NADPH in ***(1988)***

(a) PS I
(b) PS II
(c) Calvin cycle
(d) noncyclic photophosphorylation.

WHERE ARE THE ATP AND NADPH USED ?

38. How many ATP and $NADPH_2$ are required for the synthesis of one molecule of glucose during Calvin cycle? ***(2023)***

(a) 12 ATP and 16 $NADPH_2$
(b) 18 ATP and 16 $NADPH_2$
(c) 12 ATP and 12 $NADPH_2$
(d) 18 ATP and 12 $NADPH_2$

39. Which of the following statements is incorrect? ***(2021)***

(a) Cyclic photophosphorylation involves both PSI and PS II.

(b) Both ATP and NADPH + H^+ are synthesised during non-cyclic photophosphorylation.

(c) Stroma lamellae have PS I only and lack NADP reductase.

(d) Grana lamellae have both PSI and PS II.

40. In photosynthesis, the light-independent reactions take place at ***(2015)***

(a) photosystem II (b) stromal matrix

(c) thylakoid lumen (d) photosystem I.

41. Which one of the following organisms is correctly matched with its three characteristics? ***(Mains 2012)***

(a) Pea: C_3 pathway, endospermic seed, vexillary aestivation

(b) Tomato: twisted aestivation, axile placentation, berry

(c) Onion: bulb, imbricate aestivation, axile placentation

(d) Maize: C_3 pathway, closed vascular bundles, scutellum

42. PGA as the first CO_2 fixation product was discovered in photosynthesis of ***(2010)***

(a) bryophyte (b) gymnosperm

(c) angiosperm (d) alga.

43. The chemiosmotic coupling hypothesis of oxidative phosphorylation proposes that adenosine triphosphate (ATP) is formed because ***(2008)***

(a) a proton gradient forms across the inner membrane

(b) there is a change in the permeability of the inner mitochondrial membrane toward adenosine diphosphate (ADP)

(c) high energy bonds are formed in mitochondrial proteins

(d) ADP is pumped out of the matrix into the intermembrane space.

44. Chemiosmotic theory of ATP synthesis in the chloroplasts and mitochondria is based on ***(2005)***

(a) membrane potential

(b) accumulation of Na^+ ions

(c) accumulation of K^+ ions

(d) proton gradient.

45. In C_3 plants, the first stable product of photosynthesis during the dark reaction is ***(2004)***

(a) malic acid

(b) oxaloacetic acid

(c) 3-phosphoglyceric acid

(d) phosphoglyceraldehyde.

46. For assimilation of one CO_2 molecule, the energy required in form of ATP and $NADPH_2$ are ***(2000)***

(a) 2 ATP and 2 $NADPH_2$

(b) 5 ATP and 3 $NADPH_2$

(c) 3 ATP and 2 $NADPH_2$

(d) 18 ATP and 12 $NADPH_2$.

47. For the synthesis of one glucose molecule the Calvin cycle operates for ***(2000)***

(a) 2 times (b) 4 times

(c) 6 times (d) 8 times.

48. Carbon dioxide acceptor in C_3-plants is ***(1999)***

(a) PGA (b) PEP

(c) RuDP (d) none of these.

49. The mechanism of ATP formation both in chloroplast and mitochondria is explained by ***(1997)***

(a) chemiosmotic theory

(b) Munch's hypothesis (mass flow model)

(c) relay pump theory of Godlewski

(d) Cholodny-Went's model.

50. What will be the number of Calvin cycles to generate one molecule of hexose? ***(1996)***

(a) 8 (b) 9 (c) 4 (d) 6

51. The primary acceptor, during CO_2 fixation in C_3 plants, is ***(1995)***

(a) phosphoenolpyruvate (PEP)

(b) ribulose 1,5-diphosphate (RuDP)

(c) phosphoglyceric acid (PGA)

(d) ribulose monophosphati (RMP).

52. The carbon dioxide acceptor in Calvin cycle/. C_3-plants is ***(1993)***
(a) phosphoenol pyruvate (PEP)
(b) ribulose 1, 5-diphosphate (RuDP)
(c) phosphoglyceric acid (PGA)
(d) ribulose monophosphate (RMP).

53. Which technique has helped in investigation of Calvin cycle? ***(1991)***
(a) X-ray crystallography
(b) X-ray technique
(c) Radioactive isotope technique
(d) Intermittent light

54. Dark reactions of photosynthesis occur in ***(1991)***
(a) granal thylakoid membranes
(b) stromal lamella membranes
(c) stroma outside photosynthetic lamellae
(d) periplastidial space

55. Carbon dioxide joins the photosynthetic pathway in ***(1988)***
(a) PS I (b) PS II
(c) light reaction (d) dark reaction.

THE C_4 PATHWAY

56. Given below are two statements : ***(2022)***

Statement I : The primary CO_2 acceptor in C_4 plants is phosphoenol pyruvate and is found in the mesophyll cells.

Statement II : Mesophyll cells of C_4 plants lack RuBisCO enzyme.

In the light of the above statements, choose the correct answer from the options given below :
(a) Both statement I and statement II are correct.
(b) Both statement I and statement II are incorrect.
(c) Statement I is correct but statement II is incorrect.
(d) Statement I is incorrect but statement II is correct.

57. What is the role of large bundle sheath cells found around the vascular bundles in C_4 plants? ***(2022)***
(a) To provide the site for photorespiratory pathway
(b) To increase the number of chloroplast for the operation of Calvin cycle
(c) To enable the plant to tolerate high temperature
(d) To protect the vascular tissue from high light intensity

58. The first stable product of CO_2 fixation in sorghum is ***(2021)***
(a) phosphoglyceric acid
(b) pyruvic acid
(c) oxaloacetic acid
(d) succinic acid.

59. Phosphoenol pyruvate (PEP) is the primary CO_2 acceptor in ***(2017)***
(a) C_4 plants (b) C_2 plants
(c) C3 and C_4 plants (d) C_3 plants.

60. A plant in your garden avoids photorespiratory losses, has improved water use efficiency, shows high rates of photosynthesis at high temperatures and has improved efficiency of nitrogen utilisation. In which of the following physiological groups would you assign this plant? ***(NEET-I 2016)***
(a) CAM (b) Nitrogen fixer
(c) C_3 (d) C_4

61. Bundle sheath cells **(Karnataka NEET 2013)**
(a) are rich in PEP carboxylase
(b) lack RuBisCO
(c) lack both RuBisCO and PEP carboxylase
(d) are rich in RuBisCO.

62. CAM helps the plants in ***(2011)***
(a) conserving water (b) secondary growth
(c) disease resistance (d) reproduction.

63. In kranz anatomy, the bundle sheath cells have ***(Mains 2011)***

(a) thin walls, many intercellular spaces and no chloroplasts
(b) thick walls, no intercellular spaces and large number of chloroplasts
(c) thin walls, no intercellular spaces and several chloroplasts
(d) thick walls, many intercellular spaces and few chloroplasts.

64. Study the pathway given below. ***(Mains 2010)***

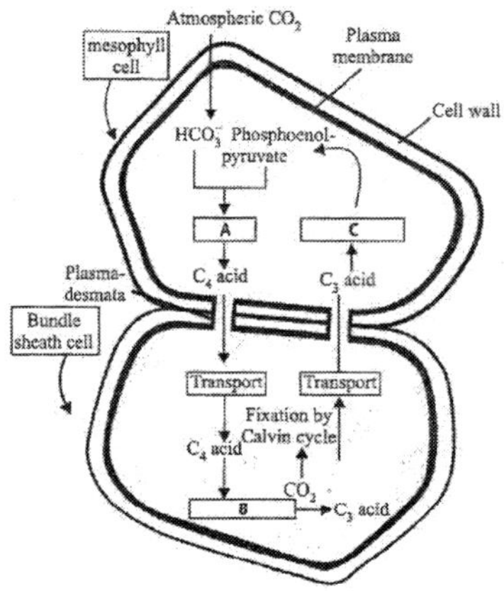

In which of the following options correct words for all the three blanks A, B and C are indicated?

	A	B	C
(a)	Decarboxylation	Reduction	Regeneration
(b)	Fixation	Transamination	Regeneration
(c)	Fixation	Decarboxylation	Regeneration
(d)	Carboxylation	Decarboxylation	Reduction

65. Kranz anatomy is one of the characteristics of the leaves of ***(Mains 2010)***

(a) potato (b) wheat
(c) sugarcane (d) mustard.

66. The C4 plants are photosynthetically more efficient than C_3 plants because ***(2008)***

(a) the CO_2 efflux is not prevented
(b) they have more chloroplasts
(c) the CO_2 compensation point is more
(d) CO_2 generated during photorespiration is trapped and recycled through PEP carboxylase.

67. In leaves of C_4 plants, malic acid synthesis during CO_2 fixation occurs in ***(2008)***

(a) bundle sheath (b) guard cells
(c) epidermal cells (d) mesophyll cells.

68. In the leaves of C4 plants, malic acid formation during CO_2 fixation occurs in the cells of ***(2007)***

(a) bundle sheath (b) phloem
(c) epidermis (d) mesophyll.

69. As compared to a C3-plant, how many additional molecules of ATP are needed for net production of one molecule of hexose sugar by C4-plants? ***(2005)***

(a) Two (b) Six
(c) Twelve (d) Zero

70. Photosynthesis in C_4 plants is relatively less limited by atmospheric CO_2 levels because (2005)

(a) effective pumping of CO_2 into bundle sheath cells
(b) RuBisCO in C_4 plants has higher affinity for CO_2
(c) four carbon acids are the primary initial CO2 fixation products
(d) the primary fixation of CO_2 is mediated via PEP carboxylase.

71. In sugarcane plant $^{14}CO_2$ is fixed to malic acid, in which the enzyme that fixes CO_2 is ***(2003)***

(a) ribulose biphosphate carboxylase
(b) phosphoenol pyruvic acid carboxylase
(c) ribulose phosphate kinase
(d) fructose phosphatase.

72. Stomata of CAM plants ***(2003)***

(a) are always open
(b) open during the day and close at night
(c) open during the night and close during the day
(d) never open.

73. Which pair is wrong? ***(2001)***

(a) C_3-maize
(b) C_4-kranz anatomy
(c) Calvin cycle-PGA
(d) Hatch and Slack cycle - OAA

74. Which is the first CO_2 acceptor enzyme in C_4 plants? ***(2000)***
(a) RuDP carboxylase (b) Phosphoric acid
(c) RuBisCO (d) PEP- carboxylase

75. In C_4 plants, CO_2 combines with ***(1996)***
(a) phosphoenol pyruvate
(b) phosphoglyceraldehyde
(c) phosphoglyceric acid
(d) ribulose diphosphate.

76. In C_4 plants, CO_2 fixation is done by ***(1996)***
(a) sclerenchyma
(b) chlorenchyma and hypodermis
(c) mesophyll cells
(d) guard cells.

77. Which one is a C_4-plant? ***(1993)***
(a) Papaya (b) Pea
(c) Potato (d) Maize/corn

78. The enzyme that catalyses carbon dioxide fixation in C_4 plants is ***(1992)***
(a) RuBP carboxylase
(b) PEP carboxylase
(c) carbonic anhydrase
(d) carboxydismutase.

79. The first carbon dioxide acceptor in C4-plants is ***(1992,1990)***
(a) phosphoenol-pyruvate
(b) ribulose 1, 5-diphosphate
(c) oxaloacetic acid
(d) phosphoglyceric acid.

80. Kranz anatomy is typical of ***(1990)***
(a) C_4 plants (b) C_3 plants
(c) C_2 plants (d) CAM plants.

81. In C_4 plants, Calvin cycle operates in ***(1989)***
(a) stroma of bundle sheath chloroplasts
(b) grana of bundle sheath chloroplasts
(c) grana of mesophyll chloroplasts
(d) stroma of mesophyll chloroplasts.

PHOTORESPIRATION

82. The oxygenation activity of RuBisCO enzyme in photorespiration leads to the formation of ***(2020)***
(a) 2 molecules of 3-C compound
(b) 1 molecule of 3-C compound
(c) 1 molecule of 6-C compound
(d) 1 molecule of 4-C compound and 1 molecule of 2-C compound

83. The process which makes major difference between C_3 and C_4 plants is ***(NEET-II 2016)***
(a) glycolysis (b) Calvin cycle
(c) photorespiration (d) respiration.

84. A process that makes important difference between C_3 and C_4 plants is ***(2012)***
(a) transpiration (b) glycolysis
(c) photosynthesis (d) photorespiration.

85. The correct sequence of cell organelles during photorespiration is ***(2012)***
(a) chloroplast, Golgi bodies, mitochondria
(b) chloroplast, rough endoplasmic reticulum, dictyosomes
(c) chloroplast, mitochondria, peroxisome
(d) chloroplast, vacuole, peroxisome.

86. C_4 plants are more efficient in photosynthesis than C_3 plants due to ***(2010)***
(a) higher leaf area
(b) presence of larger number of chloroplasts in the leaf cells
(c) presence of thin cuticle
(d) lower rate of photorespiration.

87. Which one of the following is wrong in relation to photorespiration? ***(2003)***
(a) It occurs in chloroplast.
(b) It occurs in day time only.
(c) It is a characteristic of C_4 plants.
(d) It is a characteristic of C_3 plants.

88. Photorespiration is favoured by ***(1996)***
(a) high temperature and low O_2
(b) high humidity and temperature
(c) high O_2 and low CO_2
(d) high CO_2 and low O_2.

89. The substrate for photorespiration is *(1989)*
(a) phosphoglyceric acid
(b) glycolate
(c) serine
(d) glycine.

FACTORS AFFECTING PHOTOSYNTHESIS

90. With reference to factors affecting the rate of photosynthesis, which of the following statements is not correct? *(2017)*
(a) Increasing atmospheric CO_2 concentration up to 0.05% can enhance CO_2 fixation rate.
(b) C_3 plants respond to higher temperature with enhanced photosynthesis while C_4 plants have much lower temperature optimum.
(c) Tomato is a greenhouse crop which can be grown in CO_2-enriched atmosphere for higher yield.
(d) Light saturation for CO_2 fixation occurs at 10% of full sunlight.

91. Plants adapted to low light intensity have *(2004)*
(a) larger photosynthetic unit size than the sun plants
(b) higher rate of CO_2 fixation than the sun plants
(c) more extended root system
(d) leaves modified to spines.

92. The rate of photosynthesis is higher in *(1999)*
(a) very high light (b) continuous light
(c) red light (d) green light.

93. 'The law of limiting factors' was proposed by *(1996)*
(a) Liebig (b) Hatch and Slack
(c) Blackman (d) Arnon.

ANSWER KEY

1.	(d)	2.	(a)	3.	(a)	4.	(a)	5.	(d)	6.	(d)	7.	(c)
8.	(d)	9.	(b)	10.	(d)	11.	(d)	12.	(c)	13.	(a)	14.	(c)
15.	(b)	16.	(a)	17.	(b)	18.	(d)	19.	(c)	20.	(c)	21.	(b)
22.	(a)	23.	(d)	24.	(a)	25.	(a)	26.	(a)	27.	(c)	28.	(a)
29.	(c)	30.	(a)	31.	(b)	32.	(b)	33.	(c)	34.	(b)	35.	(b)
36.	(c)	37.	(d)	38.	(d)	39.	(a)	40.	(b)	41.	(c)	42.	(d)
43.	(a)	44.	(d)	45.	(c)	46.	(c)	47.	(c)	48.	(c)	49.	(a)
50.	(d)	51.	(b)	52.	(b)	53.	(c)	54.	(c)	55.	(d)	56.	(a)
57.	(b)	58.	(c)	59.	(a)	60.	(d)	61.	(d)	62.	(a)	63.	(b)
64.	(c)	65.	(c)	66.	(b)	67.	(d)	68.	(d)	69.	(c)	70.	(d)
71.	(b)	72.	(c)	73.	(a)	74.	(d)	75.	(a)	76.	(c)	77.	(d)
78.	(b)	79.	(a)	80.	(a)	81.	(a)	82.	(b)	83.	(c)	84.	(d)
85.	(c)	86.	(d)	87.	(c)	88.	(c)	89.	(b)	90.	(b)	91.	(a)
92.	(c)	93.	(c)										

HINTS & EXPLANATIONS

1. (d)

2. (a) : Green sulphur bacteria do not have the ability to use water as an electron donor (or cannot oxidise water), instead they perform photosynthesis using sulfide. Therefore, they do not evolve oxygen during photosynthesis.

3.(a) : In Rhodospirillum, electron donor is organic compound instead of water hence no oxygen is released, i.e, anoxygenic photosynthesis occurs. In other plants water is used as electron donor and H^+ and O_2 are produced during photolysis of water.

4. (a) : Oscillatoria is a filamentous cyanobacteria which performs oxygenic photosynthesis because of the presence of chlorophyll-a like eukaryotic algae and higher plants. Others are examples of sulphur bacteria.

5. (d): The dark reactions of photosynthesis are purely enzymatic and slower than the primary photochemical reaction. They take place in stroma portion of the chloroplast and are independent of light, i.e,, they can occur either in presence or in absence of light provided that assimilatory power is available.

6. (d): Emerson et al. (1957) found that if light of shorter wavelengths was provided at the same time as the longer red wavelengths, photosynthesis was even faster than the sum of the two rates with either colour alone. This synergism or enhancement became known as the Emerson enhancement effect. The two separate groups of pigments or photosystems cooperate in photosynthesis-long red wavelengths are absorbed only by one photosystem, called photosystem I (PS I) and the second photosystem, photosystem II (PS II), absorbs wavelengths shorter than 690 nm, and for maximum photosynthesis wavelengths absorbed by both systems must function together. The two photosystems normally cooperate to cause photosynthesis at all wavelengths shorter than 690 nm, because both photosystems absorb those wavelengths. The importance of Emerson's work is that it suggested the presence of two distinct photosystems.

7.(c) : Chromatophores are the internal membrane systems of photosynthetic forms which possess photosynthetic pigments. They occur in photoautotrophic bacteria, e.g., purple bacteria and green bacteria.

8. (d) : Carotenoids of higher plants are fat soluble compounds that include carotenes and xanthophylls. Most of them absorb light of violet and blue range. Green light is absorbed in less amount.

9. (b) : Chlorophyll is the green pigment present in plants and some photosynthetic bacteria. The empirical formula of chlorophyll-a molecule is $C_{55}H_{72}O_5N_4Mg$. It consist of a porphyrin head and a phytol tail. Porphyrin is a cyclic tetrapyrrole structure, having a magnesium atom in the centre. Tail consists of phytol alcohol and it is attached with one of the pyrrole rings.

10. (d) : The empirical formula of chlorophyll a molecule is $C_{55}H_{72}O_5N_4Mg$. It has tadpole like configuration. It consisis of a porphyrin head and a phytol tail. Porphyrin is a cyclic tetrapyrrole structure, having a magnesium atom in the centre. In chlorophyll a, a methyl group (CH_3) is attached to the third carbon in the porphyrin head.

11. (d)

12.(c) : Chlorophyll-a occurs in all photosynthesizing plants except bacteria. Chlorophyll-a is common to all organisms that possess chlorophyll (the only one in blue green algae) and is believed to be specifically required. In a few photosynthetic bacteria other kinds of chlorophyll, bacteriochlorophylls occur.

13.(a) : Photosynthetic pigments are found in the thylakoid membrane of chloroplasts. The grana lamellae are paired to form sac like structures and form thylakoids. Chlorophylls and other photosynthetic pigments are confined to grana.

14.(c) : PS II has an absorption maxima at 680 nm and is called P680. In PS II, the reaction centre chlorophyll a absorbs 680 nm wavelength of red light causing electrons to become excited and jump into an orbit farther from atomic nucleus.

15.(b) :In light reaction of photosynthesis, ATP, NADPH and oxygen are produced. NADPH participates in anabolic reactions (e.g., photosynthesis) that consume energy in order to build up larger molecules. NADH participates in catabolic reactions (e.g., respiration) that break down molecules to release energy.

16.(a) :Photosynthesis occurs in chloroplasts that contain photosynthetic pigments - chlorophylls, carotenoids, etc. The light energy required for photosynthesis comes from sunlight. The sunlight travels in the form of small particles called photons. Each photon has a quantum of energy. This quantum of energy is absorbed by a single antenna chlorophyll and then migrates from one molecule to the other till it reaches the reaction center of photosystems. The reaction center is also P700 chlorophyll molecule that releases electron as a result of transferred energy. This electron is transferred between various acceptors and generates ATP and NADPH2 in the light reaction of photosynthesis.

17.(b) : The process of photosynthesis involves two steps-

(i) Light dependent phase or photochemical reaction.

(ii) Light independent phase or dark reaction.

Light reaction occurs in grana fraction of chloroplast and in this reaction are included those activities, which are dependent on light.

The grana of chloroplasts contains many collaborating molecules of pigment. A quantum of light is absorbed by a single antenna chlorophyll, then it migrates from one molecule to the other till it reaches the reaction center. This quantum of light is used for generating ATP and NADPH, which is later consumed in dark reactions produce sugars by fixing CO_2 molecules.

18. (d)

19.(c) : There are two photochemical complexes, known as photosystem I and II. PSII absorbs far red light of wavelengths greater than $680 nm$ and PSI absorbs red light of wavelengths greater than 700 nm. Both these complexes are involved in light reactions of photosynthesis.

20.(c) : Chemiosmosis requires a membrane, a proton pump, a proton gradient and ATP synthase.

21. (b)

22.(a) After excitement, e– is passed from PS-II (P680) to primary electron acceptor (Pheophytin). From primary e^- acceptor, e^- is passed to plastoquinone. Plastoquinone (PQ) in turn transfer its e^- to $Cytb_6f$ complex. Therefore plastoquinone facilitiates the transfer of electrons from PS-II to Cyt b_6 f complex.

23. (d)

24.(a) : Polyandrous condition (having large and indefinite number of stamens) is present in Gloriosa (Family Liliaceae) and Petunia (Family Solanaceae).

Nitrogen fixation is the conversion of inert atmospheric nitrogen into utilisable compounds of nitrogen like nitrate, ammonia, amino acids, etc. Biological nitrogen fixation is performed by free living and symbiotic bacteria and cyanobacteria. Symbiotic nitrogen fixers occur in association with roots of higher plants. For example Rhizobium is nitrogen fixing bacterial symbiont of papilionaceous roots and Frankia is symbiont in root nodules of several non-leguminous plants like Casuarina. Both Rhizobium and Frankia live free as aerobes in the soil and develop the ability to fix nitrogen only as symbionts when they become anaerobic.

25.(a) : Manganese (Mn^{2+}) is used for photolysis of water to produce oxygen and electrons during light reaction of photosynthesis. It is the phenomenon of breaking up of water into hydrogen and oxygen in the illuminated chloroplast.

26. (a): Z scheme involves both PSI and PSII to transfer electron excited by light starting from PSII uphill to the acceptor, down to the electron transport chain to PSI, which further comprise of excitation of electrons, transfer to another acceptor and finally down hill to NADP+ causing reduction of it to NADPH + H^+. Cyclic photophosphorylation results only in synthesis of ATP not of NADPH + H^+. Stroma lamella contains PSI only.

27. (c)

28.(a) : The electrons released during photolysis of water are picked up by P680 photocentre of photosystem II. The electron extruded by the photocentre of photosystem II picked up by the quencher phaeophytin. From here the electron passes over a series of carriers in a downhill journey losing its energy at every step. The major carriers are plastoquinone (PQ), cytochrome b-f complex and plastocyanin (PC). While passing over cytochrome complex, the electron loses sufficient energy for the creation of proton gradient and synthesis of ATP from ADP and inorganic phosphate. The process is called photophosphorylation (noncyclic).

29. (c)

30. (a)

31.(b) : The light dependent production of ATP from ADP+Pi in the chloroplasts is called photophosphorylation. Photophosphorylation is of 2 types - Cyclic photophosphorylation - It involves only PS-I, water is not utilised and so no oxygen is evolved. Here two ATP molecules are produced. Non-cyclic photophosphorylation - It involves both PS-I and PS-II, water is utilised and so oxygen is evolved. Here one ATP molecule and one $NADPH_2$ molecule are produced.

32. (b): Photosynthesis consists of light dependent phase and light independent phase or dark reaction. Light dependent phase occurs in grana fraction of chloroplast. It involves cyclic and non-cyclic photophosphorylation where assimilatory powers (ATP and NADPH2) are produced. In dark reaction, which occurs in stroma fraction of chloroplast, actual reduction of CO_2 to carbohydrates takes place using the assimilatory powers (ATP and $NADPH_2$) produced in the light dependent phase. It needs 18ATP and 12NADPH2 molecules to produce one molecule of glucose.

33.(c) : Emerson and Lewis worked on Chlorella and calculated the quantum yield for different wavelengths. Emerson observed that rate of photosynthesis declines in the red region of the spectrum. This decline in photosynthesis is called "Red drop". It was observed that the quantum yield falls when the light of wavelengths more than 680 or 690 nm are supplied. As the PS-II P680 is driven by red light, so it remains inactive during red drop.

34. (b)

35.(b) : Water molecule breaks up into hydrogen and oxygen in the illuminated chloroplasts. This is called photolysis of water. If a photosynthesising plant is releasing ^{18}O more than the normal, the plant must have been supplied with H_2O with ^{18}O.

36.(c) : Photosystem II has almost equal number of chlorophyll a and chlorophyll b molecules. It is dark green in colour and located mostly in the appressed parts of grana thylakoids towards the inner surface of membranes.

37.(d) : Non-cyclic photophosphorylation involves both PS-I and PS-II. Here electrons are not cycled back and are used in the reduction of NADP to $NADPH_2$. The electrons generated by PSII are passed over a series of electron carriers in a downhill journey and handed over to reaction centre of PSI. PSI again passes the electrons to $NADP^+$ which combines with H^+ ions to form NADPH.

38.(d) : In Calvin cycle, 3 molecules of ATP and 2NADPH2 are required for every CO_2 molecules for entering the cycle. For one molecule of glucose, 6 turns of the cycle are required. Thus, 18ATP and $12NADPH_2$ are required for the synthesis of one molecule of glucose during Calvin cycle.

39.(a) :Non-cyclic photophosphorylation involves both PSI and PSII.

40.(b) :The light-independent reactions (dark or Blackman's reactions) of photosynthesis take place in stroma or matrix of chloroplasts. These reactions are enzymatic reactions which catalyse assimilation of CO_2 into carbohydrates.

41. (c)

42.(d) : Calvin, Benson and their colleagues in California, U.S.A. fed Chlorella and Scenedesmus with radioactive ^{14}C in carbon dioxide. Radioactive carbon, ^{14}C has a half life of 5568 years. Therefore, the path of CO_2 fixation can be easily traced with its help. Algal suspension, illuminated and carrying out photosynthesis with normal carbon dioxide, was supplied $^{14}CO_2$. The alga was killed at intervals in near boiling methanol. It immediately stopped photosynthesis activity due to denaturation of enzymes. Alcohol was evaporated and after crushing the alga, the product was made into paste. The paste was placed on paper chromatogram and the different compounds were separated by two dimensional chromatography. The radioactive compounds were identified by comparing their position on the chromatogram with standard chemicals. Calvin and co-workers found that after three seconds, radioactivity appeared in phosphoglyceric acid or PGA. Phosphoglyceric acid is, therefore, the first stable product of photosynthesis.

43.(a) : The chemiosmotic coupling hypothesis of oxidative phosphorylation proposed by Mitchell, explains the process of ATP formation and states that it is linked to development of a proton gradient across a membrane. ATP synthase, required for ATP synthesis is located in F1 particles present in the inner mitochondrial membrane and becomes active only when there is high concentration of proton on F0 side as compared to F1 side. The flow of proton through F0 channel induces F1 particle to function as ATP synthase and the energy of proton gradient produces ATP by attaching a phosphate radical to ADP.

44.(d) : Chemiosmotic coupling hypothesis is the most widely accepted explanation for oxidative phosphorylation in mitochondria and photophosphorylation in thylakoid membranes. Mitchell proposed the idea of chemiosmotic coupling. He suggested that a concentration gradient of protons is established across the mitochondrial membrane because there is an accumulation of hydrogen ions on one side of the mitochondrial membrane. The proton accumulation is necessary for energy transfer to the endergonic ADP phosphorylation process.

45.(c) : The Calvin cycle is also known as C_3 cycle because CO2 reduction is cyclic process and first stable product in this cycle is a 3-C compound (i.e., 3-phosphoglyceric acid or 3-PGA). In this cycle, CO_2 acceptor molecule is RuBP or RuDP (i.e., Ribulose 1, 5-biphosphate or Ribulose 1, 5-diphosphate). There occurs covalent bonding of CO_2 to RuBP and the enzyme catalyzing this reaction is RuBP-carboxylase/oxygenase (RuBisCO).

46.(c) : In Calvin cycle, CO_2 acceptor molecule is RuBP or RuDP. The enzyme catalyzing this reaction is RuBPcarboxylase/oxygenase (RuBisCO). As Calvin cycle takes in only one carbon (as CO_2) at a time, so it takes six turns of the cycle to produce a net gain of six carbons (i.e., hexose or glucose). In this cycle, for formation of one mole of hexose sugar (Glucose), 18ATP and 12NADPH$_2$ are used. For 6 molecules of CO_2 it needs 18ATP and 12NADPH$_2$ molecules so for assimilation of one molecule of CO_2 it needs 3 ATP and 2NADPH$_2$ molecules.

47. (c)

48.(c) : The Calvin cycle is also known as C_3 cycle because CO_2 reduction is cyclic process and first stable product in this cycle is a 3-C compound (i.e., 3-phosphoglyceric acid or 3 -PGA). In this cycle, CO_2 acceptor molecule is RuBP or RuDP (i.e., Ribulose 1, 5-biphosphate or Ribulose 1, 5-diphosphate). There occurs covalent bonding of CO_2 to RuBP and the enzyme catalyzing this reaction is RuBP-carboxylase/oxygenase (RuBisCO).

49. (a)

50. (d)

51. (b)

52. (b)

53.(c) : By employing ^{14}C labelled carbon dioxide $^{14}CO_2$ in photosynthesis and observing the appearance of characteristic radiations in different reaction intermediates and product in different experiments, Calvin and his co-workers were able to formulate the complete metabolic path of carbon assimilation in the form of cycle which is called Calvin cycle.

54.(c) : The dark reactions of photosynthesis are purely enzymatic and slower than the primary photochemical reaction. They take place in stroma portion of the chloroplast and independent of light, i.e., they can occur either in presence or in absence of light provided that assimilatory power is available.

55. (d): The dark reactions or Blackman's reactions or biosynthetic phase involves three steps:

(i) Fixation of CO_2, (ii) Reduction of CO_2 and (iii) Synthesis of other compound from glucose. It is independent of light. Pigment System I is relatively very weakly fluorescent while pigment system II is strongly fluorescent. Light energy absorbed by pigment in the two systems is ultimately trapped by the P_{700} and P_{680}. Light reaction is associated with the grana of the chloroplasts. It takes place in the presence of light only.

56.(a) : In C_4 plants, the primary CO_2 acceptor is a 3-carbon molecule phosphoenol pyruvate (PEP) and is present in the mesophyll cells. The enzyme responsible for the fixation is PEP carboxylase or PEPcase. Mesophyll cells of C_4 plants lack RuBisCO enzyme whereas bundle sheath cells are rich in an enzyme ribulose bisphosphate carboxylase- oxygenase (RuBisCO).

57. (b)

58. (c) : Sorghum is an example of C_4 plant, so the first stable product of CO_2 fixation in this plant is oxaloacetic acid.

59. (a)

60. (d)

61. (d)

62.(a) : Crassulacean acid metabolism (CAM) is photosynthesis by the C_4 pathway in which carbon- dioxide is taken up during the night, when the plant's stomata are open and fixed into malic acid. During the day, when the stomata are closed, carbon dioxide is released from malic acid for use in the Calvin cycle. This is important for plants that live in arid conditions as it enables them to keep their stomata closed during the day to reduce water loss from evaporation. Crassulacean acid metabolism is common in succulent plants of desert regions, including cacti and in certain ferns.

63.(b) : The C_4 plants are adapted to dry tropical regions and have greater productivity of biomass. They have special type of leaf anatomy known as kranz anatomy. In this type of anatomy the bundle sheath cells form several layers around the vascular bundles; they are characterised by having a large number of chloroplasts, thick walls impervious to gaseous exchange and no intercellular spaces

64. (c)

65. (c): In kranz anatomy, the mesophyll is undifferentiated and its cells occur in concentric layers around vascular bundles Vascular bundles are surrounded by large sized bundle sheath cells which are arranged in a wreath-like manner in one to several layers. C_4 plants, both monocots and dicots, such as sugarcane, maize, sorghum have kranz anatomy in leaf.

66.(b) : C_4 plants are photosynthetically more efficient than C_3 plants because C_4 plants contain two types of chloroplast, i.e., bundle sheath chloroplast and mesophyll chloroplast. So such plants operate a dicarboxylic acid cycle in addition to Calvin cycle. CO_2 acceptor molecule (PEP) is present in large bundle sheath cell which has higher efficiency in picking up CO_2. Thus, photosynthesis continues even at low CO_2 concentration and the rate of photorespiration is also negligible.

67.(d) :C_4 plants show kranz anatomy, i.e., the mesophyll is undifferentiated and its cells occur in concentric layers around vascular bundle, which is surrounded by large sized bundle sheath cells, in a wreath like manner. In this type of plants, the initial fixation of CO_2 occur in mesophyll cell. The primary acceptor (phosphoenol pyruvate) combines with CO_2 to form oxaloacetic acid which later reduces to malic acid. Malic acid is then translocated to bundle sheath cell for further decarboxylation.

68. (d)

69.(c) : In C_4 plants, 12 ATP molecules are required for producing one hexose sugar. In the bundle sheath cells, C_3 cycle operates which requires 18ATP and 12NADPH$_2$ molecules. So total 30ATP and 12NADPH$_2$ molecules are required in C_4 cycle, whereas in C_3 cycle 18ATP and 12NADPH$_2$ molecules are required.

70. (d)

71.(b) :C_4 pathway was first reported in members of Family Gramineae (grasses) like sugarcane, maize, sorghum, etc. In C_4 plants, PEP case (PEP carboxylase) is the key enzyme used to fix CO_2 in C_4 plants. Oxaloacetic acid is a 4-C compound and is the first stable product so this pathway is known as C_4 cycle.

Phosphoenol pyruvic acid + Carbon dioxide

$$\xrightarrow{\text{PEP-carboxylase}} \text{Oxaloacetic acid}$$

72.(c) : Stomata of most plants open at sunrise and close in darkness to allow the entry of CO_2 needed for photosynthesis during the daytime. Certain succulents that are native to hot, dry conditions (e.g., cacti, Kalanchoe, and Bryophyllum) act in an opposite manner. They open their stomata at night, fix carbon dioxide into organic acids in the dark, and close their stomata during the day. This is an appropriate way to absorb CO_2 through open stomata at night, when transpiration stress is low, and conserve water during the heat of the day. These plants show Crassulacean Acid Metabolism (CAM).

73.(a) :C_4 pathway was first reported in members of Family Gramineae (grasses) like sugarcane, maize, sorghum, etc.

74.(d) : In C_4 plants, PEP case (PEP carboxylase) is the key enzyme used to fix CO_2 in C4 plants. Oxaloacetic acid is a 4 -C compound and is the first stable product so this pathway is known as C_4 cycle.

Phosphoenol pyruvic acid + Carbon dioxide

$$\xrightarrow{\text{PEP-carboxylase}} \text{Oxaloacetic acid}$$

75. (a)

76.(c) : The C_4 plants have a characteristic leaf anatomy called kranz anatomy. Here two types of chloroplasts are present - bundle sheath chloroplasts and mesophyll chloroplasts. In C_4 plants, there are two carboxylation reactions which occur first in mesophyll chloroplasts and then in bundle sheath chloroplasts. CO_2 acceptor molecule in mesophyll chloroplasts is PEP (Phosphoenol pyruvate) and not Ribulose 1, 5-biphosphate. Further it has enzyme PEP-carboxylase for initial CO_2 fixation. RuBP-carboxylase is absent in mesophyll chloroplasts but is present in bundle sheath chloroplasts. The first product formed is oxaloacetic acid and hence it is known as C_4 cycle. Bundle sheath cells fix CO_2 through C_3 cycle.

77. (d)

78. (b)

79.(a) :In C_4 cycle, CO_2 combines with phosphoenol pyruvic acid to form oxaloacetic acid with the help of enzyme phosphoenol pyruvate carboxylase (PEPcase). The oxaloacetic acid breaks up into pyruvic acid and CO_2 combines with RuBP to form PGA as in Calvin cycle.

80. (a)

81. (a)

82.(b) :During photorespiration in C_3 plants, some O_2 does bind to RuBisCO and RuBP instead of being converted to 2 molecules of PGA binds with O_2 to form one molecule of phosphoglycerate (3 Carbon) and phosphoglycolate (2 Carbon).

83.(c) :Photorespiration is the light dependent process of oxygenation of ribulose biphosphate (RuBP) and release of carbon dioxide by the photosynthetic organs of a plant. It leads to oxidation of considerable amount of photosynthetic products to CO_2 and H_2O without the production of useful energy. Photorespiration occurs only in C_3 plants because at high temperature and high oxygen concentration RuBP carboxylase changes to

RuBP oxygenase. Photorespiration is absent in C_4 plants. Peroxisome and mitochondria are required for completing the process.

84. (d)

85. (c)

86. (d) : Rate of net photosynthesis in C_3 plants is 15-35mg CO_2 dm2/hr while in C_4 plants is 40-80 mg CO/dm2/hr. This variation in rate is due to photorespiration. Photorespiration is an inhibitory process which decreases the rate of photosynthesis. In excess of oxygen RuBP carboxylase converts to RuBP oxygenase. As a result glycolate synthesis is enhanced and leads to begin photorespiration. Photorespiration is negligible or absent in C_4 plants and present only in C_3 plants. So C_4 plants are photosynthetically more efficient.

87. (c)

88. (c)

89. (b)

90.(b) : C_4 plants respond to higher temperature with enhanced photosynthesis while C_3 plants have lower temperature optimum.

91.(a) :To absorb more sunlight (quantitatively), the plants growing in low light conditions have larger photosynthetic unit size. It means that they have more number of chlorophyll molecules per reaction center to trap more light energy available to them.

92.(c) :Plants can use a small portion of light which falls upon them. Chlorophyll- a and chlorophyll- b absorb too much light in the blue and red region. Carotenoids absorb light mostly in the blue region of spectrum of light. In monochromatic lights, maximum photosynthesis occurs in red light, followed by blue light and poor photosynthesis in green light. Under very high light intensity solarisation phenomenon occurs. It involves photooxidation of different cellular components including chlorophyll.

93.(c) :Blackman (1905) gave the law of limiting factors which states that when a process is conditioned as to its rapidity by a number of separate factors, the rate of the process is limited by the pace of the slowest process. It is the factor which is present in minimum amount.

Chapter : 12 RESPIRATION IN PLANTS

GLYCOLYSIS

1. Given below are two statements : One is labelled as Assertion (A) and the other is labelled as Reason (R) : Assertion (A) : ATP is used at two steps in glycolysis. Reason (R) : First ATP is used in converting glucose into glucose-6-phosphate and second ATP is used in conversion of fructose-6-phosphate into fructose-1-6-diphosphate.

   In the light of the above statements, choose the correct answer from the options given below: ***(2023)***

   (a) (A) is true but (R) is false.
   (b) (A) is false but (R) is true.
   (c) Both (A) and (R) are true and (R) is the correct explanation of (A).
   (d) Both (A) and (R) are true but (R) is not the correct explanation of (A).

2. Conversion of glucose to glucose-6-phosphate, the first irreversible reaction of glycolysis, is catalysed by ***(2019)***
   (a) phosphofructokinase
   (b) aldolase
   (c) hexokinase
   (d) enolase.

3. What is the role of NAD+ in cellular respiration? ***(2019)***
   (a) It functions as an enzyme.
   (b) It functions as an electron carrier.
   (c) It is a nucleotide source for ATP synthesis.
   (d) It is the final electron acceptor for anaerobic respiration.

4. In glycolysis, during oxidation electrons are removed by ***(2004)***
   (a) ATP
   (b) glyceraldehyde-3-phosphate
   (c) NAD+
   (d) molecular oxygen.

5. At the end of glycolysis, six carbon compound ultimately changes into ***(1996)***
   (a) ethyl alcohol (b) acetyl Co-A
   (c) pyruvic acid (d) ATP.

6. The first phase in the breakdown of glucose, in animal cell, is ***(1994)***
   (a) fermentation (b) Krebs' cycle
   (c) glycolysis (d) ETS

7. End product of glycolysis is ***(1990)***
   (a) acetyl CoA
   (b) pyruvic acid
   (c) glucose 1-phosphate
   (d) fructose 1-phosphate.

FERMENTATION

8. What amount of energy is released from glucose during lactic acid fermentation? ***(2022)***
   (a) Approximately 15% (b) More than 18%
   (c) About 10% (d) Less than 7%

9. In which one of the following processes CO_2 is not released? ***(2014)***
   (a) Aerobic respiration in plants
   (b) Aerobic respiration in animals
   (c) Alcoholic fermentation
   (d) Lactate fermentation

10. The energy-releasing metabolic process in which substrate is oxidised without an external electron acceptor is called ***(2010, 2008)***
    (a) glycolysis (b) fermentation
    (c) aerobic respiration (d) photorespiration.

11. In alcohol fermentation ***(2003)***
    (a) triose phosphate is the electron donor while acetaldehyde is the electron acceptor
    (b) triose phosphate is the electron donor while pyruvic acid is the electron acceptor
    (c) there is no electron donor
    (d) oxygen is the electron acceptor.

12. The end product of fermentation are ***(1997)***

(a) O_2 and C_2H_5 OH

(b) CO_2 and acetaldehyde

(c) CO_2 and O_2

(d) CO_2 and C2 H_5 OH.

13. Which of the following products are obtained by anaerobic respiration from yeast? ***(1996)***

(a) Beer and wine (b) Alcohols

(c) CO_2 (d) All of these

14. When yeast ferments glucose, the products obtained are ***(1994)***

(a) ethanol and CO_2 (b) methanol and CO_2

(c) ethanol and water (d) water and CO_2

AEROBIC RESPIRATION

15. Match List I with List II : ***(2023)***

List I	List II
A. Oxidative decarboxylation	I. Citrate synthase
B. Glycolysis	II. Pyruvate dehydrogenase
C. Oxidative phosphorylation	III. Electron transport system
D. Tricarboxylic acid cycle	IV. EMP pathway

Choose the correct answer from the options given below:

(a) A-III, B-I, C-II, D-IV (b) A-II, B-IV, C-III, D-I

(c) A-III, B-IV, C-II, D-I (d) A-II, B-IV, C-I, D-III

16. The number of substrate level phosphorylations in one turn of citric acid cycle is ***(2020)***

(a) zero (b) one

(c) two (d) three.

17. Where is respiratory electron transport system (ETS) located in plants ? ***(Odisha NEET 2019)***

(a) Mitochondrial matrix

(b) Outer mitochondrial membrane

(c) Inner mitochondrial membrane

(d) Intermembrane space

18. Which of these statements is incorrect? (2018)

(a) Enzymes of TCA cycle are present in mitochondrial matrix.

(b) Glycolysis occurs in cytosol.

(c) Glycolysis operates as long as it is supplied with NAD that can pick up hydrogen atoms.

(d) Oxidative phosphorylation takes place in (outer mitochondrial membrane.

19. Which statement is wrong for Krebs' cycle? ***(2017)***

(a) There is one point in the cycle where FAD+ is reduced to $FADH_2$.

(b) During conversion of succinyl CoA to succinic acid, a molecule of GTP is synthesised.

(c) The cycle starts with condensation of acetyl group (acetyl CoA) with pyruvic acid to yield citric acid.

(d) There are three points in the cycle where NAD^+ is reduced to $NADH+H^+$.

20. Oxidative phosphorylation is ***(NEET-II 2016)***

(a) formation of ATP by transfer of phosphate group from a substrate to ADP

(b) oxidation of phosphate group in ATP

(c) addition of phosphate group to ATP

(d) formation of ATP by energy released from electrons removed during substrate oxidation.

21. Cytochromes are found in ***(2015 Cancelled)***

(a) cristae of mitochondria

(b) lysosomes

(c) matrix of mitochondria

(d) outer wall of mitochondria.

22. In mitochondria, protons accumulate in the ***(Mains 2011)***

(a) outer membrane

(b) inner membrane

(c) intermembrane space

(d) matrix.

23. All enzymes of TCA cycle are located in the mitochondrial matrix except one which is located in inner mitochondrial membranes in eukaryotes and in cytosol in prokaryotes. This enzyme is ***(2007)***

(a) isocitrate dehydrogenase
(b) malate dehydrogenase
(c) succinate dehydrogenase
(d) lactate dehydrogenase.

24. In which one of the following do the two names refer to one and the same thing? ***(2003)***
(a) Krebs' cycle and Calvin cycle
(b) Tricarboxylic acid cycle and citric acid cycle
(c) Citric acid cycle and Calvin cycle
(d) Tricarboxylic acid cycle and urea cycle

25. Cytochrome is ***(2001)***

(a) metallo flavo protein
(b) Fe containing porphyrin pigment
(c) glycoprotein
(d) lipid.

26. Which of the following is the key intermediate compound linking glycolysis to the Krebs' cycle? ***(1997)***

(a) Malic acid (b) Acetyl CoA
(c) NADH (d) ATP

27. In Krebs' cycle, the FAD precipitates as electron acceptor during the conversion of ***(1997)***

(a) fumaric acid to malic acid
(b) succinic acid to fumaric acid
(c) succinyl CoA to succinic acid
(d) α-ketoglutarate to succinyl CoA.

28. The correct sequence of electron acceptor in ATP synthesis is ***(1997)***
(a) Cyt. b, c, a3,a (b) Cyt. c,b,a,a3
(c) Cyt. a,a,b,c (d) Cyt. b, c, a, a a3.

29. End product of citric acid cycle/Krebs' cycle is ***(1993)***

(a) citric acid (b) lactic acid
(c) pyruvic acid (d) CO_2 +H_2O.

30. Oxidative phosphorylation is production of ***(1992)***

(a) ATP in photosynthesis
(b) NADPH in photosynthesis
(c) ATP in respiration
(d) NADH in respiration.

31. End products of aerobic respiration are ***(1992)***

(a) sugar and oxygen
(b) water and energy
(c) carbon dioxide, water and energy
(d) carbon dioxide and energy.

32. Terminal cytochrome of respiratory chain which donates electrons to oxygen is ***(1992)***

(a) Cyt b (b) Cyt c
(c) Cyt a1 (d) Cyt a3.

33. Connecting link between glycolysis and Krebs' cycle before pyruvate entering Krebs' cycle is changed to ***(1990)***

(a) oxaloacetate (b) PEP
(c) pyruvate (d) acetyl CoA.

THE RESPIRATORY BALANCE SHEET

34. What is the net gain of ATP when each molecule of glucose is converted to two molecules of pyruvic acid? ***(2022)***

(a) Four (b) Six
(c) Two (d) Eight

35. Which of the following statements is incorrect? ***(2021)***

(a) Oxidation-reduction reactions produce proton gradient in respiration.
(b) During aerobic respiration, role of oxygen is limited to the terminal stage.
(c) In ETC (Electron Transport Chain), one molecule of NADH + H^+ gives rise to 2 ATP molecules, and one $FADH_2$ gives rise to 3 ATP molecules.
(d) ATP is synthesised through complex V.

36. The three boxes in this diagram represent the three major biosynthetic pathways in aerobic respiration. Arrows represent net reactants or products. ***(2007)***

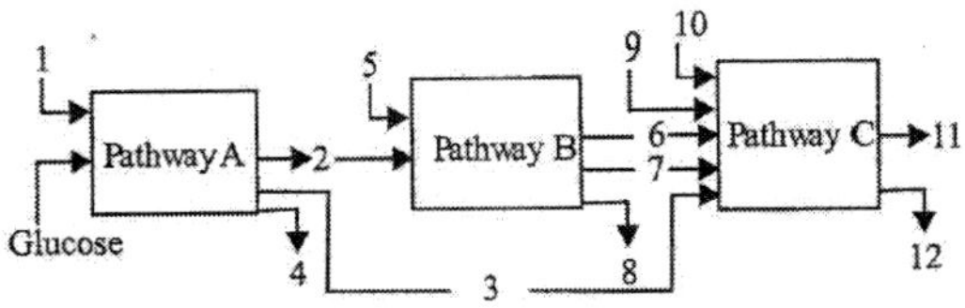

Arrows numbered 4, 8 and 12 can all be

(a) H_2O (b) FAD^+ or $FADH_2$
(c) NADH (d) ATP.

37. The overall goal of glycolysis, Krebs' cycle and the electron transport system is the formation of ***(2007)***

(a) ATP in one large oxidation reaction
(b) sugars
(c) nucleic acids
(d) ATP in small stepwise units.

38. How many ATP molecules could maximally be generated from one molecule of glucose, if the complete oxidation of one mole of glucose to CO_2 and H_2O yields 686 kcal and the useful chemical energy available in the high energy phosphate bond of one mole of ATP is 12kcal ? ***(2006)***

(a) 1 (b) 2
(c) 30 (d) 57

39. During which stage in the complete oxidation of glucose are the greatest number of ATP molecules formed from ADP? ***(2005)***

(a) Glycolysis
(b) Krebs' cycle
(c) Conversion of pyruvic acid to acetyl CoA
(d) Electron transport chain

40. How many ATP molecules are produced by aerobic oxidation of one molecule of glucose? ***(2002)***

(a) 2 (b) 4
(c) 38 (d) 34

41. When one molecule of ATP is disintegrated, what amount of energy is liberated? ***(1996)***

(a) 8kcal (b) 38kcal
(c) 7kcal (d) 4.5kcal

42. The ultimate respiratory substrate, yielding maximum number of ATP molecules, is (1994)

(a) glycogen
(b) ketogenic amino acid
(c) glucose
(d) amylose.

43. Out of 38 ATP molecules produced per glucose, 32 ATP molecules are formed from NADH/FADH F2 in ***(1993)***

(a) respiratory chain
(b) Krebs' cycle
(c) oxidative decarboxylation
(d) EMP.

44. When one glucose molecule is completely oxidised, it changes ***(1992)***

(a) 36ADP molecules into 36ATP molecules
(b) 38ADP molecules into 38ATP molecules
(c) 30ADP molecules into 30ATP molecules
(d) 32ADP molecules into 32ATP molecules.

45. Out of 36 ATP molecules produced per glucose molecule during respiration ***(1992)***

(a) 2 are produced outside glycolysis and 34 during respiratory chain
(b) 2 are produced outside mitochondria and 34 inside mitochondria
(c) 2 during glycolysis and 34 during Krebs' cycle
(d) all are formed inside mitochondria.

AMPHIBOLIC PATHWAY

46. Which of the following biomolecules is common to respiration-mediated breakdown of fats, carbohydrates and proteins? (NEET-II 2016)

(a) Glucose-6-phosphate
(b) Fructose 1, 6-bisphosphate
(c) Pyruvic acid
(d) Acetyl CoA

47. Which of the metabolites is common to respirationmediated breakdown of fats, carbohydrates and proteins? ***(2013)***
(a) Pyruvic acid
(b) Acetyl CoA
(c) Glucose - 6 - phosphate
(d) Fructose 1,6- bisphosphate

48. Aerobic respiratory pathway is appropriately termed ***(2009)***
(a) parabolic(b) amphibolic
(c) anabolic(d) catabolic

49. Plants, but not animals, can convert fatty acids to sugars by a series of reactions called ***(1994)***
(a) photosynthesis (b) Kreb's cycle
(c) glycolysis (d) glyoxylate cycle.

50. Link between glycolysis, Krebs' cycle and β-oxidation of fatty acid or carbohydrate and fat metabolism is ***(1992)***
(a) oxaloacetic acid (b) succinic acid
(c) citric acid (d) acetyl CoA.

RESPIRATORY QUOTIENT

51. Respiratory Quotient (RQ) value of tripalmitin is ***(2019)***
(a) 0.09 (b) 0.9
(c) 0.7 (d) 0.07

52. Apparatus to measure rate of respiration and R.Q. is ***(1992)***
(a) auxanometer (b) potometer
(c) respirometer (d) manometer.

53. R.Q. is ratio of ***(1990)***
(a) CO_2 produced to substrate consumed
(b) CO_2 produced to O_2 consumed
(c) oxygen consumed to water produced
(d) oxygen consumed to CO_2 produced.

ANSWER KEY

1.	(c)	2.	(c)	3.	(b)	4.	(c)	5.	(c)	6.	(c)	7.	(b)
8.	(d)	9.	(d)	10.	(b)	11.	(a)	12.	(d)	13.	(d)	14.	(a)
15.	(b)	16.	(b)	17.	(c)	18.	(d)	19.	(c)	20.	(d)	21.	(a)
22.	(c)	23.	(c)	24.	(b)	25.	(b)	26.	(b)	27.	(b)	28.	(d)
29.	(d)	30.	(c)	31.	(c)	32.	(d)	33.	(d)	34.	(c)	35.	(c)
36.	(d)	37.	(d)	38.	(d)	39.	(d)	40.	(c)	41.	(c)	42.	(c)
43.	(a)	44.	(b)	45.	(b)	46.	(d)	47.	(b)	48.	(b)	49.	(d)
50.	(d)	51.	(c)	52.	(c)	53.	(b)						

HINTS & EXPLANATIONS

1. **(c)** : In glycolysis, ATP is used at two steps : first in the conversion of glucose into glucose-6-phosphate and second in the conversion of fructose 6 phosphate to fructose-1, 6-bisphosphate.

2. **(c)**: Glucose is phosphorylated to glucose-6-phosphate by ATP in presence of enzyme hexokinase and Mg^{2+}.

3. **(b)**: NAD+ is a coenzyme and an electron carrier. It acts as an electron acceptor in glycolysis and Kreb's cycle through dehydrogenation processes and is then reduced to NADH. NAD^+ acts as electron carrier which is later used to generate proton gradient across the inner mitochondrial membrane and produce energy in the form of ATP.

4. **(c)** : During glycolysis, NAD^+ (Nicotinamide adenine dinucleotide) removes electrons from 1, 3-diphosphoglyceric acid using diphosphoglyceraldehyde dehydrogenase. NAD+ changes to $NADH_2$ and this is either utilised as such in anaerobic respiration or in the presence of oxygen.

5. **(c)**: Glycolysis or EMP pathway is the breakdown of glucose to two molecules of pyruvic acid through a series of enzyme mediated reaction releasing energy. Pyruvic acid is a 3-carbon compound. In glycolysis net gain of 2ATP and 2 NADH2 molecules occurs.

   It can be represented in equation form as -

$$C_6H_{12}O_6 + 2ADP + 2Pi + 2NAD \rightarrow$$
$$2CH_3COCOOH + 2ATP + 2NADH_2$$

6. (c): Glycolysis is the first step of glucose breakdown in both animals and plants. During glycolysis 6-carbon glucose molecule is converted into 2 molecules of 2 carbon pyruvic acid. In this process net gain of 2 ATP and 2 $NADH_2$ occurs. It is a common pathway for both aerobic and anaerobic modes of respiration.

7. **(b)**

8. **(d)**: Less than seven percent of the energy in glucose is released from lactic acid fermentation and moreover not all of it is stored as ATP.

9. **(d)**: Anaerobic respiration or fermentation can be of two types, i.e., lactate fermentation and ethanol fermentation. Lactate fermentation produces lactic acid only as pyruvic acid produced in glycolysis is directly reduced by NADH to form lactic acid and no CO_2 is produced. Alcoholic (ethanol) fermentation involves conversion of pyruvate to acetaldehyde, hence, CO_2 is released.

10. **(b)**: Fermentation is the process of deriving energy from the oxidation of organic compounds such as carbohydrates and using an endogenous electron acceptor not external or exogenous, which is usually an organic compound, as opposed to aerobic respiration where electrons are donated to an exogenous electron acceptor, such as oxygen via an electron transport chain.

11. **(a)** :When oxygen is not available (anaerobic condition) yeast and some other microbes convert pyruvic acid into ethyl alcohol. It is a two step process.

    In the first step pyruvic acid is decarboxylated to yield acetaldehyde and CO_2. Pyruvic acid is a 3-C compound and acts as electron donor while acetaldehyde is the electron acceptor.

$$CH_3COCOOH \xrightarrow[\text{carboxylase}]{\text{Pyruvic}} CH_3CHO + CO_2$$

    In the second step acetaldehyde is reduced to ethyl alcohol by $NADH_2$ formed in the glycolysis.

$$CH_3CHO + NADH_2 \xrightarrow[\text{dehydrogenase}]{\text{Alcoholic}} C_2H_5OH + NAD$$

12. (d)

13. (d): In the absence of O_2, fermentation or anaerobic respiration occurs. In this process pyruvic acid forms ethyl alcohol and CO_2.

14.(a) :When oxygen is not available (anaerobic condition) yeast and some other microbes convert pyruvic acid into ethyl alcohol. It is a two step process.

In the first step pyruvic acid is decarboxylated to yield acetaldehyde and CO_2. Pyruvic acid is a 3-C compound and acts as electron donor while acetaldehyde is the electron accceptor.

$$CH_3COCOOH \xrightarrow[\text{carboxylase}]{\text{Pyruvic}} CH_3CHO + CO_2$$

In the second step acetaldehyde is reduced to ethyl alcohol by $NADH_2$ formed in the glycolysis.

$$CH_3CHO + NADH_2 \xrightarrow[\text{dehydrogenase}]{\text{Alcoholic}} C_2H_5OH + NAD$$

15. (b)

16. (b): In citric acid cycle, during the conversion of succinyl-CoA to succinic acid a molecule of GTP is synthesized which is called substrate level phosphorylation.

17. (c)

18. (d) :Oxidative phosphorylation is the synthesis of energy rich ATP molecules with the help of energy liberated during oxidation of reduced coenzymes (NADH, $FADH_2$) produced in respiration. The enzyme required for this synthesis is ATP synthase. It is located in F1 or head piece of F0– F1 or elementary particles present on the inner mitochondrial membrane.

19. (c): Krebs' cycle starts with condensation of acetyl group (acetyl CoA) with oxaloacetate to form a tricarboxylic, 6-carbon compound called citric acid.

20. (d) :Oxidative phosphorylation is the synthesis of energy rich ATP molecules with the help of energy liberated during oxidation of reduced co-enzymes $(NADH, FADH_2)$ produced in respiration.

The enzyme required for this synthesis is called ATP synthase. It is located in F_1 or head piece of F_0– F_1 or elementary particles present in the inner mitochondrial membrane. F_1 particle is capable of ATP synthesis.

ATP synthase becomes active in ATP formation only when there is a proton gradient having higher concentration of H^+ or protons on the F0 side as compared to F1 side. This higher concentration creates an electric potential across the mitochondrial membrane. The proton gradient and membrane electric potential together form proton motive force (PMF). The flow of protons through the F0 channel which induces F1 particle to function as ATP synthase. The energy of the proton gradient is used in attaching a phosphate radicle to ADP by high-energy bond. This produces ATP.

21. (a): Cytochrome is a group of proteins, each with an iron containing haeme group. They are a part of electron transport chain in mitochondria (present in cristae) and chloroplasts (in thylakoids).

22. (c): In respiration, protons accumulate in the intermembrane space of the mitochondria when electrons move through the ETS.

23. (c): Mitochondrion is the organelle which bears various enzymes participating in Krebs' cycle. Each mitochondrion is covered by double membrane. The inner membrane is selectively permeable and forms foldings called cristae. The inner membrane bears oxysomes, enzymes of fatty acids, succinate dehydrogenase (of Krebs' cycle) and electron transport system. All other enzymes of Krebs' cycle are present in the mitochondrial matrix.

24. (b): The reactions of Krebs' cycle were worked out by Sir Hans Krebs, hence the name Krebs' cycle. It involves many 3-C compounds such as citric acid, cis-aconitic acid and iso-citric acid etc., so it is also called TCA cycle or tricarboxylic acid, cycle. It involves formation of citric acid as its first product so it is called citric acid cycle. It involves production of 24 ATP molecules.

25. (b): Cytochromes are electron transferring proteins often regarded as enzymes. They contain iron porphyrin or copper porphyrin as prosthetic groups. Cytochrome a, b and c are harmo-chromogens widely occurring in cells and acting as oxygen carriers during cellular respiration.

26. (b): During glycolysis pyruvic acid is produced from glucose and is oxidatively decarboxylated to form acetyl CoA. This formation of acetyl CoA from pyruvic acid needs a multienzyme complex and 5 essential cofactors, i.e, lipoic acid, CoA, Mg^{2+}, NAD and TPP (thiamine pyrophosphate). It results in production of 2 molecules of CO_2 and 2 molecules of $NADH_2$. This acetyl CoA enters mitochondria and is completely oxidised during Krebs' cycle. Thus acetyl CoA acts as the linker of glycolysis and Krebs' cycle.

27. (b): During Krebs' cycle when succinic acid is oxidised to fumaric acid then the precipitation of FAD as electron acceptor occurs. It is the only Krebs' cycle oxidation that does not employ a pyridine nucleotide. In this, succinate is dehydrogenated by succinate dehydrogenase. This enzyme removes two hydrogen ions and two electrons from succinate and these are then used to reduce FAD to FADH2.

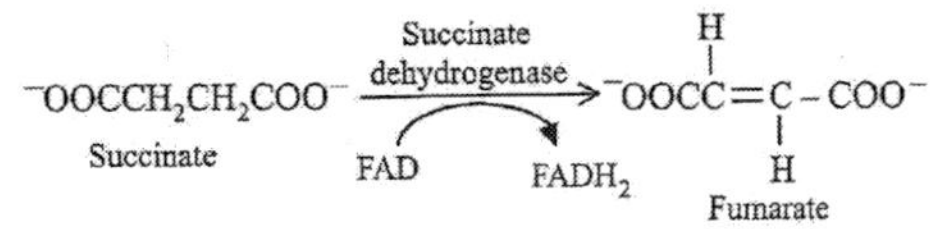

28. (d): Last step of aerobic respiration is oxidation of reduced co-enzymes, i.e., $NADH_2$ and $FADH_2$ by molecular oxygen through FAD, CoQ (ubiquinone), Cyt. b, Cyt. c1, Cyt. c, Cyt. a and Cyt a3. Two hydrogen atoms or electrons move from NADH2 and travel through this ETS chain and finally combine with half molecule of O_2 to form water. During this electron transport F A D and F of different cytochromes are successively reduced and oxidised and at certain points, enough energy is released which is used to bind ADP with Pi to form ATP.

29. (d): The end product of glycolysis is pyruvic acid whereas acetyl CoA is the connecting link between glycolysis and Krebs' cycle. The TCA cycle is a process in which acetyl CoA is oxidised to CO_2 and water. Acetyl CoA combines with oxalo acetic acid to form citric acid. After a series of cyclic reactions OAA is recycled back.

30. (c)

31.(c) :Respiration is an energy liberating enzymatically controlled multistep catabolic process of stepwise breakdown of organic substances (hexose sugar) inside the living cells. Aerobic respiration includes the 3 major process, glycolysis, Krebs' cycle and electrons transport chain. The substrate is completely broken down to form CO_2 and water. A large amount of energy is released stepwise in the form of ATP.

32. (d) : Cytochrome a3 helps in transfer of electron to oxygen. The oxygen has great affinity to accept the electrons and in presence of protons a water molecule is formed.

33. (d)

34. (c): In glycolysis, two molecules of ATP are consumed during two phosphorylation reactions to form fructose 1, 6-bisphosphate. In return, four molecules of ATP are produced by substrate level phosphorylation (conversion of 1, 3-bisphosphoglycerate to 3-phosphoglycerate and phosphoenol pyruvate to pyruvate).

35. (c): In electron transport system, the number of ATF molecules synthesised depends on the nature of electron donor. Oxidation of me molecule of NADH gives rise to 3 molecules of ATP, while one molecule of FADH2 produces 2 molecules of ATP.

36. (d) In the given diagram, pathway A represents glycolysis, pathway B represents Krebs' cycle and pathway C represents oxidative phosphorylation. Arrows numbered 4, and 12 can all be ATP.

37. (d)

38. (d) One mole of ATP liberates 12 kcal of energy. So 686 kcal will be liberated by 686 / 12 = 57.1 ATP molecules.

39. (d) :The last step of aerobic respiration is the oxidation of reduced coenzymes, i.e, NADH2 and FADH2 by molecular oxygen through FAD, ubiquinone, Cyt b, Cyt c, Cyt c1, Cyt a and Cyt a3, By oxidation of 1 molecule of NADH2, 3 ATP molecules are produced and by oxidation of 1 molecule of FADH2, 2 ATP molecules are produced. In glycolysis 2 ATP molecules ard produced from ADP. Further 2 NADH2 produced, give $2 \times 3 =$ 6 ATP, on oxidative phosphorylation. Similarly in Krebs' cycle 2 ATP molecules are produced. So the greatest number of ATA molecules are produced in the electron transport chain.

40.(c) : Energy gain in one complete cycle of aerobi respiration is :

Glycolysis → 2 ATP + $2NADH_2$ = 8 ATP
(or EMP) ↓ ETS
6 ATP
Intermediate step = 2 $NADH_2$ $\xrightarrow{ETS}$ = 6 ATP
Krebs' cycle = 6 $NADH_2$ + 2 $FADH_2$ + 2 ATP = 24 ATP
ETS ↓ ↓ ETS
18 ATP 4 ATP
Total = 38 ATP

In aerobic respiration complete oxidation of one glucose molecule produces 38 ATP molecules. But the number of ATP molecules so produced may vary depending upon the mode of entry of $NADH_2$ in the mitochondria. If the electrons of NADH2 are accepted by malate then each molecule of $NADH_2$ yields 3 ATP molecules and the total would be 38 ATP molecules. But if the electrons of $NADH_2$ are accepted by FAD it yields only 2 ATP molecules making the total of 36 ATP molecules. This type of shuttle occurs in most of the eukaryotic cells.

41.(c) : ATP is adenosine triphosphate. It was discovered by Lohmann in 1929. It consists of a purine, adenine, a pentose sugar (ribose) and a row of three phosphates out of which the last two are attached by high energy bonds. The last phosphate bond yields an energy equivalent of 7 kcal.

42. (c): Glucose is the chief respiratory substrate which yields maximum number of ATP molecules. Glucose is the most common substrate in glycolysis. Any other carbohydrate is first converted into glucose. During glycolysis it changes to pyruvic acid and net gain is of 2 ATP and 2 $NADH_2$ molecules. And later on during Krebs' cycle 30 molecules of ATP are produced. So a total of 38 ATP molecules are produced from 1 mol of glucose during aerobic respiration.

43. (a): During respiratory chain, complete degradation of one glucose molecule produced 38 ATP molecules. NAD and FAD is reduced to NADH / $FADH_2$.

44. (b)

45. (b): During respiration, 36 ATP molecules are produced per glucose molecule. 2 molecules of ATP are produced outside mitochondria, i.e, during glycolysis and other 34 molecules of ATP are produced inside mitochondria from Krebs' cycle.

46. (d): Carbohydrates are usually first converted into glucose before they are used for respiration. Fats are broken down into glycerol and fatty acids first. If fatty acids were to be respired they would first be degraded to acetyl CoA and enter the pathway. Glycerol would enter the pathway after being converted to 3-phosphoglyceraldehyde (PGAL). The proteins are degraded by proteases to individual amino acids (after deamination) and depending on their structure enter the pathway within the Krebs' cycle or as pyruvate or acetyl CoA. Thus, acetyl CoA is the common metabolite of all the three (carbohydrates, proteins and fats).

The given flowchart shows these interrelationships:

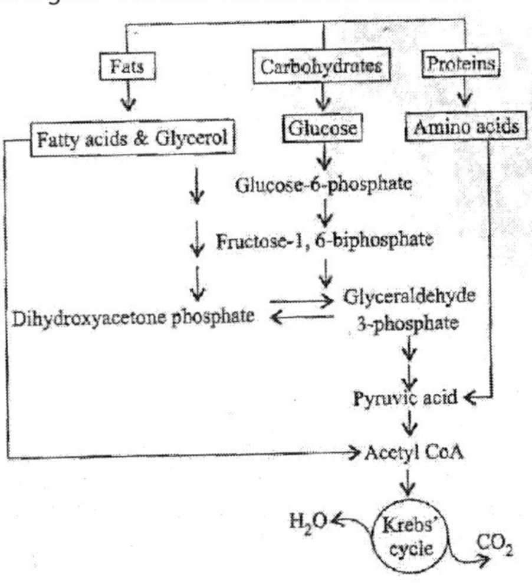

47. (b)

48. (b): A biochemical pathway that serves both anabolic and catabolic process is known as amphibolic pathway. The aerobic respiration involves both catabolism of carbohydrates and fatty acids and the synthesis of anabolic precursors for amino acid synthesis, various intermediatory metabolic products and secondary metabolites. Thus it is called as amphibolic pathway rather than a catabolic pathway.

49. (d): Kornberg and Krebs (1957) gave glyoxylate cycle in Pseudomonas bacteria. It involves conversion of insoluble fats into soluble sugars. This occurs in germinating fatty seeds because plants are not able to transport fats from the endosperm to the root and shoot tissues of the germinating seedling, so they must convert stored lipids to a more mobile form of carbon, generally sucrose.

50. (d): Krebs' cycle is intimately related with fat metabolism. Dihydroxyacetone phosphate produced in glycolysis may be converted into glycerol via glycerol - 3 - phosphate and vice-versa. Glycerol is important constituent of fats. After β-oxidation, fatty acids give rise to active 2-C units, the acetylCoA which may enter the Krebs' cycle. Thus, acetyl-CoA is a link between glycolysis, Krebs' cycle and β-oxidation of fatty acid or carbohydrate and fat metabolism.

51. (c): Respiratory Quotient (RQ) is the ratio of the volume of carbon dioxide produced to the volume of oxygen consumed in respiration over a period of time.

$$RQ = \frac{\text{Volume of } CO_2 \text{ evolved}}{\text{Volume of } O_2 \text{ absorbed}};$$

RQ for fats is about 0.7 .

Tripalmitin $= C_{51}H_{98}O_6$

$$2(C_{51}H_{98}O_6) + 145O_2 \longrightarrow 102CO_2 + 98H_2O$$

$$RQ = 102CO_2 / 145O_2 = 0.7$$

52. (c): Respirometer is an instrument used for measuring R.Q. and rate of respiration. The apparatus consists of a graduated tube attached at right angles to a bulbous respiratory chamber in its upper end. Desired plant material whose R.Q. is to be determined is placed in the respiratory chamber.

53. (b)

Chapter : 13 PLANT GROWTH AND DEVELOPMENT

GROWTH

1. The process of growth is maximum during (2020)
(a) log phase (b) lag phase
(c) senescence (d) dormancy.

2. Typical growth curve in plants is ***(2015 Cancelled)***
(a) stair-steps shaped (b) parabolic
(c) sigmoid (d) linear.

DIFFERENTIATION, DEDIFFERENTIATION AND REDIFFERENTIATION

3. In tissue culture experiments, leaf mesophyll cells are put in a culture medium to form callus. This phenomenon may be called as ***(2023)***
(a) development (b) senescence
(c) differentiation (d) dedifferentiation.

DEVELOPMENT

4. Which one of the following plants does not show plasticity? ***(2022)***
(a) Cotton (b) Coriander
(c) Buttercup (d) Maize

5. Plants follow different pathways in response to environment or phases of life to form different kinds of structures. This ability is called ***(2021)***
(a) maturity (b) elasticity
(c) flexibility (d) plasticity.

6. Senescence as an active developmental cellular process in the growth and functioning of a flowering plant, is indicated in ***(2008)***
(a) annual plants
(b) floral parts
(c) vessels and tracheid differentiation
(d) leaf abscission.

PLANT GROWTH REGULATORS

7. Which hormone promotes internode/petiole elongation in deep water rice? ***(2023)***
(a) Ethylene (b) 2,4-D
(c) GA_3 (d) Kinetin

8. Spraying of which of the following phytohormone on juvenile conifers helps in hastening the maturity period, that leads to early seed production? ***(2023)***
(a) Zeatin
(b) Abscisic Acid
(c) Indole-3-butyric Acid
(d) Gibberellic Acid

9. The gaseous plant growth regulator is used in plants to ***(2022)***
(a) speed up the malting process
(b) promote root growth and root hair formation to increase the absorption surface
(c) help overcome apical dominance
(d) kill dicotyledonous weeds in the fields.

10. Production of cucumber has increased manifold in recent years. Application of which of the following phytohormones has resulted in this increased yield as the hormone is known to produce female flowers in the plants (2022)
(a) ABA (b) gibberellin
(c) ethylene (d) cytokinin

11. The plant hormone used to destroy weeds in a field is ***(2021)***
(a) IBA (b) IAA
(c) NAA (d) 2, 4-D.

12. Name the plant growth regulator which upon spraying on sugarcane crop, increases the length of stem, thus increasing the yield of sugarcane crop. ***(2020)***
(a) Cytokinin (b) Gibberellin
(c) Ethylene (d) Abscisic acid

13. Which of the following is not an inhibitory substance governing seed dormancy? ***(2020)***
(a) Gibberellic acid (b) Abscisic acid
(c) Phenolic acid (d) Para-ascorbic acid

14. It takes very long time for pineapple plants to produce flowers. Which combination of hormones can be applied to artificially induce flowering in pineapple plants throughout the year to increase yield? ***(2019)***
(a) Cytokinin and Abscisic acid
(b) Auxin and Ethylene
(c) Gibberellin and Cytokinin
(d) Gibberellin and Abscisic acid

15. Fruit and leaf drop at early stages can be prevented by the application of ***(2017)***
(a) ethylene (b) auxins
(c) gibberellic acid (d) cytokinins.

16. You are given a tissue with its potential for differentiation in an artificial culture. Which of the following pairs of hormones would you add to the medium to secure shoots as well as roots? ***(NEET-II 2016)***
(a) IAA and gibberellin
(b) Auxin and cytokinin
(c) Auxin and abscisic acid
(d) Gibberellin and abscisic acid

17. The Avena curvature is used for bioassay of ***(NEET-I 2016)***
(a) IAA (b) ethylene
(c) ABA (d) GA_3.

18. Auxin can be bioassayed by ***(2015)***
(a) potometer
(b) lettuce hypocotyl elongation
(c) Avena coleoptile curvature
(d) hydroponics.

19. What causes a green plant exposed to the light, on only one side, to bend towards the source of light as it grows? ***(2015 Cancelled)***
(a) Light stimulates plant cells on the lighted side to grow faster.
(b) Auxin accumulates on the shaded side, stimulating greater cell elongation there.
(c) Green plants need light to perform photosynthesis.
(d) Green plants seek light because they are phototropic.

20. Dr. F. Went noted that if coleoptile tips were removed and placed on agar for one hour, the agar would produce a bending when placed on one side of freshly-cut coleoptile stumps. Of what significance is this experiment? ***(2014)***
(a) It made possible the isolation and exact identification of auxin.
(b) It is the basis for quantitative determination of small amounts of growth-promoting substances.
(c) It supports the hypothesis that IAA is auxin.
(d) It demonstrated polar movement of auxins.

21. Which one of the following growth regulators is known as 'stress hormone'? ***(2014)***
(a) Abscisic acid (b) Ethylene
(c) GA_3 (d) Indole acetic acid

22. During seed germination, its stored food is mobilized by ***(2013)***
(a) ABA (b) gibberellin
(c) ethylene (d) cytokinin.

23. The pineapple which under natural condition is difficult to blossom has been made to produce fruits throughout the year by application of ***(Karnataka NEET 2013)***
(a) NAA, 2, 4-D (b) Phenyl acetic acid
(c) Cytokinin (d) IAA, IBA.

24. Through their effects on plant growth regulators, what do the temperature and light control in the plants? ***(Mains 2012)***
(a) Apical dominance (b) Flowering
(c) Closure of stomata (d) Fruit elongation

25. Which one of the following generally acts as an antagonist to gibberellins? ***(Mains 2012)***
(a) Zeatin (b) Ethylene
(c) ABA (d) IAA

26. Phototropic curvature is the result of uneven distribution of ***(2010)***
(a) gibberellin (b) phytochrome
(c) cytokinins (d) auxin.

27. One of the commonly used plant growth hormone in tea plantations is ***(Mains 2010)***
(a) ethylene (b) abscisic acid
(c) zeatin (d) indole-3-acetic acid.

28. Root development is promoted by ***(Mains 2010)***
(a) abscisic acid (b) auxin
(c) gibberellin (d) ethylene

29. One of the synthetic auxin is ***(2009)***
(a) IAA (b) GA
(c) IBA (d) NAA.

30. Which one of the following acids is a derivative of carotenoids? ***(2009)***
(a) Indole-3-acetic acid (b) Gibberellic acid
(c) Abscisic acid (d) Indole butyric acid

31. Which one of the following pairs, is not correctly matched? ***(2007)***
(a) Gibberellic acid - Leaf fall
(b) Cytokinin - Cell division
(c) IAA - Cell wall elongation
(d) Abscissic acid - Stomatal closure

32. Parthenocarpic tomato fruits can be produced by ***(2006)***
(a) treating the plants with phenylmercuric acetate
(b) removing androecium of flowers before pollen grains are released
(c) treating the plants with low concentrations of gibberellic acid and auxins
(d) raising the plants from vernalized seeds.

33. How does pruning help in making the hedge dense? ***(2006)***
(a) It releases wound hormones.
(b) It induces the differentiation of new shoots from the rootstock.
(c) It frees axillary buds from apical dominance.
(d) The apical shoot grows faster after pruning.

34. Cell elongation in internodal regions of the green plants takes place due to ***(2004)***
(a) indole acetic acid (b) cytokinins
(c) gibberellins (d) ethylene.

35. Coconut milk factor is ***(2003)***
(a) an auxin (b) a gibberellin
(c) abscisic acid (d) cytokinin.

36. Plants deficient of element zinc, show its effect on the biosynthesis of plant growth hormone ***(2003)***
(a) auxin (b) cytokinin
(c) ethylene (d) abscisic acid.

37. Differentiation of shoot is controlled by ***(2003)***
(a) high auxin : cytokinin ratio
(b) high cytokinin : auxin ratio
(c) high gibberellin : auxin ration
(d) high gibberellin : cytokinin ratio.

38. Dwarfness can be controlled by treating the plant with ***(2002,1992)***
(a) cytokinin (b) gibberellic acid
(c) auxin (d) anti-gibberellin.

39. Which of the following prevents the fall of fruits? ***(2001)***
(a) GA_3 (b) NAA
(c) Ethylene (d) Zeatin

40. Hormone responsible for senescence is ***(2001)***
(a) ABA (b) auxin
(c) GA (d) cytokinin.

41. Which hormone breaks dormancy of potato tuber? ***(2001)***
(a) Gibberellin (b) IAA
(c) ABA (d) Zeatin

42. If the apical bud has been removed then we observe ***(2000)***
(a) more lateral branches
(b) more axillary buds
(c) plant growth stops
(d) flowering stops.

43. Which hormone is responsible for fruit ripening? ***(2000)***
(a) Ethylene (b) Auxin
(c) Ethyl chloride (d) Cytokinin

44. ABA is involved in ***(1999)***
(a) shoot elongation
(b) increased cell division
(c) dormancy of seeds
(d) root elongation.

45. A plant hormone used for inducing morphogenesis in plant tissue culture is ***(1998)***
(a) cytokinins (b) ethylene
(c) abscisic acid (d) gibberellins.

47. If the growing plant is decapitated, then ***(1994)***
(a) its growth stops
(b) leaves become yellow and fall down
(c) axillary buds are inactivated
(d) axillary buds are activated.

48. Removal of apical bud results in ***(1993)***
(a) formation of new apical bud
(b) elongation of main stem
(c) death of plant
(d) formation of lateral branching.

49. The regulator which retards ageing/senescence of plant parts is ***(1993)***
(a) cytokinin (b) auxin
(c) gibberellin (d) abscisic acid.

50. The hormone produced during adverse environmental conditions is ***(1993)***
(a) benzyl aminopurine
(b) bichlorophenoxy acetic acid
(c) ethylene
(d) abscisic acid.

51. Which is produced during water stress that brings stomatal closure? ***(1993)***
(a) Ethylene (b) Abscisic acid
(c) Ferulic acid (d) Coumarin

52. Apical dominance is caused by ***(1992)***
(a) abscisic acid in lateral bud
(b) cytokinin in leaf tip
(c) gibberellin in lateral buds
(d) auxin in shoot tip.

53. Cytokinins ***(1992)***
(a) promote abscission
(b) influence water movement
(c) help retain chlorophyll
(d) inhibit protoplasmic streaming.

54. Which is employed for artificial ripening of banana fruits? ***(1992)***
(a) Auxin (b) Coumarin
(c) Ethylene (d) Cytokinin

55. Abscisic acid causes ***(1991)***
(a) stomatal closure (b) stem elongation
(c) leaf expansion (d) root elongation.

56. The hormone responsible for apical dominance is ***(1991)***
(a) IAA (b) GA
(c) ABA (d) Florigen.

57. Hormone primarily connected with cell division is ***(1991,1988)***
(a) IAA (b) NAA
(c) cytokinin/zeatin (d) gibberellic acid.

58. Highest auxin concentration occurs ***(1990)***
(a) in growing tips
(b) in leaves
(c) at base of plant organs
(d) in xylem and phloem.

59. Phytohormones are ***(1990)***
(a) chemical regulating flowering
(b) chemical regulating secondary growth
(c) hormones regulating growth from seed to adulthood
(d) regulators synthesised by plants and influencing physiological processes.

60. Abscisic acid controls ***(1990)***
(a) cell division
(b) leaf fall and dormancy
(c) shoot elongation
(d) cell elongation and wall formation.

61. Phototropic and geotropic movements are linked to ***(1990)***
(a) gibberellins (b) enzymes
(c) auxin (d) cytokinins.

62. Leaf fall can be prevented with the help of ***(1989)***
(a) abscisic acid (b) auxins
(c) florigen (d) cytokinins.

63. Mowing grass lawn facilitates better maintenance because ***(1989)***
(a) wounding stimulates regeneration
(b) removal of apical dominance and stimulation of intercalary meristem
(c) removal of apical dominance
(d) removal of apical dominance and promotion of lateral meristem.

64. Cut or excised leaves remain green for long if induced to root or dipped in ***(1988)***
(a) gibberellins (b) cytokinins
(c) auxins (d) ethylene.

65. Gibberellins promote ***(1988)***
(a) seed germination (b) seed dormancy
(c) leaf fall (d) root elongation.

ANSWER KEY

1.	(a)	2.	(c)	3.	(d)	4.	(d)	5.	(d)	6.	(d)	7.	(a)
8.	(d)	9.	(b)	10.	(c)	11.	(d)	12.	(b)	13.	(a)	14.	(b)
15.	(b)	16.	(b)	17.	(a)	18.	(c)	19.	(b)	20.	(d)	21.	(a)
22.	(b)	23.	(a)	24.	(b)	25.	(c)	26.	(d)	27.	(d)	28.	(d)
29.	(d)	30.	(c)	31.	(a)	32.	(c)	33.	(c)	34.	(c)	35.	(d)
36.	(a)	37.	(b)	38.	(b)	39.	(b)	40.	(a)	41.	(a)	42.	(a)
43.	(a)	44.	(c)	45.	(a)	47.	(d)	48.	(d)	49.	(a)	50.	(d)
51.	(b)	52.	(d)	53.	(c)	54.	(c)	55.	(a)	56.	(a)	57.	(c)
58.	(a)	59.	(d)	60.	(b)	61.	(c)	62.	(d)	63.	(b)	64.	(b)
65.	(a)												

HINTS & EXPLANATIONS

1. **(a)**: In most systems, the initial growth is slow i.e., lag phase, and it increases rapidly thereafter - at an exponential rate i.e., log or exponential phase.

2. **(c)**: Geometric growth cannot be sustained for long in natural condition. Limited nutrient availability slows down the growth. It leads to a stationary phase or even a decline. Plotting the growth against time, gives a typical sigmoid or S-curve. Sigmoid curve of growth is typical of most organisms in their natural environment including plants. An idealised sigmoid growth curve is shown below:

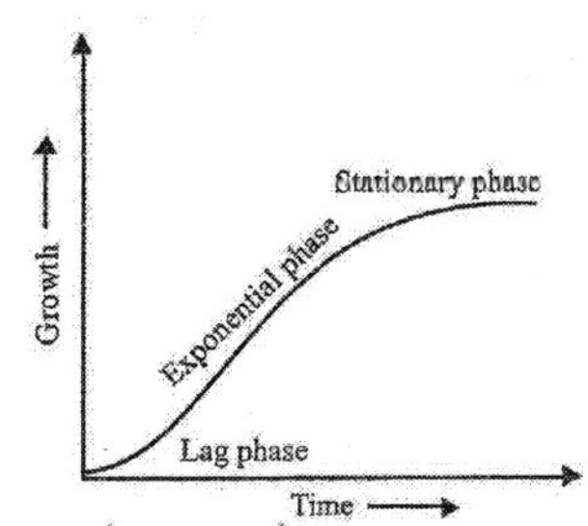

3. **(d)**

4. **(d)** : The ability of plants to follow different pathway in response to environment or phases of life to form different kinds of structures is called plasticity, e.g., heterophylly in cotton, coriander and larkspur.

5.(d) : Plants follow different pathways in response to environment or phases of life to form different kinds of structures. This ability is called plasticity, e.g. heterophylly in cotton, coriander and larkspur.

6. **(d)** :The period between reproductive maturity and death of the plant part is known as senescence. It is indicated in leaf abscission. The leaves of the plant are shed first with the onset of senescence.

7. **(a)**: Ethylene promotes rapid internode/petiole elongation in deep water rice plants. It helps leaves/upper parts of the shoot to remain above water

8. **(d)**: Gibberellins are one of the promotory plant growth regulators. Spraying juvenile conifers with gibberellic acids hastens the maturity period, thus leading to early seed production.

9. **(b)**: Ethylene is gaseous plant growth regulator that promotes root growth and root hair formation thus helping the plants to increase the absorption surface. Gibberellic acid (GA_2) is used to speed up malting process in brewing industry. Cytokinin helps to overcome apical dominance. Auxin kills dicotyledonous weeds in the field.

10. **(c)**: Ethylene is gaseous hormone that promotes female flowers in cucumbers thereby increasing the yield.

11.(d) Auxins like 2,4-D acts as weedicides by being selectively harmful to broad leaved dicot weeds.

12. **(b)**:Spraying sugarcane crop with gibberellins increases the length of the stem and increasing the yield by as much as 20 tonnes per acre.

13. **(a)**: Gibberellic acid involved in growth promoting activities, such as cell division, cell enlargement, pattern formation, tropic growth, flowering, fruiting and seed formation and is called plant growth promoters. It breaks seed dormancy which is antagonistic to abscisic acid.

14. **(b)**: Synthetic auxins like NAA and 2, 4-D are often employed for inducing flowering in pineapple. Ethylene also stimulates flowering in pineapple and related plants. Hence, both auxin and ethylene can be applied artificially to induce flowering in pineapple plants throughout the year to increase yield.

15. **(b)**: In low concentrations, auxins such as 2, 4 –D (2, 4 Dichlorophenoxy acetic acid) is useful in preventing preharvest fruit drop and leaf drop.

16. **(b)**: Cytokinin and auxin are two plant hormones that are supplied to the tissue culture medium in definite proportions. They bring about cell division and differentiation of callus. A low auxin to cytokinin ratio promotes shoot formation whereas a high auxin to cytokinin ratio promotes rooting of callus.

17. **(a)**: Avena curvature test is a test based on the experiments of Went (1928) which can measure auxin upto 300 mg/ litre. Indole 3-acetic acid (IAA) is a universal natural auxin and Avena curvature test serves as an accurate bioassay for this plant hormone.

18. **(c)**: Auxin bioassay is a quantitative test as it measures concentration of auxin to produce the effect and the amount of the effect. Avena curvature is based upon experiments of Went (1928). 10° curvature is produced by auxin concentration of 150mg /litre at 25°C and 90% relative humidity. The test can measure auxin upto 300mg/litre. Auxin from a shoot tip or any other plant organ is allowed to diffuse in a standard size agar block (generally 2× 2×1 mm). Auxin can also be dissolved directly in agar. 15 – 30mm long oat coleoptile grown in dark is held vertically over water. 1 mm tip of coleoptile is removed without injuring the primary leaf. After 3 hours a second decapitation is carried out for a distance of 4 mm. Primary leaf is now pulled loose and agar block supported against it at the tip of decapitated coleoptile. After 90-110 minutes, the coleoptile is found to have bent. The curvature is measured. It can also be photographed and the curvature known from shadow graph.

19. **(b)**: uxins induce cell elongation. In a differentially illuminated plant, they accumulate in the shaded part, causing elongation of the cells in the shaded part. This unequal elongation on two sides causes the plant to curve or bend towards the light source, i.e., phototropic curvature.

20. **(d)**

21. **(a)**: Abscisic acid prepares plants to cope with stress conditions like drought, etc. by inducing stomatal closure and other reactions. Hence, it is named stress hormone.

22. **(b)**: Gibberellins are plant growth substances chemically related to terpenes and occurring naturally in plants and fungi. They promote elongation of stems, e.g., bolting in cabbage plants and the mobilization of food reserves in germinating seeds. They are influential in inducing flowering and fruit development.

23. **(a)**: NAA (a-Naphthalene acetic acid) and 2, 4D (2, 4 dichlorophenoxy acetic acid) are synthetic auxins. In pineapple, application of auxin promotes flowering and thus pineapple which under natural conditions is difficult to blossom has been made to produce fruits throughout the year by application of synthetic auxins such as NAA and 2, 4, D.

24. **(b)**: Light and temperature may affect flowering in plants in various ways. The effect of photoperiods or daily duration of light hours (and dark periods) on flowering is called photoperiodism. For example, in short day plants flowering occurs when day length is below critical period, e.g., dahlia, rice, etc. In long day plants, flowering occurs when day length is above critical period, e.g., spinach, lettuce, etc. In short-long day plants, short photoperiod is required for floral initiation and long photoperiod is required for blossoming and vice-versa for long-short day plants. Hence, flowering in certain plants not only depends on a combination of light and dark exposures but also on their relative durations. Similarly, there are plants for which flowering is either quantitatively or qualitatively dependent on exposure to low temperature. This phenomenon is termed as vernalisation. It prevents precocious reproductive development late in the growing season and enables the plant to have sufficient time to reach maturity. Thus, many plants require a warm-cold-warm sequence to complete their annual cycle.

25. **(c)**: Abscisic acid or ABA is an antagonist to gibberellins. The given table tabulated the antagonistic effect of ABA and gibberellic acid :

S. No.	Abscisic acid	Gibberellic acid
(i)	It inhibits growth.	It promotes growth.
(ii)	It promotes the dormancy of seeds, buds and tubers.	It overcomes the natural dormancy of seeds, tubers, etc.
(iii)	It inhibits the synthesis of RNA and proteins.	It promotes the synthesis of RNA and proteins.
(iv)	It causes abscission of flowers and fruits.	It promotes development of fruits.

(v)	It promotes leaf senescence.	It prevents leaf senescence.
(vi)	It promotes stomatal closure.	It promotes stomatal opening.
(vii)	It prevents amylase activity.	It promotes amylase activity during seed germination.

26. (d): Phototropic curvature is the result of uneven distribution of auxin. Charles Darwin and his son Francis Darwin observed that the coleoptiles of canary grass responded to unilateral illmination by growing towards the light source (phototropism). After a series of experiments, it was concluded that the tip of coleoptile contains auxin that caused the bending of the entire coleoptile in relation to the direction of light.

27. (d): Indole-3-acetic acid (auxin) is a phytohormone which is generally produced by the growing apices of the stems and roots, from where they migrate to the regions of their action. It is observed that the growing apical bud inhibits the growth of the lateral (axillary) bud (apical dominance). Since apical meristem is the site of auxin synthesis, it is the physiological effect of the auxin which results in the phenomenon of apical dominance. When shoot tip is removed it usually results in the growth of lateral buds. This phenomenon is widely applied in tea plantations and hedge-making because as in tea plantation and industries, the apical bud is plucked for tea processing which results in more lateral buds thus enhancing plantation and further industrial purposes.

28. (d): Ethylene promotes root growth and root hair formation. In low concentration, ethylene is used for initiation of roots and also of lateral roots.

29. (d): Many auxins have been synthesized which have similar properties with natural auxin and some examples of synthetic auxins are indole-3-butyric acid (IBA), naphthalene acetic acid (NAA), 2,4-dichlorophenoxy acetic acid (2,4-D), 2,4,5-trichlorophenoxyacetic acid (2, 4, 5 – T).

30. (c): Biosynthesis of abscisic acid (ABA) in most plants occur indirectly by degradation of certain carotenoids present in chloroplasts or other plastids. The biosynthetic pathway follow mevalonic acid pathway for their synthesis. The sites of synthesis are fruits, tissues, leaves, roots and seeds.

31. (a): Gibberellic acid is a simple weakly acidic plant growth hormone which promotes cell elongation of both leaves and stems in general and internodal length of genetically dwarf plants in particular. It is in general a growth promoting hormone and does not inhibit growth. So, leaf abscission is not associated with gibberellic acid but with abscisic acid.

32. (c): Development of fruits without fertilization is called parthenocarpy and such fruits are called parthenocarpic fruits Parthenocarpic fruits are seedless. A flower is emasculated and auxins are applied to the stigma of the flower, it forms a parthenocarpic fruit. For parthenocarpy induction by auxins, these should be applied after anthesis (first opening of flower) and by gibberellins, these should be applied earlier, i.e., at anthesis.

33. (c): Prunning is the process of cutting shoot tips to promote lateral growth of branches. Removal of shoot tips involves removal of apical buds. In the shoot tips auxins are produced. Auxins are growth promoting phytohormones. They cause apical dominance by promoting the growth of apical buds and suppressing the growth of axillary buds. So when the auxins produced in the shoot tips are removed by decapitation it results in lateral growth and plants thus show bushy appearance. This is because of a relatively high concentration of auxin in the apical bud than in the lateral buds.

34. (c): Gibberellins play a role in the elongation of internodes in 'rosette' plants. Before reproductive stage there is too much elongation of internodes but there is less leaf formation. An elongated internode without leaves in called a "bolt" like structure and the process is called "bolting". Flowering takes place after bolting. Gibberellins induce cell division and cell elongation, when bolting takes place.

35. (d): Many experiments were done to sustain the proliferation of normal stem tissues in culture. The growth of culture was most dramatic when the liquid endosperm of coconut, also known as coconut milk, was added to the culture medium. This finding indicated that coconut milk contains a substance or substances that stimulate mature cells to enter and remain in the cell division cycle. Eventually coconut milk was shown to contain the cytokinin zeatin, but this finding was not obtained until several years after the discovery of the cytokinins. The first cytokinin to be discovered was the synthetic analog kinetin.

36. (a): Zinc is available to the plants for absorption in the divalent form. It occurs in the form of minerals as hornblende, magnetite, biotite, etc., from where it is released by weathering. It is involved in the synthesis of Indole-acetic acid in plants. It is an activator in the enzyme tryptophan synthetase. Tryptophan is the precursor of Indole-acetic acid.

37. (b): The major physiological function of cytokinin is to enhance cell division. In tissue culture the undifferentiated mass of cells formed in the culture tubes is called callus. The callus may remain in the undifferentiated condition or differentiation may take place in this. If it is differentiated, then root and shoot may be formed.

Skoog and Miller had reported that cytokinins induce shoot formation and auxins induce root formation.

38. (b): Gibberellins helps in the reversal of dwarfism in many genetically dwarf plants. External supply of gibberellic acid causes rapid elongation, e.g., rosette plants of sugarbeet when treated with GA_3 undergo marked longitudinal growth of axis.

39. (b): a-Naphthalene acetic acid (NAA) is a synthetic or exogenous auxin. It prevents the formation of abscission layer, which is a layer of dead cells in the petiole and pedicel that causes fall of leaf or fruit. NAA prevents formation of this layer and so it prevents fall of leaf or fruit.

40. (a): Abscisic acid is a growth inhibiting phyto-hormone. It induces senescence in leaves by promoting the degradation of chlorophyll and proteins.

41. (a): Gibberellin is the hormone that breaks seed/bud dormancy. The tubers of potato reproduce vegetatively to give rise to new plants. So the dormancy of these tubers can be overcome by applying gibberellins.

42. (a): Apical dominance is the phenomenon by which presence of apical bud does not allow the nearby lateral buds to grow. When apical bud is removed, the lateral buds sprout.

43. (a): Ethylene is largely a growth inhibiting phytohormone but is also involved in some growth promotion activities. It has been established that ethylene is a fruit ripening hormone. Ethylene stimulates all the biochemical changes which take place at the time of fruit ripening.

44. (c)

45. (a): Cytokinins are growth promoting phytohomones. Cytokinin plays an important role in organ formation (morphogenesis) with auxin. Different auxin/cytokinin ratio decides the development of root/shoot ratio. The major physiological function of cytokinin is to enhance cell division. If cytokinin to auxin ratio is low, then root formation takes place but if the ratio of cytokinin to auxin is high, then, there is formation of meristematic cells in the callus.

47. (d): Decapitating a growing plant means removing shoot apex of the plant. Auxin, a growth promoting phytohormone present in apex inhibits the growth of axillary buds so that only the apex continues to grow. When the apex containing auxin is removed or decapitation is done, then axillary or lateral buds show their growth, this is because the apical dominance is removed. This practice of removal of apical dominance is applied in tea gardens, hedges, rose gardens, etc.

48. (d)

49. (a): Richmond and Lang, 1967 observed that degradation of protein and chlorophyll was delayed in the detached leaves, if there was cytokinin in the medium. The senescence in the detached leaves was controlled by cytokinin first by keeping the stomata open thus allowing more CO_2 to enter. This suppresses the action of ethylene which promotes senescence.

50. (d): Abscisic acid is a hormone which is produced during adverse environmental conditions. It also causes the closure of stomata under conditions of water stress and also under high concentration of CO_2 in the guard cells. ABA plays an important role in plants during water stress and drought conditions. The concentration of ABA increases in the leaves of plants facing such stresses, hence it is called as a stress hormone.

51. (b): Abscisic acid is produced during water stress that brings stomatal closure. Abscisic acid is a stress hormone and it is produced during water scarcity, when the transpiration rate exceeds absorption, the plant faces water stress condition. As a result, incipient wilting occurs. Under water stress condition ABA increases which induces stomatal closure.

52. (d)

53. (c)

54. (c): Ethylene is a hormone which is used for ripening of fruit. In case of unripe banana, it can be made to ripe before proper time if they are kept in ethylene atmosphere. Uncontrolled application of this gas may spoil the fruits. Ethylene is produced in mature but unripe fruits and then it initiates a chain of reactions that finally lead to ripening.

55. (a): Abscisic acid is a hormone produced during adverse environmental condition. It also causes the closure of stomata under conditions of water stress and also under high concentration of CO_2 in the guard cells. Abscisic acid inhibits the K^+ uptake by guard cells and promotes the leakage of malic acid. It results in reduction of osmotically active solutes so that the guard cells become flaccid and stomata get closed.

56. (a)

57. (c): Cytokinin has a very specific effect on cell division (cytokinesis), hence the name cytokinin. They contain kinetin and related compound generally called kinins. Chemically, cytokinins are degradation product of adenine, ATP, NAD and NADP. Cytokinins are essential for cytokinesis though chromosome doubling can occur in their absence. Cytokinins bring about division even in permanent cells.

58. (a): Auxins are well known to promote elongation of stem and coleoptile. However when exogenous auxin is given to intact plants this is not observed because the required amount of auxin is already present in plants. When the apex of shoot is removed, then the exogenous application of auxin promotes growth, this clearly indicates that growing apex, having meristematic cells, is the site where endogenous auxins are present in sufficient amount, once the apex is removed the source of auxin is also removed.

59. (d): Growth hormones or phytohormones are defined as organic substances which are synthesized in minute quantities in one part of the plant body and transported to another part where they influence specific physiological processes. Phytohormones are chemical substances which are synthesized by plants and are naturally occurring.

60. (b): Before a leaf fall, a special zone of cells is formed at the base of the pedicel or petiole. This zone is called abscission zone. It is delimited by a protection layer on the stem side and a separation layer on the organ side. The leaf is ultimately separated and phenomenon is called abscission. ABA is also a growth inhibitor. It regulates the dormancy of seeds and buds perhaps by inhibiting the growth process. The ABA level decreases in the whole seed as their dormancy is broken.

61. (c) : Auxin regulates some of the important plant growth movements like photoropism and geotropism. Phototropism means growth of plants in response to light and geotropism means growth of plants towards gravity.

62. (d)

63. (b): Mowing grass lawn facilitates better maintenance because of removal of apical dominance and stimulation of intercalary meristem.

64. (b) : Cytokinins are plant growth hormones which are basic in nature. Cytokinins induce formation of new leaves, chloroplasts in leaves, which in turn keeps the leaves green for a longer duration of time. Cytokinins applied to marketed vegetables can keep them fresh for several days. Shelf life of cut shoots and flowers is prolonged by employing the hormones.

65. (a): Gibberellins promote seed germination. Gibberellins are weakly acidic growth hormones having ring structure and cause cell elongation of intact plants in general and increased internodal length of genetically dwarfed plants. Gibberellins are synthesized in the apical shoot buds, root tips and developing seeds. During seed germination, especially of cereals gibberellin stimulates the production of some messenger RNAs and then hydrolytic enzymes like amylases, lipases, proteases. The enzymes solubilize the reserve food of the seed.

Chapter : 14 BREATHING AND EXCHANGE OF GASES

RESPIRATORY ORGANS

1. Which of the following is not the function of conducting part of respiratory system ? ***(2022)***
(a) It clears inhaled air from foreign particles
(b) Inhaled air is humidified
(c) Temperature of inhaled air is brought to body temperature
(d) Provides surface for diffusion of O_2 and CO_2

2. The figure shows a diagrammatic view of human respiratory system with labels A, B, C and D. Select the option which gives correct identification and main function and / or characteristic. ***(2013)***

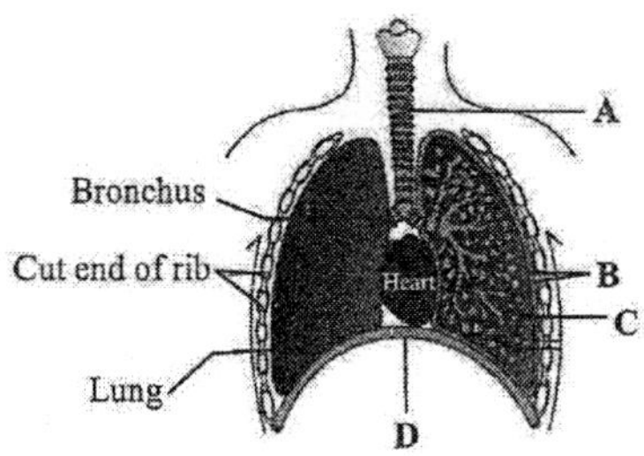

(a) C - Alveoli - Thin walled vascular bag like structures for exchange of gases.
(b) D - Lower end of lungs - Diaphragm pulls it down during inspiration.
(c) A - Trachea - Long tube supported by complete cartilaginous rings for conducting inspired air.
(d) B - Pleural membrane - Surround ribs on both sides to provide cushion against rubbing.

3. Lungs are enclosed in ***(1996)***
(a) periosteum (b) perichondrium
(c) pericardium (d) pleural membrane.

4. Skin is an accessory organ of respiration in ***(1990)***
(a) humans (b) frog
(c) rabbit (d) lizard.

MECHANISM OF BREATHING

5. Vital capacity of lung is (2023)
(a) IRV + ERV + TV - RV
(b) IRV + ERV + TV
(c) IRV + ERV
(d) IRV + ERV + TV + RV

6. Select the correct events that occur during inspiration. ***(2020)***
(1) Contraction of diaphragm
(2) Contraction of external inter-costal muscles
(3) Pulmonary volume decreases
(4) Intra pulmonary pressure increases
(a) (1) and (2) (b) (3) and (4)
(c) (1), (2) and (4)(d) only (4)

7. Tidal volume and expiratory reserve volume of an athlete is 500 mL and 1000 mL respectively. What will be his expiratory capacity if the residual volume is 1200 mL ? ***(2019)***
(a) 2700 mL (b) 1500 mL
(c) 1700 mL (d) 2200 mL

8. Select the correct statement. ***(Odisha NEET 2019)***
(a) Expiration occurs due to external intercostal muscles.
(b) Intrapulmonary pressure is lower than the atmospheric pressure during inspiration.
(c) Inspiration occurs when atmospheric pressure is less than intrapulmonary pressure.
(d) Expiration is initiated due to contraction of diaphragm.

9. Match the items given in column I with those in column II and select the correct option given below. ***(2018)***

Column I	Column II
(A) Tidal volume	(i) 2500-3000 mL
(B) Inspiratory reserve volume	(ii) 1100-1200 mL
(C) Expiratory reserve volume	(iii) 500-550 mL
(D) Residual volume	(iv) 1000-1100 mL

	A	B	C	D
(a)	(iii)	(ii)	(i)	(iv)
(b)	(iii)	(i)	(iv)	(ii)
(c)	(i)	(iv)	(ii)	(iii)
(d)	(iv)	(iii)	(ii)	(i)

10. Lungs are made up of air-filled sacs, the alveoli. They do not collapse even after forceful expiration, because of ***(2017)***

(a) inspiratory reserve volume
(b) tidal volume
(c) expiratory reserve volume
(d) residual volume.

11. Lungs do not collapse between breaths and some air always remains in the lungs which can never be expelled because ***(NEET-II 2016)***

(a) there is a negative pressure in the lungs
(b) there is a negative intrapleural pressure pulling at the lung walls
(c) there is a positive intrapleural pressure
(d) pressure in the lungs is higher than the atmospheric pressure.

12. Which one of the following is a possibility for most of us in regard to breathing, by making a conscious effort? ***(Mains 2011)***

(a) One can breathe out air totally without oxygen.
(b) One can breathe out air through Eustachian tube by closing both nose and mouth.
(c) One can consciously breathe in and breathe out by moving the diaphragm alone, without moving the ribs at all.
(d) The lungs can be made fully empty by forcefully breathing out all air from them.

13. Listed below are four respiratory capacities (i-iv) and four jumbled respiratory volumes of a normal human adult. ***(2010)***

Respiratory capacities	Respiratory volumes
(i) Residual volume	2500 mL
(ii) Vital capacity	3500 mL
(iii) Inspiratory reserve volume	1200 mL
(iv) Inspiratory capacity	4500 mL

Which one of the following is the correct matching of two capacities and volumes?

(a) (ii) 2500 mL, (iii) 4500 mL
(b) (iii) 1200 mL, (iv) 2500 mL
(c) (iv) 3500 mL, (i) 1200 mL
(d) (i) 4500 mL, (ii) 3500 mL

14. What is vital capacity of our lungs? ***(2009)***

(a) Inspiratory reserve volume plus expiratory reserve volume
(b) Total lung capacity minus residual volume
(c) Inspiratory reserve volume plus tidal volume
(d) Total lung capacity minus expiratory reserve volume

15. Which one of the following statements is incorrect? ***(2006)***

(a) The principle of countercurrent flow facilitates efficient respiration in gills of fishes.
(b) The residual air in lungs slightly decreases the efficiency of respiration in mammals.
(c) The presence of non-respiratory air sacs, increases the efficiency of respiration in birds.
(d) In insects, circulating body fluids serve to distribute oxygen to tissues.

16. The ventilation movements of the lungs in mammals are governed by ***(1995)***

(a) muscular walls of lung
(b) diaphragm
(c) intercostal muscles
(d) both (b) and (c).

17. In man and mammals, air passes from outside into the lungs through ***(1994)***
(a) nasal cavity, larynx, pharynx, trachea, bronchi, alveoli
(b) nasal cavity, larynx, pharynx, trachea, bronchioles, alveoli
(c) nasal cavity, pharynx, larynx, trachea, bronchioles, bronchi, alveoli
(d) nasal cavity, pharynx, larynx, trachea, bronchi, bronchioles, alveoli.

EXCHANGE OF GASES

18. The partial pressures (in mmHg) of oxygen (O_2) and carbon dioxide (CO_2) at alveoli (the site of diffusion) are ***(2021)***
(a) $pO_2 = 159$ and $pCO_2 = 0.3$
(b) $pO_2 = 104$ and $pCO_2 = 40$
(c) $pO_2 = 40$ and $pCO_2 = 45$
(d) $pO_2 = 95$ and $pCO_2 = 40$

19. The partial pressure of oxygen in the alveoli of the lungs is ***(NEET-II 2016)***
(a) equal to that in the blood
(b) more than that in the blood
(c) less than that in the blood
(d) less than that of carbon dioxide.

20. The figure given below shows a small part of human lung where exchange of gases takes place. Select the option which represents labelled part (A, B, C or D) correctly identified along with its function. ***(2011)***

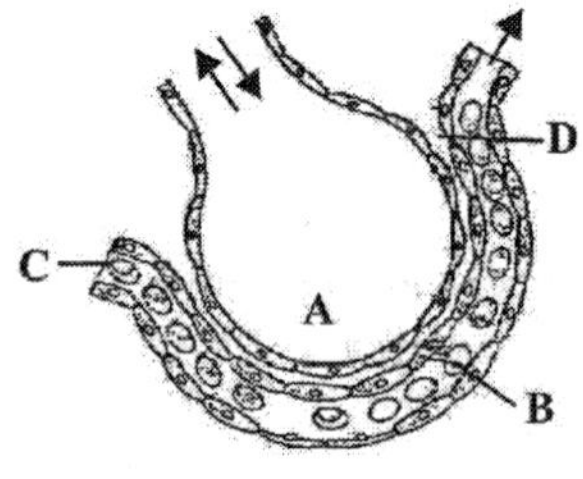

(a) C : Arterial capillary - Passes oxygen to tissues
(b) A : Alveolar cavity - Main site of exchange of respiratory gases
(c) D : Capillary wall - Exchange of O_2 and CO_2 takes place here
(d) B : Red blood cells - Transport of CO_2 mainly

21. The exchange of gases in the alveoli of the lungs takes place by ***(1998)***
(a) passive transport (b) active transport
(c) osmosis (d) simple diffusion.

TRANSPORT OF GASES

22. Under normal physiological conditions in human being every 100ml of oxygenated blood can deliver ***(2022)***
(a) 2ml ml of O_2 to the tissues
(b) 5ml
(c) 4ml
(d) 10ml

23. Select the favourable conditions required for the formation of oxyhaemoglobin at the alveoli. ***(2021)***
(a) Low pO_2, low pCO_2, more H^+, higher temperature
(b) High pO_2, low pCO_2, less H^+, lower temperature
(c) Low pO_2, high pCO_2, more H^+, higher temperature
(d) High pO_2, high pCO_2, less H^+, higher temperature

24. Identify the wrong statement with reference to transport of oxygen. ***(2020)***
(a) Binding of oxygen with haemoglobin is mainly related to partial pressure of O_2.
(b) Partial pressure of CO_2 can interfere with O_2 binding with haemoglobin.
(c) Higher H^+ conc. in alveoli favours the formation of oxyhaemoglobin.
(d) Low pCO_2 in alveoli favours the formation of oxyhaemoglobin.

25. Reduction in pH of blood will ***(NEET-I 2016)***
(a) decrease the affinity of haemoglobin with oxygen
(b) release bicarbonate ions by the liver
(c) reduce the rate of heartbeat
(d) reduce the blood supply to the brain.

26. Approximately seventy percent of carbon dioxide absorbed by the blood will be transported to the lungs ***(2014)***
(a) as bicarbonate ions
(b) in the form of dissolved gas molecules
(c) by binding to RBC
(d) as carbamino - haemoglobin.

27. A large proportion of oxygen remains unused in the human blood even after its uptake by the body tissues. This O_2 ***(2011)***
(a) acts as a reserve during muscular exercise
(b) raises the pCO_2 of blood to 75"" mm of Hg
(c) is enough to keep oxyhaemoglobin saturation at 96%
(d) helps in releasing more O_2 to the epithelial tissues.

28. Bulk of carbon dioxide (CO_2) released from body tissues into the blood is present as ***(Mains 2011)***
(a) bicarbonate in blood plasma and RBCs
(b) free CO_2 in blood plasma
(c) 70% carbamino-haemoglobin and 30% as bicarbonate
(d) carbamino-haemoglobin in RBCs.

29. What is true about RBCs in humans? ***(2010)***
(a) They carry about 20-25 percent of CO_2.
(b) They transport 99.5 percent of O_2.
(c) They transport about 80 percent oxygen only and the rest 20 percent of it is transported in dissolved state in blood plasma.
(d) They do not carry CO_2 at all.

30. The haemoglobin of a human fetus ***(2009)***
(a) has only 2 protein subunits instead of 4
(b) has a higher affinity for oxygen than that of an adult
(c) has a lower affinity for oxygen than that of the adult
(d) its affinity for oxygen is the same as that of an adult.

31. The majority of carbon dioxide produced by our body cells is transported to the lungs as ***(2006)***
(a) attached to haemoglobin
(b) dissolved in the blood
(c) as bicarbonates(d) as carbonates.

32. Haemoglobin is a type of ***(1999)***
(a) carbohydrate (b) respiratory pigment
(c) vitamin (d) skin pigment.

33. How the transport of O_2 and CO_2 by blood happens? ***(1996)***
(a) With the help of WBCs and blood serum
(b) With the help of platelets and corpuscles
(c) With the help of RBCs and blood plasma
(d) With the help of RBCs and WBCs

34. At high altitude, the RBCs in the human blood will ***(1995)***
(a) increase in number (b) decrease in number
(c) increase in size (d) decrease in size.

35. The carbon dioxide is transported via blood to lungs mostly ***(1995)***
(a) in combination with haemoglobin only
(b) dissolved in blood plasma
(c) in the form of bicarbonate ions
(d) as carbamino-haemoglobin and as carbonic acid.

36. Carbon dioxide is transported from tissues to respiratory surface by only ***(1993)***
(a) plasma and erythrocytes
(b) plasma
(c) erythrocytes
(d) erythrocytes and leucocytes.

REGULATION OF RESPIRATION

37. When you hold your breath, which of the following gas changes in blood would first lead to the urge to breathe? ***(2015 Cancelled)***
(a) Falling CO_2 concentration
(b) Rising CO_2 and falling O2 concentration
(c) Falling O_2 concentration
(d) Rising CO_2 concentration

38. The respiratory centres, which control inspiration and expiration, are located in ***(1999)***
(a) diencephalon (b) medulla oblongata
(c) cerebellum (d) spinal cord.

39. The respiratory centre which regulates respiration is located in ***(1994)***
(a) cerebellum (b) medulla oblongata
(c) cerebral peduncle (d) the vagus nerve.

DISORDERS OF RESPIRATORY SYSTEM

40. Due to increasing air-borne allergens and pollutants, many people in urban areas are suffering from respiratory disorder that cause wheezing due to ***(2019)***
(a) reduction in the secretion of surfactant by pneumocytes
(b) benign growth on mucous lining of nasal cavity
(c) inflammation of bronchi and bronchioles
(d) proliferation of fibrous tissues and damage of the alveolar walls.

41. Which of the following options correctly represents the lung conditions in asthma and emphysema, respectively? ***(2018)***
(a) Inflammation of bronchioles; Decreased respiratory surface
(b) Increased number of bronchioles; Increased respiratory surface
(c) Increased respiratory surface; Inflammation of bronchioles
(d) Decreased respiratory surface; Inflammation of bronchioles

42. Which of the following is an occupational respiratory disorder? ***(2018)***
(a) Anthracis (b) Silicosis
(c) Botulism (d) Emphysema

43. Name the chronic respiratory disorder caused mainly by cigarette smoking. ***(NEET-I 2016)***
(a) Respiratory acidosis
(b) Respiratory alkalosis
(c) Emphysema
(d) Asthma

44. Asthma may be attributed to ***(NEET-I 2016)***
(a) inflammation of the trachea
(b) accumulation of fluid in the lungs
(c) bacterial infection of the lungs
(d) allergic reaction of the mast cells in the lungs.

45. Name the pulmonary disease in which alveolar surface area involved in gas exchange is drastically reduced due to damage in the alveolar walls. ***(2015)***
(a) Pneumonia (b) Asthma
(c) Pleurisy (d) Emphysema

46. Which one of the following is the correct statement for respiration in humans? ***(2012)***
(a) Cigarette smoking may lead to inflammation of bronchi.
(b) Neural signals from pneumotoxic centre in pons region of brain can increase the duration of inspiration.
(c) Workers in grinding and stone-breaking industries may suffer from lung fibrosis.
(d) About 90% of carbon dioxide (CO_2) is carried by haemoglobin as carbaminohaemoglobin.

47. Blood analysis of a patient reveals an unusually high quantity of carboxyhaemoglobin content. Which of the following conclusions is most likely to be correct? ***(2004)***

The patient has been inhaling polluted air containing unusually high content of
(a) carbon disulphide (b) chloroform
(c) carbon dioxide (d) carbon monoxide.

48. When CO_2 concentration in blood increases breathing becomes ***(2004)***
(a) shallower and slow
(b) there is no effect on breathing
(c) slow and deep
(d) faster and deeper

ANSWER KEY

1.	(d)	2.	(a)	3.	(d)	4.	(b)	5.	(b)	6.	(a)	7.	(b)
8.	(b)	9.	(b)	10.	(d)	11.	(b)	12.	(b)	13.	(c)	14.	(b)
15.	(b)	16.	(d)	17.	(d)	18.	(b)	19.	(b)	20.	(b)	21.	(d)
22.	(b)	23.	(b)	24.	(c)	25.	(a)	26.	(a)	27.	(a)	28.	(a)
29.	(a)	30.	(b)	31.	(c)	32.	(b)	33.	(c)	34.	(a)	35.	(c)
36.	(a)	37.	(d)	38.	(b)	39.	(b)	40.	(c)	41.	(a)	42.	(b)
43.	(c)	44.	(d)	45.	(d)	46.	(c)	47.	(d)	48.	(d)		

HINTS & EXPLANATIONS

1. **(d)**: Exchange or respiratory part of respiratory system is the site of actual diffusion of O_2 and CO_2 between blood and atmospheric air.

2. **(a)** In the given figure, A is trachea. It is supported by incomplete cartilaginous rings which prevent its collapse during inspiration. B is pleural membrane and it encloses lungs. C is alveoli that are thin walled sacs having extensive network of capillaries for gaseous exchange. D is diaphragm.

3. **(d)**: Each lung is enclosed in two membranes, the pleura. The inner membrane is called the visceral pleuron and the outer membrane is called parietal pleuron. A very narrow space exists between the two pleura. It is called the pleural cavity and contains a watery fluid called the pleural fluid that lubricates the pleura. Periosteum is the outer membrane of the bone.

   Perichondrium is a layer that surrounds the cartilage and pericardium is the membrane that encloses the pericardial cavity, containing the vertebrate heart.

4. **(b)**: In addition to lungs, skin is also an organ of respiration in frog. It is practically the only mode of respiration when the frog is under water or hibernating. Skin is richly supplied with blood and is permeable to gases. That is why frogs always stay near water to keep their skin moist. It is further kept moist by secretion of mucus from its glands and does not become dry out of water.

5. **(b)**: Vital capacity (VC) is the maximum volume of air a person can breathe in after forced expiration or maximum volume of air a person can breathe out after forced inspiration. This includes ERV, TV and IRV.

6. **(a)**: Inspiration is initiated by the contraction of diaphragm that increases the volume of thoracic chamber in the antero-posterior axis. The contraction of external intercostal muscles lifts up the ribs and the sternum causing an increase in the volume of the thoracic chamber in the dorsoventral axis. The overall increase in the thoracic volume causes a similar increase in pulmonary volume. An increase in pulmonary volume decreases the intra-pulmonary pressure to less than the atmospheric pressure which forces the air from outside to move into the lungs.

7. **(b)**: Expiratory capacity is the total volume of air a person can expire after normal inspiration.

It includes tidal volume (TV) and expiratory reserve volume (ERV).

EC = TV + ERV = 500 mL + 1000 mL = 1500 mL

8. **(b)**

9. **(b)**

10. **(d)** : Residual volume is the volume of air which remains in the lungs after the most forceful expiration. This residual air enables the lungs to continue exchange of gases even after maximum exhalation. Due to this, lungs do not collapse even after forceful expiration.

11. **(b)**: Intrapleural pressure is the pressure of air within the pleural cavity. Intrapleural pressure is always negative, which acts like a suction to keep the lungs inflated and prevent them from collapsing. The negative intrapleural pressure is due to three main factors: surface tension of the alveolar fluid elasticity of lungs; elasticity of thoracic wall. Normally, there is a difference between intrapleural and intrapulmonary pressure, which is called transpulmonary pressure. This transpulmonary pressure creates the suction to keep the lungs inflated. If there is no pressure difference, there is no suction and lungs will collapse.

12. **(b)**

13. **(c)**

14. **(b)**: TLC = VC + RV. So, vital capacity is also total lung capacity (TLC) - residual volume (RV).

15. **(b)**

16. **(d)**: The ventilation movements of the lungs in mammals are governed by diaphragm and intercostal muscles (between the ribs).

17. **(d)**: Air passes from the external nares into the nasal cavity where the dust particles are trapped. From nasal cavity, the air moves into pharynx which is a short, vertical tube. It further leads into two tubes, trachea and oesophagus. Larynx is the upper part of trachea. Besides forming a part of the respiratory tract, it also serves as the voice box. Trachea is a thin walled tube that extends downward through the neck. It divides into two primary bronchi which on entering the lungs divide into fine branches called bronchioles which enter the alveoli. Exchange of gases occur in alveoli.

18. **(b)**: The partial pressure (in mm Hg) of oxygen and carbon dioxide at alveoli are 104 and 40 respectively.

19. **(b)**: The partial pressure of oxygen in alveolar air is 104 mm Hg whereas it is 40 mmHg in deoxygenated blood and 95 mmHg in oxygenated blood.

20. **(b)**

21. **(d)**: Diffusion is the net flow of a substance from a region of higher concentration to a region of lower concentration. The exchange of gases between the alveoli and blood in the lung is the result of difference in partial pressure of respiratory gases. The partial pressure of oxygen (pO_2) of the alveolar air is higher than the pO_2 of blood in alveolar capillaries, thus O_2 diffuses rapidly from the alveolar air into the blood of alveolar capillaries. The PCO_2 of blood reaching the alveolar capillaries is higher than the pCO_2 of alveolar air. Therefore, CO_2 diffuses into the alveolar air.

22. **(b)**

23. **(b)**: In the alveoli, high pO_2, low pCO_2, less H^+ concentration and low temperature are the favourable conditions required for formation of oxyhaemoglobin. This means oxygen gets bound to haemoglobin in the lung surface.

24. **(c)**: Binding of oxygen with haemoglobin is related to partial pressure of O_2, partial pressure

of CO_2, hydrogen ion concentration and temperature. In the alveoli, high pO_2, low pCO_2, lesser H^+ concentration and lower temperature are factors favourable for the formation of oxyhaemoglobin, whereas in the tissues, low pO_2, high pCO_2, high H^+ concentration and high temperature are favourable for dissociation of oxygen from the oxyhaemoglobin.

25. **(a)**:Reduction in pH of blood causes oxygenhaemoglobin dissociation curve to shift to right which indicates dissociation of oxygen from haemoglobin. This decreases affinity of haemoglobin for oxygen.

26. **(a)**: About 70% of CO_2 (about 2.5 mL per 100 mL of blood), received by blood from the tissues, enters the RBCs where it reacts with water to form carbonic acid ($H_2\,CO_3$). Carbonic anhydrase, exclusively found in RBCs, speeds up the formation of $H_2\,CO_3$ and rapidly converts it back to carbon dioxide and water when blood reaches the lungs. Almost as rapidly as formed, all carbonic acid of RBCs– dissociates into hydrogen (H^+)and bicarbonate ions (HCO_3^-)

27. **(a)**

28. **(a)**: At the tissue site where partial pressure of CO_2 is high due to catabolism, CO_2 diffuses into blood (RBCs and plasma) and forms HCO_2^- and H^+. At the alveolar site where pCO_2 is low, the reaction proceeds in the opposite direction leading to the formation of CO_2 and H_2O. Thus, CO_2 trapped as bicarbonate at the tissue level and transported to the alveoli is released out as CO_2.

29.(a) Blood is the medium of transport for O_2 and CO_2. About 97 percent of O_2 is transported by RBCs in the blood. The remaining 3 percent of O_2 is carried in a dissolved state through the plasma. Nearly 20-25 percent of CO_2 is transported by RBCs whereas 70 percent of it is carried as bicarbonate. About 7 percent of CO_2 is carried in a dissolved state through plasma.

30. **(b)**: Oxygen is needed for aerobic respiration and diffuses from a region of high to low concentration from the mother's blood to the blood of the fetus. The haemoglobin of the fetus has a higher affinity for oxygen than that of adult haemoglobin and so the efficiency of exchange is increased. Carbon dioxide, a waste product of aerobic respiration diffuses in the opposite direction.

31. **(c)**: When systemic arterial blood flows through capillaries, carbon dioxide diffuses from the tissues intit the blood. Some carbon dioxide is dissolved in the blood Some carbon dioxide reacts with haemoglobin to form carbaminohaemoglobin. The remaining carbon dioxide is converted to bicarbonate and hydrogen ions. Most carbot dioxide is transported through the blood in the form bicarbonate ions.

32. **(b)**: Haemoglobin (Hb) is a conjugated protein. It consists of a basic protein globin joined to a nonprotein group heme. Heme is an iron-porphyrin ring. A mammalian Hb molecule is a complex of 4 heme molecules joined with 4 globin molecules. It is present in RBC and carries O2 from the lungs to the tissues and transports CO2 from the tissues to the lungs.

33. **(c)**: The transport of O_2 and CO_2 occurs with the help of RBCs and blood plasma. 97% of O_2 is transported by RBCs and 3% of O_2 is carried by plasma. About 7% of CO_2 is transported in plasma and rest by RBCs (23%) by binding with Hb and 70% reacts with water to form carbonic acid in RBCs.

34. **(a)**

35. (c)

36. (a): Carbon dioxide is carried by the blood in three forms : physical solution, bicarbonate ions and carbaminohaemoglobin. A very small amount of carbon dioxide dissolves in the plasma and is carried as a physical solution. About 70% of carbon dioxide released by respiring tissue cells diffuses into the plasma and then into the erythrocytes (red blood corpuscles). Here, CO_2 combines with water to form carbonic acid. Carbonic acid dissociates into bicarbonate and hydrogen ions.

37. (d)

38. (b): The respiratory centre is located in the medulla oblongata, that regulates the rate and depth of breathing. The dorsal group of neurons located in the dorsal portion of medulla oblongata regulates inspiration and ventral group of neurons located in the ventrolateral part of medulla oblongata regulates both inspiration and expiration.

39. (b)

40. (c): Allergens cause bronchial asthma that stimulates release of histamine from mast cells. Symptoms of bronchial asthma are coughing, wheezing (breathing noisily), difficulty in breathing due to inflammation of bronchi and bronchioles.

41. (a): Asthma is a difficulty in breathing causing wheezing due to inflammation of bronchi and bronchioles. Emphysema is a chronic disorder in which abnormal distension of the bronchioles or alveolar sacs of the lungs occurs due to which respiratory surface is decreased for the exchange of oxygen and carbon dioxide.

42. (b): Occupational respiratory disorders are due to the occupation of the individual. Silicosis is an occupational disease that occurs due to the excessive inhalation of silica dust by the workers of mining industry. Long exposure can cause proliferation of fibrous connective tissue (fibrosis) of upper part of lungs causing inflammation. Anthrax and botulism are bacterial diseases of humans caused by Bacillus anthracis and Clostridium botulinum respectively. Emphysema is an abnormal distension of the bronchioles or alveolar sacs of the lungs.

43. (c): Emphysema is a chronic obstructive pulmonary disease (COPD) caused due to cigarette smoking. It is an inflation or abnormal distention of the bronchioles or alveolar sacs of the lungs which causes irreversible distension and loss of elasticity in the walls of alveolar sacs of the lungs.

44.(d) Asthma is an allergic condition in which the tissue surrounding the bronchioles of the lungs swell up and compress the bronchioles thus causing difficulty in breathing. This allergy mainly involves IgE antibodies and chemicals like histamine and serotonin from the mast cells.

45. (d)

46. (c): In certain industries, especially those involving grinding or stone breaking so much dust is produced that the defense mechanism of the body cannot fully cope with the situation. Long exposure can give rise to inflammation leading to fibrosis (proliferation of fibrous tissues) and thus causing serious lung damage. Workers in such industries should wear protective masks.

47. (d): Carboxyhaemoglobin, a stable compound, is formed when haemoglobin readily combines with carbon monoxide. Carbon monoxide converts iron (II) to iron (III) in its reaction with haemoglobin. In this form haemoglobin does not carry oxygen resulting in its (oxygen) starvation and leads to asphyxiation and in extreme cases to death. The affinity of haemoglobin for CO is 250 times its affinity for O_2 and COHb liberates CO very slowly and also due to that compound the dissociation curve of the remaining HbO_2 shifts to the left, decreasing the amount of O_2 released.

48. **(d)**: The effect of rising CO_2 tension is to decrease the affinity of Hb for O_2. Thus, when CO_2 concentration in blood increases, breathing becomes faster and deeper.

Chapter : 15

BODY FLUIDS AND CIRCULATION

BLOOD

1. Which of the following statements are correct? **(2023)**

A. Basophils are most abundant cells of the total WBCs.

B. Basophils secrete histamine, serotonin and heparin.

C. Basophils are involved in inflammatory response.

D. Basophils have kidney-shaped nucleus.

E. Basophils are agranulocytes.

Choose the correct answer from the options given below.

(a) B and C only (b) A and B only
(c) D and E only (d) C and E only

2. Given below are two statements. **(2022)**

Statement I: The coagulum is formed of network of threads called thrombins.

Statement II: Spleen is the graveyard of erythrocytes. In the light of the above statements, choose the most appropriate answer from the options given below.

(a) Both statement I and Statement II are correct
(b) Both Statement I and Statement II are incorrect
(c) Statement I is correct but Statement II is incorrect
(d) Statement I is incorrect but Statement II is correct

3. Persons with 'AB' blood group are called as "Universal recipients". This is due to **(2021)**

(a) absence of antibodies, anti-A and anti-B, in plasma
(b) absence of antigens A and B on the surface of RBCs
(c) absence of antigens A and B in plasma
(d) presence of antibodies, anti-A and anti-B, on RBCs.

4. Which enzyme is responsible for the conversion of inactive fibrinogens to fibrins? **(2021)**

(a) Thrombokinase (b) Thrombin
(c) Renin (d) Epinephrine

5. Match the following columns and select the correct option. **(2020)**

Column-I	Column - II
(A) Eosinophils	(i) Immune response
(B) Basophils	(ii) Phagocytosis
(C) Neutrophils	(iii) Release histaminase, destructive enzymes
(D) Lymphocytes	(iv) Release granules containing histamine

	A	B	C	D
(a)	(iii)	(iv)	(ii)	(i)
(b)	(iv)	(i)	(ii)	(iii)
(c)	(i)	(ii)	(iv)	(iii)
(d)	(ii)	(i)	(iii)	(iv)

6. Match the items given in column I with those in column II and select the correct option given below. **(2018)**

Column I	Column II
A. Fibrinogen	(i) Osmotic balance
B. Globulin	(ii) Blood clotting
C. Albumin	(iii) Defence mechanism

	A	B	C
(a)	(iii)	(ii)	(i)
(b)	(i)	(ii)	(iii)
(c)	(i)	(iii)	(ii)
(d)	(ii)	(iii)	(i)

7. Adult human RBCs are enucleate. Which of the following statement(s) is/are most appropriate explanation for this feature? ***(2017)***

(1) They do not need to reproduce.

(2) They are somatic cells.

(3) They do not metabolise.

(4) All their internal space is available for oxygen transport.

(a) Only (1) (b) (1), (3) and (4)
(c) (2) and (3) (d) Only (4)

8. Name the blood cells, whose reduction in number can cause clotting disorder, leading to excessive loss of blood from the body. ***(NEET-II 2016)***

(a) Erythrocytes (b) Leucocytes
(c) Neutrophils (d) Thrombocytes

9. Serum differs from blood in ***(NEET-II 2016)***
(a) lacking globulins
(b) lacking albumins
(c) lacking clotting factors
(d) lacking antibodies.

10. Erythropoiesis starts in ***(2015 Cancelled)***
(a) spleen (b) red bone marrow
(c) kidney (d) liver

11. Person with blood group AB is considered as universal recipient because he has ***(2014)***
(a) both A and B antigens on RBC but no antibodies in the plasma
(b) both A and B antibodies in the plasma
(c) no antigen on RBC and no antibody in the plasma
(d) both A and B antigens in the plasma but no antibodies.

12. The figure shows a human blood cell. Identify it and give its characteristics.

(Karnataka NEET 2013)

	Blood cell	Characteristics
(a)	Basophil	Secretes serotonin, inflammatory response
(b)	B-lymphocyte	Forms about 20% of blood cells involved in immune response
(c)	Neutrophil	Most abundant blood cells, phagocytic
(d)	Monocyte	Lifespan of 3 days, produces antibodies

13. A certain road accident patient with unknown blood group needs immediate blood transfusion. His one doctor friend at once offers his blood. What was the blood group of the donor? ***(2012)***
(a) Blood group B (b) Blood group AB
(c) Blood group O (d) Blood group A

14. Which one of the following human organs is often called the "graveyard" of RBCs?

(Mains 2012)

(a) Gall bladder (b) Kidney
(c) Spleen (d) Liver

15. Which one of the following plasma proteins is involved in the coagulation of blood? ***(2011)***
(a) Albumin (b) Serum amylase
(c) Globulin (d) Fibrinogen

16. A person with unknown blood group under ABO system, has suffered much blood loss in an accident and needs immediate blood transfusion. His friend who has valid certificate of his own blood type, offers for blood donation without delay. What would have been the type of blood group of the donor friend? ***(2011)***
(a) Type B (b) Type AB
(c) Type O (d) Type A

17. Which two of the following changes (i -iv) usually tend to occur in the plain dwellers when they move to high altitudes (3,500 m or more)?

(2010)

(i) Increase in red blood cell size

(ii) Increase in red blood cell production

(iii) Increased breathing rate

(iv) Increase in thrombocyte count

Changes occurring are
(a) (ii) and (iii) (b) (iii) and (iv)
(c) (i) and (iv) (d) (i) and (ii).

18. The haemoglobin content per 100 mL of blood of a normal healthy human adult is ***(Mains 2010)***
(a) 5-11mg (b) 25-30mg
(c) 17-20mg (d) 12-16mg.

19. There is no DNA in ***(2009)***
(a) mature RBCs
(b) a mature spermatozoan
(c) hair root
(d) an enucleated ovum.

20. Globulins contained in human blood plasma are primarily involved in ***(2009)***
(a) osmotic balance of body fluids
(b) oxygen transport in the blood
(c) clotting of blood
(d) defence mechanisms of body.

21. The most popularly known blood grouping is the ABO grouping. It is named ABO and not ABC, because "O" in it refers to having ***(2009)***
(a) overdominance of this type on the genes for A and B types
(b) one antibody only - either anti - A or anti - B on the RBCs
(c) no antigens A and B on RBCs
(d) other antigens besides A and B on RBCs.

22. The most active phagocytic white blood cells are ***(2008)***
(a) eosinophils and lymphocytes
(b) neutrophils and monocytes
(c) neutrophils and eosinophils
(d) lymphocytes and macrophages.

23. Which type of white blood cells are concerned with the release of histamine and the natural anticoagulant heparin? ***(2008)***
(a) Eosinophils(b) Monocytes
(c) Neutrophils(d) Basophils

24. A drop of each of the following, is placed separately on four slides. Which of them will not coagulate? ***(2007)***
(a) Blood serum
(b) Sample from the thoracic duct of lymphatic system
(c) Whole blood from pulmonary vein
(d) Blood plasma

25. You are required to draw blood from a patient and to keep it in a test tube for analysis of blood corpuscles and plasma. You are also provided with the following four types of test tubes. Which of these you will not use for the purpose? ***(2004)***
(a) Test tube containing calcium bicarbonate
(b) Chilled test tube
(c) Test tube containing heparin
(d) Test tube containing sodium oxalate

26. In the ABO system of blood groups, if both antigens are present but no antibody, the blood group of the individual would be ***(2003)***
(a) B (b) O
(c) AB (d) A.

27. What is correct for blood group O? ***(2001)***
(a) No antigens but both a and b antibodies are present.
(b) A antigen and b antibody present.
(c) Antigen and antibody both absent.
(d) A and B antigens and a, b antibodies present.

28. Erythroblastosis fetalis is caused when fertilisation takes place between gametes of ***(2000)***
(a) Rh^- female and Rh^+ male
(b) Rh^+ female and Rh^- male
(c) Rh^+ female and Rh^+ male
(d) Rh^- female and Rh^- male.

29. Which statement is true for WBC? ***(2000)***
(a) Non-nucleated
(b) In deficiency, cancer is caused
(c) Manufactured in thymus
(d) Can squeeze through blood capillaries

30. Which is the principal cation in the plasma of the blood? ***(1999)***
(a) Potassium (b) Magnesium
(c) Calcium (d) Sodium

31. The blood group, with antibody-A and antibody-B is ***(1999)***
(a) O (b) B
(c) A (d) AB

32. The problem, due to Rh– factor arises when the blood of two (Rh+ and –Rh–) mix up ***(1999)***
(a) during pregnancy
(b) in a test tube
(c) through transfusion
(d) both (a) and (c).

33. Which of the following is agranulocyte? ***(1997)***
(a) Basophil (b) Neutrophil
(c) Lymphocyte (d) Eosinophil

34. The life span of human WBC is approximately ***(1997)***
(a) between 2 to 3 months
(b) more than 4 months
(c) less than 10 days
(d) between 20 to 30 days.

35. Vitamin K is required for ***(1993)***
(a) change of prothrombin into thrombin
(b) synthesis of prothrombin
(c) change of fibrinogen to fibrin
(d) formation of thromboplastin.

36. Cells formed in bone marrow include ***(1992)***
(a) RBCs
(b) RBCs and leucocytes
(c) leucocytes
(d) lymphocytes.

37. Component of blood responsible for producing antibodies is ***(1992)***
(a) thrombocytes (b) monocytes
(c) erythrocytes (d) lymphocytes.

38. Blood group AB has ***(1991)***
(a) no antigen
(b) no antibody
(c) neither antigen nor antibody
(d) both antigen and antibody.

39. Carbonic anhydrase occurs in ***(1991)***
(a) lymphocytes (b) blood plasma
(c) RBCs (d) leucocytes.

40. Removal of calcium from freshly collected blood would ***(1989)***
(a) cause delayed clotting
(b) prevent clotting
(c) cause immediate clotting
(d) prevent destruction of haemoglobin

41. A person with blood group A requires blood. The blood group which can be given is ***(1989)***
(a) A and B (b) A and AB
(c) A and O (d) A, B, AB and O.

42. Which one engulfs pathogens rapidly? ***(1989)***
(a) Acidophils (b) Monocytes
(c) Basophils (d) Neutrophils

43. Child death may occur in the marriage of ***(1988)***
(a) Rh^+ man and Rh^+ woman
(b) Rh^+ man and Rh^- woman
(c) Rh^- man and Rh^- woman
(d) Rh^- man and Rh^+ woman.

44. Breakdown product of haemoglobin is ***(1988)***
(a) bilirubin (b) iron
(c) biliverdin (d) calcium.

LYMPH (TISSUE FLUID)

45. Which one of the following is correct? **(2015 cancelled)**
(a) Lymph = Plasma + RBC + WBC
(b) Blood = Plasma + RBC + WBC + Platelets
(c) Plasma = Blood - Lymphocytes
(d) Serum = Blood + Fibrinogen

46. Compared to blood our lymph has **(2009)**
(a) plasma without proteins
(b) more WBCs and no RBCs
(c) more RBCs and less WBCs
(d) no plasma.

47. Which of the following statements is true for lymph? **(2002)**
(a) WBC + serum
(b) Blood – RBCs and some proteins
(c) RBCs + WBCs + plasma
(d) RBCs + proteins + platelets

48. Which of the following is not the main function of lymph glands? **(1998)**
(a) Forming RBCs (b) Destroying bacteria
(c) Forming WBCs (d) Forming antibodies

49. The lymph serves to **(1995)**
(a) return the interstitial fluid to the blood
(b) return the WBCs and RBCs to the lymph nodes
(c) transport CO_2 to the lungs
(d) transport O_2 to the brain.

CIRCULATORY PATHWAYS

50. Match List I with List II. **(2023)**

List I	List II
A. P-wave	I. Beginning of systole
B. Q-wave	II. Repolarisation of ventricles
C. QRS complex	III. Depolarisation of atria
D. T-wave	IV. Depolarisation of ventricles

Choose the correct answer from the options given below.
(a) A-II, B-IV, C-I, D-III
(b) A-I, B-II, C-III, D-IV
(c) A-III, B-I, C-IV, D-II
(d) A-IV, B-III, C-II, D-I

51. Which one of the following statements is correct ? **(2022)**
(a) The atrio-ventricular node (AVN) generates an action potential to stimulate atrial contraction.
(b) The tricuspid and the bicuspid valves open due to the pressure exerted by the simultaneous contraction of the atria.
(c) Blood moves freely from atrium to the ventricle during joint diastole.
(d) Increased ventricular pressure causes closing of the semilunar valves.

52. The QRS complex in a standard ECG represents **(2020)**
(a) repolarisation of auricles
(b) depolarisation of auricles
(c) depolarisation of ventricles
(d) repolarisation of ventricles.

53. Match the column - I with column - II. **(2019)**

Column-I	Column-II
(A) P-wave	(i) Depolarisation of ventricles
(B) QRS complex	(ii) Repolarisation of ventricles
(C) T-wave	(iii) Coronary ischaemia
(D) Reduction in the size of T- wave	(iv) Depolarisation of atria
	(v) Repolarisation of atria

Select the correct option.

	(A)	(B)	(C)	(D)
(a)	(ii)	(iii)	(v)	(iv)
(b)	(iv)	(i)	(ii)	(iii)
(c)	(iv)	(i)	(ii)	(v)
(d)	(ii)	(i)	(v)	(iii)

54. What would be the heart rate of a person if the cardiac output is 5 L, blood volume in the ventricles at the end of diastole is 100"" mL and at the end of ventricular systole is 50 mL ? **(2019)**
(a) 125 beats per minute
(b) 50 beats per minute
(c) 75 beats per minute
(d) 100 beats per minute

55. Match the items given in column I with those in column II and select the correct option given below. **(2018)**

Column I	Column II
A. Tricuspid valve	(i) Between left atrium and left ventricle
B. Bicuspid valve	(ii) Between right ventricle and pulmonary artery
C. Semilunar valve	(iii) Between right atrium and right ventricle

	A	B	C
(a)	(iii)	(i)	(ii)
(b)	(i)	(iii)	(ii)
(c)	(i)	(ii)	(iii)
(d)	(ii)	(i)	(iii)

56. Doctors use stethoscope to hear the sounds produced during each cardiac cycle. The second sound is heard when ***(2015)***

(a) AV node receives signal from SA node
(b) AV valves open up
(c) Ventricular walls vibrate due to gushing in of blood from atria
(d) Semilunar valves close down after the blood flows into vessels from ventricles.

57. Blood pressure in the mammalian aorta is maximum during ***(2015 Cancelled)***

(a) systole of the left ventricle
(b) diastole of the right atrium
(c) systole of the left atrium
(d) diastole of the right ventricle.

58. The diagram given here is the standard ECG of a normal person. The P-wave represents the ***(2013)***

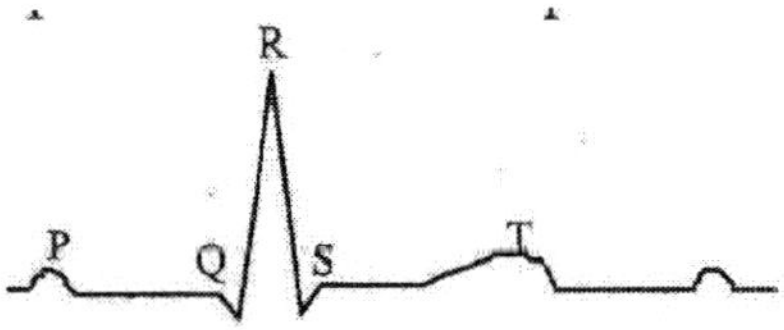

(a) beginning of the systole
(b) end of systole
(c) contraction of both the atria
(d) initiation of the ventricular contraction.

59. 'Bundle of His' is a part of which one of the following organs in humans? ***(2011)***

(a) Brain (b) Heart
(c) Kidney (d) Pancreas

60. Given below is the ECG of a normal human. Which one of its components is correctly interpreted below? ***(Mains 2011)***

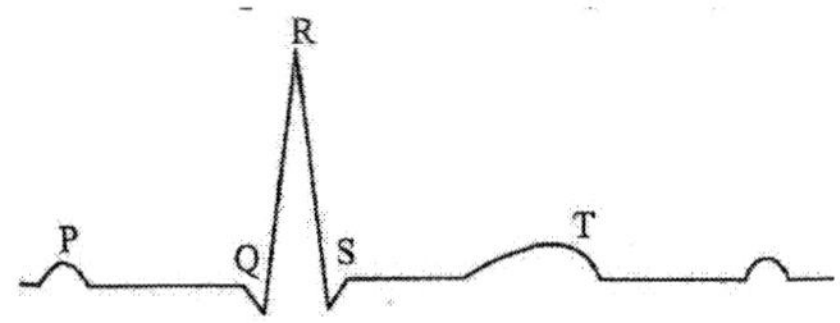

(a) Complex QRS - one complete pulse
(b) Peak T - initiation of total cardiac contraction
(c) Peak P and peak R together - systolic and diastolic blood pressures
(d) Peak P- initiation of left atrial contraction only

61. If due to some injury the chordae tendinae of the tricuspid valve of the human heart is partially nonfunctional, what will be the immediate effect? ***(2010)***

(a) The flow of blood into the aorta will be slowed down.
(b) The 'pacemaker' will stop working.
(c) The blood will tend to flow back into the left atrium.
(d) The flow of blood into the pulmonary artery will be reduced.

62. In a standard ECG which one of the following alphabets is the correct representation of the respective activity of the human heart? ***(2009)***

(a) S - start of systole
(b) T - end of diastole
(c) P - depolarisation of the atria
(d) R - repolarisation of ventricles

63. In humans, blood passes from the post caval to the diastolic right atrium of heart due to ***(2008)***

(a) stimulation of the sino auricular node
(b) pressure difference between the post caval and atrium
(c) pushing open of the venous valves
(d) suction pull.

64. Which one of the following has an open circulatory system? ***(2006)***
(a) Octopus (b) Pheretima
(c) Periplaneta (d) Hirudinaria

65. Bundle of His is a network of ***(2003)***
(a) muscle fibres distributed throughout the heart walls
(b) muscle fibres found only in the ventricle wall
(c) nerve fibres distributed in ventricles
(d) nerve fibres found throughout the heart.

66. Systemic heart refers to ***(2003)***
(a) the heart that contracts under stimulation from nervous system
(b) left auricle and left ventricle in higher vertebrates
(c) entire heart in lower vertebrates
(d) the two ventricles together in humans.

67. Impulse of heart beat originates from ***(2002)***
(a) SA node (b) AV node
(c) vagus nerve (d) cardiac nerve.

68. Rate of heart beat is determined by ***(1999)***
(a) Purkinje fibres (b) papillary muscles
(c) AV node (d) SA node.

69. The correct route through which pulse-making impulse travels in the heart is ***(1995)***
(a) SA node → Purkinje fibres → bundle of His→AV node → heart muscles
(b) SA node → AV node → bundle of His → Purkinje fibres → heart muscles
(c) AV node → bundle of His → SA node → Purkinje fibres → heart muscles
(d) AV node → SA node → Purkinje fibres → bundle of His → heart muscles.

70. The neurogenic heart is the characteristic feature of ***(1995)***
(a) humans (b) arthropods
(c) rabbits (d) rats.

71. The heart sound 'dup' is produced when ***(1994)***
(a) mitral valve is closed
(b) semi-lunar valves at the base of aorta get closed
(c) tricuspid valve is opened
(d) mitral valve is opened.

72. Tricuspid valve is found in between ***(1989)***
(a) sinus venosus and right auricle
(b) right auricle and right ventricle
(c) left ventricle and left auricle
(d) ventricle and aorta.

DOUBLE CIRCULATION

73. The hepatic portal vein drains blood to liver from ***(2017)***
(a) stomach (b) kidneys
(c) intestine (d) heart.

74. Blood pressure in the pulmonary artery is ***(NEET-I 2016)***
(a) more than that in the pulmonary vein
(b) less than that in the venae cavae
(c) same as that in the aorta
(d) more than that in the carotid.

75. In mammals, which blood vessel would normally carry largest amount of urea? ***(NEET-I 2016)***
(a) Hepatic vein (b) Hepatic portal vein
(c) Renal vein (d) Dorsal aorta

76. Which one of the following animals has two separate circulatory pathways? ***(2015)***
(a) Whale (b) Shark
(c) Frog (d) Lizard

77. The given figure shows schematic plan of blood circulation in humans with labels A to D. Identify the label and give its functions. ***(2013)***

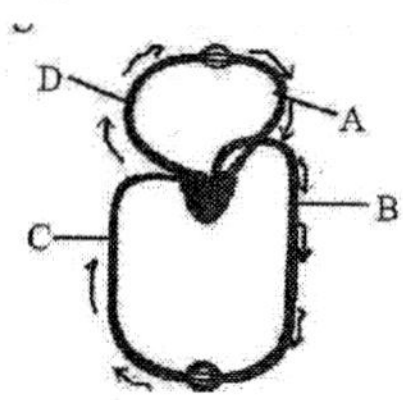

(a) C - Vena cava - Takes blood from body parts to right auricle, $pCO_2 = 45$ mmHg
(b) D - Dorsal aorta - Takes blood from heart to body parts, $pO_2 = 95$ mmHg
(c) A - Pulmonary vein - Takes impure blood from body parts, $pO_2 = 60$ mmHg
(d) B - Pulmonary artery - Takes blood from heart to lungs, $pO_2 = 90$ mmHg

78. The figure shows blood circulation in humans with labels A to D. Select the option which gives correct identification of label and functions of the part. ***(Karnataka NEET 2013)***

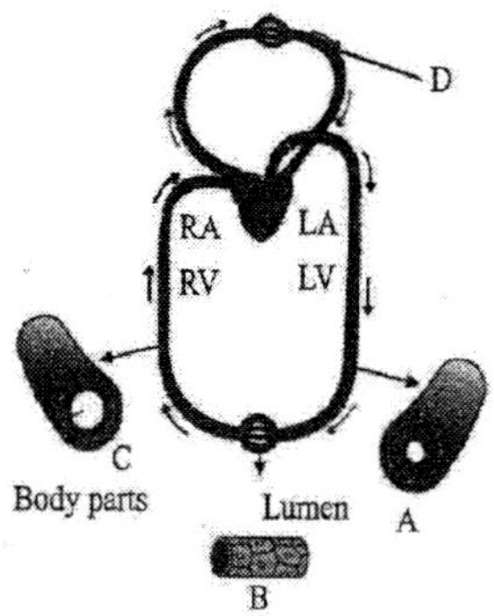

(a) B - Capillary-Thin without muscle layer and wall two cell layers thick
(b) C - Vein-Thin walled and blood flows in jerks/ spurts
(c) D - Pulmonary vein-Takes oxygenated blood to heart, $pO_2 = 95$ mmHg
(d) A - Artery-Thick walled and blood flows evenly

79. Arteries are best defined as the vessels which ***(2011)***
(a) supply oxygenated blood to the different organs
(b) carry blood away from the heart to different organs
(c) break up into capillaries which reunite to form a vein
(d) carry blood from one visceral organ to another visceral organ.

80. Fastest distribution of some injectible material/ medicine and with no risk of any kind can be achieved by injecting it into the ***(Mains 2010)***
(a) muscles (b) arteries
(c) veins (d) lymph vessels.

81. Difference between pulmonary artery and pulmonary vein is that, the pulmonary artery has ***(2000)***
(a) no endothelium (b) valves
(c) thicker walls (d) oxygenated blood

82. In which point, pulmonary artery is different from pulmonary vein? ***(2000)***
(a) Its lumen is broad.
(b) Its wall is thick.
(c) It has valves.
(d) It does not possess endothelium.

83. Which vertebrate organ receives only oxygenated blood? ***(1996)***
(a) Spleen (b) Liver
(c) Gill (d) Lung

84. In veins, valves are present to check backward flow of blood flowing at ***(1995)***
(a) atmospheric pressure
(b) high pressure
(c) low pressure
(d) all of these.

85. Blood capillaries are made of ***(1993)***
(a) endothelium, connective tissue and muscle fibres
(b) endothelium and muscle fibres
(c) endothelium and connective tissue
(d) endothelium only.

86. Wall of blood capillary is formed of ***(1991)***
(a) haemocytes (b) parietal cells
(c) endothelial cells (d) oxyntic cells.

87. Arteries carry oxygenated blood except ***(1989)***
(a) pulmonary (b) cardiac
(c) hepatic (d) systemic.

REGULATION OF CARDIAC ACTIVITY

88. How do parasympathetic neural signals affect the working of the heart? ***(2014)***
(a) Reduce both heart rate and cardiac output.
(b) Heart rate is increased without affecting the cardiac output.
(c) Both heart rate and cardiac output increase
(d) Heart rate decreases but cardiac output increases.

DISORDERS OF CIRCULATORY SYSTEM

89. Which one of the following statements is correct regarding blood pressure? ***(2011)***

(a) 130/90 mmHg is considered high and requires treatment.

(b) 100/55 mmHg is considered an ideal blood pressure.

(c) 105/50 mmHg makes one very active.

(d) 190/110 mm Hg may harm vital organs like brain and kidney.

90. Given below are four statements (i-iv) regarding human blood circulatory system. (Mains 2010)

(i) Arteries are thick-walled and have narrow lumen as compared to veins.

(ii) Angina is acute chest pain when the blood circulation to the brain is reduced.

(iii) Persons with blood group AB can donate blood to any person with any blood group under ABO system.

(iv) Calcium ions play a very important role in blood clotting.

Which two of the above statements are correct?

(a) (i) and (iv) (b) (i) and (ii)

(c) (ii) and (iii) (d) (iii) and (iv)

91. The thickening of walls of arteries is called ***(1999)***

(a) arteriosclerosis (b) arthritis

(c) aneurysm (d) both (b) and (c)

92. An adult human with average health has systolic and diastolic pressures as ***(1998)***

(a) 120 mmHg and 80 mmHg

(b) 50 mmHg and 80 mmHg

(c) 80 mmHg and 80 mmHg

(d) 70 mmHg and 120 mmHg.

ANSWER KEY

1.	(a)	2.	(d)	3.	(a)	4.	(b)	5.	(a)	6.	(d)	7.	(d)
8.	(d)	9.	(c)	10.	(b)	11.	(a)	12.	(a)	13.	(c)	14.	(c)
15.	(d)	16.	(c)	17.	(a)	18.	(d)	19.	(a)	20.	(d)	21.	(c)
22.	(b)	23.	(d)	24.	(a)	25.	(a)	26.	(c)	27.	(a)	28.	(a)
29.	(d)	30.	(d)	31.	(a)	32.	(d)	33.	(c)	34.	(c)	35.	(b)
36.	(b)	37.	(d)	38.	(b)	39.	(c)	40.	(b)	41.	(c)	42.	(d)
43.	(b)	44.	(a, b)	45.	(b)	46.	(b)	47.	(b)	48.	(a)	49.	(a)
50.	(c)	51.	(c)	52.	(c)	53.	(b)	54.	(d)	55.	(a)	56.	(d)
57.	(a)	58.	(c)	59.	(b)	60.	(a)	61.	(d)	62.	(c)	63.	(b)
64.	(c)	65.	(b)	66.	(b)	67.	(a)	68.	(d)	69.	(b)	70.	(b)
71.	(b)	72.	(b)	73.	(a,c)	74.	(a)	75.	(a)	76.	(a)	77.	(a)
78.	(c)	79.	(b)	80.	(c)	81.	(c)	82.	(c)	83.	(a)	84.	(c)
85.	(d)	86.	(c)	87.	(a)	88.	(a)	89.	(d)	90.	(a)	91.	(a)
92.	(a)												

HINTS & EXPLANATIONS

1. **(a)**: Basophils are least (0.5-1 percent) among the total WBCs. They usually have three lobed nucleus and are granulocytes.

2. **(d)**: Clot or coagulum is formed mainly of network of threads called fibrins in which dead and damaged formed elements of blood are trapped.

3. **(a)** : AB blood group has A and B antigens on RBCs and no antibodies in plasma. So, these persons can accept blood from person with AB as well as the other groups of blood. Therefore, such persons are called universal recipients.

4. **(b)**: Fibrins are formed by the conversion of inactive fibrinogen in the plasma by the enzyme thrombin and thrombins are formed from an another inactive substance present in plasma i.e., prothrombin.

5. **(a)**

6. (d)

7. **(d)**: Red blood cells of adult humans do not have cell organelles including nucleus, Golgi bodies, mitochondria, ribosomes, etc. It increases the surface area of RBCs and enables them to contain more haemoglobin (the oxygen carrying pigment).

8. **(d)**: Thrombocytes are called blood platelets. They are minute disc-shaped cell fragments in mammalian blood. They are formed as fragments of larger cells found in red bone marrow; they have no nucleus. They play an important role in blood clotting and release thromboxane A_2, serotonin and other chemicals, which cause a chain of events leading to the formation of a plug at the site of the damage, thus preventing further blood loss. A reduction in their number can lead to clotting factors which will lead to excessive loss of blood from the body.

9. **(c)**: Serum is the fluid that separates from blood plasma on centrifugation. Serum is essentially similar in composition to plasma but lacks fibrinogen and other substances that are used in the coagulation process.

10. **(b)**: Erythropoiesis is the formation of red blood cells (erythrocytes) which occurs in the red bone marrow.

11. **(a)**: Individuals with *AB* blood group have both antigen *A* and *B* on their RBCs, and no antibodies for either of the antigen in their plasma. Type *O* individuals are without *A* and *B* antigens on their RBCs, but have antibodies for both these antigens in their plasma. Individuals with blood group *AB* can receive blood of A, B or O group, while those with blood group *O* can donate blood to anyone.

12. **(a)**: Basophils have nucleus which is three-lobed and have less number of coarse granules. Their granules take basic stain and release heparin, histamine and serotonin.

13. **(c)**: The blood group was O. The person having O blood group is universal donor. It lacks both antigens 'A' and 'B' thus does not cause agglutination or clumping of blood cells when transfused into person with any of the four blood groups.

14. **(c)**: Spleen is a vertebrate organ, lying behind the stomach, that is basically a collection of lymphoid tissue. Its functions include producing lymphocytes and destroying foreign particles. It acts as a reservoir for RBCs and can regulate the number in circulation. It is also the site for the breakdown of worn out RBCs and thus is known as "graveyard" of RBCs.

15. **(d)**: Blood plasma is a faint yellow, slightly alkaline and somewhat viscous fluid. The plasma contains a number of proteins: serum albumin, serum globulins, properdin, prothrombin and fibrinogen. Prothrombin and fibrinogen play an important role in blood clotting.

16. **(c)**: The blood group was O. The person having O blood group is universal donor. It lacks both antigens 'A' and 'B' thus does not cause agglutination or clumping of blood cells when transfused into person with any of the four blood groups.

17. **(a)**: The body undergoes numerous changes at higher elevation in order to increase oxygen delivery to cells and improve efficiency of oxygen use. The early changes include increased breathing rate, increased heart rate and fluid shifts. The later changes includes increased red blood cell production, increased 2, 3 DPG production and increased number of capillaries.

18. **(d)**

19. **(a)**

20. **(d)**: Globulins in human blood plasma are primarily involved in defence mechanisms of body. Globulins like immunoglobulins act as antibodies that destroy bacteria, viruses and toxic substances that may enter into the blood from outside.

21. **(c)**: In ABO blood group, O refers to O blood group. It has no antigen (A and B) on RBCs.

22. **(b)**: Phagocytes are cells that are able to engulf and breakdown foreign particles, cell debris and disease producing microorganisms. Neutrophils and monocytes (type of white blood cells) are the most active phagocytic cells.

23. **(d)**: Basophils have nucleus which is three-lobed and have less number of coarse granules. Their granules take basic stain and release heparin, histamine and serotonin.

24. (a): Blood serum is blood plasma from which the fibrin and clotting factors have been removed by centrifugation or vigorous stirring, so that it cannot clot. Serum containing a specific antibody or antitoxin may be used in the treatment or prevention of certain infections. Such serum is generally derived from a non-human mammal (e.g., a horse).

25. (a)

26. (c): Individuals with AB blood group have both antigen A and B on their RBCs, and no antibodies for either of the antigen in their plasma. Type O individuals are without A and B antigens on their RBCs, but have antibodies for both these antigens in their plasma. Individuals with blood group AB can receive blood of A,B or O group, while those with blood group O can donate blood to anyone.

27. (a)

28. (a): If fertilisation takes place between gametes of Rh^- female and Rh^+ male then the resulting fetus' blood is Rh^+. The Rh^+ blood of the fetus stimulates the formation of anti Rh factors in the mother's blood. In second pregnancy (with Rh^+ fetus), the anti Rh factors of the mother's blood destroy the fetal red blood corpuscles. This is called erythroblastosis fetalis. New born may survive but it is often anaemic. The Rh^-child does not suffer.

29. (d): WBCs are the colourless nucleated amoeboid cells that can squeeze through blood capillaries by a process known as diapedesis. The increase in their number causes leukemia, a cancer. WBCs are of two types, granulocytes (formed in bone marrow) and agranulocytes (formed in bone marrow and thymus).

30. (d): Blood consists of a watery fluid called plasma. Plasma is a faint yellow, slightly alkaline, viscous fluid. It consists of 90% water, 1% inorganic salts, 7% or 8% proteins and 1% of other substances. The inorganic salts in plasma occur as ions. Sodium is the main cation of plasma and chloride, the main anion. Potassium, calcium and magnesium occur in small amount.

31. (a)

32. (d): The first blood transfusion of Rh^+ blood to the person with Rh^- blood causes no harm because the Rh^-person develops anti Rh factors or antibodies in his/her blood. In second blood transfusion of Rh^+ blood to the Rh^- person, the latter's anti Rh factors attack and destroy the red blood corpuscles of the donor. If father's blood is Rh^+, mother's blood is Rh^- and fetus' blood is Rh^+. Then in second pregnancy (with Rh^+ fetus), the anti Rh factors of the mother's blood destroy the fetal red blood corpuscles.

33. (c): Agranulocytes are leucocytes that lack granules in the cytoplasm. They are formed in spleen and lymph nodes and bone marrow. Since lymphocyte does not have granules in their cytoplasm so it is called agranulocyte. Lymphocytes are important in the body's defence and are responsible for immune reactions as the presence of antigens stimulates them to produce antibodies. Another type of agranulocyte is monocyte. The other three are granulocytes which are produced in red bone marrow.

34. (c): WBCs (also called leucocytes) are rounded or irregular colourless cells with a nucleus. They can change their shape and are capable of amoeboid movement. Leucocytes, formed in lymph nodes and red bone marrow, can produce antibodies and move through the walls of vessels to migrate to the sites of injuries, where they surround and isolate dead tissue, foreign bodies and bacteria. They survive for a few days generally 3-4 days after which they die and get phagocytised in blood, liver and lymph nodes.

35. (b): Vitamin K is essential for blood clotting as it is necessary for the synthesis of prothrombin in the liver.

36. (b): In the embryo and fetal stage of vertebrates, RBCs and leucocytes are formed in the bone marrow, lymph nodes, yolk sac, liver, spleen and thymus but after birth they are formed in red bone marrow only.

37. (d): Lymphocytes have a very large, rounded nucleus and scanty cytoplasm. They are nonmotile and nonphagocytic. They secrete antibodies to destory microbes and their toxins, reject grafts and kill tumour cells. They also help in healing of injuries. Thrombocytes aid in clotting of blood. Monocytes are phagocytic in nature and erythrocytes (RBCs) transport gases in the body.

38. (b)

39. (c): During transport of CO_2 in the blood, about 70% of CO_2 released by respiring tissue cells is transported as bicarbonate ions. It diffuses into the plasma and then into the RBCs. Here, CO_2 combines with water to form carbonic acid. This reaction is catalyzed by a zinc containing enzyme carbonic anhydrase. Carbonic acid dissociates into bicarbonate and hydrogen ions. A small amount of bicarbonate ions is transported in the RBCs, whereas most of them diffuse into the plasma to be carried by it.

40. (b): Thromboplastin, a lipoprotein, helps in clot formation. Thromboplastin helps in the formation of an enzyme prothrombinase. This enzyme inactivates heparin and it also converts the inactive plasma protein prothrombin into its active form, thrombin. Both the changes require calcium ions. Thrombin converts fibrinogen molecule to insoluble fibrin. The fibrin monomers polymerise to form long, sticky fibres. The fibrin threads form a fine network over the wound and trap blood corpuscles (RBCs, WBCs, platelets) to form a crust, the clot. Thus, if calcium is removed from the blood, clotting process will not occur.

41. (c)

42. (d): Neutrophils, are the most abundant type of white blood cells and form an integral part of the immune system. These phagocytes are normally found in the blood stream. However, during the acute phase of inflammation, particularly as a result of bacterial infection, neutrophils leave the vasculature and migrate toward the site of inflammation in a process called chemotaxis. They are the predominant cells in pus, accounting for its whitish/yellowish appearance. Neutrophils react within an hour of tissue injury and are the hallmark of acute inflammation. Monocytes are also phagocytes but take 7-8 hours to reach at the site of injury. Acidophils and basophils are not phagocytic in nature.

43. (b): Rh factor plays a crucial role in child's birth born out of a marriage between Rh^- woman and Rh^+ man. In such a case, the mother becomes sensitive while carrying a first Rh^+ child within her womb. The reason for such sensitivity is that some of the RBCs from the developing embryo get into the blood stream of the mother during development, causing her to produce anti-Rh antibodies. In fact, the first child of such parents is nearly normal and is delivered safely. However, if such a mother gets pregnant again, the subsequent Rh+ foetuses will be exposed to the anti-Rh antibodies produced by the mother. As a result serious damage to the red blood cells of the developing embryo will occur causing haemolytic disease of the newborn (HDN) or erythroblastosis fetalis. This disease leads to the death of the developing embryo before birth or after parturition.

44. **(a, b)**: The haemoglobin is broken down into haem i.e., iron and globin protein which is then converted into yellowish substance bilirubin which is extracted by the liver cells from the blood and stored in the form of bile in gall bladder.

45.(b) : Lymph = Plasma + WBC

Plasma = Blood - Cellular components

Serum = Plasma - Clotting factors

46. **(b)**

47. **(b)**

48. **(a)**: Formation of WBCs, antibodies and destruction of bacteria occur in lymph glands while formation of RBCs occur in bone marrow. Lymph gland is a rounded mass of lymphatic tissue that is surrounded by a capsule of connective tissue. Lymph glands filter lymph (lymphatic fluid) and they store lymphocytes (white blood cells). They are located along lymphatic vessels. They are also called lymph node.

49. **(a)**: Lymph (also called tissue fluid in the intercellular spaces) is the colourless liquid found within the lymphatic system. An important function of lymph is to return interstitial fluid back to the blood. The interstitial fluid is the filtered form of the blood without the cellular components and plasma proteins. It consists of water containing dissolved materials. It receives CO2, nitrogenous waste products, hormones and other synthetic substances from the tissue cells and enters the lymph capillaries to discharge them into blood.

50. **(c)**: The P-wave represents the electrical excitation (or depolarisation) of the atria which leads to the contraction of both the atria. The QRS complex represents the depolarisation of the ventricles which initiates the contraction of ventricles. The contraction starts shortly after Q and marks the beginning of the systole. The T-wave represents the return of the ventricles from excited to normal state (repolarisation). The end of the T-wave marks the end of systole.

51. **(c)**

52. **(c)**: The QRS complex represents the depolarisation of the ventricles, that initiates the ventricular contraction.

53. **(b)**: A normal electrocardiogram or ECG comprises of a P wave, a QRS wave complex and a T wave in which P wave represents depolarisation of the atria, QRS wave complex represents depolarisation of the ventricles and T wave represents ventricular repolarisation. Myocardial ischaemia can affect morphology of T-wave in a variety of ways, i.e., T-wave may become tall, flattened, inverted or biphasic. Flattened T-waves is common in patient with myocardial ischaemia.

54. **(d)**: Stroke volume

= End diastolic volume – End systolic volume

$= 100 - 50 = 50$ mL

Cardiac output = Heart beat × Stroke volume

$\therefore$ Heart beat = Cardiac output/Stroke volume

$= 5000 / 50 = 100$ beats per minute

55. **(a)**

56. **(d)**: Second heart sound i.e., dup is caused by the closure of the semilunar valves and marks the end of ventricular systole.

57. (a): The temporary rise in blood pressure during the contraction of the heart is called systolic pressure and the temporary fall in blood pressure during relaxation of the heart is called diastolic pressure. Blood pressure is expressed as the ratio of the systolic pressure over the diastolic pressure. For a healthy resting adult person, the average systolic/diastolic pressures are 120/80mmHg. Aorta is directly supplied by left ventricle thus, the blood pressure in aorta is highest during systole of left ventricle. During it, left ventricle contracts and pushes blood into aorta.

58. (c): In the given diagram the P-wave represents the electrical excitation (or depolarisation) of the atria, which leads to the contraction of both the atria. The QRS complex represents the depolarisation of the ventricles, which initiates the ventricular contraction. The contraction starts shortly after Q and marks the beginning of the systole. The T-wave represents the return of the ventricles from excited to normal state (repolarisation). The end of the T-wave marks the end of systole.

59. (b): 'Bundle of His' is a part of heart. A bundle of nodal fibres, atrioventricular bundle (AV bundle), continues from the atrioventricular node (AVN) and passes through the atrioventricular septa. It emerges on the top of the interventricular septum and immediately divides into a right and left bundle, which give rise to minute fibres throughout the ventricular musculature of the respective sides called Purkinje fibres. These fibres along with right and left bundles are known as Bundle of His.

60. (a): By counting the number of QRS complexes that occur in a given time period, one can determine the heart beat rate (pulse) of an individual. The QRS complex represents the depolarisation of the ventricles, which initiates the ventricular contraction.

61. (d): Tricuspid valve is the valve in the heart between the right atrium and right ventricle. It consists of three cusps that channel the flow of blood from the atrium to the ventricle. When the right ventricle contracts, forcing blood into the pulmonary artery, the tricuspid valve closes the aperture to the atrium, thereby preventing any backflow of blood. The valve reopens to allow blood to flow from the atrium into the ventricle. Thus, if tricuspid valve is partially non-functional the flow of blood into the pulmonary artery will be reduced.

62. (c)

63. (b): Due to the pressure difference between the post caval and atrium, the blood passes from the post caval to the diastolic right atrium. Diastolic right atrium has less pressure and post caval has high pressure, thus blood moves from post caval to right atrium.

64. (c): Periplaneta has open circulatory system, i.e., the blood does not flow in blood vessels but flows in a haemocoel (body cavity). The circulatory systems of all vertebrates, as well as of annelids (for example, earthworms) and cephalopods (squid and Octopus) are closed, in which the blood never leaves the system of blood vessels consisting of arteries, capillaries and veins.

65. (b): Bundle of His is a part of heart. A bundle of nodal fibres, atrioventricular bundle (AV bundle), continues from the atrioventricular node (AVN) and passes through the atrioventricular septa. It emerges on the top of the interventricular septum and immediately divides into a right and left bundle, which give rise to minute fibres throughout the ventricular musculature of the respective sides called Purkinje fibres. These fibres along with right and left bundles are known as Bundle of His.

66. (b)

67. (a): SA (sinoatrial) node is a specialised bundle of neurons located in the upper part of the right atrium of the heart. SA node is the natural cardiac pacemaker from which the heart beat originates.

68. (d)

69. (b)

70. (b): The neurogenic heart is a characteristic feature of most arthropods and some annelids. In this, the heart beat is initiated by a nerve impulse coming from a nerve ganglion situated near the heart. The myogenic heart is a characteristic feature of molluscs and vertebrates. In this, heart beat is initiated by a patch of modified heart muscle itself. So, humans, rabbits and rats have myogenic heart.

71. (b)

72. (b)

73. (a, c): Blood enters the liver from two sources. From the hepatic artery, it gets oxygenated blood and from the hepatic portal vein, it receives deoxygenated blood. Blood in the hepatic artery comes from the aorta. Blood in the hepatic portal vein comes directly from the intestine containing newly absorbed nutrients, stomach, etc.

74. (a)

75. (a): Hepatic vein carries largest amount of urea. Urea is produced in liver. Hepatic vein transports liver's deoxygenated blood to heart for oxygenation.

76. (a): Whale is a mammal and in mammals, two separate circulatory pathways are found - systemic circulation and pulmonary circulation. Oxygenated and deoxygenated bloods received by the left and right atria respectively pass on to the left and right ventricles. Thus, oxygenated and deoxygenated bloods are not mixed. This is referred to as double circulation.

77. (a): In the given figure, A is pulmonary vein which brings pure blood from lungs to left atrium, B is dorsal aorta which carries blood from heart to body parts, C is vena cava which carries impure blood from body parts to right auricle and D is pulmonary artery which takes impure blood from heart to lungs.

78. (c): A- Artery : Carries blood from heart to different body parts. It is thick-walled and elastic. The flow of blood in it is intermittent.

B - Capillary : Nutrients, hormones, gases, etc., can diffuse into tissue cells through capillaries and vice versa. It is thin-walled and only one layer thick resting on basement membrane.

C - Vein : Brings blood from different body parts to the heart. It is thin-walled and acts as low-resistance conduct for blood flow.

D - Pulmonary vein : Two pulmonary veins from each lung transport the oxygenated blood to the left atrium.

79. (b): Arteries and veins are main blood vessels. Arteries carry blood from the heart to different body parts. Veins bring blood from different body parts to the heart.

80. (c): Intravenous injection is given for rapid distribution of drugs/substance. Intra-muscular injection is given for producing local effect.

81. (c): An artery has thick and more elastic wall but its lumen is narrow as compared to vein. Pulmonary artery carries deoxygenated blood from the right ventricle to the lungs for oxygenation. Pulmonary vein carries oxygenated blood from the lungs to the left auricle.

82. (c)

83. (a): Spleen receives only oxygenated blood from the heart through splenic artery. The liver receives a blood supply from two sources. The first is the hepatic artery which delivers oxygenated blood from the general circulation. The second is the hepatic portal vein delivering deoxygenated blood from the small intestine containing nutrients. The blood flows through the liver tissue to the hepatic cells where many metabolic functions take place. The blood drains out of the liver via the hepatic vein. Gill and lung receive deoxygenated blood as these are the organs where oxygenation of blood takes place.

84. (c): Veins carry blood at low pressure as compared to blood carried by arteries. Arteries carry blood from the heart whose function is to pump blood at high pressure so that blood can reach each and every part of the body. Veins carry blood from tissues to the heart, so they carry blood at low pressure. Valves are present in the veins to prevent backflow of blood due to force of gravity.

85. (d): The wall of capillaries is very thin (usually less than one micron) and have numerous minute pores and made up of only endothelium. Exchange of material takes place between blood and tissue fluid across the endothelial membrane of capillaries through active diffusion.

86. (c)

87. (a): Pulmonary artery carries the blood from the right ventricle of the heart to the lungs for oxygenation so it carries deoxygenated blood.

88. (a): A special neural centre in medulla oblongata can moderate the cardiac function through autonomic nervous system (ANS). Neural signals through the sympathetic nerves (part of ANS) can increase the rate of heart beat, the strength of ventricular contraction and thereby the cardiac output. Parasympathetic neural signals (component of ANS) decrease the rate of heart beat, speed of conduction of action potential and thereby the cardiac output.

89. (d): If repeated checks of blood pressure of an individual is 140/90"" mmHg or higher, it shows hypertension or high blood pressure. It leads to heart diseases and also affects vital organs like brain and kidney.

90. (a): The term angina means chest pain. In this disease, enough oxygen does not reach the heart muscles. The patient experiences heart pain usually in front of the chest.

AB blood group person have both antigens A and B, but do not have antibodies in the plasma. Due to the presence of both the antigens, AB blood group person cannot donate blood to anyone. However, the person can receive blood from any blood group as it has no antibodies. Thus, AB blood group is a universal recepient.

91. (a): Arteriosclerosis is the hardening of arteries and arterioles due to thickening of the fibrous tissue, and the consequent loss of elasticity. In this disease, calcium salts precipitate with the cholesterol. This calcification ultimately makes the wall of arteries stiff and rigid.

92.(a) : The temporary rise in blood pressure during the contraction of the heart is called systolic pressure and the temporary fall in blood pressure during relaxation of the heart is called diastolic pressure. Blood pressure is expressed as the ratio of the systolic pressure over the diastolic pressure. For a healthy resting adult person, the average systolic/diastolic pressures are 120/80 mmHg. Aorta is directly supplied by left ventricle thus, the blood pressure in aorta is highest during systole of left ventricle. During it, left ventricle contracts and pushes blood into aorta.

Chapter : 16 EXCRETORY PRODUCTS AND THEIR ELIMINATION

INTRODUCTION

1. Nitrogenous waste is excreted in the form of pellet or paste by: ***(2022)***
(a) Ornithorhynchus (b) Salamandra
(c) Hippocampus (d) Pavo

2. Select the option which shows correct matching of animal with its excretory organ and excretory product. ***(Karnataka NEET 2013)***

	Animal	Excretory organ	Excretory product
(a)	Labeo (Rohu)	Nephridial tubes	Ammonia
(b)	Salamander	Kidneys	Urea
(c)	Peacock	Kidneys	Urea
(d)	Housefly	Renal tubules	Uric acid

3. Which one of the following options gives the correct categorization of six animals according to the type of nitrogenous waste they give out? ***(Mains 2012)***

	Ammonotelic	Ureotelic	Uricotelic
(a)	Pigeon, humans	Aquatic amphibia, lizards	Cockroach, frog
(b)	Frog, lizards	Aquatic amphibia, humans	Cockroach pigeon
(c)	Aquatic amphibia	Frog, humans	Pigeon, lizards, cockroach
(d)	Aquatic amphibia	Cockroach, humans	Frog, pigeon, lizards

4. Which one of the following characteristics is common both in humans and adult frogs? ***(Mains 2012)***
(a) Four chambered heart
(b) Internal fertilisation
(c) Nucleated RBCs
(d) Ureotelic mode of excretion

5. Uricotelic mode of excreting nitrogenous wastes is found in ***(Mains 2011)***
(a) reptiles and birds
(b) birds and annelids
(c) amphibians and reptiles
(d) insects and amphibians.

6. The principal nitrogenous excretory compound in humans is synthesised ***(2010)***
(a) in kidneys but eliminated mostly through liver
(b) in kidneys as well as eliminated by kidneys
(c) in liver and also eliminated by the same through bile
(d) in the liver, but eliminated mostly through kidneys.

7. Uric acid is the chief nitrogenous component of the excretory products of ***(2009)***
(a) earthworm (b) cockroach
(c) frog (d) man.

8. In ornithine cycle, which of the following wastes are removed from the blood? ***(2005)***
(a) CO_2 and urea
(b) Ammonia and urea
(c) CO_2 and ammonia
(d) Urea and urine

9. Uricotelism is found in ***(2004)***
(a) mammals and birds
(b) fish and fresh water protozoans
(c) birds, land reptiles and insects
(d) frogs and toads.

10. Conversion of ammonia to urea is done by ***(2000)***
(a) ornithine cycle (b) arginine cycle
(c) fumaric cycle (d) citrulline cycle.

11. In ureotelic animals, urea is formed by ***(1997)***
(a) Krebs' cycle (b) EM pathway
(c) Ornithine cycle (d) Cori cycle.

12. The ornithine cycle removes two waste products from the blood in liver. These products are ***(1996)***

(a) CO_2 and ammonia
(b) ammonia and uric acid
(c) CO_2 and urea
(d) ammonia and urea

13. Two examples in which the nitrogenous wastes are excreted from body in the form of uric acid are ***(1994)***

(a) birds and lizards
(b) frogs and cartilaginous fish
(c) insects and bony fish
(d) mammals and molluscs.

14. Nitrogenous waste products are eliminated mainly as ***(1991)***

(a) urea in tadpole and ammonia in adult frog
(b) ammonia in tadpole and urea in adult frog
(c) urea in both tadpole and adult frog
(d) urea in tadpole and uric acid in adult frog.

HUMAN EXCRETORY SYSTEM

15. Given below are statements. ***(2023)***

One is labelled as Assertion (A) and the other is labelled as Reason (R).

Assertion (A) : Nephrons are of two types: Cortical and Juxtamedullary, based on their relative position in cortex and medulla.

Reason (R) : Juxtamedullary nephrons have short loop of Henle whereas, cortical nephrons have longer loop of Henle.

In the light of the above statements, choose the correct answer from the options given below.

(a) (A) is true but (R) is false.
(b) (A) is false but (R) is true.
(c) Both (A) and (R) are true and (R) is the correct explanation of (A).
(d) Both (A) and (R) are true but (R) is not the correct explanation of (A).

16. Figure shows human urinary system with structures labelled A to D. Select option which correctly identifies them and gives their characteristic and/ or functions. ***(2013)***

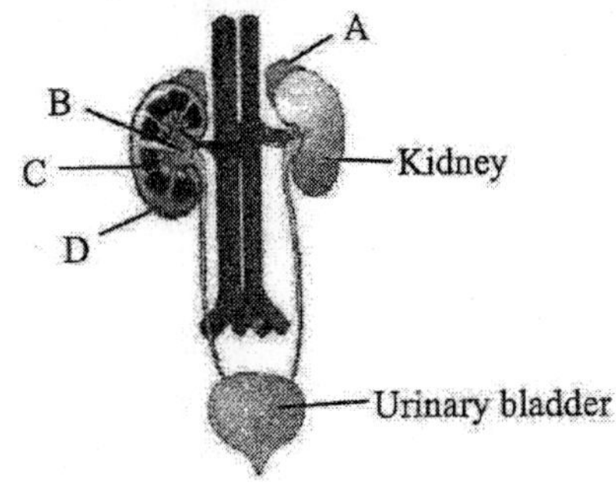

(a) C - Medulla - inner zone of kidney and contains complete nephrons.
(b) D - Cortex - outer part of kidney and do not contain any part of nephrons.
(c) A - Adrenal gland - located at the anterior part of kidney. Secrete catecholamines which stimulate glycogen breakdown.
(d) B - Pelvis - broad funnel shaped space inner to hilum, directly connected to loops of Henle.

17. Which one of the following is not a part of a renal pyramid? ***(Mains 2011)***

(a) Peritubular capillaries
(b) Convoluted tubules
(c) Collecting ducts
(d) Loop of Henle

18. The basic functional unit of human kidney is ***(1997)***

(a) nephridia (b) Henle's loop
(c) nephron (d) pyramid.

19. Which one of the four parts mentioned below does not constitute a part of single uriniferous tubule? ***(1994)***

(a) Distal convoluted tubule
(b) Collecting duct
(c) Bowman's capsule
(d) Loop of Henle

FUNCTION OF THE TUBULES

20. Which of the following statements is correct? ***(2017)***

(a) The descending limb of loop of Henle is impermeable to water.

(b) The ascending limb of loop of Henle is permeable to water.

(c) The descending limb of loop of Henle is permeable to electrolytes.

(d) The ascending limb of loop of Henle is impermeable to water.

21. The part of nephron involved in active reabsorption of sodium is ***(NEET-II 2016)***

(a) distal convoluted tubule
(b) proximal convoluted tubule
(c) Bowman's capsule
(d) descending limb of Henle's loop.

22. Removal of proximal convoluted tubule from the nephron will result in ***(2015 Cancelled)***

(a) no change in quality and quantity of urine
(b) no urine formation
(c) more diluted urine
(d) more concentrated urine.

23. The maximum amount of electrolytes and water (70 - 80 percent) from the glomerular filtrate is reabsorbed in which part of the nephron? ***(2012)***

(a) Ascending limb of loop of Henle
(b) Distal convoluted tubule
(c) Proximal convoluted tubule
(d) Descending limb of loop of Henle

24. Which one of the following correctly explains the function of a specific part of the human nephron? ***(Mains 2011)***

(a) Podocytes : create minute spaces (slit pores) for the filtration of blood into the Bowman's capsule

(b) Henle's loop : most reabsorption of the major substances from the glomerular filtrate

(c) Distal convoluted tubule : reabsorption of K^+ ions into the surrounding blood capillaries

(d) Afferent arteriole : carries the blood away from the glomerulus towards renal vein.

25. Which one of the following statements in regard to the excretion by the human kidneys is correct? ***(2010)***

(a) Descending limb of loop of Henle is impermeable to water.

(b) Distal convoluted tubule is incapable of reabsorbing HCO_3^-.

(c) Nearly 99 per cent of the glomerular filtrate is reabsorbed by the renal tubules.

(d) Ascending limb of loop of Henle is impermeable to electrolytes.

26. Glucose is taken back from glomerular filtrate through ***(1993)***

(a) active transport (c) osmosis
(b) passive transport (d) diffusion.

27. Under normal conditions which one is completely reabsorbed in the renal tubule? ***(1991)***

(a) Urea (b) Uric acid
(c) Salts (d) Glucose

28. Brush border is characteristic of ***(1990)***

(a) neck of nephron
(b) collecting tube
(c) proximal convoluted tubule
(d) all of these

29. Reabsorption of useful substances from glomerular filtrate occurs in ***(1989)***

(a) collecting tube
(b) loop of Henle
(c) proximal convoluted tubule
(d) distal convoluted tubule.

MECHANISM OF CONCENTRATION OF THE FILTRATE

30. Which of the following factors is responsible for the formation of concentrated urine? ***(2019)***

(a) Hydrostatic pressure during glomerular filtration.

(b) Low levels of antidiuretic hormone.

(c) Maintaining hyperosmolarity towards the medullary interstitium in the kidneys.

(d) Secretion of erythropoietin by Juxtaglomerular complex.

31. If Henle's loop were absent from mammalian nephron, which one of the following is to be expected? ***(2003)***

(a) There will be no urine formation.
(b) There will be hardly any change in the quality and quantity of urine formed
(c) The urine will be more concentrated.
(d) The urine will be more dilute.

32. Concentration of urine depends upon which organ? ***(2000)***

(a) Bowman's capsule
(b) Length of Henle's loop
(c) PCT
(d) Network of capillaries arising from glomerulus

REGULATION OF KIDNEY FUNCTION

33. Which of the following statements are correct? ***(2023)***

A. An excessive loss of body fluid from the body switches off osmoreceptors.

B. ADH facilitates water reabsorption to prevent diuresis.

C. ANF causes vasodilation.

D. ADH causes increase in blood pressure.

E. ADH is responsible for decrease in GFR.

Choose the correct answer from the options given below.

(a) A, B and E only (b) C, D and E only
(c) A and B only (d) B, C and D only

34. Which of the following would help in prevention of diuresis? ***(2020)***

(a) More water reabsorption due to undersecretion of ADH.
(b) Reabsorption of Na^+ and water from renal tubules due to aldosterone.
(c) Atrial natriuretic factor causes vasoconstriction
(d) Decrease in secretion of renin by JG cells.

35. A decrease in blood pressure/volume will not cause the release of **(2017)**

(a) atrial natriuretic factor(b) aldosterone
(c) ADH(d) renin.

36. Which of the following causes an increase in sodium reabsorption in the distal convoluted tubule? ***(2014)***

(a) Increase in aldosterone levels
(b) Increase in antidiuretic hormone levels
(c) Decrease in aldosterone levels
(d) Decrease in antidiuretic hormone levels

37. A fall in glomerular filtration rate (GFR) activates ***(Mains 2012)***

(a) juxtaglomerular cells to release renin
(b) adrenal cortex to release aldosterone
(c) adrenal medulla to release adrenaline
(d) posterior pituitary to release vasopressin.

38. Which one of the following statements is correct with respect to kidney function regulation? ***(Mains 2011)***

(a) When someone drinks lot of water, ADH release is suppressed.
(b) Exposure to cold temperature stimulates ADH release.
(c) An increase in glomerular blood flow stimulates formation of angiotensin II.
(d) During summer when body loses lot of water by evaporation, the release of ADH is suppressed.

39. Angiotensinogen is a protein produced and secreted by ***(2006)***

(a) juxtaglomerular (JG) cells
(b) macula densa cells
(c) endothelial cells (cells lining the blood vessels)
(d) liver cells.

40. If excess water passes out from the tissue without being restored by the kidneys, the cells would ***(1994)***
(a) burst open and die
(b) take water from the plasma
(c) not be affected at all
(d) shrivel and die.

MICTURITION

41. Match the items given in column I with those in column II and select the correct option given below. ***(2018)***

Column I (Function)	Column II (Part of excretory system)
A. Ultrafiltration	(i) Henle's loop
B. Concentration of urine	(ii) Ureter
C. Transport of urine	(iii) Urinary bladder
D. Storage of urine	(iv) Malpighian corpuscle
	(v) Proximal convoluted tubule

	A	B	C	D
(a)	(iv)	(v)	(ii)	(iii)
(b)	(iv)	(i)	(ii)	(iii)
(c)	(v)	(iv)	(i)	(ii)
(d)	(v)	(iv)	(i)	(iii)

42. Human urine is usually acidic because ***(2015)***
(a) potassium and sodium exchange generates acidity
(b) hydrogen ions are actively secreted into the filtrate
(c) the sodium transporter exchanges one hydrogen ion for each sodium ion, in peritubular capillaries
(d) excreted plasma proteins are acidic.

43. Which of the following does not favour the formation of large quantities of dilute urine? ***(2015 Cancelled)***
(a) Renin
(b) Atrial-natriuretic factor
(c) Alcohol (d) Caffeine

44. What will happen if the stretch receptors of the urinary bladder wall are totally removed? ***(2009)***
(a) Micturition will continue.
(b) Urine will continue to collect normally in the bladder.
(c) There will be no micturition.
(d) Urine will not collect in the bladder.

45. A person who is on a long hunger strike and is surviving only on water, will have ***(2007)***
(a) less amino acids in his urine
(b) more glucose in his blood
(c) less urea in his urine
(d) more sodium in his urine.

46. A person is undergoing prolonged fasting. His urine will be found to contain abnormal quantities of ***(2005)***
(a) fats (b) amino acids
(c) glucose (d) ketones.

DISORDERS OF THE EXCRETORY SYSTEM

47. Use of an artificial kidney during hemodialysis may result in ***(2019)***

(A) Nitrogenous waste build-up in the body

(B) Non-elimination of excess potassium ions

(C) Reduced absorption of calcium ions from gastro-intestinal tract

(D) Reduced RBC production.

Which of the following options is the most appropriate ?
(a) (A) and (D) are correct
(b) (A) and (B) are correct
(c) (B) and (C) are correct
(d) (C) and (D) are correct

48. Match the items given in column I with those in column II and select the correct option given below. ***(2018)***

Column I	Column II
A. Glycosuria	(i) Accumulation of uric acid in joints
B. Gout	(ii) Mass of crystallised salts within the kidney
C. Renal calculi	(iii) Inflammation in glomeruli
D.Glomerular nephrit	(iv) Presence of glucose in urine

	A	B	C	D
(a)	(iii)	(ii)	(iv)	(i)
(b)	(i)	(ii)	(iii)	(iv)
(c)	(ii)	(iii)	(i)	(iv)
(d)	(iv)	(i)	(ii)	(iii)

49. A condition of failure of kidney to form urine is called ***1998)***

(a) anuria (b) deamination
(c) uremia (d) none of these.

50. Presence of RBC in urine is ***(1988)***

(a) alkaptonuria (b) urothiasis
(c) hematuria (d) proteinuria

ANSWER KEY

1.	(d)	2.	(b)	3.	(c)	4.	(d)	5.	(a)	6.	(d)	7.	(b)
8.	(c)	9.	(c)	10.	(a)	11.	(c)	12.	(a)	13.	(a)	14.	(b)
15.	(a)	16.	(c)	17.	(b)	18.	(c)	19.	(b)	20.	(d)	21.	(b)
22.	(c)	23.	(c)	24.	(a)	25.	(c)	26.	(a)	27.	(d)	28.	(c)
29.	(c)	30.	(c)	31.	(d)	32.	(b)	33.	(d)	34.	(b)	35.	(a)
36.	(a)	37.	(a)	38.	(a)	39.	(d)	40.	(d)	41.	(b)	42.	(b)
43.	(a)	44.	(c)	45.	(c)	46.	(d)	47.	(d)	48.	(d)	49.	(a)
50.	(c)												

HINTS & EXPLANATIONS

1. **(d)**: Pavo belongs to Class Aves, so, excrete nitrogenous wastes as uric acid in the form of pellet or paste.

2. **(b)**: In salamander, kidneys (mesonepheric) are the excretory organs and the excretory matter is urea. In Labeo, mesonephric kidney is the excretory organ and excretion is ammonotelic. Peacock has metanephric kidneys with excretory matter being uric acid. In housefly, excretion takes place by Malpighian tubules. Excretory waste is uric acid chiefly.

3. **(c)**

4. **(d)**: Excretion of urea is known as ureotelism and the animals which excrete urea are called ureotelic. Ureotelic animals include marine fishes, semi-aquatic amphibians such as frogs and toads, aquatic or semi-aquatic reptiles like turtles, terrapins and alligators, and man and all other mammals. Urea is less toxic and less soluble in water than ammonia. Hence, it can stay for some time in the body. Amphibian tadpole (e.g., tadpole of frog) excrete ammonia but after metamorphosis, frog excretes urea.

5. **(a)**: Reptiles, birds, land snails and insects excrete nitrogenous wastes as uric acid in the form of pellet or paste with a minimum loss of water and are called uricotelic animals.

6. **(d)**: The principle nitrogenous excretory compound in humans is urea. Urea is produced in a series of reactions (urea cycle) which take place in the mitochondrial matrix and cytosol of liver cells. Urea cycle (ornithine cycle) is the series of biochemical reactions that converts ammonia, which is highly toxic and carbon dioxide to the much less toxic urea during the excretion of metabolic nitrogen derived from the deamination of excess amino acids. The urea is ultimately excreted in solution in urine..

7. **(b)**: Cockroach shows uricotelism. Excretion of uric acid is known as uricotelism and the animals which excrete uric acid are called uricotelic. Animals which live in dry conditions have to conserve water in their bodies. Therefore, they synthesise crystals of uric acid from ammonia. Uric acid crystals are non-toxic and almost insoluble in water. Hence, these can be retained in the body for a considerable time. Uricotelic animals include most insects, (e.g., cockroach), land reptiles (e.g., lizards and snakes) and birds.

8. **(c)**

9. **(c)**: Uricotelism means excretion of uric acid. Uric acid excretion occurs in organisms which develop in an enclosed egg (where water is severely limited) or which normally experience very dry terrestrial environment as adult organisms. Uric acid is discharged as thick paste or as solid pellet. Examples: terrestrial reptiles, birds, insects, gastropod mollusc, etc.

10. **(a)**

11. **(c)**: Urea is formed of two molecules of ammonia and one molecule of CO_2. During catabolism, proteins break up into amino acids. The amino acids are converted into keto-acids (such as a-keto-glutaric acid) with the removal of ammonia (deamination). The keto-acid enters the Krebs cycle to yield energy. Carbon dioxide is formed during decarboxylation.

    Ornithine (amino acid) combines with one molecule of NH_3 and CO_2 producing citrulline (amino acid) and water. Citrulline combines with another molecule of ammonia and forms arginine (essential amino acid) and water. Arginine is broken into urea and ornithine in the presence of an enzyme arginase and water. Thus the cycle is repeated. This is called urea or ornithine or Krebs'-Henseleit cycle after the names of its discoverers.

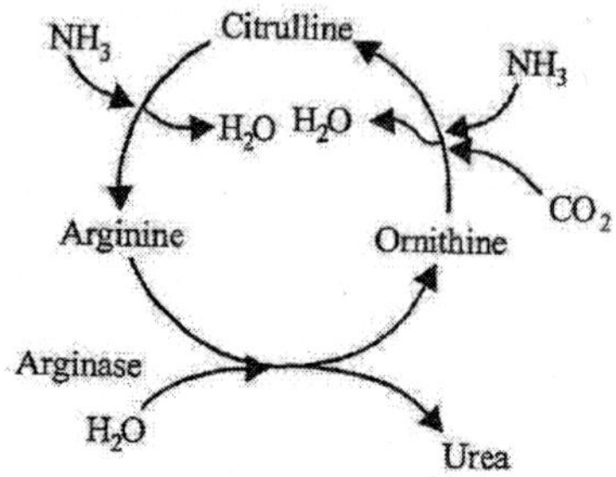

Most of the urea is produced in the liver. The liver cells continuously release urea into the blood and kidneys withdraw it from the blood to excrete it in urine.

12. (a)

13. (a): Birds and lizards are uricotelic. Uricotelic animals are those that excrete nitrogenous waste in the form of uric acid. It is being insoluble in water, does not require water for its elimination. Frogs and cartilaginous fish are ureotelic, that is they excrete nitrogenous waste in the form of urea. The main excretory matter of insects is uric acid and of bony fish is ammonia (ammonotelic). Molluscs may be ammonotelic or uricotelic. Mammals are ureotelic (excretory matter is urea).

14. (b): Ammonia is highly soluble in water, so in aquatic animals, e.g., tadpole of frog, the nitrogenous waste products are excreted in the form of ammonia. In terrestrial animals, e.g., adult frog, these wastes are excreted in the form of urea.

15. (a): In juxtamedullary nephrons, loop of Henle is very long and runs deep into medulla. In cortical nephrons, loop of Henle is short and extends very little into the medulla.

16. (c): In the given figure, A is adrenal gland which secretes two catecholamines; adrenaline (epinephrine) and noradrenaline (norepinephrine). Adrenaline increases the conversion of glycogen to glucose providing quick energy for "fight or flight" response. B is renal pelvis which is a sac like cavity of the kidney leading to ureters, is not directly connected to loop of Henle. C is medulla, the inner region of kidney containing loop of Henle, collecting ducts and ducts of Bellini. D is cortex which has proximal and distal convoluted tubules and contains Malpighian corpuscles.

17. (b): The medulla of kidney is divided into a number of conical areas, the medulla pyramids or renal pyramids. Peritubular capillaries, loop of Henle and collecting ducts lie in the medulla (renal pyramids) while convoluted tubules lie in the cortex of kidney.

18. (c): A nephron is a unit of structure and function in a kidney. A kidney contains about a million nephrons, each approximately 3 cm. long. A nephron is a long tubule differentiated into four regions having different anatomical features and physiological role : Bowman's capsule, proximal convoluted tubule (PCT), loop of Henle, and distal convoluted tubule (DCT). The latter opens into one of the collecting ducts. Nephridia are the excretory organs of annelids.

19. (b)

20. (d): Descending limb of loop of Henle is permeable to water but almost impermeable to electrolytes. Ascending limb of loop of Henle is impermeable to water but permeable to electrolytes.

21. (b): From the Bowman's capsule, a glomerular filtrate enters the proximal convoluted tubule. Absorption of selected materials takes place from the filtrate into the blood of the peritubular capillaries or vasa recta. It is termed the tubular reabsorption. Reabsorption involves both passive and active transport across the tubular epithelium. About 65 per cent of the glomerular filtrate is normally reabsorbed in the proximal convoluted tubule before reaching the loop of Henle. Glucose, amino acids, vitamins, hormones, sodium, potassium, chlorides, phosphates, bicarbonates, much of water and some urea from the filtrate are absorbed. Sodium and potassium are reabsorbed by primary active transport.

22. (c)

23. (c)

24. (a): The visceral layer of Bowman's capsule surrounds the glomerulus and is composed of special type of cells, the podocytes. The podocytes are so called because they possess foot like processes (projection), the pedicels. The space between pedicels are called slit pores (= filtration slits) through which the glomerular filtrate filters.

25. (c): Urine formation involves three main processes namely, glomerular filtration, reabsorption and secretion, that takes place in different parts of the nephron. A comparison of the volume of the filtrate formed per day (180 litres per day) with that of the urine released (1.5 litres), suggest that nearly 99 percent of the filtrate is reabsorbed by the renal tubules. The descending limb of loop of Henle is permeable to water but almost impermeable to electrolytes. The ascending limb is impermeable to water but allows transport of electrolytes actively or passively. Conditional reabsorption of Na+ and water takes place in distal convoluted tubule. It is also capable of reabsorption of HCO_3^-.

26. (a) :Glucose is taken back from the glomerular filtrate by the proximal convoluted tubule by active transport.

27. (d) : The cells lining the proximal convoluted tubule are well adapted for reabsorption of materials from the filtrate. They have abundant mitochondria and bear numerous microvilli on the free side thus giving brush border appearance. The cells reabsorb entire glucose, amino acids, most of the inorganic ions, much of the water as well as some urea from the filtrate.

28. (c)

29. (c)

30.(c) :The counter current mechanism helps to maintain a concentration gradient in the medullary interstitium. The proximity between the Henle's loop and vasa recta, as well as the counter current in them help in maintaining an increasing osmolarity towards the inner medullary interstitium, i.e., from 300mOsmolL^{-1} in the cortex to about 1200mOsmolL^{-1} in the inner medulla. This gradient is mainly caused by NaCl and urea. Presence of such interstitial gradient helps in an easy passage of water from the collecting tubule thereby concentrating the filtrate (urine).

31. (d): Reabsorption is a process by which useful constituents of glomerular filtrate are returned into the blood streams. It occurs in convoluted tubules (proximal convoluted tubule) as well as loop of Henle. Basically loop of Henle, in association with vasa rectae, plays an important role in the counter current mechanism (the process which makes urine hypertonic, i.e., more concentrated). Therefore, if Henle's loop was absent from mammalian nephron the urine will be more dilute.

32. (b): Concentration of urine depends upon the length of Henle's loop. Loop of Henle is the hairpin shaped section of a kidney tubule situated between the proximal and distal tubules in the nephron. It consists of a thin descending limb which is permeable to water and a thick ascending limb which is impermeable to water, complex movements of ions and water across the walls of the loop enable it to function as a countercurrent multiplier, resulting in the production of concentrated urine in the collecting duct.

33. (d): An excessive loss of fluid from the body can activate osmoreceptors which stimulate the hypothalamus to release antidiuretic hormone (ADH) or vasopressin from the neurohypophysis. ADH facilitates water reabsorption from latter parts of the tubule, thereby preventing diuresis. An increase in body fluid volume can switch off the osmoreceptors and suppress the ADH release to complete the feedback. ADH can also affect the kidney function by its constrictory effects on blood vessels. This causes an increase in blood pressure. An increase in blood pressure can increase the glomerular blood flow and thereby the GFR.

34. (b): Aldosterone acts mainly at the renal tubules and stimulates the reabsorption of Na+ and water and excretion of K+ and phosphate ions. Thus, aldosterone helps in prevention of diuresis.

35. (a): Atrial natriuretic factor (ANF) is responsible for lowering of blood pressure and volume. The walls of the atria of the heart release ANF in response to an increase in blood volume and pressure. It opposes regulation by RAAS. It inhibits release of renin from JGA thereby inhibiting NaCl reabsorption by the collecting duct and reduces aldosterone release from adrenal gland.

36. (a): Aldosterone is a hormone secreted by the outer layer of the adrenal gland (cortex part). Decreased blood volume and interstitial fluid level, results in decreased blood pressure, trigger aldosterone secretion. When aldosterone is present in the blood, reabsorption of Na+ in the filtrate is increased by the epithelial cells of the collecting duct. Retaining Na+, raises the osmotic pressure of the blood and reduces water loss from the body. When aldosterone is absent; some Na+ remains in the filtrate and is excreted with the urine.

37. (a): The amount of the filtrate formed by the kidneys per minute is called glomerular filtration rate (GFR). GFR in a healthy individual is approximately 125 mL/ minute, i.e. 180 litres per day. The kidneys have built-in mechanisms for the regulation of glomerular filtration rate. One such efficient mechanism is carried out by juxtaglomerular apparatus (JGA). JGA is a special sensitive region formed by cellular modifications in the distal convoluted tubule and the afferent arteriole at the location of their contact. A fall in GFR can activate the JG cells to release renin which can stimulate the glomerular blood flow and thereby the GFR come back to normal.

38. (a): Antidiuretic hormone (ADH) or vasopressin increases the reabsorption of water in the distal convoluted tubule, collecting tubules and collecting ducts of the nephrons of the kidneys. As a result, the reabsorption of water from the glomerular filtrate is increased. When someone drinks lot of water, requirement of absorption of water decreases, so ADH release is suppressed.

39. (d): Juxtaglomerular cells secrete an enzyme renin into blood. Renin changes plasma protein angiotensinogen to a peptide called angiotensin II. It increases the blood volume : (i) by inducing proximal convoluted tubules to reabsorb more NaCl and water (ii) stimulates the adrenal glands to release a hormone, called aldosterone which induces the distal convoluted tubule to absorb more Na^+ and water Angiotensinogen is an a-globulin protein produced by liver. Renin serves as an enzyme in the conversion of the plasma protein angiotensinogen into angiotensin. This protein stimulates the adrenal cortex to produce aldosterone which acts on the cells of the ascending limb of the loop of Henle and increases the rate of reabsorption of Na^+. Reabsorption of Na^+ brings about the uptake of an osmotically equivalent amount of water. Absorption of sodium and water increases blood volume and pressure.

40. **(d)**: Kidney's main function is to maintain water balance in blood plasma by reabsorbing water. If the excess amount of water will move out of tissue without being restored in kidneys, cell will shrivel due to dehydration and ultimately die.

41. **(b)**

42. **(b)**

43.(a) : Juxtaglomerular cells secrete an enzyme renin into blood. Renin changes plasma protein angiotensinogen to a peptide called angiotensin. 11. It increases the blood volume (i) by inducing proximal convoluted tubules to reabsorb more NaCl and water (ii) stimulates the adrenal glands to release a hormone called aldosterone which induces the distal convoluted tubule to absorb more Na+ and water.

44. **(c)**: Micturition is the expulsion of urine from the urinary bladder. Sensory stretch receptors are responsible for the stretch reflex. If these are removed then there will be no Micturition.

45. **(c)**: Due to a long hunger strike and survival on water, a person will have less urea in his urine, because it is formed the breakdown of proteins, and there is no intake of proteins during fasting.

46. **(d)**: Under fasting conditions which are associated with high rate of fatty acid oxidation, the liver produces large amount of ketone bodies viz. acetoacetate, b-hydroxybutyrate and acetone. The normal level of ketone blood level is 0.2 mmol/L. Presence of excess ketone bodies in urine is termed as ketonuria.

47. **(d)**: Since both kidneys are non-functional thus absorption of Ca^{2+} from small intestine will be affected as coversion of vitamin D to calcitriol will not take place which is needed for calcium absorption from small intestine(GI tract). Erythropoietin production will also be affected, thus RBC production will be reduced

48. **(d)**

49. **(a)**: Anuria is the complete suppression of urine formation by the kidney. In this case most of the nephrons are destroyed. Uremia is the presence of an excessive amount of urea in the blood. Deamination is the removal of ammonia from amino acids.

50. **(c)**: Presence of RBCs in the blood is known as hematuria. Alkaptonuria is the excretion of large amount of alkapton in urine which when comes in contact with air turns black. Proteinuria is the presence of proteins in the blood.

Chapter : 17 LOCOMOTION AND MOVEMENT

MUSCLE

1. Which of the following statements are correct regarding skeletal muscle? ***(2023)***

A. Muscle bundles are held together by collagenous connective tissue layer called fascicle.

B. Sarcoplasmic reticulum of muscle fibre is a store house of calcium ions.

C. Striated appearance of skeletal muscle fibre is due to distribution pattern of actin and myosin proteins.

D. M line is considered as functional unit of contraction called sarcomere.

Choose the most appropriate answer from the options given below:

(a) A, C and D only (b) C and D only
(c) A, B and C only (d) B and C only

2. During muscular contraction which of the following events occur? ***(2021)***

(A) 'H' zone disappears.

(B) 'A' band widens.

(C) 'I' band reduces in width.

(D) Myosine hydrolyzes ATP, releasing the ADP and P_i.

(E) Z-lines attached to actins are pulled inwards.

Choose the correct answer from the options given below.

(a) (B), (D), (E), (A) only
(b) (A), (C), (D), (E) only
(c) (A), (B), (C), (D) only
(d) (B), (C), (D), (E) only

3. Calcium is important in skeletal muscle contraction because it ***(2018)***

(a) binds to troponin to remove the masking of active sites on actin for myosin
(b) activates the myosin ATPase by binding to it
(c) detaches the myosin head from the actin filament
(d) prevents the formation of bonds between the myosin cross bridges and the actin filament.

4. Name the ion responsible for unmasking of active sites for myosin for cross-bridge activity during muscle contraction. ***(NEET-II 2016)***

(a) Calcium (b) Magnesium
(c) Sodium (d) Potassium

5. Lack of relaxation between successive stimuli in sustained muscle contraction is known as ***(NEET-I 2016)***

(a) tetanus (b) tonus
(c) spasm (d) fatigue.

6. Sliding filament theory can be best explained as ***(2015 Cancelled)***

(a) actin and myosin filaments do not shorten but rather slide pass each other
(b) when myofilaments slide pass each other, myosin filaments shorten while actin filaments do not shorten
(c) when myofilaments slide pass each other actin filaments shorten while myosin filaments do not shorten
(d) actin and myosin filaments shorten and slide pass each other.

7. Stimulation of a muscle fibre by a motor neuron occurs at ***(2014)***

(a) the neuro-muscular junction
(b) the transverse tubules
(c) the myofibril
(d) the sacroplasmic reticulum.

8. The H-zone in the skeletal muscle fibre is due to ***(2013)***

(a) the central gap between actin filaments extending through myosin filaments in the A-band
(b) extension of myosin filaments in the central portion of the A-band
(c) the absence of myofibrils in the central portion of A-band
(d) the central gap between myosin filaments in the A-band.

9. During muscle contraction in humans, the ***(Karnataka NEET 2013)***
(a) sarcomere does not shorten
(b) A band remains same
(c) A, H and I bands shorten
(d) actin filaments shorten.

10. The type of muscle present in our ***(2011)***
(a) heart is involuntary and unstriated smooth muscle
(b) intestine is striated and involuntary
(c) thigh is striated and voluntary
(d) upper arm is smooth muscle and fusiform in shape.

11. The contractile protein of skeletal muscle involving ATPase activity is ***(2006)***
(a) troponin (b) tropomyosin
(c) myosin (d) a-actinin.

12. Which statement is correct for muscle contraction? ***(2001)***
(a) Length of H-zone decreases.
(b) Length of A-band remains constant.
(c) Length of I-band increases.
(d) Length of two Z-line increases.

13. What is sarcomere? ***(2001)***
(a) Part between two H-line
(b) Part between two A-line
(c) Part between two I-band
(d) Part between two Z line

14. The functional unit of contractile system in striated muscle is ***(1998)***
(a) sarcomere (b) Z-band
(c) cross bridges (d) myofibril.

SKELETAL SYSTEM

15. Match the following columns and select the correct option. ***(2020)***

Column-I	Column-II
(A) Floating ribs	(i) Located between second and seventh ribs
(B) Acromion	(ii) Head of the humerus
(C) Scapula	(iii) Clavicle
(D) Glenoid cavity	(iv) Do not connect with the sternum

	(A)	(B)	(C)	(D)
(a)	(ii)	(iv)	(i)	(iii)
(b)	(i)	(iii)	(ii)	(iv)
(c)	(iii)	(ii)	(iv)	(i)
(d)	(iv)	(iii)	(i)	(ii)

16. Select the correct option. ***(2019)***
(a) There are seven pairs of vertebrosternal, three pairs of vertebrochondral and two pairs of vertebral ribs.
(b) 8th, 9th and 10th pairs of ribs articulate directly with the sternum.
(c) 11th and 12th pairs of ribs are connected to the sternum with the help of hyaline cartilage.
(d) Each rib is a flat thin bone and all the ribs are connected dorsally to the thoracic vertebrae and ventrally to the sternum.

17. Out of 'X' pairs of ribs in humans only 'Y' pairs are true ribs. Select the option that correctly represents values of X and Y and provides their explanation. ***(2017)***

(a)	X = 12, Y = 5	True ribs are attached dorsally to vertebral column and sternum on the two ends
(b)	X = 24, Y= 2	The true ribs are dorsally attached to vertebral column but are free on ventral side
(c)	X = 24, Y = 12	True ribs are dorsally attached to vertebral column but are free on ventral side
(d)	X = 12, Y = 7	True ribs are attached dorsally to vertebral column and ventrally to the sternum

18. Which of the following is not a function of the skeletal system? ***(2015)***
(a) Production of body heat
(b) Locomotion
(c) Production of erythrocytes
(d) Storage of minerals

19. Glenoid cavity articulates ***(2015 Cancelled)***
(a) clavicle with scapula
(b) humerus with scapula
(c) clavicle with acromion
(d) scapula with acromion.

20. Three of the following pairs of the human skeletal parts are correctly matched with their respective inclusive skeletal category and one pair is not matched. Identify the non-matching pair. ***(2011)***

Pair of skeletal parts	Category
(a) Sternum and ribs	Axial skeleton
(b) Clavicle and glenoid cavity	Pelvic girdle
(c) Humerus and ulna	Appendicular skeleton
(d) Malleus and stapes	Ear ossicles

21. Which one of the following is the correct matching of three items and their grouping category? ***(2009)***
(a) Cytosine, uracil, thiamine – Pyrimidines
(b) Malleus, incus, cochlea – Ear ossicles
(c) Ilium, ischium, pubis – Coxal bones of pelvic girdle
(d) Actin, myosin, rhodopsin -- Muscle proteins

22. Which one of the following items gives its correct total number? ***(2007)***
(a) Types of diabetes-3
(b) Cervical vertebrae in humans- 8
(c) Floating ribs in humans-4
(d) Amino acids found in proteins-16

23. In human body, which one of the following is anatomically correct? ***(2007)***
(a) Collar bones - 3 pairs
(b) Salivary glands - 1 pair
(c) Cranial nerves - 10 pairs
(d) Floating ribs - 2 pairs

24. An acromion process is characteristically found in the ***(2005)***
(a) pelvic girdle of mammals
(b) pectoral girdle of mammals
(c) skull of frog
(d) sperm of mammals.

25. What will happen if ligaments are torn? ***(2002)***
(a) Bones will move freely at joint and no pain.
(b) Bone less movable at joint and pain.
(c) Bone will become unfixed.
(d) Bone will become fixed.

26. Sternum is connected to ribs by ***(2000)***
(a) bony matter
(b) white fibrous cartilage
(c) hyaline cartilage
(d) areolar tissue.

27. Total number of bones in each limb of a man is ***(1998)***
(a) 24 (b) 30 (c) 14 (d) 21

28. The number of floating ribs in the human body is ***(1995)***
(a) 3 pairs (b) 2 pairs
(c) 6 pairs (d) 5 pairs.

29. Which of the following components is a part of the pectoral girdle? ***(1994)***
(a) Sternum (b) Acetabulum
(c) Glenoid cavity (d) Ilium

30. The cervical vertebrae in human is ***(1993)***
(a) same as in whale
(b) more than that in rabbit
(c) double than that of horse
(d) less than that in giraffe.

31. Long bones function in ***(1993)***
(a) support
(b) support, erythrocyte and leucocyte synthesis
(c) support and erythrocyte synthesis
(d) erythrocyte formation.

32. Number of cervical vertebrae in camel is (1993)
(a) more than that of rabbit
(b) less than that of rabbit
(c) same as that of whale
(d) more than that of horse

JOINTS

33. Match List I with List II. ***(2023)***

List I (Type of Joint)	List II (Found between)
A. Cartilaginous Joint	I. Between flat skull bones
B. Ball and Socket Joint II.	II. Between adjacent vertebrae in vertebral column
C. Fibrous Joint	III. Between carpal and metacarpal of thumb
D. Saddle Joint	IV.Between humerus and pectoral girdle

Choose the correct answer from the options given below:

(a) A-I, B-IV, C-III, D-II (b) A-II, B-IV, C-III, D-I
(c) A-III, B-I, C-II, D-IV (d) A-II, B-IV, C-I, D-III

34. Match List-I with List-II. ***(2021)***

List-I	List-II
(p) Scapula	(i) Cartilaginous joints
(q) Cranium	(ii) Flat bone
(r) Sternum	(iii) Fibrous joints
(s) Vertebral column	(iv) Triangular flat bone

Choose the correct answer from the options given below.

	p	q	r	s
(a)	(iv)	(iii)	(ii)	(i)
(b)	(i)	(iii)	(ii)	(iv)
(c)	(ii)	(iii)	(iv)	(i)
(d)	(iv)	(ii)	(iii)	(i)

35. Match the following joints with the bones involved: ***(Odisha NEET 2019)***

(1) Gliding joint	(i) Between carpal and metacarpal of thumb
(2) Hinge joint	(ii) Between atlas and axis
(3) Pivot joint	(iii) Between the carpals
(4) Saddle joint	(iv) Between humerus and ulna

Select the correct option from the following:

(a) (1)-(iii), (2)-(iv), (3)-(ii), (4)-(i)
(b) (1)-(iv), (2)-(i), (3)-(ii), (4)-(iii)
(c) (1)-(iv), (2)-(ii), (3)-(iii), (4)-(i)
(d) (1)-(i), (2)-(iii), (3)-(ii), (4)-(iv)

36. The pivot joint between atlas and axis is a type of ***(2017)***

(a) cartilaginous joint (b) synovial joint
(c) saddle joint (d) fibrous joint.

37. Which of the following joints would allow no movements? ***(2015)***

(a) Synovial joint (b) Ball and socket joint
(c) Fibrous joint (d) Cartilaginous joint

38. Select the correct matching of the type of the joint with the example in human skeletal system. ***(2014)***

Type of joint		Example
(a) Cartilaginous	-	Between frontal and joint parietal
(b) Pivot joint	-	Between third and fourth cervical vertebrae
(c) Hinge joint	-	Between humerus and pectoral girdle
(d) Gliding joint	-	Between carpals

39. The characteristic and an example of a synovial joint in humans is ***(2013)***

Characteristics	Examples
(a) Fluid filled synovial cavity between two bones	Joint between atlas and axis
(b) Lymph filled between two bones, limited movement	Gliding joint between carpals
(c) Fluid cartilage between two bones, limited movements	Knee joint
(d) Fluid filled between two joints, provides cushion	Skull bones

40. Which one of the following is the correct description of a certain part of a normal human skeleton? ***(2010)***

(a) Parietal bone and the temporal bone of the skull are joined fibrous joint.
(b) First vertebra is axis which articulates with the occipital condyles.
(c) The 9th and 10th pairs of ribs are called the floating ribs.
(d) Glenoid cavity is a depression to which the thigh bone articulates.

41. Elbow joint is an example of ***(2009)***
(a) hinge joint
(b) gliding joint
(c) ball and socket joint
(d) pivot joint.

42. Which of the following pairs is correctly matched? ***(2005)***

(a) Hinge joint	–	Between vertebrae
(b) Gliding joint	–	Between zygapophyses of the successive vertebrae
(c) Cartilaginous joint	–	Skull bones
(d) Fibrous joint	–	Between phalanges

43. What is the name of joint between ribs and sternum? ***(2000)***
(a) Cartilaginous joint (b) Angular joint
(c) Gliding joint (d) Fibrous joint

44. The joint between atlas and axis is called ***(1999)***
(a) angular joint (b) hinge joint
(c) pivot joint (d) saddle joint.

45. The type of joint between the human skull bones is called ***(1994)***
(a) cartilaginous joint (b) hinge joint
(c) fibrous joint (d) synovial joint.

DISORDERS OF MUSCULAR AND SKELETAL SYSTEM

46. Given below are two statements: one is labelled as Assertion (A) and the other is labelled as reason (R).

Assertion (A) : Osteoporosis is characterised by decreased bone mass and increased chances of fractures.

Reason (R) : Common cause of osteoporosis is increased levels of estrogen.

In the light of the above statements, choose the appropriate answer from the options given below. ***(2022)***

(a) Both (A) and (R) are correct but (R) is not the correct explanation of (A)
(b) (A) is correct but (R) is not correct
(c) (A) is not correct but (R) is correct
(d) Both (A) and (R) are correct and (R) is correct explanation of (A)

47. Which of the following is a correct match for disease and its symptoms? ***(2022)***
(a) Arthritis-Inflammed joints
(b) Tetany - High Ca^{2+} level causing rapid spasms
(c) Myasthenia gravis - Genetic disorder resulting in weakening and paralysis of skeletal muscle
(d) Muscular dystrophy - An autoimmune disorder causing progressive degeneration of skeletal muscle

48. Chronic autoimmune disorder affecting neuro muscular junction leading to fatigue, weakening and paralysis of skeletal muscle is called as ***(2021)***
(a) gout
(b) arthritis
(c) muscular dystrophy
(d) myasthenia gravis.

49. Which of the following muscular disorders is inherited? ***(2019)***
(a) Botulism
(b) Tetany
(c) Muscular dystrophy
(d) Myasthenia gravis

50. Osteoporosis, an age-related disease of skeletal system, may occur due to ***(NEET-II 2016)***
(a) immune disorder affecting neuromuscular junction leading to fatigue
(b) high concentration of Ca^{++} and Na^{+}
(c) decreased level of estrogen
(d) accumulation of uric acid leading to inflammation of joints.

51. Select the correct statement with respect to locomotion in humans. ***(2013)***

(a) The vertebral column has 10 thoracic vertebrae.

(b) The joint between adjacent vertebrae is a fibrous joint.

(c) A decreased level of progesterone causes osteoporosis in old people.

(d) Accumulation of uric acid crystals in joints causes their inflammation.

52. Select the correct statement with respect to disorders of muscles in humans. ***(Karnataka NEET 2013)***

(a) Failure of neuromuscular transmission in myasthenia gravis can prevent normal swallowing.

(b) Accumulation of urea and creatine in the joints causes their inflammation.

(c) An overdose of vitamin D causes osteoporosis.

(d) Rapid contractions of skeletal muscles cause muscle dystrophy.

53. Select the correct statement regarding the specific disorder of muscular or skeletal system. ***(2012)***

(a) Muscular dystrophy - Age related shortening of muscles

(b) Osteoporosis - Decrease in bone mass and higher chances of fractures with advancing age

(c) Myasthenia gravis - Autoimmune disorder which inhibits sliding of myosin filaments

(d) Gout - Inflammation of joints due to extra deposition of calcium

ANSWER KEY

1.	(d)	2.	(b)	3.	(a)	4.	(a)	5.	(a)	6.	(a)	7.	(a)
8.	(a)	9.	(b)	10.	(c)	11.	(c)	12.	(a,b)	13.	(d)	14.	(a)
15.	(d)	16.	(a)	17.	(d)	18.	(a)	19.	(b)	20.	(b)	21.	(c)
22.	(c)	23.	(d)	24.	(b)	25.	(b)	26.	(c)	27.	(b)	28.	(b)
29.	(c)	30.	(a)	31.	(b)	32.	(c)	33.	(d)	34.	(a)	35.	(a)
36.	(b)	37.	(c)	38.	(d)	39.	(a)	40.	(a)	41.	(a)	42.	(b)
43.	(a)	44.	(c)	45.	(c)	46.	(b)	47.	(a)	48.	(d)	49.	(c)
50.	(c)	51.	(d)	52.	(a)	53.	(b)						

HINTS & EXPLANATIONS

1. **(d)**: Each organised skeletal muscle in our body is made of a number of muscle bundles or fascicles held together by a common collagenous connective tissue layer called fascia. The portion of the myofibril between two successive ' Z ' lines is considered as the functional unit of contraction and is called a sarcomere.

2. **(b)**: During muscle contraction, the thin myofilaments i.e, actin slide inwards towards the H-zone. As the thin myofilaments move past the thick myofilaments, the H-zone narrows and even disappears during contraction. Utilising the energy from ATP hydrolysis, the myosin head now binds to the exposed active sites on actin to form cross bridge. The 'Z' line attached to these actins are pulled inwards thereby causing shortening of the sarcomere. Size of I-bands shorten, but the width of the A-band remains constant.

3. **(a)**: Calcium ion plays an important role in skeletal muscle contraction. Muscle contraction is initiated by signal sent by the central nervous system. The neural signal further spreads through the muscle fibre and causes the release of calcium ions. Increase in calcium ion levels lead to the binding of calcium with a subunit of troponin on actin filaments and thereby remove the masking of active sites for myosin.

4. **(a)**: Calcium ion plays an important role in muscle contraction. Calcium ions bind to troponin causing a change in its shape and position. Thus, in turn alters shape and position of tropomyosin to which troponin binds. This shift exposes the active sites on F-actin molecules. Myosin cross-bridge are then able to bind to these active sites.

5. **(a)**: Tetanus refers to continued state of contraction of a muscle resulting from the summation of a series of rapid muscular contractions (twitches) that are induced by repeated stimulation of the muscle.

6. **(a)**: During muscle contraction, the laterally projecting heads (cross bridges) of the thick myosin myofilaments come in contact with the thin actin myofilaments and rotate on them. This pulls the thin myofilaments toward the middle of the sarcomere, past the thick myofilaments. The Z lines come closer together and the sarcomere becomes shorter. Length of the A band remains constant. Myofilaments (both actin and myosin) stay the same length. Free ends of actin myofilaments move closer to the centre of the sarcomere, bringing Z lines closer together. I bands shorten and H zone narrows. A similar action in all the sarcomeres results in shortening of the entire myofibril and thereby of the whole fibre and the whole muscle.

7. **(a)**: A neuron that transmits a stimulus to muscle tissue is called motor neuron. A motor unit consists of a single motor neuron (nerve cell) and the muscle fibres innervates it. The portion of the muscle plasma membrane (sarcolemma) that lies beneath the nerve endings (axon terminals) is called the motor end plate. The axon terminals and the motor end plate together constitute the neuro-muscular junction or neuromotor junction.

8. **(a)**: Each muscle fibre has many parallelly arranged myofibrils. Each myofibril contains many serially arranged units called sarcomere which are the functional units. Each sarcomere has a central 'A' band made of thick myosin filaments and two half 'I' bands made of thin actin filaments on either side of it marked by 'Z' lines. In a resting state, the edges of thin

filaments on either side of the thick filaments partially overlap the free ends of the thick filaments leaving the central part of the thick filaments. This central part of thick filament, not overlapped by thin filaments is called the 'H' zone.

9. **(b)**: According to sliding-filament theory of muscle contraction, the actin and myosin filaments slide past each other with the help of cross-bridge to reduce the length of the sarcomeres. The smallest unit of muscle contraction is a sarcomere (which is delineated by Z-lines). As a muscle contracts, the Z lines come closer together (shortening sarcomere), the width of the I bands decreases, the width of the H zones decreases, but there is no change in the width of the A band. During relaxation, cross-bridges disappear and actin filaments slide back from A-bands, the width of the I bands and H zones increases, but there is still no change in the width of the A band.

10. **(c)**: Cardiac muscles are found in the wall of the heart. It is involuntary and slightly striated. Smooth muscles are found in gastrointestinal tract. These are non-striated and involuntary. Striated (or skeletal) muscles are found in the limbs and body walls. These muscles are voluntary (under the control of animals' will) and show dark and light bands thus are striated.

11. **(c)**: Myosin is a contractile protein that interacts with actin to bring about contraction of muscle or cell movement. The type of myosin molecule found in muscle fibres consists of a tail, by which it aggregates with other myosin molecules to form so-called thick filaments and a globular head, which has sites for the attachment of actin and ATP molecule. Troponin, tropomyosin and α-actinin are the actin in the thin filament.

12. **(a,b)**

13. **(d)**: A striated muscle fibre is bounded by sarcolemma. It shows alternating dark and light cross bands, the striations. Dark band is called A band which has at its middle a light zone termed H zone. Light band is known as I band which is crossed through its centre by a dark membrane called Z line. The part of the muscle fibre between two successive Z lines functions as a contractile unit called sarcomere.

14. **(a)** The part of the muscle fibre between two successive Z lines functions as a contractile unit called sarcomere.

15. **(d)**

16. **(a)** Ribs 1-7 are classified as true ribs (vertebrosternal ribs), ribs 8-10 are false ribs (vertebrochondral ribs) and ribs 11 and 12 are floating ribs (vertebral ribs).

17. **(d)**

18. **(a)**

19. **(b)**: Upper rounded end of the humerus (bone of arm) is called head that articulates into the glenoid cavity of the pectoral girdle (shoulder girdle) of scapula or shoulder blade bone.

20. **(b)**: Each pectoral girdle consists of two bones, clavicle and scapula. The scapula (shoulder blade) consists of a sharp ridge, the spine and a triangular body. The end of the spine projects as a flattened and expanded process called acromion. This process articulates with the clavicle. At the lateral end of the superior of the scapula there is projection of the anterior surface called the coracoid process, to which the tendons of the muscles attach. At the point where the superior and lateral borders of the scapula meet there is the lateral angle which presents a shallow articular surface termed as glenoid cavity into which the head of the humerus is articulated.

21. (c): The pelvic girdle is formed by two innominate bones (hip bones). Each innominate bones consists of three separate bones, ilium, ischium and the pubis.
Thiamine is a vitamin and thymine is a pyrimidine.

22. (c): There are twelve pairs of ribs which form the bony lateral walls of the thoracic cage. The first seven pairs are called true ribs; eighth, ninth and tenth pairs are called false ribs. The last two pairs of ribs are called floating ribs because their anterior ends are not attached either to the sternum or to the cartilage of another rib. The floating ribs protect the kidneys.

23. (d): Collar bones (Clavicle) – 2 pairs
Salivary glands – 3 pairs
Cranial nerves – 12 pairs

24. (b): Each half of pectoral girdle is made up of two bones scapula and clavicle. At the outer angle of scapula is present a shallow socket known as glenoid cavity into which head of humerus bone fits to form a shoulder joint. Above glenoid cavity project two processes - acromion process and coracoid process. Acromion process extends over the glenoid cavity and articulates with clavicle to form shoulder girdle. Coracoid process is like a hook and is smaller than acromion process.

25. (b): Ligaments join a bone with another bone in movable/synovial joints. Torn ligaments make movement at joints very painful and restricted.

26. (c): Sternum is connected to ribs by hyaline cartilage (= giving a shiny glass like appearance and gives flexibility and support at the joints). Sternum is also called breast bone. It is a narrow, elongated and flattened structure, present just under the skin in the middle of front of the chest. It consists of three parts - manubrium, mesosternum and xiphoid process.

27. (b)

28. (b)

29. (c): The pectoral girdle lies on the posterolateral aspect of the upper region of the thorax. It consists of 2 bones : scapula and clavicle. The scapula, also called shoulder blade, is a large, flat, triangular bone placed at the back of the shoulder. It has at its lateral angle a shallow concavity, the glenoid cavity, for the articulation of the head of the humerus. Acetabulum and ilium are parts of pelvic girdle. Sternum is a long, narrow, flat vertical bone in the middle of the front wall of the chest.

30. (a): The number of cervical vertebrae are same in man and whale that is 7 in number.

31. (b): Long bones strengthen the legs and arms, provide support and also synthesise erythrocytes and leucocytes due to presence of bone marrow in their cavities.

32. (c): The vast majority of mammals have seven cervical vertebrae (neck bones), including camel, bats, giraffes, whales and humans. The few exceptions include the manatee and the two-toed sloth, both have only six cervical vertebrae and the three-toed sloth with nine cervical vertebrae.

33. (d): Cartilaginous joint → Between adjacent vertebrae in vertebral column Ball and Socket joint → Between Humerus and Pectoral girdle Fibrous joint → Between flat skull bones Saddle joint → Between carpal and metacarpal of thumb

34. (a): Scapula is a large triangular flat bone situated in the dorsal part of the thorax between the second and the seventh ribs. Cranium shows fibrous joints which do not allow any movement. Sternum is a flat bone on the ventral midline of thorax. Vertebral column involves cartilaginous joints in which bones are joined with the help of cartilages.

35. (a)

36. (b)

37. (c): Fibrous or immovable joints are the joints in which no movement occurs between the bones concerned. White fibrous tissue is present between the ends of the bones. Fibrous joint occurs between the bones of the skull called sutures and the joints between the teeth and the maxilla and the teeth and the mandible.

38. (d)

Cartilaginous joint	–	Between the adjacent vertebrae in vertebral column
Pivot joint	–	Between atlas and axis
Hinge joint	–	Knee joint
Ball and socket joint	–	Between head of humerus and glenoid cavity of pectoral girdle
Fibrous joint	–	Between frontal and parietal bones of skull (sutures)

39. (a) : Joint between atlas and axis is a pivot joint, a type of synovial joint. Synovial joints are characterised by presence of fluid filled cavity between the articulating surface of the two bones.

40. (a): The bones of skulls are joined by white fibrous tissue which sustain no movement between the skull bones. This kind of joint is classified as fibrous or immovable joints. Thus, parietal and temporal bone of the skull are joined by fibrous joints.

First cervical vertebra, atlas, joins the second cervical vertebra axis to form a joint (pivot joint) which allows movement in one plane. The atlas supports the head and allows movement of head over neck.

The last two pairs of ribs (11th and (12th) are called floating ribs because their anterior ends are not attached to either the sternum or the cartilage of anterior rib.

Glenoid cavity is a depression to which humerus articulates.

41. (a): Hinge joint is a form of diarthrosis (freely movable joint) that allows angular movement in one plane only, increasing or decreasing the angle between the bones. Examples are - knee joint and elbow joint.

42. (b): Gliding joint permits sliding movements of two bones over each other. Hinge joint allows movements in one plane only. Knee joint, elbow joint, ankle joint are of this type. Cartilaginous joint is a slightly movable joint and is found between the centre of vertebrae, at the pubic symphysis and between ribs and sternum. Fibrous joint is an immovable joint which occur between the bones of cranium.

43.(a) : Cartilaginous joint is present between ribs and sternum. It allows only limited movement. An angular joint allows movement in two directions - side to side and back and forth. Wrist and metacarpophalangeal joints are of this type. Gliding joint permits sliding movements of two bones over each other, e.g., joints between sternum and clavicles. Fibrous joints do not allow movement and are present between the bones of cranium.

44. (c): Pivot joint is present between atlas and the axis in humans. In this joint, articular end of one bone is fixed while the other can rotate over it. In angular joint, an oval condyle of one bone fits into an elliptical concavity of the other, e.g. wrist and meta-carpophalangeal joints. Hinge joint allows movements in one plane only, e.g., knee joint. In saddle joint, small projection of one bone fits into a saddle-like depression of another bone.

45. (c): Fibrous joint is present between the human skull bones. It does not allow movement because the bones are held firmly together by bundles of strong white collagen fibres. Cartilaginous joints are present between the centre of vertebrae, at the pubic symphysis and between ribs and sternum. Knee joint, elbow joint and ankle joint are types of hinge joint. Synovial joint occurs between limbs and bones.

46.(b) : Osteoporosis is a disease characterised by low bone mass and loss of bone tissue that may lead to weak and fragile bones. Decreased levels of estrogen is a common cause for osteoporosis.

47. (a): Arthritis is inflammation of joints. Tetany is a muscular disorder that causes rapid spasms in muscles, which occur due to less calcium in body fluid. Myasthenia gravis is an autoimmune disorder affecting neuromuscular junction leading to fatigue, weakening and paralysis of skeletal muscle. Muscular dystrophy is the progressive degeneration of skeletal muscle mostly due to genetic disorder.

48. (d): Myasthenia gravis is an autoimmune disorder affecting neuromuscular junction leading to fatigue, weakening and paralysis of skeletal muscle.

49.(c) : Muscular dystrophy is a group of muscle diseases, marked by weakness and wasting of skeletal muscles, in which there is a recognizable pattern of inheritance. In this disorder, the mutated gene on middle of the short arm of X-chromosome is unable to produce a protein dystrophin in skeletal muscles. It is common in males, female heterozygous carriers are normal.

50. (c): Osteoporosis is reduction in bone mineral density, resulting in bones that are brittle and liable to fracture. Infection, injury and synovitis can cause localised osteoporosis of adjacent bone. Generalised osteoporosis is common in the elderly and in women after menopause. After menopause the estrogen level in blood plasma are much reduced. Estrogen helps to regulate bone cells called osteoclasts which are responsible for building new bone. When estrogen level drop fewer osteoclasts are produced resulting in osteoporosis.

51. (d): Thoracic vertebrae are 12 in numbers. Joints between adjacent vertebrae are cartilaginous joints and the opposing surfaces are connected by fibrocartilage which allows very little movement. Osteoporosis is a disease characterised by low bone mass and loss of bone tissue that may lead to weak and fragile bones. Osteoporosis occurs when there is an imbalance between new bone formation and old bone resorption. Generalised osteoporosis is common in elderly people and in women following menopause. In osteoporosis, the osteoblastic (bone forming) activity in the bone usually is less than normal and consequently the rate of bone deposition is depressed. Estrogen inhibit osteoclastic (bone resorption) activity in the bones and therefore stimulate bone growth. After menopause, almost no estrogens are secreted by ovaries. This estrogen deficiency leads to increased osteoclastic activity in the bones, decreased bone matrix and decreased deposition of bone calcium and phosphate. In some women, this effect result in osteoporosis.

52.(a) : Myasthenia gravis is an autoimmune disorder in which autoantibodies bind to cholinergic receptors on muscle cells and impairs the ability of the neurotransmitter acetylcholine to induce muscular contraction. This leads to fatigue, weakening and paralysis of skeletal muscles of mouth and throat which may prevent normal swallowing. Gouty arthritis is caused either due to excessive formation of uric acid or inability to excrete it. It gets deposited in synovial joints and causes inflammation. Osteoporosis is a disease in which bone loses minerals and fibres from its matrix. Major causative factors of osteoporosis are imbalances of hormones like calcitonin of thyroid, parathormone of parathyroids, sex hormones and deficiencies of calcium and vitamin D. Muscular dystrophy is inborn abnormality of muscles associated with dysfunction and ultimately with deterioration.

53. (b): Muscular dystrophy is characterised by progressive skeletal muscle weakness, defects in muscle proteins and the death of muscle cells and tissue.

Myasthenia gravis is an auto-immune neuromuscular disease in which muscle becomes weak, which is caused by circulating antibodies that block acetylcholine receptors at the postsynaptic neuromuscular junction inhibiting the excitatory effects of the acetylcholine.

Gout is inflammation of joints which is caused by elevated levels of uric acid in the blood which crystallises and the crystals are deposited in joints, tendons and surrounding tissues.

Chapter : 18 NEURAL CONTROL AND COORDINATION

HUMAN NEURAL SYSTEM

1. In a man, abducens nerve is injured. Which one of the following functions will be affected? ***(2005)***

(a) Movement of the eyeball
(b) Movement of the tongue
(c) Swallowing
(d) Movement of the neck

2. Injury to vagus nerve in humans is not likely to affect ***(2004)***

(a) tongue movements
(b) gastrointestinal movements
(c) pancreatic secretion
(d) cardiac movements.

3. Sympathetic nervous system induces ***(1999)***

(a) secretion of digestive juices
(b) heart beat
(c) secretion of saliva
(d) all of these.

4. Afferent nerve fibres carry impulses from ***(1992)***

(a) effector organs to CNS
(b) receptors to CNS
(c) CNS to receptors
(d) CNS to muscles

5. Vagus nerve is ***(1992)***

(a) X (b) IX (c) VII (d) V

6. One function of parasympathetic nervous system is ***(1990)***

(a) contraction of hair muscles
(b) stimulation of sweat glands
(c) acceleration of heart beat
(d) constriction of pupil.

NEURON AS STRUCTURAL AND FUNCTIONA UNIT OF NEURAL SYSTEM

7. Select the incorrect statement regarding synapses. ***(2022)***

(a) The membranes of presynaptic and postsynaptic neurons are in close proximity in an electrical synapse.
(b) Electrical current can flow directly from one neuron into the other across the electrical synapse.
(c) Chemical synapses use neurotransmitters.
(d) Impulse transmission across a chemical synapse is always faster than that across an electrical synapse.

8. Nissl's bodies are mainly composed of ***(2018)***

(a) proteins and lipids
(b) DNA and RNA
(c) nucleic acids and SER
(d) free ribosomes and RER.

9. Myelin sheath is produced by ***(2017)***

(a) astrocytes and Schwann cells
(b) oligodendrocytes and osteoclasts
(c) osteoclasts and astrocytes
(d) Schwann cells and oligodendrocytes.

10. Receptor sites for neurotransmitters are present on ***(2017)***

(a) pre-synaptic membrane
(b) tips of axons
(c) post-synaptic membrane
(d) membranes of synaptic vesicles.

11. The most abundant intracellular cation is ***(2013)***

(a) H^+ (b) K^+ (c) Na^+ (d) Ca^{++}

12. A diagram showing axon terminal and synapse is given. Identify correctly at least two of A - D. ***(2013)***

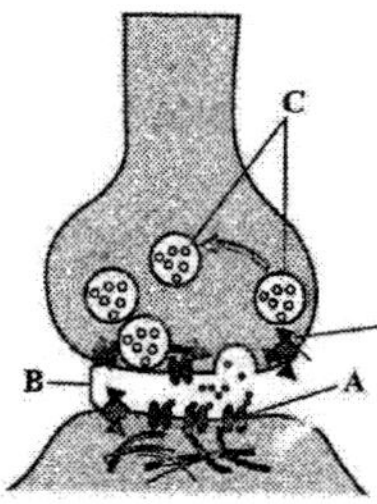

(a) A - Neurotransmitter, B - Synaptic cleft
(b) C - Neurotransmitter, D - Ca^{++}
(c) A - Receptor, C - Synaptic vesicles
(d) B - Synaptic connection, D – K^+

13. The figure shows an axon terminal and synapse. Select the option giving correct identification of labels A-D. ***(Karnataka NEET 2013)***

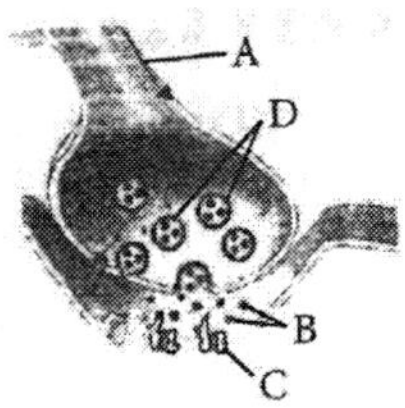

(a) A-Action potential, C-Neurotransmitter
(b) B-Neurotransmitter, D- Receptor capsules
(c) C-Receptor, D-Synaptic vesicles
(d) A-Axon terminal, B- Serotonin complex

14. When a neuron is in resting state i.e., not conducting any impulse, the axonal membrane is ***(2011)***
(a) comparatively more permeable to Na+ ions and nearly impermeable to K^+ ions
(b) equally permeable to both Na^+ and K+ ions
(c) impermeable to both Na^+ and K^+ ions
(d) comparatively more permeable to K^+ ions and nearly impermeable to Na^+ ions.

15. Alzheimer's disease in humans is associated with the deficiency of ***(2009)***
(a) glutamic acid
(b) acetylcholine
(c) gamma aminobutyric acid (GABA)
(d) dopamine.

16. During the propagation of a nerve impulse, the action potential results from the movement of ***(2008)***
(a) K^+ ions from intracellular fluid to extracellular fluid
(b) Na^+ ions from extracellular fluid to intracellular fluid
(c) K^+ ions from extracellular fluid to intracellular fluid
(d) Na^+ ions from intracellular fluid to extracellular fluid.

17. During the transmission of nerve impulse through a nerve fibre, the potential on the inner side of the plasma membrane has which type of electric charge? ***(2007)***
(a) First positive, then negative and continue to be negative
(b) First negative, then positive and continue to be positive
(c) First positive, then negative and again back to positive
(d) First negative, then positive and again back to negative.

18. Which one of the following does not act as a neurotransmitter? ***(2006)***
(a) Cortisone (b) Acetylcholine
(c) Epinephrine (d) Norepinephrine

19. Parkinson's disease (characterized by tremors and progressive rigidity of limbs) is caused by degeneration of brain neurons that are involved in movement control and make use of neurotransmitter ***(2005)***
(a) acetylcholine (b) norepinephrine
(c) dopamine (d) GABA.

20. In the resting state of the neural membrane, diffusion due to concentration gradients, if allowed, would drive ***(2004)***
(a) K^+ into the cell
(b) K^+ and Na^+ out of the cell
(c) Na^+ into the cell
(d) Na^+ out of the cell.

21. What used to be described as Nissl's granules in a nerve cell are now identified as *(2003)*

(a) cell metabolites (b) fat granules
(c) ribosomes (d) mitochondria.

22. Which of the following statement is correct for node of Ranvier of nerve? *(2002)*

(a) Neurilemma is discontinuous.
(b) Myelin sheath is discontinuous.
(c) Both neurilemma and myelin sheath are discontinuous.
(d) Covered by myelin sheath.

23. Depolarization of axolemma during nerve conduction takes place because of *(2000)*

(a) equal amount of Na^+ and K^+ move out across axolemma
(b) Na^+ move inside and K^+ move more outside
(c) more Na+ outside
(d) none of these.

24. The junction between the axon of one neuron and the dendrite of the next is called *(1999)*

(a) constant bridge (b) junction point
(c) a joint (d) a synapse.

25. Which of the following is regarded as a unit of nervous tissue? *(1999)*

(a) Neurons (b) Myelin sheath
(c) Axons (d) Dendrites

26. The Nissl's granules of nerves cell are made up of *(1997)*

(a) DNA (b) RNA
(c) ribosome (d) protein.

CENTRAL NEURAL SYSTEM

27. The parts of human brain that helps in regulation of sexual behaviour, expression of excitement, pleasure, rage, fear etc. are: **(2023)**

(a) Brain stem & epithalamus
(b) Corpus callosum and thalamus
(c) Limbic system & hypothalamus
(d) Corpora quadrigemina & hippocampus

28. Which part of the brain is responsible for thermoregulation? *(2019)*

(a) Medulla oblongata (b) Cerebrum
(c) Hypothalamus (d) Corpus callosum

29. Which of the following structures or regions is incorrectly paired with its functions? *(2018)*

(a) Medulla: Controls respiration oblongata and cardiovascular reflexes
(b) Limbic : Consists of fibre tracts system that interconnect different regions of brain, controls movement
(c) Hypothalamus : Production of releasing hormones and regulation of temperature, hunger and thirst
(d) Corpus callosum: Band of fibers connecting left and right cerebral hemispheres

30. Which of the following regions of the brain is incorrectly paired with its function? *(2015 Cancelled)*

(a) Corpus callosum - communication between the left and right cerebral cortices
(b) Cerebrum - calculation and contemplation
(c) Medulla oblongata - homeostatic control
(d) Cerebellum - language comprehension

31. Injury localized to the hypothalamus would most likely disrupt *(2014)*

(a) short - term memory
(b) co-ordination during locomotion
(c) executive functions, such as decision making
(d) regulation of body temperature.

32. A sagittal section of human brain is shown here. Identify at least two labels from A-D. *(Karnataka NEET 2013)*

(a) C-Midbrain, D-Cerebellum
(b) A-Cerebrum, C-Pons
(c) B-Corpus callosum, D-Medulla
(d) A-Cerebral hemispheres, B-Cerebellum

33. The human hind brain comprises three parts, one of which is *(2012)*

(a) spinal cord (b) corpus callosum
(c) cerebellum (d) hypothalamus.

34. The nerve centres which control the body temperature and the urge for eating are contained in ***(2010)***
(a) hypothalamus (b) pons
(c) cerebellum (d) thalamus.

35. Which part of human brain is concerned with the regulation of body temperature? ***(2009)***
(a) Cerebellum (b) Cerebrum
(c) Hypothalamus (d) Medulla oblongata

ANSWER KEY

1.	(a)	2.	(a)	3.	(b)	4.	(b)	5.	(a)	6.	(d)	7.	(d)
8.	(d)	9.	(d)	10.	(c)	11.	(b)	12.	(c)	13.	(c)	14.	(d)
15.	(b)	16.	(b)	17.	(d)	18.	(a)	19.	(c)	20.	(c)	21.	(c)
22.	(b)	23.	(b)	24.	(d)	25.	(a)	26.	(c)	27.	(c)	28.	(c)
29.	(b)	30.	(d)	31.	(d)	32.	(b)	33.	(c)	34.	(a)	35.	(c)

HINTS & EXPLANATIONS

1. **(a)** : Abducens is the sixth cranial nerve which innervates the external rectus muscle of the eye ball. It is responsible for turning the eye outwards. Movement of the tongue is controlled by the hypoglossal nerve. Neck movements is controlled by the facial nerve. Swallowing is controlled by glossopharyngeal nerves.

2. **(a)**: Vagus nerve arises from the side of medulla oblongata. It innervates the larynx, trachea, oesophagus, stomach, lungs, heart and intestines. It is a mixed nerve. It controls the visceral sensations and visceral movements, i.e., heart beat, respiratory movements, peristalsis, sound production, etc. Movement of the tongue is controlled by hypoglossal nerve as it innervates the muscles of the tongue.

3. **(b)**: Sympathetic nervous system is a component of autonomic nervous system consisting of a pair of sympathetic trunks, preganglionic sympathetic fibres, postganglionic sympathetic fibres and collateral ganglia. It quickens rate and force of heart beat while it inhibits secretion of saliva and gastric juice.

4. **(b)**: Afferent nerve fibres carry impulses from the receptors to the central nervous system. Efferent nerve fibres conduct nerve impulses from the central nervous system to the effector organs such as muscles and glands.

5. **(a)**

6. **(d)**: The action of the parasympathetic nervous system is opposite to that of the sympathetic nervous system. If the sympathetic nervous system accelerates an action, the parasympathetic nervous system slows it. The parasympathetic fibres constrict the pupil, decrease the rate and force of heart beat, dilate many blood vessels, lower the arterial blood pressure, quicken the peristaltic movements and contract the urinary bladder.

7. **(d)**: Impulse transmission across an electrical synapse is always faster than that across chemical synapse.

8. **(d)**: Nissl's bodies, also known as Nissl's granules are irregular masses of rough endoplasmic reticulum (RER) with numerous as well as free ribosomes and polysomes, found in cell body or cyton of a neuron. These probably synthesise proteins for the nerve cell.

9. **(d)**: Schwann cells and oligodendrocytes form myelin sheath around the axon. Myelin sheath serves as an insulating layer, preventing loss of energy of the nerve impulse during its passage along the fibre.

10. **(c)**: Neurotransmitter is a chemical substance responsible for transmission of nerve impulse across synapse. It is released by synaptic vesicle into the synaptic cleft. Neurotransmitter binds with protein receptor molecule present on post synaptic membrane causing its depolarisation and generation of action potential.

11. **(b)**: K^+ ions predominate in the intracellular fluid whereas Na+ ions predominate in extracellular fluid.

12. **(c)**

13. **(c)**

14. **(d)**: When a neuron is not conducting any impulse, i.e., resting, the axonal membrane is comparatively more permeable to potassium ions (K^+)and nearly impermeable to sodium ions (Na^+).

15. **(b)**: Alzheimer's disease is a neurological disease characterized by progressive loss of intellectual ability. The disease, which is named after German physician Alois Alzheimer (1864-1915), is associated with general shrinkage of the brain tissue, with deposits of β-amyloid protein and abnormal filaments composed of tau protein in the brain, and changes in the neurotransmitter systems within the brain that include a loss in the activity of cholinergic neurons (neurons releasing acetylcholine). Some inherited forms are associated with a genetic locus on chromosome 21 .

16. **(b)**: Action potential is the change in electrical potential that occurs across a plasma membrane during the passage of a nerve impulse. As an impulse travels in a wave-like manner along the axon of a nerve, it causes a localized and transient switch in electric potential across the membrane from -60mV (millivolts; the resting potential) to +45mV. It is due to the fact that the sodium channels open and the potassium channels remain closed. As a result, sodium channels permit the influx of Na^+ diffusion from extracellular fluid to intracellular fluid.

17. **(d)**: The signal that travels along the length of a nerve fibre and is the means by which information is transmitted through the nervous system is called nerve impulse. During resting phase, inside of the plasma membrane is negatively charged (polarized, -70mv, resting potential). As the stimulus reaches it becomes positively charged (+45mV, action potential). This condition is known as depolarization of nerve fibres. As impulse passes away, it regains its original ionic distribution and becomes repolarized.

18. **(a)**: Neurotransmitters are chemicals that are used to relay, amplify and modulate electrical signals between a neuron and another cell. Substances that act as neurotransmitters can be categorized into three major groups: (i) amino acids (primarily glutamic acid, GABA, aspartic acid and glycine), (ii) peptides (vasopressin, somatostatin, neurotensin, etc.), and (iii) monoamines (norepinephrine, dopamine and

serotonin) plus acetylcholine. Cortisone is a glucocorticoid steroid hormone, produced by the adrenal glands and has antiinflammatory and immune-system suppressing properties.

19. **(c)**: Parkinson's disease is caused by degeneration of neurons in substantia nigra tract which are essentially dopaminergic. This striatum controls muscle tones and coordinates movements. An imbalance is caused by deficiency of dopamine (an inhibitory neurotransmitter) vis-a-vis.

20. **(c)**: In the resting nerve fibre, in the external medium (tissue fluid), sodium ions (Na^+) predominate, whereas within the fibre (intracellular fluid) potassium ions (K^+) predominate. Due to different concentrations of ions on the two sides of the membrane, sodium ions tend to passively diffuse into the nerve fibre and potassium ions tend to diffuse out of the nerve fibre down their electrochemical gradients. The membrane of a resting nerve fibre is, however, more permeable to potassium than to sodium. Because of this selective permeability of the membrane, potassium leaves the nerve fibre faster than sodium enters it. This makes the membrane of the resting nerve fibre polarized, extracellular fluid outside it being electropositive (positively charged) with respect to the cell contents inside it.

21. **(c)**: Cell body of a nerve cell contains basophilic granules called Nissl's granules. These granules appear to be cisternae of rough endoplasmic reticulum with numerous attached and free ribosomes. They probably synthesise proteins for the cell.

22. **(b)**: At the level of node of Ranvier the myelin sheath is discontinuous but not the neurilemma lining. Actually myelin sheath is an integral part of Schwann cell which form a continuous neurilemmal covering. Each Schwann cell wrap-around the neurite to form concentric layers of plasma membrane. But at the level of junction between two Schwann cells myelin cannot be formed and thus a gap appears.

23. **(b)**: Depolarization of a nerve cell membrane occurs during the passage of an action potential along the axon where the nerve is transmitting an impulse. During depolarization, the activation gates of Na^+ channels open and the K^+ channels remain closed. Na^+ rush into the axon. Entry of sodium ions leads to depolarization (reversal of polarity) of the nerve membrane, so that the nerve fibre contents become electropositive with respect to the extracellular fluid.

24. **(d)**: Synapse is the close proximity of the axon of one neuron and the dendrite or cyton of another neuron with a gap of just about 200 Å in between. A nerve impulse is transmitted across the synapse by the release from the presynaptic membrane of neurotransmitter, which diffuses across the synaptic cleft to the post synaptic membrane. This triggers the propagation of the impulse from the dendrite along the length of the post synaptic neuron.

25. **(a)**: Neurons or nerve cells are the structural and functional unit of nervous system. These have a special structure but vary greatly in size and shape. Each neuron has a cell body which encloses cytoplasm and has a nucleus. A number of processes arise from the cell body. There is usually a single axon and a variable number of dendrites. The medullated nerve fibres is composed of a shining, white, fatty substance called myelin.

26. **(c)**

27. **(c)**: Limbic system or limbic lobe along with hypothalamus is involved in the regulation of sexual behaviour, expression of emotional reactions, such as excitement, pleasure, rage, fear, motivation, etc.

28. (c): Hypothalamus is thermoregulatory centre. Hence it is called "thermostat" of the body. It keeps body temperature at roughly 37° C by means of a complex thermostat system.

29. (b): Certain components of the cerebrum and diencephalon constitute the limbic system. It is sometimes called the emotional brain because it controls emotional behaviour expressed in the form of joy, sorrow, fear, fight, friendship, liking and disliking. It also controls food habits and sex behaviours necessary for survival of the individual.

30. (d): Language comprehension is a function of cerebrum Cerebellum coordinates and controls rapid muscular activities such as running, typing, etc. Although it does not initiate such voluntary movements, but it is an important centre for coordinating movements and for controlling posture and balance. Cerebellum's function is almost exclusively motor; but it is also implicated in some forms of learning.

31. (d): Hypothalamus lies at the base of the thalamus. It provides anatomical connection between the nervous and endocrine systems by its relationship to the pituitary gland. Hypothalamus is thermoregulatory centre. Hence, it is called "thermostat" of the body. It keeps body temperature at roughly 37°C by means of a complex thermostat system. Any localised injury to hypothalamus will, hence, disrupt regulation of body temperature.

32. (b): A - Cerebrum

B - Thalamus

C - Pons varolii

D - Cerebellum

33. (c): Brain is the anterior most part of central nervous system. Human brain can be divided into three parts: forebrain, midbrain and hindbrain. Human hindbrain comprises of pons, cerebellum and medulla (also called the medulla oblongata).

34. (a)

35. (c)

Chapter : 19

CHEMICAL COORDINATION AND INTEGRATION

INTRODUCTION

1. Which one of the following statements is correct? ***(2006)***
   (a) Endocrine glands regulate neural activity, but not vice versa.
   (b) Neurons regulate endocrine activity, but not vice versa.
   (c) Endocrine glands regulate neural activity and nervous system regulates endocrine glands.
   (d) Neither hormones control neural activity nor the neurons control endocrine activity.

HUMAN ENDOCRINE SYSTEM

2. Which of the following are not under the control of thyroid hormone? ***(2023)***

   A. Maintenance of water and electrolyte balance

   B. Regulation of basal metabolic rate

   C. Normal rhythm of sleep-wake cycle

   D. Development of immune system

   E. Support the process of RBCs formation

   Choose the correct answer from the options given below.
   (a) C and D only (b) D and E only
   (c) A and D only (d) B and C only

3. Which of the following are not the effects of parathyroid hormone? ***(2022)***
   (A) Stimulates the process of bone resorption
   (B) Decreases Ca^{2+} level in blood
   (C) Reabsorption of Ca^{2+} by renal tubules
   (D) Decreases the absorption of Ca^{2+} from digested food
   (E) Increases metabolism of carbohydrates

   Choose the most appropriate answer from the options given below.
   (a) (A) and (C) only (b) (B), (D) and (E) only
   (c) (A) and (E) only (d) (B) and (C) only

4. Presence of which of the following conditions in urine are indicative of diabetes mellitus? ***(2020)***
   (a) Uremia and Ketonuria
   (b) Uremia and Renal Calculi
   (c) Ketonuria and Glycosuria
   (d) Renal calculi and Hyperglycaemia

5. Match the following columns and select the correct option. ***(2020)***

Column-I	Column-II
(A) Pituitary gland	(i) Grave's disease
(B) Thyroid gland	(ii) Diabetes mellitus
(C) Adrenal gland	(iii) Diabetes insipidus
(D) Pancreas	(iv) Addison's disease

	(A)	(B)	(C)	(D)
(a)	(iv)	(iii)	(i)	(ii)
(b)	(iii)	(ii)	(i)	(iv)
(c)	(iii)	(i)	(iv)	(ii)
(d)	(ii)	(i)	(iv)	(iii)

6. Select the correct statement. ***(2020)***
   (a) Glucocorticoids stimulate gluconeogenesis
   (b) Glucagon is associated with hypoglycemia.
   (c) Insulin acts on pancreatic cells and adipocytes.
   (d) Insulin is associated with hyperglycemia.

7. Match the following hormones with their respective disease. ***(2019)***

Column-I	Column-II
(A) Insulin	(i) Addison's disease
(B) Thyroxin	(ii) Diabetes insipidus
(C) Corticoids	(iii) Acromegaly
(D) Growth hormone	(iv) Goitre
	(v) Diabetes mellitus

	(A)	(B)	(C)	(D)
(a)	(ii)	(iv)	(i)	(iii)
(b)	(v)	(i)	(ii)	(iii)
(c)	(ii)	(iv)	(iii)	(i)
(d)	(v)	(iv)	(i)	(iii)

8. Which of the following hormones can play a significant role in osteoporosis? ***(2018)***
(a) Aldosterone and prolactin
(b) Progesterone and aldosterone
(c) Estrogen and parathyroid hormone
(d) Parathyroid hormone and prolactin

9. GnRH, a hypothalamic hormone, needed in reproduction, acts on ***(2017)***
(a) anterior pituitary gland and stimulates secretion of LH and FSH
(b) posterior pituitary gland and stimulates secretion of oxytocin and FSH
(c) posterior pituitary gland and stimulates secretion of LH and relaxin
(d) anterior pituitary gland and stimulates secretion of LH and oxytocin.

10. Hypersecretion of growth hormone in adults does not cause further increase in height, because ***(2017)***
(a) epiphyseal plates close after adolescence
(b) bones loose their sensitivity to growth hormone in adults
(c) muscle fibres do not grow in size after birth
(d) growth hormone becomes inactive in adults.

11. A temporary endocrine gland in the human body is ***(2017)***
(a) corpus cardiacum (b) corpus luteum
(c) corpus allatum (d) pineal gland.

12. Graves' disease is caused due to ***(NEET-II 2016)***
(a) hyposecretion of thyroid gland
(b) hypersecretion of thyroid gland
(c) hyposecretion of adrenal gland
(d) hypersecretion of adrenal gland.

13. Name a peptide hormone which acts mainly on hepatocytes, adipocytes and enhances cellular glucose uptake and utilisation. ***(NEET-II 2016)***
(a) Insulin (b) Glucagon
(c) Secretin (d) Gastrin

14. The posterior pituitary gland is not a 'true' endocrine gland because ***(NEET-II 2016)***
(a) it is provided with a duct
(b) it only stores and releases hormones
(c) it is under the regulation of hypothalamus
(d) it secretes enzymes.

15. Which of the following pairs of hormones are not antagonistic (having opposite effects) to each other? ***(NEET-I 2016)***

(a) Aldosterone	Atrial Natriuretic Factor
(b) Relaxin	Inhibin
(c) Parathormone	Calcitonin
(d) Insulin	Glucagon

16. Which one of the following hormones is not involved in sugar metabolism? ***(2015)***
(a) Insulin (b) Glucagon
(c) Cortisone (d) Aldosterone

17. Which one of the following hormones though synthesised elsewhere, is stored and released by the master gland? ***(2015)***
(a) Prolactin
(b) Melanocyte stimulating hormone
(c) Antidiuretic hormone
(d) Luteinising hormone

18. Fight-or-flight reactions cause activation of ***(2014)***
(a) the parathyroid glands, leading to increased metabolic rate
(b) the kidney, leading to suppression of reninangiotensin-aldosterone pathway
(c) the adrenal medulla, leading to increased secretion of epinephrine and norepinephrine
(d) the pancreas leading to a reduction in the blood sugar levels.

19. A pregnant female delivers a baby who suffers from stunted growth, mental retardation, low intelligence quotient and abnormal skin. ***(2013)***

This is the result of
(a) cancer of the thyroid gland
(b) oversecretion of pars distalis
(c) deficiency of iodine in diet
(d) low secretion of growth hormone.

20. Select the answer which correctly matches the endocrine gland with the hormone it secretes and its function/deficiency symptom. ***(NEET 2013)***

Endocrine gland	**Hormone**	**Function/ Deficiency symptoms**
(a) Thyroid gland	Thyroxine	Lack of iodine in diet results in goitre
(b) Corpus luteum	Testosterone	Stimulates spermatogenesis
(c) Anterior pituitary	Oxytocin	Stimulates uterus contraction during child birth
(d) Posterior pituitary	Growth hormone (GH)	Oversecretion stimulates abnormal growth

21. Select the option which correctly matches the endocrine gland with its hormone and its function. ***(Karnataka NEET 2013)***

	Endocrine gland	Hormone	Function
(a)	Placenta	Estrogen	Initiates secretion of the milk
(b)	Corpus luteum	Estrogen	Essential for maintenance of endometrium
(c)	Leydig's cells	Androgen	Initiates the production of sperms
(d)	Ovary	FSH	Stimulates follicular development and the secretion of estrogens

22. Nor-epinephrine ***(Karnataka NEET 2013)***

(i) is released by sympathetic fibers

(ii) is released by parasympathetic fibers

(iii) increases the heart rate

(iv) decreases blood pressure.

Which of the above statements are correct?

(a) (i) and (iii) (b) (ii) and (iii)
(c) (ii) and (iv) (d) (i) and (iv)

23. Which of the following represents the action of insulin? ***(Karnataka NEET 2013)***

(a) Increases blood glucose level by stimulating glucagon production.
(b) Decreases blood glucose levels by forming glycogen.
(c) Increases blood glucose levels by promoting cellular uptake of glucose.
(d) Increases blood glucose levels by hydrolysis of glycogen.

24. A person entering an empty room suddenly finds a snake right in front on opening the door. Which one of the following is likely to happen in his neurohormonal control system? ***(2012)***

(a) Sympathetic nervous system is activated releasing epinephrine and norepinephrine from adrenal medulla.
(b) Neurotransmitters diffuse rapidly across the cleft and transmit a nerve impulse.
(c) Hypothalamus activates the parasympathetic division of brain.
(d) Sympathetic nervous system is activated releasing epinephrine and norepinephrine from adrenal cortex.

25. The 24 hour (diurnal) rhythm of our body such as the sleep-wake cycle is regulated by the hormone ***(Mains 2011)***

(a) calcitonin (b) prolactin
(c) adrenaline (d) melatonin.

26. Match the source gland with its respective hormone and function and select the correct option. ***(2011)***

	Source gland	**Hormone**	**Function**
(a)	Anterior pituitary	Oxytocin	Contraction of uterus muscles during child birth
(b)	Posterior pituitary	Vasopressin	Stimulates reabsorption of water in the distal tubules in the nephron
(c)	Corpus luteum	Estrogen	Supports pregnancy
(d)	Thyroid	Thyroxine	Regulates blood calcium level

27. Given below is an incomplete table on hormones, their source glands and one major effect of each human body. Identify the option representing correct grouping of hormone its gland and effect. ***(2011)***

Gland	**Secretion**	**Effect on body**
A	Estrogen	Maintenance of secondary sexual characters
Alpha cells of Islets of Langerhans	B	Raises blood sugar level
Anterior pituitary	C	Over secretion leads to gigantism

	A	**B**	**C**
(a)	Ovary	Glucagon	Growth hormone
(b)	Placenta	Insulin	Vasopressin
(c)	Ovary	Insulin	Calcitonin
(d)	Placenta	Glucagon	Calcitonin

28. Injury to adrenal cortex is not likely to affect the secretion of which one of the following? (2010)
(a) Aldosterone
(b) Both androstenedione and dehydroepiandrosterone
(c) Adrenaline
(d) Cortisol

29. Which one of the following pairs is incorrectly matched? ***(2010)***
(a) Glucagon - Beta cells (source)
(b) Somatostatin - Delta cells (source)
(c) Corpus luteum - Relaxin (secretion)
(d) Insulin - Diabetes mellitus (disease)

30. Toxic agents present in food which interfere with thyroxine synthesis lead to the development of ***(2010)***
(a) toxic goitre (b) cretinism
(c) simple goitre (d) thyrotoxicosis.

31. Select the correct matching of a hormone, its source and function.

	Hormone	Source	Function
(a)	Vasopressin	Posterior pituitary	Increases loss of water through urine
(b)	Norepinephrine	Adrenal medulla	Increases heart beat, rate of respiration and alterness
(c)	Glucagon	Beta-cells of Islets of Langerhans	Stimulates glycogenolysis
(d)	Prolactin	Posterior pituitary	Regulates growth of mammary glands and milk formation in females

32. A health disorder that results from the deficiency of thyroxine in adults and characterised by (i) a low metabolic rate, (ii) increase in body weight and (iii) tendency to retain water in tissues is ***(2009)***
(a) simple goitre (b) myxoedema
(c) cretinism (d) hypothyroidism.

33. Which one of the following pair of organs includes only the endocrine glands? ***(2008)***
(a) Thymus and testes
(b) Adrenal and ovary
(c) Parathyroid and adrenal
(d) Pancreas and parathyroid

34. The blood calcium level is lowered by the deficiency of ***(2008)***
(a) both calcitonin and parathormone
(b) calcitonin
(c) parathormone
(d) thyroxine.

35. Feeling the tremors of an earthquake a scared resident of seventh floor of a multistoryed building starts climbing down the stairs rapidly. ***(2007)***

Which hormone initiated this action?
(a) Adrenaline (b) Glucagon
(c) Gastrin (d) Thyroxine

36. A person is having problems with calcium and phosphorus metabolism in his body. Which one of the following glands may not be functioning properly? ***(2007)***
(a) Parotid (b) Pancreas
(c) Thyroid (d) Parathyroid

37. Which hormone causes dilation of blood vessels, increased oxygen consumption and glucogenesis? ***(2006)***
(a) Glucagon (b) ACTH
(c) Insulin (d) Adrenaline

38. Which of the following is an accumulation and release centre of neurohormones? ***(2006)***
(a) Anterior pituitary lobe
(b) Posterior pituitary lobe
(c) Intermediate lobe of the pituitary
(d) Hypothalamus

39. A steroid hormone which regulates glucose metabolism is ***(2006)***
(a) cortisone
(b) cortisol
(c) corticosterone
(d) 11-deoxycorticosterone.

40. Which one of the following pairs correctly matches a hormone with a disease resulting from its deficiency? ***(2003)***

(a)	Luteinising hormone	-	Failure of ovulation
(b)	Insulin	-	Diabetes insipidus
(c)	Thyroxine	-	Tetany
(d)	Parathyroid hormone	-	Diabetes mellitus

41. Which one of the following pairs correctly matches a hormone with a disease resulting from its deficiency? ***(2003)***
(a) Relaxin - Gigantism
(b) Prolactin - Cretinism
(c) Parathyroid hormone - Tetany
(d) Insulin - Diabetes insipidus

42. Acromegaly is caused by ***(2002)***
(a) excess of STH
(b) excess of thyroxine
(c) deficiency of thyroxine
(d) excess of adrenaline.

43. Adrenaline directly affects on ***(2002)***
(a) SA node
(b) b-cells of Langerhans
(c) dorsal root of spinal nerve
(d) epithelial cells of stomach.

44. When both ovaries are removed from rat then which hormone is decreased in blood? ***(2002)***
(a) Oxytocin (b) Prolactin
(c) Estrogen
(d) Gonadotropin releasing factor

45. Mainly which type of hormones control the menstrual cycle in human beings? ***(2002)***
(a) FSH (b) LH
(c) FSH, LH, estrogen (d) progesterone

46. Which set is similar? ***(2001)***
(a) Corpus luteum - Graafian follicles
(b) Sebum - Sweat
(c) Bundle of His - Pace maker
(d) Vitamin B7 - Niacin

47. Melatonin is secreted by ***(2000)***
(a) pineal body (b) skin
(c) pituitary gland (d) thyroid.

48. Which gland secretes odorous secretion in mammals? ***(2000)***
(a) Bartholins (b) Prostate
(c) Anal gland (d) Liver

49. MSH is secreted by ***(2000)***
(a) anterior lobe of pituitary
(b) middle lobe of pituitary
(c) posterior lobe of pituitary
(d) endostyle.

50. The function of oxytocin is to help in ***(1999)***
(a) child birth (b) gametogenesis
(c) growth (d) lactation.

51. Secretion of progesterone by corpus luteum is initiated by ***(1999)***
(a) testosterone (b) thyroxine
(c) MSH (d) LH

52. The gonadotrophic hormones are secreted by ***(1999)***
(a) anterior lobe of pituitary
(b) interstitial cells of testes
(c) adrenal cortex
(d) posterior part of thyroid.

53. Diabetes is due to ***(1999)***
(a) enzyme deficiency
(b) iodine deficiency
(c) Na_+ deficiency
(d) hormonal deficiency.

54. Calcitonin is a thyroid hormone which ***(1998)***
(a) elevates calcium level in blood
(b) has no effect on calcium
(c) elevates potassium level in blood
(d) lowers calcium level in blood.

55. The hormone which regulates the basal metabolism in our body is secreted from ***(1998)***
(a) adrenal cortex (b) pancreas
(c) pituitary (d) thyroid.

56. Which hormone stimulates the secretion of milk from female? ***(1996)***
(a) Oxytocin (b) Progesterone
(c) LH (d) Prolactin

57. The immediate cause of induction of ovulation in human female is the large plasma surge of ***(1994)***
(a) LH
(b) FSH
(c) progesterone
(d) estradiol.

58. Testosterone is produced by ***(1993)***
(a) sertoli cells
(b) Leydig's cells
(c) oxyntic cells
(d) pituitary gland.

59. ADH or vasopressin is ***(1991)***
(a) enzyme that hydrolyses peptides
(b) hormone secreted by pituitary that promotes reabsorption of water from glomerular filtrate
(c) hormone that promotes glycogenolysis
(d) energy rich compound connected with muscle contraction.

60. Occurrence of Leydig's cells and their secretion is ***(1991)***
(a) ovary and estrogen
(b) liver and cholesterol
(c) pancreas and glucagon
(d) testis and testosterone.

61. Insulin is a ***(1990)***
(a) vitamin (b) lipid
(c) hormone (d) enzyme.

62. Which hormone possesses anti-insulin effect? ***(1988)***
(a) Cortisol
(b) Calcitonin
(c) Oxytocin
(d) Aldosterone

63. MSH of pars intermedia of middle pituitary is responsible for ***(1988)***
(a) darkening of skin in lower vertebrates
(b) light colouration of skin in lower vertebrates
(c) both A and B
(d) darkening of skin in human beings.

HORMONES OF HEART, KIDNEY AND GASTROINTESTINAL TRACT

64. Match List I with List II. (2023)

List I	List II
A. CCK	I. Kidney
B. GIP	II. Heart
C. ANF	III. Gastric gland
D. ADH	IV. Pancreas

Choose the correct answer from the options given below.
(a) A-II, B-IV, C-I, D-III (b) A-IV, B-II, C-III, D-I
(c) A-IV, B-III, C-II, D-I (d) A-III, B-II, C-IV, D-I

65. Erythropoietin hormone which stimulates RBC formation is produced by ***(2021)***
(a) juxtaglomerular ceils of the kidney
(b) alpha cells of pancreas
(c) the cells of rostral adenohypophysis
(d) the cells of bone marrow.

66. Identify the hormone with its correct matching of source and function. ***(2014)***
(a) Oxytocin - posterior pituitary, growth and maintenance of mammary glands.
(b) Melatonin - pineal gland, regulates the normal rhythm of sleepwake cycle.
(c) Progesterone - corpus luteum, stimulation of growth and activities of female secondary sex organs.
(d) Atrial natriuretic factor - ventricular wall, increases the blood pressure.

67. Which of the following statements is correct in relation to the endocrine system? ***(2013)***
(a) Non-nutrient chemicals produced by the body in trace amounts that act as intercellular messenger are known as hormones.
(b) Releasing and inhibitory hormones are produced by the pituitary gland.
(c) Adenohypophysis is under direct neural regulation of the hypothalamus.
(d) Organs in the body like gastrointestinal tract, heart, kidney and liver do not produce any hormones.

68. Cholecystokinin and duocrinin are secreted by ***(1999)***
(a) adrenal cortex (b) thyroid gland
(c) intestine (d) pancreas.

69. The hormone that stimulates the stomach to secrete gastric juice is ***(1998)***
(a) enterokinase (b) enterogastrone
(c) gastrin (d) renin.

70. The contraction of gall bladder is due to ***(1998)***
(a) cholecystokinin (b) enterogastrone
(c) gastrin (d) secretin

71. Gastric secretion is stopped by hormone ***(1993)***
(a) enterogastrone (b) gastrin
(c) pancreozymin (d) cholecystokinin.

MECHANISM OF HORMONE ACTION

72. How does steroid hormone influence the cellular activities? ***(2019)***
(a) Using aquaporin channels 'as second messenger'
(b) Changing the permeability of the cell membrane
(c) Binding to DNA and forming a gene-hormone complex
(d) Activating cyclic AMP located on the cell membrane

73. Identify A, B and C in the diagramatic representation of the mechanism of hormone action. ***(Odisha NEET 2019)***

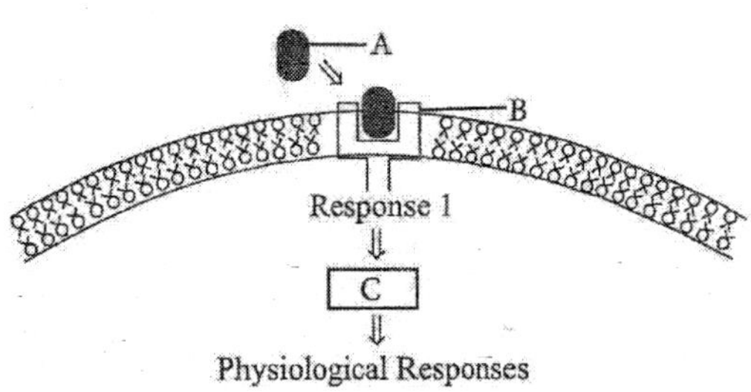

Select the correct option from the following.

(a) A-Steroid Hormone; B-Hormone-receptor Complex; C-Protein

(b) A-Protein Hormone; B-Receptor; C-Cyclic AMP

(c) A-Steroid Hormone; B-Receptor; C - Second Messenger

(d) A-Protein Hormone; B-Cyclic AMP; C-Hormone-receptor Complex

74. Which of the following is an amino acid derived hormone? ***(2018)***

(a) Epinephrine (b) Ecdysone
(c) Estradiol (d) Estriol

75. The amino acid tryptophan is the precursor for the synthesis of ***(NEET-I 2016)***

(a) estrogen and progesterone
(b) cortisol and cortisone
(c) melatonin and serotonin
(d) thyroxine and triiodothyronine.

76. Which of the following best illustrates "feedback" in development? ***(Karnataka NEET 2013)***

(a) Tissue X secretes RNA which changes the development of tissue Y.

(b) As tissue X develops, it secretes enzymes that inhibit the development of tissue Y.

(c) As tissue X develops, it secretes something that induces tissue Y to develop.

(d) As tissue X develops, it secretes something that slows down the growth of tissue Y.

77. Which one of the following pairs of hormones are the examples of those that can easily pass through the cell membrane of the target cell and bind to a receptor inside it (mostly in the nucleus)? ***(2012)***

(a) Insulin, glucagon
(b) Thyroxine, insulin
(c) Somatostatin, oxytocin
(d) Cortisol, testosterone

78. What is correct to say about the hormone action in humans? ***(2012)***

(a) Glucagon is secreted by β-cells of islets of Langerhans and stimulates glycogenolysis.

(b) Secretion of thymosins is stimulated with aging.

(c) In females, FSH first binds with specific receptors on ovarian cell membrane

(d) FSH stimulates the secretion of estrogen and progesterone.

79. Which one of the following pairs of chemical substances, is correctly categorised? ***(2012)***

(a)	Calcitonin and thymosin	– Thyroid hormones
(b)	Pepsin and prolactin	– Two digestive enzymes secreted in stomach
(c)	Troponin and myosin	– Complex proteins in striated muscles
(d)	Secretin and rhodopsin	– Polypeptide hormones

80. Which one of the following is not a secondary messenger in hormone action? ***(2006)***

(a) cAMP (b) cGMP
(c) Calcium (d) Sodium

81. Which one of the following hormones is modified amino acid? ***(2004)***

(a) Epinephrine (b) Progesterone
(c) Prostaglandin (d) Estrogen

82. Chemically hormones are ***(2004)***

(a) biogenic amines only
(b) proteins, steroids and biogenic amines
(c) proteins only
(d) steroids only.

83. Hormones thyroxine, adrenaline and the pigment melanin are formed from ***(1997)***

(a) tyrosine (b) proline
(c) tryptophan (d) glycine.

84. Which one of the following endocrine glands stores its secretion in the extracellular space before discharging it into the blood? ***(1995)***

(a) Testis (b) Thyroid
(c) Pancreas (d) Adrenal

85. According to the accepted concept of hormone action, if receptor molecules are removed from target organs, then the target organ will (1995)
(a) continue to respond to the hormone without any difference
(b) not respond to the hormone
(c) continue to respond to the hormone but will require higher concentration
(d) continue to respond to the hormone but in the opposite way.

ANSWER KEY

1.	(c)	2.	(a)	3.	(b)	4.	(c)	5.	(c)	6.	(a)	7.	(d)
8.	(c)	9.	(a)	10.	(a)	11.	(b)	12.	(b)	13.	(a)	14.	(b)
15.	(b)	16.	(d)	17.	(c)	18.	(c)	19.	(c)	20.	(a)	21.	(c)
22.	(a)	23.	(b)	24.	(a)	25.	(d)	26.	(b)	27.	(a)	28.	(c)
29.	(a)	30.	(c)	31.	(b)	32.	(b)	33.	(c)	34.	(c)	35.	(a)
36.	(d)	37.	(d)	38.	(d)	39.	(b)	40.	(a)	41.	(c)	42.	(a)
43.	(a)	44.	(c)	45.	(c)	46.	(a)	47.	(a)	48.	(c)	49.	(b)
50.	(a)	51.	(d)	52.	(a)	53.	(d)	54.	(d)	55.	(d)	56.	(d)
57.	(a)	58.	(b)	59.	(b)	60.	(d)	61.	(c)	62.	(a)	63.	(a)
64.	(c)	65.	(a)	66.	(b)	67.	(a)	68.	(c)	69.	(c)	70.	(a)
71.	(a)	72.	(c)	73.	(b)	74.	(a)	75.	(c)	76.	(c)	77.	(d)
78.	(c)	79.	(c)	80.	(d)	81.	(a)	82.	(b)	83.	(a)	84.	(b)
85.	(b)												

HINTS & EXPLANATIONS

1. (c): The endocrine system links the brain to the organs that control body metabolism, growth and development, and reproduction. The endocrine system is regulated by feedback. For example, the hormones that are regulated by the pituitary gland, a signal is sent from the hypothalamus to the pituitary gland in the form of a "releasing hormone," which stimulates the pituitary to secrete a "stimulating hormone" into the circulation. The stimulating hormone then signals the target gland to secrete its hormone. As the level of this hormone rises in the circulation, the hypothalamus and the pituitary gland shut down secretion of the releasing hormone and the stimulating hormone, which in turn slows the secretion by the target gland. This system results in stable blood concentrations of the hormones that are regulated by the pituitary gland.

2. (a)

3.(b) : Parathyroid hormone (PTH) increases Ca^{2+} levels in the blood. It increases Ca^{2+} absorption from digested food. Thyroid hormones control metabolism of carbohydrates.

4. (c): Diabetes mellitus is associated with formation of harmful compounds known as ketone bodies, i.e., ketonuria and loss of glucose through urine, i.e.,glycosuria.

5. **(c)**

6. **(a)**: Glucocorticoids also stimulates gluconeogenesis, lipolysis and proteolysis; and inhibit cellular uptake and utilisation of amino acids. Insulin acts on hepatocytes and adipocytes. Glucagon is associated with hyperglycemia while insulin is associated with hypoglycemia.

7. **(d)**

8. **(c)**: Estrogen plays a central role in control of bone strength. In a healthy individual, bone mass is maintained by balanced activity of bone forming osteoblasts and bone resorbing osteoclasts. Both these cell types are reported to respond to estrogen. Estrogen promotes the activity of osteoblast and induces osteoclast apoptosis. After menopause the level of this hormone declines. Hence, in an ageing female osteoporosis occurs. Parathormone promotes mobilisation of calcium from bone into blood. Excessive activity of parathormone causes demineralisation of bone leading to osteoporosis.

9. **(a)**: Gonadotropin releasing hormone (GnRH) is secreted by the hypothalamus which stimulates the anterior lobe of pituitary gland to secrete luteinising hormone (LH) and Follicle Stimulating Hormone (FSH).

10. **(a)**:Epiphyseal plate is a hyaline cartilage plate in the metaphysis at each end of long bone. It is part of long bone where new bone growth takes place. In adults, elevated levels of GH results in acromegaly where no increase in height occurs because of ossified epiphyseal plate.

11. **(b)**: Corpus luteum is a temporary endocrine gland in human females. It secretes progesterone which stimulates the uterine glands to produce increased amount of watery mucus and is also essential for maintenance of endothelium. In absence of fertilisation, corpus luteum disintegrate leading to menstruation.

12. **(b)**: Exophthalmic goitre or Graves' disease is a thyroid enlargement (goitre) in which the thyroid secretes excessive amount of thyroid hormone. It is characterised by exophthalmia (protrusion of eye balls because of fluid accumulation behind them), loss of weight, slightly rise in the body temperature, excitability, rapid heart beat, nervousness and restlessness.

13. **(a)**: Insulin is a peptide hormone, secreted by the β cells of the islets of Langerhans in the pancreas, that promotes the uptake of glucose by body cells, particularly in the liver (hepatocytes) and muscles (adipocytes) and thereby controls its concentration in the blood.

14. **(b)**: Posterior lobe of pituitary gland does not secrete any hormone. Its hormones are synthesised by the hypothalamus. It only stores and releases these hormones. Hence, it cannot be considered as true gland.

15. **(b)**: Relaxin hormone is secreted by ovary and placenta during pregnancy, which relaxes ligaments in pelvis and softens and widens cervix during childbirth. Inhibin secreted by granulosa cells in the ovaries inhibits secretion of FSH by anterior pituitary. Thus, relaxin and inhibin have different functions and are not antagonistic.

16. **(d)**: Aldosterone (salt-retaining hormone) is the principal mineralocorticoid in humans, secreted by adrenal cortex. Its main function is to regulate sodium content of the body.

17. **(c)**: Two hormones viz oxytocin (OT) and antidiuretic hormone (ADH) are synthesised in the hypothalamus, but stored and released by the posterior lobe of pituitary gland.

18. **(c)**: Hormones epinephrine and norepinephrine are secreted from adrenal medulla. They are emergency hormones released in condition of stress, emergency, etc. Epinephrine and norepinephrine are also released by adrenergic nerve fibres of sympathetic nervous system where they act as neurotransmitters.

19. **(c)**: Iodine is needed for the synthesis of T3 and T4. Iodine binds to the tyrosine residues in thyroglobulin, which is then hydrolysed into iodotyrosines that combine to form triiodothyronine (T3) or thyroxine (tetra-iodothyronine or T4). Therefore, deficiency of iodine in the diet of a pregnant female will lead to improper synthesis of thyroid hormones in newly borne infant. The deficiency of thyroid hormones in infants causes 'cretinism' whose symptoms are slow heart beat, lower blood pressure, decrease in temperature, stunted growth, low intelligence quotient and abnormal skin.

20. **(a)**: Iodine is required for production of thyroxine, thus lack of iodine results in hyposecretion of thyroxine. To compensate, thyroid gland enlarges and the condition is known as goitre. Corpus luteum secretes progesterone which maintains uterine endothelium and mucus secretion in uterus, fallopian tubes and vagina. Oxytocin stimulates uterine contractions but is secreted by posterior pituitary. Anterior pituitary secretes GH, whose oversecretion causes abnormal growth.

21. **(c)**: Interstitial cells (or Leydig's cells) are the cells interspersed between the seminiferous tubules of the testis. They secrete androgens including testosterone in response to stimulation by luteinising hormone from the anterior pituitary gland. Androgens produce and maintain male characteristics and stimulate germinal epithelium to undergo spermatogenesis.

22. **(a)**: Nor-epinephrine is secreted by some neurons of the sympathetic nervous system and also by adrenal medulla. It accelerates heart rate.

23. **(b)**

24. **(a)**

25. **(d)**: Melatonin is a hormone secreted by the pineal gland and retinas of vertebrates. Melatonin secretion by the pineal gland is linked to the dark-light cycle of the organism's environment, being greatest at night and lowest by day. The hormone is involved in regulating certain diurnal and seasonal changes in the body, such as the reproductive cycle in seasonally breeding animals. It is used as a drug to treat sleep disorders and symptoms of jet lag.

26. **(b)**: Posterior lobe of pituitary stores and releases two hormones, called oxytocin and vasopressin. These hormones are actually produced by the neurosecretary cells in the hypothalamus and stand in the terminals of their axons that pass into the posterior lobe through a stalk. They are released via posterior lobe when required. Vasopressin is also called antidiuretic hormone (ADH). It decreases the loss of water in the urine by increasing reabsorption of water in the distal convoluted tubules, collecting tubules and collecting ducts in the kidneys.

27. **(a)**: The correct option for the three blanks A, B and C are ovary, glucagon and growth hormone respectively.

28. **(c)**: Adrenal glands or (suprarenal glands) are two triangular endocrine glands, each of which covers the superior surface of a kidney. Each gland has two parts, the medulla and cortex. The medulla forms the grey core of the gland; it consists mainly of chromaffin tissue and is stimulated by the sympathetic nervous system to produce adrenaline and noradrenaline. The cortex is a yellowish tissue surrounding the medulla. It is stimulated by pituitary hormones (principally ACTH) to produce three kinds of corticosteroid hormones, which affect carbohydrate metabolism (e.g., cortisol), electrolyte metabolism (e.g., aldosterone), and the sex glands (estrogens and androgens). Thus injury to adrenal cortex is not likely to affect the secretion of adrenaline.

29. (a): Glucagon is a hormone, secreted by the a-cells of the islets of Langerhans in the pancreas, that increases the concentration of glucose in the blood by stimulating the metabolic breakdown of glycogen. It thus antagonizes the effects of insulin.

30. (c)

31. (b): asopressin reduces water loss through urine by stimulating resorption of water by the distal tubules of the kidney. Glucagon is released from α-cells. Prolactin is produced from anterior pituitary.

32. (b): Myxoedema is caused by deficiency of thyroid hormone or thyroxine in adults. It is characterised by low metabolic rate, body gain, puffy appearance, low body temperature, etc. This disease can be treated by administration of thyroid hormones.

33. (c): Parathyroid and adrenal glands are the endocrine glands because they manufacture hormones and secretes them directly into the blood stream to act at distant sites in the body. Thyroid and pituitary are its other examples.

34. (c) : Parathormone is secreted by chief cells of the parathyroid that regulates the metabolism of calcium and phosphate. It increases calcium absorption from the intestine and also increases calcium resorption from the nephrons of the kidneys. So, its deficiency leads to low blood calcium level.

35. (a): Adrenaline (epinephrine), also called emergency hormone, is a hormone, produced by the medulla of the adrenal glands, that increases heart activity, improves the power and prolongs the action of muscles and increases the rate and depth of breathing to prepare the body for 'fright, flight or fight'. At the same time it inhibits digestion and excretion. Similar effects are produced by stimulation of the sympathetic nervous system.

36. (d)

37. (d): Adrenaline is the hormone secreted by adrenal medulla. It prepares the animal to face special conditions created by physical stress. All these conditions require more energy which is provided by increasing heart beat, blood pressure, respiratory rate, sugar level of blood, blood supply of heart and skeletal muscles and brain through dilation of their small arteries and oxidative metabolism. It also stimulates the breakdown of liver and muscle glycogen (glucogenesis) to provide glucose for respiration.

38. (d): Releasing and inhibiting factors are released by hypothalamus. The hypothalamus is connected to adenohypophysis by hypophysial portal vein and is connected to the neurohypophysis by axons of neurosecretory cells. Hence, neurohypophysis is directly under the neural control.

39. (b)

40. (a): Ovulation occurs under the influence of LH (luteinising hormone) and FSH (follicle stimulating hormone) of anterior pituitary gland. Thus, deficiency of luteinising hormone results in failure of ovulation.

41. (c): Tetany is usually caused by reduction in the blood calcium level, which may be due to underactive parathyroid glands.

42. (a): Acromegaly is caused by excess of STH (somatotrophic hormone), released by anterior lobe of pituitary after adolescence. The bones of the lower jaw and limbs become abnormally enlarge but the body does not attain a giant stature. Excess of thyroxine causes cretinism and myxoedema. Excess of adrenaline causes increased BMR (Basal Metabolic Rate), heart beat, excitement, etc.

43. (a): Adrenaline directly affects the SA node to increase rate of heartbeat. Adrenaline prepares the body for emergency reactions like fight and flight. Thus there is increase in heart rate, breathing rate, blood pressure, glucose level in blood, peripheral circulation, etc.

44. (c): Ovary secretes two hormones. Estrogen before ovulation and progesterone after ovulation. Oxytocin, prolaction are pituitary hormones and gonadotropin releasing factor is secreted by hypothalamus of brain to stimulate pituitary for the secretion of gonadotropic hormones.

45. (c): Menstrual cycle is controlled by several endocrinal parameters.

In beginning of the cycle FSH (follicle stimulating hormone) of pituitary initiates development of an ovarian follicle. A growing ovarian follicle gradually secretes increasing amount of estrogen. This in turn leads to sudden surge of LH secretion by the pituitary. As the LH (luteinising hormone) level in blood suddenly increases there is ovulation.

Thus only FSH or LH cannot control all the events of menstrual cycle. Progesterone is released by a corpus luteum after ovulation which actually prepares the uterus for a possible pregnancy.

46. (a): After ovulation many of the follicular cells remain in the collapsed Graafian follicle on the surface of the ovary. The antrum (cavity) of the collapsed follicle fills with a partially clotted fluid. The follicular cells enlarge and fill with a yellow pigment, lutein. Such a follicle is called a corpus luteum.

47. (a)

48. (c): The anal glands are small paired sacs located on either side of the anus between the external and internal sphincter muscles. These sebaceous glands within the lining secrete a foul smelling liquid that is used for identification of members within a species. These glands are found in all carnivora except bears.

49. (b): Middle lobe of pituitary secretes a hormone named melanocyte-stimulating hormone. It stimulates the synthesis of black pigment melanin in the skin and also causes dispersal of melanin granules in the pigment cells, thereby darkening the colour in certain animals (fishes, amphibians). In man it has no such role. Anterior lobe of pituitary secretes FSH, LH, TSH, ACTH and STH. Posterior lobe of pituitary secretes oxytocin and vasopressin.

50. (a)

51. (d): Luteinising Hormone (LH) in the male, induces the interstitial cells of the testes to produce male sex hormones named androgens such as testosterone. In the female, the luteinising hormone causes ovulation, secretion of female sex hormone, estrogen from the maturing ovarian follicle and progesterone by the corpus luteum.

52. (a): Gonadotrophic hormones are secreted by anterior lobe of pituitary gland. They are as follows:

(i) Follicle-stimulating hormone (FSH): It stimulates growth of ovarian follicles and their secretion of estrogens in the female and spermatogenesis (formation of sperms) in the male.

(ii) Interstitial cell stimulating hormone (ICSH): It activates the Leydig's (interstitial) cells of the testis to secrete androgens. In female, it stimulates the corpus luteum of the ovary to secrete progesterone. In female it is termed luteinising hormone (LH).

53. (d): Diabetes mellitus is caused by the deficiency of hormone insulin which is secreted by pancreas. Insulin lowers the blood-glucose level. Deficiency of antidiuretic hormone (ADH) leads to diabetes insipidus.

54. (d): Calcitonin is secreted by the C cells. It regulates the concentration of calcium and phosphorus in the blood. It is under the feedback control of plasma calcium concentration and is secreted when concentration of calcium rises in the blood. It then lowers the concentration of calcium and phosphorus in the plasma by decreasing their release from the bones.

55. (d): The basal metabolism is the minimum amount of energy the body uses in order to maintain vital processes of the body. Generally, this expenditure of energy is expressed in terms of heat production per unit of body surface per day on the basal metabolic rate (BMR). Thyroid is the largest endocrine gland secreting three hormones : thyroxine, triiodothyronine and calcitonin. Thyroxine and triiodothyronine control BMR of the body by regulating the rate of oxidation and production of energy.

56. (d): Prolactin hormone stimulates the growth of milk glands during pregnancy and the secretion of milk after delivery. Oxytocin causes release of milk during sucking by the infant. LH causes ovulation and secretion of estrogen and progesterone from ovarian follicle and corpus luteum respectively. Oxytocin, LH and prolactin are released by anterior lobe of pituitary gland. Progesterone is secreted by corpus luteum.

57. (a)

58. (b)

59.(b) : ADH or vasopressin is a hormone secreted by pituitary that promotes reabsorption of water from glomerular filtrate.

60. (d)

61. (c): Insulin is a peptide hormone, secreted by the β cells of the islets of Langerhans in the pancreas. It plays a major role in the regulation of glucose homeostasis.

62. (a): Insulin decreases the level of glucose in the blood while cortisol (secreted by middle region of adrenal cortex) increases the blood-glucose level by converting proteins and fats into carbohydrates which are, in turn, converted to glucose.

63. (a): Pars intermedia is the boundary between the anterior and posterior lobes of the pituitary. It contains three types of cells - basophils, chromophobes and colloid-filled cysts. This area produces melanocyte stimulating hormone or MSH. It stimulates the synthesis of black pigment melanin in the skin and also causes dispersion of melanin granules in the pigment cells, thereby darkening the colour in certain animals (fishes; amphibians). In man it has no such role.

64. (c): CCK $\rightarrow$ pancreas

GIP $\rightarrow$ Gastric gland

ANF $\rightarrow$ Heart

ADH $\rightarrow$ Kidney

65. (a): The juxtaglomerular cells of kidney produce

a peptide hormone called erythropoietin which stimulates erythropoiesis i.e., formation of RBC.

66. (b): Oxytocin is produced by hypothalamus and generally secreted by posterior pituitary. It stimulates ejection of milk from mammary glands; causes contraction of uterus at the time of child birth.

Progesterone is secreted by corpus luteum. It stimulates uterus for pregnancy, implantation, formation of placenta and development of mammary glands.

Atrial natriuretic factor is secreted by atrial wall in response to an increased return of the venous blood. This hormone reduces blood pressure.

67.(a) : Releasing and inhibiting factors are released by hypothalamus. The hypothalamus is connected to adenohypophysis by hypophysial portal vein and is connected to the neurohypophysis by axons of neurosecretory cells. Hence, neurohypophysis is directly under the neural control. The cardiocytes of atria of the heart secrete peptide hormone, called atrial natriuretic factor (ANF) in response to an increased return of the deoxygenated (venous) blood. The liver produces angiotensinogen which is changed to angiotensin II by an enzyme renin secreted by juxtaglomerular apparatus (JGA).

68. (c): Cholecystokinin and duocrinin are secreted by intestine. It stimulates pancreas to release enzymes in pancreatic juice and stimulates gall bladder to release bile. Duocrinin causes release of viscous mucus from Brunner's glands into intestinal juice.

69. (c): Gastrin hormone is secreted by mucosa of stomach and it stimulates secretion of gastric juice. Enterogastrone is secreted by duodenal epithelium. Enterokinase is an enzyme that converts trypsinogen into trypsin. Renin is secreted by kidneys. It acts on angiotensinogen to form angiotensin-II.

70. (a)

71. (a): Enterogastrone is secreted by duodenal epithelium and it slows gastric contractions to delay its emptying and also stops secretion of gastric juice. Gastrin stimulates secretion of gastric juice. Cholecystokinin stimulates release of enzymes in pancreatic juice and release of bile from gall bladder. Cholecystokinin is also known as pancreozymin.

72. (c): Steroid hormones are lipid-soluble and easily pass through the cell membrane of a target cell into the cytoplasm where they bind to specific intracellular receptors (proteins) to form a hormone receptor complex that enters the nucleus. In the nucleus, hormone which interact with intracellular receptors mostly regulate gene expression or chromosome function by the interaction of hormone-receptor complex with the genome. Biochemical actions result in physiological and developmental effects.

73. (b)

74. (a): Epinephrine which triggers the flight or fight response is derived from amino acid tyrosine. It is synthesised in the medulla of the adrenal glands.

75. (c): Tryptophan is an essential amino acid which is precursor for the synthesis of melatonin and serotonin.

76. (c): As tissue X develops, It secretes something that induces tissue Y to develop indicating positive feedback mechanism.

77. (d): Steroid hormones such as cortisol, testosterone, estradiol and progesterone, mostly regulate gene expression or chromosome function by the interaction of hormone-receptor complex with the genome. So, these easily pass through the cell membrane of the target cell and bind to a receptor inside it.

78. **(c)**: Hormone action involves their reception by target cells. Specific proteins called hormone receptors that are located in target tissues only bind with these hormones. Hormone receptor may be of two types: membrane bound receptor and intracellular receptors. Steroid hormones, bind with intracellular receptors while some hormones e.g., pituitary hormones like FSH bind with membrane bound receptors.

79. **(c)**: Skeletal muscle fibres occur in bundles and are normally attached to the skeleton. Each muscle fibre is an elongated cell surrounded externally by a delicate membrane, the sarcolemma. Just beneath the sarcolemma in each fibre many nuclei occur at irregular intervals. Thus, these fibres are mutlinucleated or syncytial in nature. The cytoplasm of each fibre (sarcoplasm) has a large number of myofibrils which are tightly packed. Each myofibril shows dark bands (A bands) containing myosin and light band (I bands) containing actin, alternating with each other. That is why these are named as striped muscle fibres.

80. **(d)**: Secondary messengers are low-weight diffusible molecules that are used to relay signals within a cell. They are synthesised or released by specific enzymatic reactions, usually as a result of an external signal that is received by a transmembrane receptor. cAMP, cGMP and $Ca(2^+)$ act as secondary messengers and are located within the cytoplasm. Sodium is an essential nutrient which helps to maintain blood volume and keeps nerves functioning.

81. **(a)**: Epinephrine is synthesized from tyrosine which is a non-essential amino acid possessing cyclic structure with a straight side chain bearing carboxylic and amino group. The conversion of tyrosine to epinephrine involves 4 steps (i) ring hydroxylation (ii) decarboxylation, (iii) side-chain hydroxylation (iv) N-methylation.

Tyrosine $\rightarrow$ DOPA $\rightarrow$ Dopamine $\rightarrow$Norepinephrine $\rightarrow$ Epinephrine.

82. **(b)**: Hormones are chemical messengers produced by the ductless glands (sometimes by neurons) and transported in the circulation to target cells. They regulate metabolic processes. Chemically hormones are of different nature like biogenic amines (like thyroxine, adrenaline, etc.), proteinaceous or polypeptide (like hypothalamic hormones) and steroids (like sex hormones and adrenocorticoids).

83. **(a)**: Hormones thyroxine, adrenaline and the pigment melanin are formed from tyrosine. Tyrosine is transformed into DOPA through the enzyme tyrosinase. Then through different metabolic pathways it produces thyroxine, adrenaline, melanin, etc.

84. **(b)**: The thyroid gland secretes three hormones: thyroxine or tetraiodothyronine (T4), triiodothyronine (T3) and calcitonin. Thyroxine and Triiodothyronine are iodinated forms of the amino acid tyrosine. They are stored in the colloid that fills the follicles and are released to the blood when needed. The storage occurs in an unusual place, the extracellular colloid.

85. **(b)**: The molecules of hormones that are amino acid derivatives, peptides or proteins are large and insoluble in lipids and cannot enter the target cell. Therefore, they act at the cell surface. They bind to specific receptor molecules located on the surface of the cell membrane. Therefore, if receptor molecules are removed from target organs, then the target organ will not respond to the hormone.

Chapter : 20 SEXUAL REPRODUCTION IN FLOWERING PLANTS

PRE-FERTILISATION: STRUCTURES AND EVENTS

1. What is the function of tassels in the corn cob? ***(2023)***

(a) To disperse pollen grains
(b) To protect seeds
(c) To attract insects
(d) To trap pollen grains

2. Large, colourful, fragrant flowers with nectar are seen in ***(2023)***

(a) bat pollinated plants
(b) wind pollinated plants
(c) insect pollinated plants
(d) bird pollinated plants.

3. Identify the incorrect statement related to pollination. ***(2022)***

(a) Pollination by water is quite rare in flowering plants.
(b) Pollination by wind is more common amongst abiotic pollination.
(c) Flowers produce foul odours to attract flies and beetles to get pollinated.
(d) Moths and butterflies are the most dominant pollinating agents among insects.

4. Given below are two statements : ***(2022)***

Statement I: Cleistogamous flowers are invariably autogamous.

Statement II : Cleistogamy is disadvantageous as there is no chance for cross pollination.

In the light of the above statements, choose the correct answer from the options given below :

(a) Both Statement I and Statement II are correct
(b) Both Statement I and Statement II are incorrect
(c) Statement I is correct but Statement II is incorrect
(d) Statement I is incorrect but Statement II is correct.

5. The term used for transfer of pollen grains from anthers of one plant to stigma of a different plant which, during pollination, brings genetically different types of pollen grains to stigma, is ***(2021)***

(a) cleistogamy (b) xenogamy
(c) geitonogamy (d) chasmogamy.

6. A typical angiosperm embryo sac at maturity is ***(2021)***

(a) 8-nucleate and 8-celled
(b) 8-nucleate and 7-celled
(c) 7-nucleate and 8-celled
(d) 7-nucleate and 7-celled.

7. In some members of which of the following pairs of families, pollen grains retain their viability for months after release? ***(2021)***

(a) Rosaceae : Leguminosae
(b) Poaceae : Rosaceae
(c) Poaceae : Leguminosae
(d) Poaceae : Solanaceae

8. The plant parts which consist of two generations one within the other ***(2020)***

(1) pollen grains inside the anther
(2) germinated pollen grain with two male gametes
(3) seed inside the fruit
(4) embryo sac inside the ovule

(a) (1) only (b) (1), (2), and (3)
(c) (3) and (4)(d) (1) and (4).

9. In water hyacinth and water lily, pollination takes place by ***(2020)***

(a) insects or wind (b) water currents only
(c) wind and water (d) insects and water.

10. Which is the most common type of embryo sac in angiosperms? ***(Odisha NEET 2019)***
(a) Tetrasporic with one mitotic stage of divisions
(b) Monosporic with three sequential mitotic divisions
(c) Monosporic with two sequential mitotic divisions
(d) Bisporic with two sequential mitotic divisions

11. What type of pollination takes place in Vallisneria? ***(Odisha NEET 2019)***
(a) Pollination occurs in submerged condition by water.
(b) Flowers emerge above surface of water, and pollination occurs by insects.
(c) Flowers emerge above water surface, and pollen is carried by wind.
(d) Male flowers are carried by water currents to female flowers at surface of water.

12. In which one of the following, both autogamy and geitonogamy are prevented? ***(Odisha NEET 2019)***
(a) Wheat (b) Papaya
(c) Castor (d) Maize

13. Pollen grains can be stored for several years in liquid nitrogen having a temperature of ***(2018)***
(a) –120° C (b) –80°C
(c) –196°C (d) –160°C.

14. Which of the following has proved helpful in preserving pollen as fossils? ***(2018)***
(a) Pollenkitt (b) Cellulosic intine
(c) Oil content (d) Sporopollenin

15. Winged pollen grains are present in ***(2018)***
(a) mustard (b) Cycas
(c) mango (d) Pinus

16. Functional megaspore in an angiosperm develops into an ***(2017)***
(a) endosperm (b) embryo sac
(c) embryo (d) ovule.

17. Attractants and rewards are required for ***(2017)***
(a) entomophily (b) hydrophily
(c) cleistogamy (d) anemophily

18. Flowers which have single ovule in the ovary and are packed into inflorescence are usually pollinated by ***(2017)***
(a) bee (b) wind
(c) bat (d) water

19. A dioecious flowering plant prevents both ***(2017)***
(a) autogamy and geitonogamy
(b) geitonogamy and xenogamy
(c) cleistogamy and xenogamy
(d) autogamy and xenogamy.

20. In majority of angiosperms, ***(NEET-II 2016)***
(a) egg has a filiform apparatus
(b) there are numerous antipodal cells
(c) reduction division occurs in the megaspore mother cells
(d) a small central cell is present in that embryo sac.

21. Pollination in water hyacinth and water lily is brought about by the agency of ***(NEET-II 2016)***
(a) water (b) insects or wind
(c) birds (d) bats

22. The ovule of an angiosperm is technically equivalent to ***(NEET-II 2016)***
(a) megasporangium
(b) megasporophyll
(c) megaspore mother cell
(d) megaspore

23. Which one of the following statements is not true? ***(NEET-I 2016)***
(a) Pollen grains of many species cause severe allergies.
(b) Stored pollen in liquid nitrogen can be used in the crop breeding programmes.
(c) Tapetum helps in the dehiscence of anther.
(d) Exine of pollen grains is made up of sporopollenin.

24. Which of the following statements is not correct? ***(NEET-I 2016)***

(a) Pollen germination and pollen tube growth are regulated by chemical components of pollen interacting with those of the pistil.

(b) Some reptiles have also been reported as pollinators in some plant species.

(c) Pollen grains of many species can germinate on the stigma of a flower, but only one pollen tube of the same species grows into the style.

(d) Insects that consume pollen or nectar without bringing about pollination are called pollen/ nectar robbers.

25. Proximal end of the filament of stamen is attached to the ***(NEET-I 2016)***

(a) placenta (b) thalamus or petal

(c) anther (d) connective.

26. Filiform apparatus is characteristic feature of ***(2015)***

(a) aleurone cell (b) synergids

(c) generative cell (d) nucellar embryo.

27. In angiosperms, microsporogenesis and megasporogenesis ***(2015)***

(a) involve meiosis

(b) occur in ovule

(c) occur in anther

(d) form gametes without further divisions.

28. Male gametophyte in angiosperms produces ***(2015)***

(a) single sperm and two vegetative cells

(b) three sperms

(c) two sperms and a vegetative cell

(d) single sperm and a vegetative cell.

29. Which of the following are the important floral rewards to the animal pollinators? ***(2015 Cancelled)***

(a) Floral fragrance and calcium crystals

(b) Protein pellicle and stigmatic exudates

(c) Colour and large size of flower

(d) Nectar and pollen grains

30. Which one of the following may require pollinators, but is genetically similar to autogamy? ***(2015 Cancelled)***

(a) Apogamy (b) Cleistogamy

(c) Geitonogamy (d) Xenogamy

31. Which one of the following statements is not tru e? ***(2015 Cancelled)***

(a) The flowers pollinated by flies and bats secrete foul odour to attract them.

(b) Honey is made by bees by digesting pollen collected from flowers.

(c) Pollen grains are rich in nutrients and they are used in the form of tablets and syrups.

(d) Pollen grains of some plants cause severe allergies and bronchial afflictions in some people.

32. The hilum is a scar on the ***(2015 Cancelled)***

(a) fruit, where style was present

(b) seed, where micropyle was present

(c) seed, where funicle was attached

(d) fruit, where it was attached to pedicel.

33. Transmission tissue is characteristic feature of ***(2015 Cancelled)***

(a) dry stigma (b) wet stigma

(c) hollow style (d) solid style.

34. Geitonogamy involves ***(2014)***

(a) fertilisation of a flower by the pollen from another flower of the same plant

(b) fertilisation of a flower by the pollen from the same flower

(c) fertilisation of a flower by the pollen from a flower of another plant in the same population

(d) fertilisation of a flower by the pollen from a flower of another plant belonging to a distant population.

35. Pollen tablets are available in the market for ***(2014)***

(a) in vitro fertilisation

(b) breeding programmes

(c) supplementing food

(d) ex situ conservation.

36. Function of filiform apparatus is to ***(2014)***
(a) recognise the suitable pollen at stigma
(b) stimulate division of generative cell
(c) produce nectar
(d) guide the entry of pollen tube.

37. Advantage of cleistogamy is ***(2013)***
(a) no dependence on pollinators
(b) vivipary
(c) higher genetic variability
(d) more vigorous offspring.

38. Megasporangium is equivalent to ***(2013)***
(a) nucellus (b) ovule
(c) embryo sac (d) fruit.

39. Which one of the following statements is correct? ***(2013)***
(a) Endothecium produces the microspores.
(b) Tapetum nourishes the developing pollen.
(c) Hard outer layer of pollen is called intine.
(d) Sporogenous tissue is haploid.

40. Animal vectors are required for pollination in ***(Karnataka NEET 2013)***
(a) Vallisneria (b) mulberry
(c) cucumber (d) maize.

41. Megaspores are produced from the megaspore mother cells after ***(Karnataka NEET 2013)***
(a) mitotic division
(b) formation of thick wall
(c) differentiation
(d) meiotic division.

42. Which one of the following statements is correct? ***(Karnataka NEET 2013)***
(a) Cleistogamous flowers are always autogamous.
(b) Xenogamy occurs only by wind pollination.
(c) Chasmogamous flowers do not open at all.
(d) Geitonogamy involves the pollen and stigma of flowers of different plants.

43. Which of the following statements is correct? ***(Karnataka NEET 2013)***
(a) Sporopollenin can be degraded by enzymes.
(b) Sporopollenin is made up of inorganic materials.
(c) Sporopollenin can withstand high temperatures as well as strong acids and alkalis.
(d) Sporopollenin can withstand high temperatures but not strong acids.

44. Both, autogamy and geitonogamy are prevented in ***(2012)***
(a) papaya (b) cucumber
(c) castor (d) maize.

45. An organic substance that can withstand environmental extremes and cannot be degraded by any enzyme is ***(2012)***
(a) cuticle (b) sporopollenin
(c) lignin (d) cellulose.

46. Even in absence of pollinating agents seed-setting is assured in ***(2012)***
(a) Commelina (b) Zostera
(c) Salvia (d) Fig

47. What is the function of germ pore? ***(Mains 2012)***
(a) Emergence of radicle
(b) Absorption of water for seed germination
(c) Initiation of pollen tube
(d) Release of male gametes

48. Plants with ovaries having only one or a few ovules, are generally pollinated by ***(Mains 2012)***
(a) bees (b) butterflies
(c) birds (d) wind.

49. Filiform apparatus is a characteristic feature of ***(2011)***
(a) suspensor (b) egg
(c) synergid (d) zygote.

50. Which one of the following pollinations is autogamous? ***(2011)***
(a) Geitonogamy (b) Xenogamy
(c) Chasmogamy (d) Cleistogamy

51. Wind pollination is common in ***(2011)***
(a) legumes (b) lilies
(c) grasses (d) orchids.

52. In angiosperms, functional megaspore develops into ***(Mains 2011)***
(a) embryo sac (b) ovule
(c) endosperm (d) pollen sac.

53. Transfer of pollen grains from the anther to the stigma of another flower of the same plant is called ***(2010)***
(a) xenogamy (b) geitonogamy
(c) karyogamy (d) autogamy.

54. Wind pollinated flowers are ***(2010)***
(a) small, brightly coloured, producing large number of pollen grains
(b) small, producing large number of dry pollen grains
(c) large producing abundant nectar and pollen
(d) small, producing nectar and dry pollen.

55. Which one of the following pairs of plant structures has haploid number of chromosomes? ***(2008)***
(a) Nucellus and antipodal cells
(b) Egg nucleus and secondary nucleus
(c) Megaspore mother cell and antipodal cells
(d) Egg cell and antipodal cells

56. What does the filiform apparatus do at the entrance into ovule? ***(2008)***
(a) It brings about opening of the pollen tube.
(b) It guides pollen tube from a synergid to egg.
(c) It helps in the entry of pollen tube into a synergid.
(d) It prevents entry of more than one pollen tube into the embryo sac.

57. Unisexuality of flowers prevents ***(2008)***
(a) geitonogamy, but not xenogamy
(b) autogamy and geitonogamy
(c) autogamy, but not geitonogamy
(d) both geitonogamy and xenogamy.

58. Which one of the following is resistant to enzyme action? ***(Mains 2008)***
(a) Pollen exine (b) Leaf cuticle
(c) Cork (d) Wood fibre

59. Male gametes in angiosperms are formed by the division of ***(2007)***
(a) generative cell
(b) vegetative cell
(c) microspore mother cell
(d) microspore.

60. Which one of the following is surrounded by a callose wall? ***(2007)***
(a) Male gamete
(b) Egg
(c) Pollen grain
(d) Microspore mother cell

61. The arrangement of the nuclei in a normal embryo sac in the dicot plants is ***(2006)***
(a) 3 + 3 + 2 (b) 2 + 4 + 2
(c) 3 + 2 + 3 (d) 2 + 3 + 3

62. Which one of the following represents an ovule, where the embryo sac becomes horse-shoe shaped and the funiculus and micropyle are close to each other? ***(2005)***
(a) Amphitropous (b) Circinotropous
(c) Atropous (d) Anatropous

63. An ovule which becomes curved so that the nucellus and embryo sac lie at right angles to the funicle is ***(2004)***
(a) hemitropous (b) campylotropous
(c) anatropous (d) orthotropous.

64. Anthesis is a phenomenon which refers to ***(2004)***
(a) reception of pollen by stigma
(b) formation of pollen
(c) development of anther
(d) opening of flower bud.

65. In a flowering plant, archesporium gives rise to ***(2003)***
(a) only the wall of the sporangium
(b) both wall and the sporogenous cells
(c) wall and the tapetum
(d) only tapetum and sporogenous cells.

66. In angiosperm, all the four microspores of tetrad are covered by a layer which is formed by ***(2002)***
(a) pectocellulose (b) callose
(c) cellulose (d) sporopollenin

67. What is the direction of micropyle in anatropous ovule? ***(2002)***
(a) Upward (b) Downward
(c) Right (d) Left

68. In grasses what happens in microspore mother cell for the formation of mature pollen grains? ***(2001)***
(a) One meiotic and two mitotic divisions
(b) One meiotic and one mitotic divisions
(c) One meiotic division
(d) One mitotic division

69. Anemophily type of pollination is found in ***(2001)***
(a) Salvia (b) bottlebrush
(c) Vallisneria (d) coconut.

70. Eight nucleated embryo sac is ***(2000)***
(a) only monosporic (b) only bisporic
(c) only tetrasporic (d) any of these.

71. If there are 4 cells in anthers, what will be the number of pollen grains? ***(1996)***
(a) 16 (b) 12 (c) 8 (d) 4

72. In an angiosperm, how many microspore mother cells are required to produce 100 pollen grains? ***(1995)***
(a) 75 (b) 100
(c) 25 (d) 50

73. When pollen of a flower is transferred to the stigma of another flower of the same plant, the pollination is referred to as ***(1994)***
(a) autogamy (b) geitonogamy
(c) xenogamy (d) allogamy.

74. Embryo sac represents ***(1994)***
(a) megaspore (b) megagametophyte
(c) megasporophyll (d) megagamete.

75. Number of meiotic divisions required to produce 200/400 seeds of pea would be ***(1993)***
(a) 200/400 (b) 400/800
(c) 300/600 (d) 250/500.

76. Ovule is straight with funiculus, embryo sac, chalaza and micropyle lying on one straight line. It is ***(1993)***
(a) orthotropous (b) anatropous
(c) campylotropous (d) amphitropous.

77. Meiosis is best observed in dividing ***(1992)***
(a) cells of apical meristem
(b) cells of lateral meristem
(c) microspores and anther wall
(d) microsporocytes.

78. Point out the odd one. ***(1991)***
(a) Nucellus (b) Embryo sac
(c) Micropyle (d) Pollen grain

79. Pollination occurs in ***(1991)***
(a) bryophytes and angiosperms
(b) pteridophytes and angiosperms
(c) angiosperms and gymnosperms
(d) angiosperms and fungi.

80. Entry of pollen tube through micropyle is ***(1990)***
(a) chalazogamy (b) mesogamy
(c) porogamy (d) pseudogamy.

81. Female gametophyte of angiosperms is represented by ***(1990)***
(a) ovule
(b) megaspore mother cell
(c) embryo sac
(d) nucellus.

82. Male gametophyte of angiosperms/monocots is ***(1990)***
(a) microsporangium (b) nucellus
(c) microspore (d) stamen.

83. Which is correct? ***(1989)***
(a) Gametes are invariably haploid.
(b) Spores are invariably haploid.
(c) Gametes are generally haploid.
(d) Both spores and gametes are invariably

haploid.

84. Generative cell was destroyed by laser but a normal pollen tube was still formed because ***(1989)***

(a) vegetative cell is not damaged
(b) contents of killed generative cell stimulate pollen growth
(c) laser beam stimulates growth of pollen tube
(d) the region of emergence of pollen tube is not harmed.

85. Total number of meiotic divisions required for forming 100 zygotes/100 grains of wheat is ***(1988)***

(a) 100 (b) 75
(c) 125 (d) 50

86. Male gametophyte of angiosperms is shed at ***(1988)***

(a) four celled pollen grain
(b) three celled pollen grain
(c) microspore mother cell
(d) anther

DOUBLE FERTILISATION

87. In angiosperm, the haploid, diploid and triploid structures of a fertilized embryo sac sequentially are ***(2023)***

(a) Synergids, zygote and primary endosperm nucleus
(b) Synergids, antipodals and polar nuclei
(c) Synergids, primary endosperm nucleus and zygote
(d) Antipodals, synergids, and primary endosperm nucleus.

88. What is the fate of the male gametes discharged in the synergid? ***(2019)***

(a) One fuses with the egg and other fuses with central cell nuclei.
(b) One fuses with the egg, other(s) degenerates in the synergid.
(c) All fuse with the egg.
(d) One fuses with the egg, other(s) fuse(s) with synergid nucleus.

89. Double fertilisation is ***(2018)***

(a) fusion of two male gametes of a pollen tube with two different eggs
(b) fusion of one male gamete with two polar nuclei
(c) fusion of two male gametes with one egg
(d) syngamy and triple fusion.

90. Double fertilisation is exhibited by ***(2017)***

(a) algae (b) fungi
(c) angiosperms (d) gymnosperms.

91. Which one of the following statements is wrong? ***(Mains 2012)***

(a) When pollen is shed at two-celled stage, double fertilisation does not take place.
(b) Vegetative cell is larger than generative cell.
(c) Pollen grains in some plants remain viable for months.
(d) Intine is made up of cellulose and pectin.

92. Through which cell of the embryo sac, does the pollen tube enter the embryo sac? ***(2005)***

(a) Egg cell
(b) Persistant synergid
(c) Degenerated synergids
(d) Central cell

93. In angiosperms, pollen tube liberate their male gametes into the ***(2002)***

(a) central cell (b) antipodal cells
(c) egg cell (d) synergids.

94. Endosperm is formed during the double fertilisation by ***(2000)***

(a) two polar nuclei and one male gamete
(b) one polar nuclei and one male gamete
(c) ovum and male gamete
(d) two polar nuclei and two male gametes.

95. The role of double fertilisation in angiosperms is to produce ***(1998,1996)***

(a) cotyledons (b) endocarp
(c) endosperm (d) integuments.

96. Double fertilisation is characteristic of ***(1993)***
(a) angiosperms (b) anatropous
(c) gymnosperms (d) bryophytes.

97. Double fertilisation is fusion of ***(1991)***
(a) two eggs
(b) two eggs and polar nuclei with pollen nuclei
(c) one male gamete with egg and other with synergid
(d) one male gamete with egg and other with secondary nucleus.

98. Syngamy means ***(1991)***
(a) fusion of gametes
(b) fusion of cytoplasms
(c) fusion of two similar spores
(d) fusion of two dissimilar spores.

99. Which of the following pair have haploid structures? ***(1991)***
(a) Nucellus and antipodal cells
(b) Antipodal cells and egg cell
(c) Antipodal cells and megaspore mother cell
(d) Nucellus and primary endosperm nucleus

100. Double fertilisation and triple fusion were discovered by ***(1988)***
(a) Hofmeister
(b) Nawaschin and Guignard
(c) Leeuwenhoek
(d) Strasburger.

POST-FERTILISATION: STRUCTURES AND EVENTS

101. Which part of the fruit, labelled in the given figure makes it a false fruit? ***(2022)***

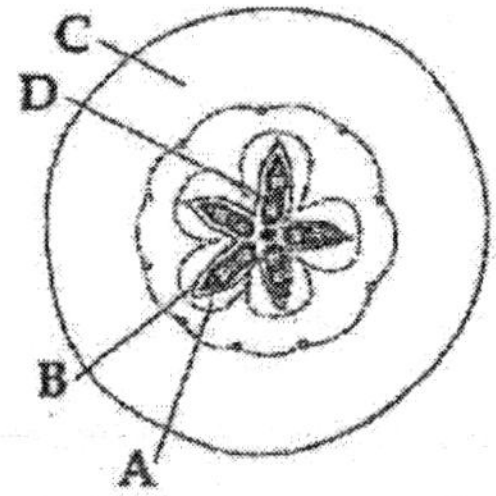

(a) A → Mesocarp (b) B → Endocarp
(c) C → Thalamus (d) D → Seed

102. Persistent nucellus in the seed is known as ***(2019)***
(a) tegmen (b) chalaza
(c) perisperm (d) hilum.

103. Which one of the following statements regarding post-fertilisation development in flowering plants is incorrect? ***(2019)***
(a) Ovules develop into embryo sac.
(b) Ovary develops into fruit.
(c) Zygote develops into embryo.
(d) Central cell develops into endosperm.

104. The coconut water from tender coconut represents ***(NEET-I 2016)***
(a) free nuclear proembryo
(b) free nuclear endosperm
(c) endocarp
(d) fleshy mesocarp.

105. Coconut water from a tender coconut is ***(2015)***
(a) innermost layers of the seed coat
(b) degenerated nucellus
(c) immature embryo
(d) free nuclear endosperm.

106. Which one of the following fruits is parthenocarpic? ***(2015)***
(a) Jackfruit (b) Banana
(c) Brinjal (d) Apple

107. Non-albuminous seed is produced in ***(2014)***
(a) maize (b) castor
(c) wheat (d) pea.

108. Seed coat is not thin, membranous in ***(2013)***
(a) groundnut (b) gram
(c) maize (d) coconut.

109. Perisperm differs from endosperm in ***(2013)***
(a) being a diploid tissue
(b) its formation by fusion of secondary nucleus with several sperms
(c) being a haploid tissue
(d) having no reserve food.

110. Albuminous seeds store their reserve food mainly in ***(Karnataka NEET 2013)***
(a) endosperm (b) cotyledons
(c) hypocotyl (d) perisperm.

111. In a cereal grain the single cotyledon of embryo is represented by ***(2006)***
(a) coleoptile (b) coleorhiza
(c) scutellum (d) prophyll.

112. The embryo in sunflower has ***(1998)***
(a) two cotyledons (b) many cotyledons
(c) no cotyledon (d) one cotyledon.

113. Embryo sac occurs in ***(1991)***
(a) embryo (b) axis part of embryo
(c) ovule (d) endosperm.

114. Perisperm is ***(1989,1988)***
(a) remnant of endosperm
(b) persistent nucellus
(c) peripheral part of endosperm
(d) disintegrated secondary nucleus.

115. Tegmen develops from ***(1990)***
(a) funiculus (b) chalaza
(c) inner integument (d) outer integument.

APOMIXIS AND POLYEMBRYONY

116. Seed formation without fertilisation in flowering plants involves the process of ***(NEET-I 2016)***
(a) somatic hybridisation
(b) apomixis
(c) sporulation
(d) budding.

117. Nucellar polyembryony is reported in species of ***(2011)***
(a) Citrus (b) Gossypium
(c) Triticum (d) Brassica

118. What is common between vegetative reproduction and apomixis? ***(Mains 2011)***
(a) Both are applicable to only dicot plants.
(b) Both bypass the flowering phase.
(c) Both occur round the year.
(d) Both produce progeny identical to the parent.

119. Apomictic embryos in Citrus arise from ***(2010)***
(a) synergids
(b) maternal sporophytic tissue in ovule
(c) antipodal cells
(d) diploid egg.

120. The polyembryony commonly occurs in ***(1995)***
(a) tomato (b) potato
(c) Citrus (d) turmeric.

121. Development of an organism from female gamete/ egg without involving fertilization is ***(1989)***
(a) adventitive embryony
(b) polyembryony
(c) parthenocarpy
(d) parthenogenesis.

ANSWER KEY

1.	(d)	2.	(c)	3.	(d)	4.	(a, c)	5.	(b)	6.	(b)	7.	(a)
8.	(d)	9.	(a)	10.	(b)	11.	(d)	12.	(b)	13.	(c)	14.	(d)
15.	(d)	16.	(b)	17.	(a)	18.	(b)	19.	(a)	20.	(c)	21.	(b)
22.	(a)	23.	(c)	24.	(c)	25.	(b)	26.	(b)	27.	(a)	28.	(c)
29.	(d)	30.	(c)	31.	(b)	32.	(c)	33.	(d)	34.	(a)	35.	(c)
36.	(d)	37.	(a)	38.	(b)	39.	(b)	40.	(c)	41.	(d)	42.	(a)
43.	(c)	44.	(a)	45.	(b)	46.	(a)	47.	(c)	48.	(d)	49.	(c)
50.	(d)	51.	(c)	52.	(a)	53.	(b)	54.	(b)	55.	(d)	56.	(b)
57.	(c)	58.	(a)	59.	(a)	60.	(d)	61.	(c)	62.	(a)	63.	(a)
64.	(d)	65.	(b)	66.	(b)	67.	(b)	68.	(b)	69.	(d)	70.	(d)
71.	(a)	72.	(c)	73.	(b)	74.	(b)	75.	(d)	76.	(a)	77.	(d)
78.	(d)	79.	(c)	80.	(c)	81.	(c)	82.	(c)	83.	(a)	84.	(a)
85.	(c)	86.	(b)	87.	(a)	88.	(a)	89.	(d)	90.	(c)	91.	(a)
92.	(c)	93.	(c)	94.	(a)	95.	(c)	96.	(a)	97.	(d)	98.	(a)
99.	(b)	100.	(b)	101.	(c)	102.	(c)	103.	(a)	104.	(b)	105.	(d)
106.	(b)	107.	(d)	108.	(d)	109.	(a)	110.	(a)	111.	(c)	112.	(a)
113.	(c)	114.	(b)	115.	(c)	116.	(b)	117.	(a)	118.	(d)	119.	(b)
120.	(c)	121.	(d)										

HINTS & EXPLANATIONS

1.(d) : The tassels in the corn cob are stigma and style that wave in the wind to trap pollen grains.

2. (c)

3.(d) : Among the animals, insects, particularly bees are the dominant biotic pollinating agents.

4. (a,c) : Cleistogamous flowers are invariably autogamous as it is closed flowers, so, there is no chance of cross-pollen to land on the stigma. Cleistogamous flowers are advantageous because they produce assured seed-set even in the absence of pollinators. Cleistogamy is disadvantageous as variability and adaptability to changed environment are reduced.

5. (b)

6.(b) : A typical angiosperm embryo sac is 7 celled and 8 nucleate structure.

7.(a) : In some members of families Rosaceae, Leguminosae and Solanaceae, pollen grains maintain viability for months.

8.(d) :

9.(a) : In many aquatic plants with emergent flowers, pollination occurs by wind or insects, e.g., lotus, water lily, water hyacinth.

10. (b)

11.(d) : In Vallisneria, the female flower reach the surface of water by the long stalk and the male flowers or pollen grains are released on to the surface of water. They are carried passively by water currents, some of them eventually reach the female flowers and the stigma.

12. (b)

13.(c) : Pollen grains can be stored for several years in liquid nitrogen at –196°C. This is also known as cryopreservation.

14.(d) : Exine of pollen grain is made up of highly resistant fatty substance called sporopollenin, which is not degraded by any enzyme. It is not affected by high temperature, strong acid or strong alkali. Because of the sporopollenin, pollen grains are well preserved as microfossils.

15.(d) : Each pollen grain of Pinus has two wing like structures which enable it to float in air, as an adaptation for dispersal by wind. Pollen grains of mustard, Cycas and mango are not winged.

16.(b) : In angiosperms, the functional megaspore is the first cell of female gametophyte. It enlarges and undergoes three nuclear mitotic divisions to form embryo sac.

17.(a) :

18.(b) : Single ovule in the ovary and flowers packed into inflorescence are characteristics of wind pollinated flowers.

19.(a) : Dioecious plants are those plants in which male flowers and female flowers are borne on different plants. Therefore, they prevent both autogamy and geitonogamy.

20. (c)

21. (b)

22.(a) : The ovule of an angiosperm is equivalent to integumented megasporangium.

23. (c): Tapetum is the innermost wall layer of microsporangium that nourishes developing pollen grains.

24. (c) : Pollen-pistil interaction is the group of events that occur from the time of pollen deposition over the stigma to the time of pollen tube entry into ovule. It is a safety measure to ensure that illegitimate crossing does not occur. Pollen grains of number of plants may settle over a stigma. The pollens belonging to same species would germinate while other fail to do so, but the pollen tube of the compatible pollen will grow through the style to reach the ovule whereas growth of incompatible pollens will be arrested at stigmatic disc or sometimes in the beginning part of style.

25. (b)

26. (b): Filiform apparatus is a mass of finger-like projections of the wall into the cytoplasm. It is present in synergids (help cells) of the embryo sac, in the micropylar region. It guides the pollen tube inside the ovule towards the embryo sac.

27.(a) : In angiosperms, microsporogenesis, i.e., formation of microspores (or pollen grains) occurs by the meiotic divisions of diploid microspore mother cells (or pollen mother cells). Microsporogenesis takes place in the anther.

Megasporogenesis, i.e., formation of megaspores occurs by the meiotic divisions of diploid megaspore mother cells. Megasporogenesis takes place in the ovule.

28.(c) : The protoplast of the male gametophyte divides mitotically to produce two unequal cells - a small generative cell and a large vegetative cell. The generative cell divides later into two non-motile male gametes (or sperms). Thus, the male gametophyte in angiosperms produces two sperms and a vegetative cell. The vegetative cell, later on, grows to produce pollen tube.

29. (d)

30. (c): Geitonogamy involves transfer of the pollen from one flower of a plant to the stigma of another flower of the same plant, e.g., in maize. As the pollen has to move from one flower to another flower, it requires a pollinating agent. Yet it is genetically similar to autogamy, as both the flowers of the plant, share the same genotype of the plant.

31.(b) : Honey is made from nectar through a process of regurgitation and evaporation. Honey bees transform saccharides (carbohydrates) into honey by regurgitating it a number of times, until it is partially digested. The bees do the regurgitation and digestion as a group. After the last regurgitation, the aqueous solution is still high in water, the process continues by evaporation of much of the water and enzymatic transformation. Honey is produced by bees as a food source.

32. (c): Ovule is an integumented megasporangium found in spermatophytes which develops into seed after fertilisation. An angiospermic ovule is typically an ovoid and whitish structure. It occurs inside ovary where it is attached to a parenchymatous cushion called placenta either singly or in a cluster. The ovule is stalked. The stalk is called funiculus or funicle. The point of attachment of the body of the ovule with the funiculus is known as hilum. It is present as a scar on a mature seed.

33.(d) : Style is traversed by the pollen tube to reach the ovule. It is of two types - hollow and solid. In hollow styles, the stylar canal is lined by glandular cells, which are usually multinucleate and polyploid whereas solid style has a core of transmitting tissue, composed of thin walled cells, through which the pollen tube moves.

34.(a) : Geitonogamy is the pollination taking place between the two flowers of the same plant or genetically similar plant. Hence, genetically it is self pollination but since the agency is involved, it is ecologically, cross pollination.

35.(c) : Pollen grains are believed to be rich in nutrients (protein 7-26 % carbohydrates 24-48%, fats 0.9-14.5%). They are taken as tablets or syrups to improve health. They also enhance performance of athletes and race horses.

36.(d) : In the ovule, the pollen tube is attracted by secretions of synergids. Usually the pollen tube enters the embryo sac by passing into one of the two synergids and is guided by the filiform apparatus of the synergids in their movement. Pollen tube then breaks open and releases its contents in the embryo sac. Antipodals and synergids later degenerate.

37.(a) : Cleistogamy is the process of pollination and fertilisation before the flower has opened. In such flowers, the anther and stigma lie close to each other. When anthers dehisce in the flower buds, pollen grains come in contact with the stigma to effect pollination. Thus, cleistogamous flowers are invariably autogamous as there is no chance of cross-pollen landing on the stigma. Cleistogamous flowers produce assured seed-set even in the absence of pollinators.

38. (b)

39. (b) : A microsporangium is generally surrounded by four wall layers - the epidermis, endothecium, middle layers and the tapetum. The outer three wall layers perfom the function of protection and help in dehiscence of anther to release the pollen. The innermost wall layer is the tapetum. It nourishes the developing pollen grains. Cells of the tapetum are food rich and possess dense cytoplasm and generally have more than one nucleus. They disintegrate to liberate the contents which is absorbed by the developing spores.

40.(c) : In Vallisneria, water pollination occurs while mulberry and maize undergo wind pollination. In cucumber, animal pollination is observed.

41.(d) : In angiosperms, microsporogenesis, i.e., formation of microspores (or pollen grains) occurs by the meiotic divisions of diploid microspore mother cells (or pollen mother cells). Microsporogenesis takes place in the anther. Megasporogenesis, i.e., formation of megaspores occurs by the meiotic divisions of diploid megaspore mother cells. Megasporogenesis takes place in the ovule.

42.(a) : In cleistogamy, as the flowers never open so there is no alternative of self pollination. It is invariably autogamous. In xenogamy, pollination takes place between two flowers of different plants (genetically and ecologically). It can ocur by. wind, water, insects and animals.

Chasmogamy occurs when the flowers expose their mature anther and stigma to the pollinating agents. Geitonogamy is the pollination taking place between the two flowers of the same plant or genetically similar plant. Genetically, it is self pollination but as the agency is involved it is ecologically cross pollination.

43. (c) : Pollen grain is a haploid, unicellular body. It is cuticularised and the cutin is of special type called sporopollenin, which is resistant to chemical and biological decomposition. It can withstand high temperatures as well as strong acids and alkalis. This is why, pollen wall is preserved for long periods in fossil deposits. In addition pollen wall possesses proteins for enzymatic and compatability reactions.

44.(a) : Autogamy and geitonogamy are two forms of self pollination. In autogamy, pollen falls on stigma of the same flower. While in geitonogamy pollens from a flower fall on the stigma of some other flower of the same plant. Papaya is a dioecious plant thus both autogamy and geitonogamy are prevented in it.

45.(b) : Sporopollenin is a major component of the tough outer (exine) walls of spores and pollen grains. It is chemically very stable and is usually well preserved in soils and sediments. It can withstand environmental extremes and cannot be degraded by enzymes and strong chemical reagents.

46.(a) : Some plants such as Viola (common pansy), Oxalis and Commelina produce two types of flowers- chasmogamous flowers which are similar to flowers of other species with exposed anthers and stigma and cleistogamous flowers which do not open at all. In such flowers, the anthers and stigma lie close to each other. When anthers dehisce in the flower buds, pollen grains come in contact with the stigma to effect pollination. Thus, cleistogamous flowers are invariably autogamous as there is no chance of cross-pollen landing on the stigma. Cleistogamous flowers produce assured seed-set even in the absence of pollinators.

47. (c): In a pollen grain, exine is thin or absent at certain places. These areas may have thickened intine or deposition of callose. They are called germ pores (if rounded) or germinal furrows (if elongated). After pollination, the pollen grain on the stigma absorbs water and nutrients from the stigmatic secretion through its germ pores. The tube or vegetative cell enlarges and comes out of pollen grains through germ pore to form a pollen tube.

48.(d) : Anemophily is an abiotic means of pollination by wind and being non-directional, a wasteful process as the pollen would reach the stigma through wind is a hit or miss affair. During the transit of pollen through wind, a considerable amount of pollen is lost because it never reaches a proper stigma. To stand this loss, anemophilous plants have to produce enormous quantities of pollen. Anemophily is also associated with reduction in the number of ovules per ovary. Some models predict that plants benefit from numerous inexpensive flowers distributed throughout the inflorescence, each with a single ovule or a few ovules. In grasses there is just one ovule per ovary. This is to increase the probability of successful pollination of each ovule.

49. (c): Filiform apparatus is a mass of finger like projections of the wall into the cytoplasm. It is present in synergids (help cells) of the embryo sac, in the micropylar region. It guides the pollen tube inside the ovule towards the embryo sac.

50.(d) : Autogamy is a kind of pollination in which the pollen from the anthers of a flower are transferred to stigma of the same flower. Cleistogamy, homogamy, bud pollination are three methods of the autogamy. Cleistogamy occurs in those plants, which never open and ensure complete self-pollination. E.g., Commelina bengalensis, Oxalis, Viola, etc.

51.(c) : Anemophily is pollination of a flower in which the pollen is carried by the wind. Examples of anemophilous flowers are those of grasses and conifers.

52.(a) : In angiosperms, the functional megaspore is the first cell of female gametophyte. It enlarges and undergoes three nuclear mitotic divisions to form embryo sac.

53.(b) : Geitonogamy involves transfer of the pollen from one flower of a plant to the stigma of another flower of the same plant, e.g., in maize. As the pollen has to move from one flower to another flower, it requires a pollinating agent. Yet it is genetically similar to autogamy, as both the flowers of the plant, share the same genotype of the plant.

54.(b) : Pollination by wind is called anemophily and such plants in which pollination occurs by wind are called anemophilous plants. Anemophilous plants are characterised by small flowers, pollens present in large number which are small, dry and light in weight (carried upto 1300 km by wind), number of ovules generally reduced in ovary (biological significance), feathery or brushy stigma (to receive the pollen). Grasses and palms are generally anemophilous.

55. (d)

56.(b) : Within the embryo sac three cells are grouped together at the micropylar end and constitute the egg apparatus. The egg apparatus, in turn, consists of two synergids and one egg cell. The synergids have special cellular thickenings at the micropylar tip called filiform apparatus, which plays an important role in guiding the pollen tubes from synergid to egg. Three cells are at the chalazal end and are called the antipodals. The large central cell, has two polar nuclei.

57.(c) : Unisexuality or dicliny is a condition in which two types of unisexual flowers are present i.e., staminate (male flower) and pistillate (female flower). The plant may be monoecious or dioecious. This is a device for cross pollination (or xenogamy). Both xenogamy and geitonogamy (i.e., transfer of pollen from anther of one flower to stigma of another flower of either the same or genetically similar plant) are included under allogamy/cross pollination. Autogamy or self pollination (i.e., transfer of pollen from anther to stigma of the same flower) occurs in bisexual flower.

58.(a) : Sporopollenin is a major component of the tough outer (exine) walls of spores and pollen grains. It is chemically very stable and is usually well preserved in soils and sediments. It can withstand environmental extremes and cannot be degraded by enzymes and strong chemical reagents.

59.(a) : In the pollen sac (microsporangium) of the anther, haploid microspores are formed by mitosis. Mitosis then follows to produce a two-celled pollen grain with a small generative cell and a large vegetative cell. This generative cell will undergo further mitosis to form two male gametes (nuclei). The pollen tube grows through a spore in the pollen grain, with the tube (vegetative) nucleus at its tips and the male nuclei behind.

60. (d) : Anther consists of microsporangia or pollen sacs. The archesporium gives rise to parietal cells and primary sporogenous tissue. Sporogenous cells divide to form pollen grain or microspore mother cells. They are diploid and connected by plasmodesmata. The microspore, mother cells consists of a callose wall inner to the cell wall. The mother cell then undergoes meiosis and forms tetrads of microspores. Finally the wall of the mother cell degenerates and pollen grains are separated.

61.(c)

62.(a) : Depending upon position of micropyle in relation to chalaza, ovules are of 6 types in angiosperms. In amphitropous type, the curvature is observed both in body of ovule and embryo sac. The embryo sac assumes horse shoeshape. Micropyle is directed downwards. It is commonly found in families Papaveraceae, Alismataceae and Butomaceae.

Circinotropous ovule is characteristic of Family Cactaceae. Here, the ovule is straight first but due to more growth on one side gets inverted and later becomes straight again.

Orthotropous ovule is the most primitive and of simplest type. It is also known as atropous or straight ovule.

Anatropous ovule is the most common type of ovule found in angiosperms. Here, the body of the ovule gets inverted and micropyle is on lower side.

63.(a) : In hemianatropous or hemitropous ovule, the nucellus and integuments are at right angles to stalk or funiculus so that the ovule becomes curved. It is commonly found is Primulaceae and Ranunculus. In campylotropous ovule, the body of the ovule gets curved and micropyle is directed downwards. Atropous (orthotropous) ovule is erect and micropyle, chalaza and funiculus are in the same straight line. Anatropous ovule is the most common type of ovule in angiosperms. In this, the body of the ovule gets inverted and the micropyle is on lower side.

64.(d) : Anthesis is the process of opening floral buds. Reception of pollen by stigma is called pollination. Formation of pollen is called microsporogenesis.

65.(b) : In flowering plants, archesporial cells are vertical rows of hypodermal cells at four angles of anther. These undergo periclinal (transverse) division to form an outer primary parietal cell and inner sporogenous cell. Primary parietal cell after few more periclinal divisions forms anther wall and sporogenous cells give rise to sporogenous tissue.

66. (b)

67.(b) : Anatropus ovule is the most common type of ovule found in angiosperms. Here, the body of the ovule gets inverted and micropyle is on lower side or downwards. It comes very close to the hilum and the chalaza is upwardly directed.

68.(b) : Grass is a monocot plant. Primary sporogenous cell gives rise to microspore mother cells or pollen mother cells. Each MMC on reduction division gives rise to 4 microspores or pollens and this formation of microspores or pollens is called microsporogenesis. Karyokinesis is of successive type. The successive type of cytokinesis is common in monocots. This leads to the formation of isobilateral tetrad. Among the four pollen grains formed, three degenerates and only one becomes functional. During the maturation of pollen grain, the microspore nucleus moves from a central position to an eccentric one, close to the wall. In this position, the first pollen mitosis occurs and gives two unequal cells. The larger one is the vegetative cells which contains a large and diffuse haploid nucleus and the other cell is generative cell with a small and condensed nucleus. Thus, in the formation of mature pollen grains from microspore mother cell, one meiotic and one mitotic divisions occur.

69.(d) : Anemophily is the pollination by wind. Anemophilous plants are characterised by small flowers, pollens present in large number which are small, dry and light in weight, number of ovules generally reduced in ovary, feathery or brushy stigma to recieve the pollen. All these features are shown by coconut flower.

In Vallisneria, pollination occurs outside water called epihydrophily. Callistemon (Bottlebrush) is pollinated by birds and is an example of ornithophily. Salvia is insect pollinated and is an example of entomophily.

70.(d) : On the basis of number of megaspore nuclei taking part in development of female gametophyte or embryo sac, there are 3 types of embryo sacs-

(i) Monosporic type - In this type the single nucleus of functional megaspore undergoes 3 mitotic divisions to form 8 nuclei, 7 cells.

(ii) Bisporic type - Here embryo sac develops from 2 megaspore nuclei out of 4 nuclei formed after reduction division of MMC. It is also 8 nucleated.

(iii) Tetrasporic type - Here all the 4 megaspore nuclei formed after reduction division of megaspore mother cell are functional and take part in development of embryo sac. It is further of different types. Fritillaria type, Plumbago type and Adoxa type are 8 nucleated.

71.(a) : Pollen grains or microspores are formed inside anther, which is the fertile portion of stamen or microsporophyll. Inside the anther, primary sporogenous cell gives rise to microspore mother cells or pollen mother cells (MMC or PMC). Each MMC on reduction division gives rise to 4 microspores or pollens. So, these four cells will give rise to $4 \times 4 = 16$ pollen grains.

72.(c) : Pollen grains or microspores are formed inside anther, which is the fertile portion of stamen or microsporophyll. The formation of microspores or pollens is called microsporogenesis. The primary sporogenous cell gives rise to microspore mother cells or pollen mother cells. Each microspore mother cell on reduction division gives rise to 4 microspores or pollens. So, for the formation of 100 pollen grains, 25 MMC are required. It involves karyokinesis followed by cytokinesis.

73.(b) : Geitonogamy involves transfer of the pollen from one flower of a plant to the stigma of another flower of the same plant, e.g., in maize. As the pollen has to move from one flower to another flower, it requires a pollinating agent. Yet it is genetically similar to autogamy, as both the flowers of the plant, share the same genotype of the plant.

74. (b)

75.(d) : Number of meiotic divisions required to produce 200/400 seeds of pea would be 250/500.200 seeds of pea would be produced from 200 pollen grains and 200 eggs. 200 pollen grains will be formed by 50 microspore mother cell while 200 eggs will be formed by 200 megaspore mother cell so 250/500.

76. (a)

77.(d) : Meiosis is best observed in dividing microsporocytes. Microsporocytes or microspore mother cell after meiosis give rise to microspore. Other cells do not divide by meiosis.

78.(d) : Pollen grain is odd one among all the other three. Pollen grain is a male gametophytic structure whereas all the other three are found inside ovule (nucellus, micropyle and embryo sac).

79.(c) : The term pollination refers to the transfer of pollen from anther to stigma. Because pollens are found only in angiosperms and gymnosperms so this phenomenon relates to angiosperms and gymnosperms only.

80.(c) : In most of the plants, the pollen tube enters the ovule through the micropyle and the phenomenon is called as porogamy. Entry through chalaza is chalazogamy and through integuments or funiculus is mesogamy.

81.(c) : Female gametophyte of angiosperms is represented by embryo sac. The polygonum type of embryo sac contains 8-nuclei and 7-cells. It is found in more than 80% plant families. The nucleus of megaspore undergoes division and give rise to embryo sac or female gametophyte by the process of megagametogenesis.

82.(c) : Male gametophyte of angiosperms is microspore. Microspore is haploid, uninucleate, minute spores produced in large numbers as a result of meiosis in microspore mother cell inside the microsporangia. These are the first cell of gametophytic generations in angiosperms.

83.(a) : Gametes are invariably haploid. Spores are formed in lower plants by mitotic division and they may be diploid but gametes are always be made by meiosis and they are always haploid.

84.(a) : Generative cell was destroyed by laser but a normal pollen tube was still formed because vegetative cell is not damaged. Each microspore divide by mitotic division making a smaller generative cell and a larger vegetative cell or tube cell. If generative cell is damaged then the normal pollen tube will be formed because pollen tube is formed by vegetative cell not by generative cell of microspore.

85.(c) : For formation of 100 zygotes, 100 male gametes and 100 female gametes (eggs) are required. 100 male gametes are developed from 100 microspores (from 25 meiotic divisions) and 100 eggs are developed from 100 megaspores (from 100 meiotic division).

Hence, number of meiotic divisions necessary for 100 zygotes formation = 25 + 100 = 125.

86.(b) : The male gametophyte or microspore Is shed at 3 -nucleate stage. The microspore undergoes only two mitotic divisions.

87.(a) : Synergids and antipodals are haploid structures. Zygote and polar nuclei are diploid structures. Primary endosperm nucleus is triploid structure of a fertilised embryo sac. In a fertilised embryo sac the haploid, diploid and triploid structures are synergids, zygote and primary endosperm nucleus, respectively.

88.(a) : During double fertilisation in angiosperms, one male gamete fuses with the egg to form the diploid zygote (syngamy or generative fertilisation). The diploid zygote finally develops into embryo. The other male gamete fuses with the two polar nuclei (or secondary nucleus) to form the triploid primary endosperm nucleus, PEN (triple fusion or vegetative fertilisation).

89.(d) : Double fertilisation is unique and universal feature of angiosperms. Total number of nuclei involved in double fertilisation is five, i.e., 2 in syngamy and 3 in triple fusion. Syngamy is fusion of one male gamete with egg to form zygote Triple fusion occurs when the second male gamete fuses with 2 polar nuclei or secondary nucleus to form triploid primary endosperm nucleus.

90. (c)

91.(a) : In 60% of flowering plants, the pollen grains are shed at two-celled stage (tube cell + generative cell). Further, development of male gametophyte (pollen grain) occurs on stigma. Pollen grain gives rise to pollen tube which absorbs nourishment from the cells of style for its growth. Generative cell divides to give rise to two male gametes. Out of these, one fuses with the egg to form diploid zygote (generative fertilisation or syngamy) whereas the second male gamete fuses with the two haploid polar nuclei or diploid secondary nucleus of the central cell to form primary endosperm nucleus (vegetative fertilisation or triple fusion). These two acts of fertilisation occur in the same embryo sac and are referred to as double fertilisation.

92.(c) : The pollen tube enters into the embryo sac at the micropylar end. This entry may be between egg and one synergid or between wall of embryo sac and synergid or through one synergid. So, one synergid is always degenerated to allow the entry of the pollen tube.

93.(c) : On reaching of pollen tube inside the embryo sac, the 2 male gametes are discharged through a sub-terminal pore in pollen tube. The contents of pollen tube are discharged in the synergid and the pollen tube does not grow beyond it in the embryo sac. Further, the cytoplasm of pollen tube is restricted to chalazal end of this synergid cell.

94.(a) : Double fertilisation is the simultaneous occurrence of syngamy and triple fusion. Syngamy involves fusion of one male gamete with egg cell to form zygote. The result of syngamy is zygote (2n) which ultimately develops into embryo.

The second male gamete fuses with 2 polar nuclei or secondary nucleus to form triploid primary endosperm nucleus and this is called triple fusion. This primary endosperm nucleus (3n) ultimately develops into a nutritive tissue for developing embryo called endosperm.

95.(c)

96.(a) : Double fertilisation is the characteristic feature of angiosperms. This phenomenon first observed by Nawaschin and Guignard, 1898 in Lilium and Fritillaria. In angiosperms one male gamete fuses with the two polar nuclei to form triploid primary endosperm nucleus. The process is called triple fusion. These two acts together are known as double fertilisation.

97.(d) : Double fertilisation is the simultaneous occurrence of syngamy and triple fusion. Syngamy involves fusion of one male gamete with egg cell to form zygote. The result of syngamy is zygote (2n) which ultimately develops into embryo.

The second male gamete fuses with 2 polar nuclei or secondary nucleus to form triploid primary endosperm nucleus and this is called triple fusion. This primary endosperm nucleus (3n) ultimately develops into a nutritive tissue for developing embryo called endosperm.

98.(a) : Syngamy means fusion of gametes. Syngamy is the phenomenon in which male gamete fuses with an egg.

99.(b) : Antipodal cells and egg cell are haploid structures as they are formed after meiosis while the others nucellus, megaspore mother cell and primary endosperm nucleus are diploid structures.

100.(b)

101.(c) : In some plants like apple, strawberry the thalamus (C) contributes in the formation of false fruits.

102.(c) : In some seeds, remains of nucellus persist. This residual nucellus which persists in the seed is called perisperm, e.g., black pepper, coffee, castor, cardamum, Nymphaea.

103.(a) : Ovules develop into seeds.

104.(b) : Coconut has multicellular endosperm (called coconut meal) in the outer part and free nuclear as well as vacuolate endosperm (called coconut milk or coconut water) in the centre.

105. (d) :

106.(b) : Parthenocarpic fruits are the fruits which are formed without fertilisation. These fruits are naturally seedless, e.g., banana.

107.(d) : In majority of dicot seeds, including pea, the endosperm is consumed during seed development and the food is stored in cotyledons and other regions. They are called non-endospermic or exalbuminous seeds.

108. (d)

109.(a) : Both perisperm and endosperm are nutritive layers Perisperm is residual persistent nucellus of seed prior to fertilisation while endosperm develops when one of the sperm cells fuses with two haploid polar nuclei. Thus, perisperm is diploid while endosperm is a triploid tissue.

110.(a) : In some seeds, the endosperm persists in the seed as food storage tissue. Such seeds are called endospermic or albuminous, e.g., castor, maize, wheat, barley, rubber, coconut.

111.(c) : The cotyledons are known as seed leaves, they are attached to the embryonic axis. Dicotyledons typically have two cotyledons and monocotyledons have only one cotyledon. The single shield shaped cotyledon in grains is known as scutellum. The scutellum does not contain food and its function is to absorb food from the endosperm and transfer it to the growing parts of the embryo. The plumule consists of growing tip of the shoot along with few young leaf primordia. It is covered by a sheath called coleoptile. The radicle which lies at the base of the grain is also covered with a sheath called coleorhiza. The hypocotyl is very short and is represented by a short axis in between radicle and plumule.

112.(a) : Sunflower (Helianthus) belongs to Family Asteraceae of dicotyledons. A dicot embryo has an embryonal axis and 2 cotyledons attached to it laterally. So the number of cotyledons in sunflower will be two.

113.(c) : Embryo sac occurs in ovule. Ovule is integumented megasporangium. It consists of nucleus covered by one or two integuments, mounted on a funicle, chalaza and micropyle. The ovule is vascularised.

114.(b) : Perisperm is persistent nucellus. Endosperm formation is accompanied by degeneration of nucellus.

115. (c)

116. (b)

117.(a) : In nucellar polyembryony, some of the nucellar cells surrounding the embryo sac start dividing. Then it protrudes into the embryo sac and develop into the embryos. In such species, each ovule contains many embryos. Occurrence of more than one embryo in a seed is referred as polyembryony. Nucellar polyembryony is found in many of the Citrus and mango varieties.

118.(d) : Apomixis is a reproductive process in plants that superficially resembles normal sexual reproduction but in which there is no fusion of gametes. The embryos develop simply by division of a diploid cell the ovule. So, the progenies produced are identical to the parent. In vegetative reproduction, the progenies produced are also identical to the parent.

119.(b) : Apomixis is abnormal kind of sexual reproduction in which egg or other cells associated with egg (synergids, antipodals, etc.) develop into embryo without fertilisation and meiosis. Development of embryos directly from sporophytic tissues like nucellus and integuments is called adventive embryony which is also a type of apoximis, e.g., Citrus, mango.

120.(c) :

121.(d) : Development of an organism from female gamete/ egg without involving fertilisation is parthenogenesis and when a fruit is developed by this technique it is called parthenocarpy.

Chapter : 21

HUMAN REPRODUCTION

THE MALE REPRODUCTIVE SYSTEM

1. Select the correct sequence for transport of sperm cells in male reproductive system. ***(2019)***
   (a) Testis → Epididymis → Vasa efferentia → Vas deferens → Ejaculatory duct → Inguinal canal → Urethra → Urethral meatus
   (b) Testis → Epididymis → Vasa efferentia → Rete testis → Inguinal canal → Urethra
   (c) Seminiferous tubules → Rete testis → Vasa efferentia → Epididymis → Vas deferens → Ejaculatory duct → Urethra → Urethral meatus
   (d) Seminiferous tubules → Vasa efferentia → Epididymis → Inguinal canal → Urethra

2. Which of the following depicts the correct pathway of transport of sperms? ***(NEET-II 2016)***
   (a) Rete testis → Efferent ductules → Epididymis → Vas deferens
   (b) Rete testis → Epididymis → Efferent ductules → Vas deferens
   (c) Rete testis → Vas deferens → Efferent ductules → Epididymis
   (d) Efferent ductules → Rete testis → Vas deferens → Epididymis

3. The shared terminal duct of the reproductive and urinary system in the human male is ***(2014)***
   (a) urethra (b) ureter
   (c) vas deferens (d) vasa efferentia.

4. The Leydig's cells as found in the human body are the secretory source of ***(2012)***
   (a) progesterone (b) intestinal mucus
   (c) glucagon (d) androgens.

5. If for some reason, the vasa efferentia in the human reproductive system get blocked, the gametes will not be transported from ***(2011)***
   (a) testes to epididymis
   (b) epididymis to vas deferens
   (c) ovary to uterus
   (d) vagina to uterus.

6. The testes in humans are situated outside the abdominal cavity inside a pouch called scrotum. The purpose served is for ***(2011)***
   (a) maintaining the scrotal temperature lower than the internal body temperature
   (b) escaping any possible compression by the visceral organs
   (c) providing more space for the growth of epididymis
   (d) providing a secondary sexual feature for exhibiting the male sex.

7. Sertoli cells are found in ***(2010)***
   (a) ovaries and secrete progesterone
   (b) adrenal cortex and secrete adrenaline
   (c) seminiferous tubules and provide nutrition to germ cells
   (d) pancreas and secrete cholecystokinin.

8. Vasa efferentia are the ductules leading from ***(2010)***
   (a) testicular lobules to rete testis
   (b) rete testis to vas deferens
   (c) vas deferens to epididymis
   (d) epididymis to urethra.

9. Seminal plasma in human males is rich in ***(2010)***
   (a) fructose and calcium
   (b) glucose and calcium
   (c) DNA and testosterone
   (d) ribose and potassium.

10. Secretions from which one of the following are rich in fructose, calcium and some enzymes? ***(Mains 2010)***
   (a) Male accessory glands
   (b) Liver
   (c) Pancreas
   (d) Salivary glands

11. Seminal plasma in humans is rich in ***(2009)***

(a) fructose and calcium but has no enzymes

(b) glucose and certain enzymes but has no calcium

(c) fructose and certain enzymes but poor in calcium

(d) fructose, calcium and certain enzymes.

12. Given below is a diagrammatic sketch of a portion of human male reproductive system. Select the correct set of the names of the parts labelled A, B, C, D. ***(2009)***

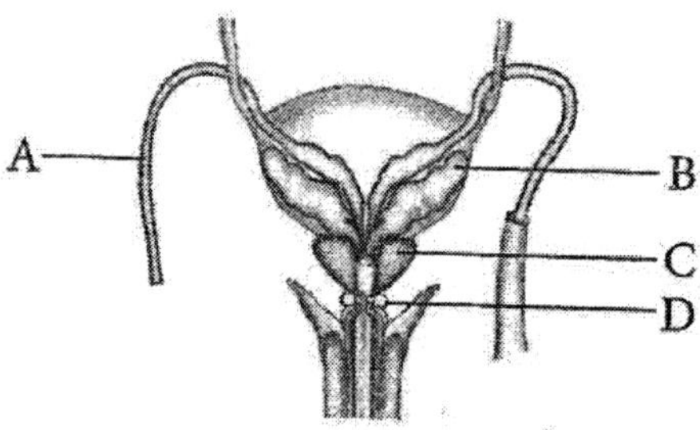

(a) A-Vas deferens, B-Seminal vesicle, C-Prostate, D-Bulbourethral gland

(b) A-Vas deferens, B-Seminal vesicle, C-Bulbourethral gland, D-Prostate

(c) A-Ureter, B-Seminal vesicle, C-Prostate, D-Bulbourethral gland

(d) A-Ureter, B-Prostate, C-Seminal vesicle, D-Bulbourethral gland

13. Male hormone is produced in the testis by cells of ***(1993)***

(a) Sertoli (b) epithelial
(c) spermatocytes (d) Leydig.

14. Location and secretion of Leydig's cells are ***(1991)***

(a) liver-cholesterol
(b) ovary-estrogen
(c) testis-testosterone
(d) pancreas-glucagon.

THE FEMALE REPRODUCTIVE SYSTEM

15. Given below are two statements: ***(2023)***

Statement I: Vas deferens receives a duct from seminal vesicle and opens into urethra as the ejaculatory duct.

Statement II: The cavity of the cervix is called cervical canal which along with vagina forms birth canal.

In the light of the above statements, choose the correct answer from the options given below:
(a) Statement I is correct but Statement II is false.
(b) Statement I incorrect but Statement II is true.
(c) Both Statement I and Statement II are true.
(d) Both Statement I and Statement II are false.

16. Hysterectomy is surgical removal of ***(2015 Cancelled)***

(a) vas deferens (b) mammary glands
(c) uterus (d) prostate gland.

17. The figure given below depicts a diagrammatic sectional view of the human female reproductive system. Which set of three parts out of I-VI have been correctly identified? ***(2011)***

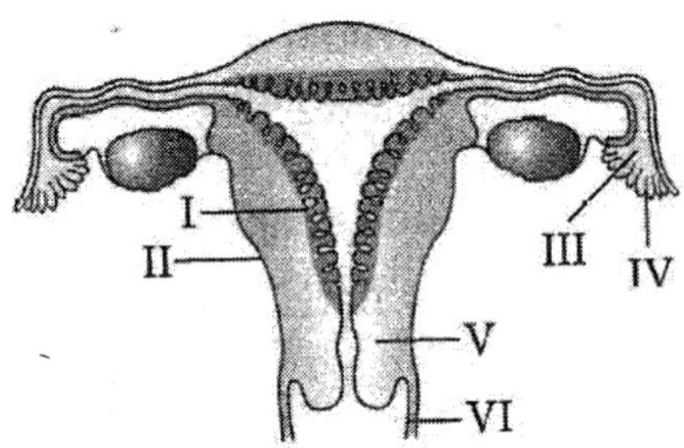

(a) (II) Endometrium, (III) Infundibulum, (IV) Fimbriae
(b) (III) Infundibulum, (IV) Fimbriae, (V) Cervix
(c) (IV) Oviducal funnel, (V) Uterus, (VI) Cervix
(d) (I) Perimetrium, (II) Myometrium, (III) Fallopian tube

18. The part of fallopian tube closest to the ovary is ***(2010)***
(a) isthmus (b) infundibulum
(c) cervix (d) ampulla.

19. Bartholin's glands are situated ***(2003)***
(a) on the sides of the head of some amphibians
(b) at the reduced tail end of birds
(c) on either side of vagina in humans
(d) on either side of vas deferens in humans.

GAMETOGENESIS

20. Given below are two statements: ***(2022)***

Statement I : The release of sperms into the seminiferous tubules is called spermiation.

Statement II : Spermiogenesis is the process of formation of sperms from spermatogonia. In the light of the above statements, choose the most appropriate answer from the options given below.
(a) Both Statement I and Statement II are correct
(b) Both Statement I and Statement II are incorrect
(c) Statement I is correct but Statement II is incorrect
(d) Statement I is incorrect but Statement II is correct

21. Which of the following statements are true for spermatogenesis but do not hold true for oogenesis? ***(2022)***

(A) It results in the formation of haploid gametes.

(B) Differentiation of gamete occurs after the completion of meiosis.

(C) Meiosis occurs continuously in a mitotically dividing stem cell population.

(D) It is controlled by the Luteinising Hormone (LH) and Follicle Stimulating Hormone (FSH) secreted by the anterior pituitary.

(E) It is initiated at puberty.

Choose the most appropriate answer from the options given below:
(a) (A) and (E) only (b) (B) and (C) only
(c) (B), (D) and (E) only (d) (B), (C) and (E) only

22. At which stage of life the oogenesis process is initiated? ***(2022)***
(a) Puberty
(b) Embryonic development stage
(c) Birth (d) Adult

23. Meiotic division of the secondary oocyte is completed ***(2020)***
(a) prior to ovulation
(b) at the time of copulation
(c) after zygote formation
(d) at the time of fusion of a sperm with an ovum.

24. The difference between spermiogenesis and spermiation is ***(2018)***
(a) in spermiogenesis spermatids are formed, while in spermiation spermatozoa are formed
(b) in spermiogenesis spermatozoa are formed, while in spermiation spermatids are formed
(c) in spermiogenesis spermatozoa from Sertoli cells are released into the cavity of seminiferous tubules, while in spermiation spermatozoa are formed
(d) in spermiogenesis spermatozoa are formed, while in spermiation spermatozoa are released from Sertoli cells into the cavity of seminiferous tubules.

25. Which of the following layers in an antral follicle is acellular? ***(2015)***
(a) Stroma (b) Zona pellucida
(c) Granulosa (d) Theca interna

26. Which of the following cells during gametogenesis is normally diploid? ***(2015 Cancelled)***
(a) Spermatogonia
(b) Secondary polar body
(c) Primary polar body
(d) Spermatid

27. What is the correct sequence of sperm formation? ***(2013)***
(a) Spermatogonia, spermatozoa, spermatocytes, spermatids
(b) Spermatogonia, spermatocytes, spermatids, spermatozoa
(c) Spermatids, spermatocytes, spermatogonia, spermatozoa
(d) Spermatogonia, spermatocytes, spermatozoa, spermatids

28. The figure shows a section of human ovary. Select the option which gives the correct identification of either A or B with function/ characteristic. ***(Karnataka NEET 2013)***

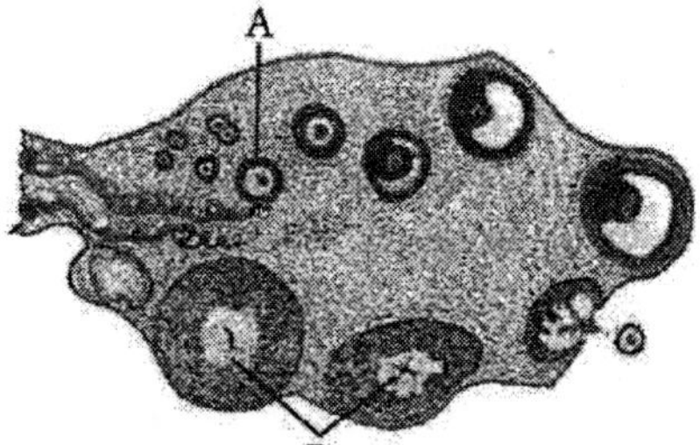

(a) B-Corpus luteum - Secretes progesterone
(b) A-Tertiary follicle - Forms Graafian follicle
(c) B-Corpus luteum - Secretes estrogen
(d) A-Primary oocyte - It is in the prophase I of the meiotic division

29. Which one of the following statements is false in respect of viability of mammalian sperm? ***(2010)***
(a) Sperm is viable for only up to 24 hours.
(b) Survival of sperm depends on the pH of the medium and is more active in alkaline medium.
(c) Viability of sperm is determined by its motility.
(d) Sperms must be concentrated in a thick suspension.

30. Which one of the following statements about human sperm is correct? ***(2010)***
(a) Acrosome has a conical pointed structure used for piercing and penetrating the egg, resulting in fertilisation.
(b) The sperm lysins in the acrosome dissolve the egg envelope facilitating fertilisation.
(c) Acrosome serves as a sensory structure leading the sperm towards the ovum.
(d) Acrosome serves no particular function.

31. The correct sequence of spermatogenetic stages leading to the formation of sperms in a mature human testis is ***(2009)***
(a) spermatogonia – spermatocyte – spermatid – sperms
(b) spermatid – spermatocyte – spermatogonia – sperms
(c) spermatogonia – spermatid – spermatocyte – sperms
(d) spermatocyte – spermatogonia – spermatid – sperms.

32. In humans, at the end of the first meiotic division, the male germ cells differentiate into the ***(2008)***
(a) spermatids
(b) spermatogonia
(c) primary spermatocytes
(d) secondary spermatocytes.

33. Sertoli cells are regulated by the pituitary hormone known as ***(2006)***
(a) LH (b) FSH
(c) GH (d) prolactin.

34. The middle piece of the sperm contains ***(1999)***
(a) proteins (b) mitochondria
(c) centriole (d) nucleus.

35. How many sperms are formed from a secondary spermatocyte? ***(1990)***
(a) 4 (b) 8 (c) 2 (d) 1

36. Egg is liberated from ovary in ***(1989)***
(a) secondary oocyte stage
(b) primary oocyte stage
(c) oogonial stage
(d) mature ovum stage.

MENSTRUAL CYCLE

37. Which of the following statements are correct regarding female reproductive cycle? ***(2023)***

A. In non-primate mammals cyclical changes during reproduction are called oestrus cycle.

B. First menstrual cycle begins at puberty and is called menopause.

C. Lack of menstruation may be indicative of pregnancy.

D. Cyclic menstruation extends between menarche and menopause.

Choose the most appropriate answer from the options given below:

(a) A, B and C only (b) A, C and D only
(c) A and D only (d) A and B only

38. Which of the following hormone levels will cause release of ovum (ovulation) from the Graafian follicle? ***(2020)***

(a) High concentration of Estrogen
(b) High concentration of Progesterone
(c) Low concentration of LH
(d) Low concentration of FSH

39. No new follicles develop in the luteal phase of the menstrual cycle because ***(Odisha NEET 2019)***

(a) follicles do not remain in the ovary after ovulation
(b) FSH levels are high in the luteal phase
(c) LH levels are high in the luteal phase
(d) both FSH and LH levels are low in the luteal phase.

40. Match the items given in column I with those in column II and select the correct option given below. ***(2018)***

Column I	Column II
A. Proliferative phase	(i) Breakdown of endometrial lining
B. Secretory phase	(ii) Follicular phase
C. Menstruation	(iii) Luteal phase

	A	B	C
(a)	(iii)	(ii)	(i)
(b)	(i)	(iii)	(ii)
(c)	(ii)	(iii)	(i)
(d)	(iii)	(i)	(ii)

41. Changes in GnRH pulse frequency in females is controlled by circulating levels of ***(NEET-I 2016)***

(a) progesterone only
(b) progesterone and inhibin
(c) estrogen and progesterone
(d) estrogen and inhibin.

42. Select the incorrect statement. ***(NEET-I 2016)***

(a) LH and FSH decrease gradually during the follicular phase.
(b) LH triggers secretion of androgens from the Leydig cells.
(c) FSH stimulates the Sertoli cells which help in spermiogenesis.
(d) LH triggers ovulation in ovary.

43. Identify the correct statement on 'inhibin'. ***(NEET-I 2016)***

(a) Is produced by granulosa cells in ovary and inhibits the secretion of LH
(b) Is produced by nurse cells in testes and inhibits the secretion of LH
(c) Inhibits the secretion of LH, FSH and prolactin
(d) Is produced by granulosa cells in ovary and inhibits the secretion of FSH

44. Which of the following events is not associated with ovulation in human female? ***(2015)***

(a) Release of secondary oocyte
(b) LH surge
(c) Decrease in estradiol
(d) Full development of Graafian follicle

45. The main function of mammalian corpus luteum is to produce ***(2014)***

(a) estrogen only
(b) progesterone
(c) human chorionic gonadotropin
(d) relaxin only.

46. Menstrual flow occurs due to lack of **(2013)**
(a) oxytocin (b) vasopressin
(c) progesterone (d) FSH.

47. The secretory phase in the human menstrual cycle is also called **(Mains 2012)**
(a) luteal phase and lasts for about 6 days
(b) follicular phase and lasts for about 6 days
(c) luteal phase and lasts for about 13 days
(d) follicular phase and lasts for about 13 days.

48. About which day in a normal human menstrual cycle does rapid secretion of LH (popularly called LH surge) normally occurs? **(Mains 2011)**
(a) 14th day (b) 20th day
(c) 5th day (d) 11th day

49. Which one of the following is the correct matching of the events occurring during menstrual cycle? **(2009)**

(a) Proliferative phase :	Rapid regeneration of myometrium and maturation of Graafian follicle
(b) Secretory phase :	Development of corpus luteum and increased secretion of progesterone
(c) Menstruation :	Breakdown of myometrium and ovum not fertilised
(d) Ovulation :	LH and FSH attain peak level and sharp fall in the secretion of progesterone

50. Which one of the following is the most likely root cause why menstruation is not taking place in regularly cycling human female? **(2009)**
(a) Maintenance of the hypertrophicalendo metriallining
(b) Maintenance of high concentration of sexhormones in the bloodstream
(c) Retention of well-developed corpus luteum
(d) Fertilisation of the ovum

51. Which one of the following statements is incorrect about menstruation? **(2008)**
(a) At menopause in the female, there is especially abrupt increase in gonadotropic hormones.
(b) The beginning of the cycle of menstruation is called menarche.
(c) During normal menstruation about 40 mL blood is lost.
(d) The menstrual fluid can easily clot.

52. Which part of ovary in mammals acts as an endocrine gland after ovulation? **(2007)**
(a) Stroma
(b) Germinal epithelium
(c) Vitelline membrane
(d) Graafian follicle

53. In the human female, menstruation can be deferred by the administration of **(2007)**
(a) combination of FSH and LH
(b) combination of estrogen and progesterone
(c) FSH only
(d) LH only.

54. Withdrawal of which of the following hormones is the immediate cause of menstruation? **(2006)**
(a) Progesterone (b) Estrogen
(c) FSH (d) FSH-RH

55. Ovulation in the human female normally takes place during the menstrual cycle **(2004)**
(a) at the mid secretory phase
(b) just before the end of the secretory phase
(c) at the beginning of the proliferative phase
(d) at the end of the proliferative phase.

56. Which set is similar? **(2001)**
(a) Corpus luteum - Graafian follicles
(b) Sebum - Sweat
(c) Bundle of His - Pacemaker
(d) Vitamin B7 - Niacin

57. After ovulation Graafian follicle regresses into **(1999)**
(a) corpus artesia (b) corpus callosum
(c) corpus luteum (d) corpus albicans.

58. In the fertile human female, approximately on which day of the menstrual cycle does ovulation take place? ***(1997)***

(a) Day 14 (b) Day 18
(c) Day 1 (d) Day 8

59. The mammalian corpus luteum produces ***(1995)***

(a) luteotrophic hormone
(b) luteinising hormone
(c) estrogen
(d) progesterone.

60. In the 28 day human ovarian cycle, the ovulation takes place typically on ***(1994)***

(a) day 14 of the cycle
(b) day 28 of the cycle
(c) day 1 of the cycle
(d) day 5 of the cycle.

FERTILISATION AND IMPLANTATION

61. Given below are two statements. ***(2023)***

One is labelled as Assertion (A) and the other is labelled as Reason (R).

Assertion (A) : Endometrium is necessary for implantation of blastocyst.

Reason (R) : In the absence of fertilization, the corpus luteum degenerates that causes disintegration of endometrium.

In the light of the above statements, choose the correct answer from the options given below:

(a) (A) Is true but (R) is false.

(b) A is false but (R) is true.

(c) Both (A) and (R) are true and (R) is the correct explanation of (A).

(d) Both (A) and (R) are true but (R) is not the correct explanation of (A).

62. Receptors for sperm binding in mammals are present on ***(2021)***

(a) zona pellucida (b) corona radiata
(c) vitelline membrane (d) perivitelline space

63. Extrusion of second polar body from egg occurs ***(2019,1993)***

(a) simultaneously with first cleavage
(b) after entry of sperm but before fertilisation
(c) after fertilisation
(d) before entry of sperm into ovum.

64. Capacitation occurs in ***(2017)***

(a) epididymis
(b) vas deferens
(c) female reproductive tract
(d) rete testis.

65. Fertilisation in humans is practically feasible only if ***(NEET-I 2016)***

(a) the ovum and sperms are transported simultaneously to ampullary-isthmic junction of the cervix

(b) the sperms are transported into cervix within 48hrs of release of ovum in uterus

(c) the sperms are transported into vagina just after the release of ovum in fallopian tube

(d) the ovum and sperms are transported simultaneously to ampullary-isthmic junction of the fallopian tube.

66. In human females, meiosis-II is not completed until ***(2015)***

(a) uterine implantation
(b) birth
(c) puberty
(d) fertilisation.

67. Capacitation refers to changes in the ***(2015 Cancelled)***

(a) ovum after fertilisation
(b) sperm after fertilisation
(c) sperm before fertilisation
(d) ovum before fertilisation.

68. In our society women are blamed for producing female children. Choose the correct answer for the sex-determination in humans. ***(Karnataka NEET 2013)***

(a) Due to some defect like aspermia in man.
(b) Due to the genetic make up of the particular sperm which fertilises the egg.
(c) Due to the genetic make up of the egg.
(d) Due to some defect in the women.

69. Identify the human developmental stage shown as well as the related right place of its occurrence in a normal pregnant woman and select the right option for the two, together. **(Mains 2012)**

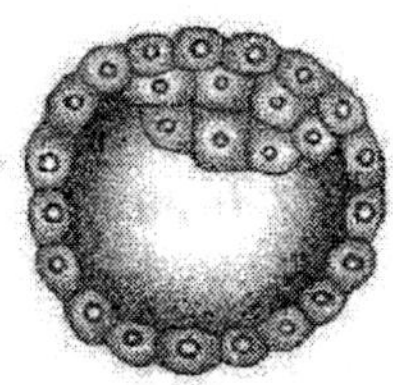

Developmental Site of occurrence stage
(a) Late morula - Middle part of fallopian tube
(b) Blastula - End part of fallopian tube
(c) Blastocyst - Uterine wall
(d) 8-celled morula - Starting point of fallopian tube

70. What happens during fertilisation in humans after many sperms reach close to the ovum? ***(Mains 2011)***

(a) Secretions of acrosome helps one sperm enter cytoplasm of ovum through zona pellucida.
(b) All sperms except the one nearest to the ovum lose their tails.
(c) Cells of corona radiata trap all the sperms except one.
(d) Only two sperms nearest the ovum penetrate zona pellucida.

71. The second maturation division of the mammalian ovum occurs ***(2010)***

(a) shortly after ovulation before the ovum makes entry into the fallopian tube
(b) until after the ovum has been penetrated by a sperm
(c) until the nucleus of the sperm has fused with that of the ovum
(d) in the Graafian follicle following the first maturation division.

72. Which one of the following statements about morula in humans is correct? ***(2010)***

(a) It has almost equal quantity of cytoplasm as an uncleaved zygote but much more DNA.
(b) It has far less cytoplasm as well as less DNA than in an uncleaved zygote.
(c) It has more or less equal quantity of cytoplasm and DNA as in uncleaved zygote.
(d) It has more cytoplasm and more DNA than an uncleaved zygote.

73. In human female, the blastocyst ***(Mains 2010)***

(a) forms placenta even before implantation
(b) gets implanted into uterus 3 days after ovulation
(c) gets nutrition from uterine endometrial secretion only after implantation
(d) gets implanted in endometrium by the trophoblast cells.

74. A change in the amount of yolk and its distribution in the egg will affect ***(2009)***

(a) pattern of cleavage
(b) number of blastomeres produced
(c) fertilisation
(d) formation of zygote.

75. What is true for cleavage? ***(2002)***

(a) Size of embryo increases
(b) Size of cells decreases
(c) Size of cells increases
(d) Size of embryo decreases

76. Fertilizin is a chemical substance produced from ***(1997,1991)***

(a) polar bodies
(b) middle piece of sperm
(c) mature eggs
(d) acrosome.

77. What is true about cleavage in the fertilised egg in humans? ***(1994)***
(a) It starts while the egg is in fallopian tube.
(b) It starts when the egg reaches uterus.
(c) It is meroblastic.
(d) It is identical to the normal mitosis.

78. During cleavage, what is true about cells? ***(1991)***
(a) Nucleocytoplasmic ratio remains unchanged.
(b) Size does not increase.
(c) There is less consumption of oxygen.
(d) The division is like meiosis.

79. Freshly released human egg has ***(1991)***
(a) one Y-chromosome
(b) one X-chromosome
(c) two X-chromosome
(d) one X-chromosome and one Y-chromosome.

80. Sperm and egg nuclei fuse due to ***(1990)***
(a) base pairing of their DNA and RNA
(b) formation of hydrogen bonds
(c) mutual attraction due to differences in electrical charges
(d) attraction of their protoplasts.

81. Cells become variable in morphology and function in different regions of the embryo. The process is ***(1989)***
(a) differentiation (b) metamorphosis
(c) organisation (d) rearrangement.

PREGNANCY AND EMBRYONIC DEVELOPMENT

82. Which of the following secretes the hormone, relaxin, during the later phase of pregnancy? ***(2021)***
(a) Uterus (b) Graafian follicle
(c) Corpus luteum (d) Fetus

83. Match the following columns and select the correct option. ***(2020)***

Column-I	Column-II
(A) Placenta	(i) Androgens
(B) Zona pellucida	(ii) Human Chorionic Gonadotropin (HCG)
(C) Bulbourethral glands	(iii) Layer of the ovum
(D) Leydig cells	(iv) Lubrication of the penis

	(A)	(B)	(C)	(D)
(a)	(iv)	(iii)	(i)	(ii)
(b)	(i)	(iv)	(ii)	(iii)
(c)	(iii)	(ii)	(iv)	(i)
(d)	(ii)	(iii)	(iv)	(i)

84. Hormones secreted by the placenta to maintain pregnancy are ***(2018)***
(a) hCG, hPL, progestogens, prolactin
(b) hCG, hPL, estrogens, relaxin, oxytocin
(c) hCG, hPL, progestogens, estrogens
(d) hCG, progestogens, estrogens, glucocorticoids.

85. The amnion of mammalian embryo is derived from ***(2018)***
(a) ectoderm and mesoderm
(b) endoderm and mesoderm
(c) mesoderm and trophoblast
(d) ectoderm and endoderm.

86. Match column I with column II and select the correct option using the given codes. ***(NEET-II 2016)***

Column I	Column II
A. Mons pubis	(i) Embryo formation
B. Antrum	(ii) Sperm
C. Trophectoderm	(iii) Female external genitalia
D. Nebenkern	(iv) Graafian follicle

(a) A-(iii), B-(iv), C-(ii), D-(i)
(b) A-(iii), B-(iv), C-(i), D-(ii)
(c) A-(iii), B-(i), C-(iv), D-(ii)
(d) A-(i), B-(iv), C-(iii), D-(ii)

87. Several hormones like hCG, hPL, estrogen, progesterone are produced by ***(NEET-II 2016)***
(a) ovary (b) placenta
(c) fallopian tube (d) pituitary.

88. Ectopic pregnancies are referred to as ***(2015)***
(a) implantation of defective embryo in the uterus
(b) pregnancies terminated due to hormonal imbalance
(c) pregnancies with genetic abnormality
(d) implantation of embryo at site other than uterus.

89. Select the correct option describing gonadotropin activity in a normal pregnant female. ***(2014,2012)***
(a) High level of FSH and LH stimulates the thickening of endometrium.
(b) High level of FSH and LH facilitates implantation of the embryo.
(c) High level of hCG stimulates the synthesis of estrogen and progesterone.
(d) High level of hCG stimulates the thickening of endometrium.

90. Which one of the following is not the function of placenta? ***(2013)***
(a) Facilitates removal of carbon dioxide and waste material from embryo
(b) Secretes oxytocin during parturition
(c) Facilitates supply of oxygen and nutrients to embryo
(d) Secretes estrogen

91. The first movements of the fetus and appearance of hair on its head are usually observed during which month of pregnancy? ***(2010)***
(a) Fourth month (b) Fifth month
(c) Sixth month (d) Third month

92. Which extra embryonic membrane in humans prevents desiccation of the embryo inside the uterus? ***(2008)***
(a) Yolk sac (b) Amnion
(c) Chorion (d) Allantosis

93. Which of the following hormones is not a secretion product of human placenta? ***(2004)***
(a) Human chorionic gonadotropin
(b) Prolactin
(c) Estrogen
(d) Progesterone

94. During embryonic development, the establishment of polarity along anterior/posterior, dorsal/ventral or medial/lateral axis is called ***(2003)***
(a) organiser phenomena
(b) axis formation
(c) anamorphosis
(d) pattern formation.

95. The extra embryonic membranes of the mammalian embryo are derived from ***(1994)***
(a) trophoblast (b) inner cell mass
(c) formative cells (d) follicle cells.

PARTURITION AND LACTATION

96. Which of these is not an important component of initiation of parturition in humans? ***(2021)***
(a) Release of prolactin
(b) Increase in estrogen and progesterone ratio
(c) Synthesis of prostaglandins
(d) Release of oxytocin

97. Which of these is not an important component of initiation of parturition in humans? ***(2015 Cancelled)***
(a) Release of oxytocin
(b) Release of prolactin
(c) Increase in estrogen and progesterone ratio
(d) Synthesis of prostaglandins

98. The fetal ejection reflex in humans triggers the release of ***(Karnataka NEET 2013)***
(a) oxytocin from fetal pituitary
(b) human chorionic gonadotropin (hCG) from placenta
(c) human placental lactogen (hPL) from placenta
(d) oxytocin from maternal pituitary.

99. Signals for parturition originate from ***(2012)***
(a) both placenta as well as fully developed fetus
(b) oxytocin released from maternal pituitary
(c) placenta only
(d) fully developed fetus only.

100. Signals from fully developed fetus and placenta ultimately lead to parturition which requires the release of ***(Mains 2010)***
(a) estrogen from placenta
(b) oxytocin from maternal pituitary
(c) oxytocin from fetal pituitary
(d) relaxin from placenta.

101. Fetal ejection reflex in human female is induced by ***(2009)***
(a) release of oxytocin from pituitary
(b) fully developed fetus and placenta
(c) differentiation of mammary glands
(d) pressure exerted by amniotic fluid.

102. In human adult females oxytocin ***(2008)***
(a) stimulates pituitary to secrete vasopressin
(b) causes strong uterine contractions during parturition
(c) is secreted by anterior pituitary
(d) stimulates growth of mammary glands.

ANSWER KEY

1.	(c)	2.	(a)	3.	(a)	4.	(d)	5.	(a)	6.	(a)	7.	(c)
8.	(b)	9.	(a)	10.	(a)	11.	(d)	12.	(a)	13.	(d)	14.	(c)
15.	(c)	16.	(c)	17.	(b)	18.	(b)	19	(c)	20.	(c)	21.	(d)
22.	(b)	23.	(d)	24.	(d)	25.	(b)	26.	(a)	27.	(b)	28.	(a)
29.	(a)	30.	(b)	31.	(a)	32.	(d)	33.	(b)	34.	(b)	35.	(c)
36.	(a)	37.	(b)	38.	(a)	39.	(d)	40.	(c)	41.	(c)	42.	(a)
43.	(d)	44.	(c)	45.	(b)	46.	(c)	47.	(c)	48.	(a)	49.	(b)
50.	(b)	51.	(d)	52.	(d)	53.	(b)	54.	(a)	55.	(d)	56.	(a)
57.	(c)	58.	(a)	59.	(d)	60.	(a)	61.	(d)	62.	(a)	63.	(b)
64.	(c)	65.	(d)	66.	(d)	67.	(c)	68.	(b)	69.	(c)	70.	(a)
71.	(b)	72.	(a)	73.	(d)	74.	(a)	75.	(b)	76.	(c)	77.	(a)
78.	(b)	79.	(b)	80.	(d)	81.	(a)	82.	(c)	83.	(d)	84.	(c)
85.	(a)	86.	(b)	87.	(b)	88.	(d)	89.	(c)	90.	(b)	91.	(b)
92.	(b)	93.	(b)	94.	(a)	95.	(a)	96.	(a)	97.	(b)	98.	(d)
99.	(a)	100.	(b)	101.	(b)	102.	(b)						

HINTS & EXPLANATIONS

1. (c)

2. (a)

3.(a) : Urethra is the urinary duct which originates from the neck of urinary bladder and opens to the exterior at the tip of penis in males. It is a common pathway for passage of urine and semen.

4.(d) : Interstitial cells or Leydig's cells are the cells interspersed between the seminiferous tubules of the testis. They secrete androgens (e.g., testosterone) in response to stimulation by luteinising hormone from the anterior pituitary gland.

5.(a) : The male sex accessory ducts include rete testis, vasa efferentia, epididymis and vas deferens. The seminiferous tubules of the testis open into the vasa efferentia through rete testis. The vasa efferentia leave the testis and open into epididymis located along the posterior surface of each testis. So, if vasa efferentia gets blocked, the gametes will not be transported from testes to epididymis.

6.(a) : The testes are situated outside the abdominal cavity within a pouch called scrotum. The scrotum helps in maintaining the low temperature of the testes (2–2.5°C lower than the normal internal body temperature) necessary for spermatogenesis.

7.(c) : Sertoli cells (named after Italian histologist Enrico Sertoli) are found in the walls of the seminiferous tubules of the testis. Compared with the germ cells they appear large and pale. They anchor and probably nourish the developing germ cells, especially the spermatids, which become partly embedded within them.

8.(b) : The seminiferous tubules are closed at one end but on the other side they join to a network the rete testis from where fine ciliated ductules, the vasa efferentia arise. Cilia help in conducting sperms. The rete testis is a network of tubules conducting sperms from the seminiferous tubules of the testis to the vasa efferentia.

9.(a) : Semen or seminal fluid or seminal plasma is the fluid ejaculated from the penis at sexual climax. Each ejaculate may contain 300-500 million spermatozoa suspended in a fluid secreted by the prostate gland and seminal vesicles with a small contribution from Cowper's glands. It is rich in fructose, calcium and certain enzymes. It provides a fluid medium for transport of sperms, nourishes and activates sperms, lubricates the reproductive tract of female and neutralizes the acidity of the vagina of female to protect the sperms.

10.(a) : The male accessory glands include paired seminal vesicles, a prostate and paired bulbourethral glands. Secretions of these glands constitute the seminal plasma which is rich in fructose, calcium and certain enzymes. The secretions of bulbourethral glands also help in the lubrication of the penis.

11. (d)

12. (a)

13. (d)

14. (c)

15. (c)

16.(c) : Hysterectomy is the surgical removal of uterus. It may also involve removal of the cervix, ovaries, fallopian tubes and other surrounding structures.

17.(b) : The oviducts (fallopian tubes), uterus and vagina constitute the female accessory ducts.

Each Fallopian tube is about 10-12 cm long and extends from the periphery of each ovary to the uterus, the part closer to the ovary is the funnel shaped infundibulum. The edges of the infundibulum possess finger-like projections called fimbriae, which help in collection of the ovum after ovulation. The uterus is single and it is also called womb, open into vagina through a narrow cervix. So, III is infundibulum, IV is fimbriae and V is cervix.

18. (b) : Each fallopian tube is about 10-12 cm long and extends from the periphery of each ovary to the uterus, the part closer to the ovary is the funnel-shaped infundibulum. The edges of the infundibulum possess finger-like projections called fimbriae, which help in collection of the ovum after ovulation. The infundibulum leads to a wider part of the oviduct called ampulla. The last part of the oviduct, isthmus has a narrow lumen and it joins the uterus.

19 (c) : Bartholin's glands are situated on either side of vagina in human females. These glands secrete a fluid that lubricates the vulva during copulation.

20.(c) : Formation of mature spermatozoa from spermatids is called spermiogenesis. Spermiation is the process by which mature spermatids are released from Sertoli cell into the seminiferous tubule lumen prior to their passage to the epididymis.

21.(d) : In both, spermatogenesis and oogenesis haploid gametes are formed. The spermatids are transformed into spermatozoa (sperms) by the process called spermiogenesis occurs in process spermatogenesis only. Spermatogenesis and oogenesis both are controlled by LH and FSH secreted by the anterior pituitary. Spermatogenesis is a continuous process that begins at puberty. Oogenesis on the other hand begins during embryonic development of the female.

22.(b) : Oogenesis is initiated during embryonic development stage when a couple of million oogonia are formed within each fetal ovary. No oogonia are formed or added after birth.

23.(d) : In humans, the secondary oocyte is produced when the primary oocyte grows in size and completes its first meiotic division. The secondary oocyte will be halted at this stage of metaphase of meiosis II until fertilisation takes place. Thus, when a sperm cell fertilises the female sex cell, the secondary oocyte rapidly completes the remaining stages of meiosis II, giving rise to ovum, with which the sperm cell unites.

24.(d) : Formation of spermatozoa from spermatids is called spermiogenesis, After spermiogenesis, sperm heads become embedded in the Sertoli cells and are finally released from the seminiferous tubules by the process called spermiation.

25. (b)

26.(a) : Spermatogonia are diploid cells which mature into primary spermatocytes (2n) by growth. They then produce two haploid secondary spermatocytes by meiosis I. Each secondary spermatocyte (n) completes the meiosis II and produces two spermatids (n). Each spermatid (n) develops into a spermatozoan or sperm (n).

27.(b) : Spermatogenesis is the process of formation of haploid spermatozoa (sperms) from diploid spermatogonia inside the testes of the male. At sexual maturity, the undifferentiated primordial germ cells divide several times by mitosis to produce a large number of spermatogonia or sperm mother cells. Each spermatogonium actively grows to a larger primary spermatocyte by obtaining nourishment from the nursing cells. The phenomenon of formation of primary spermatocytes from spermatogonia, is called spermatocytogenesis. Each primary spermatocyte undergoes two successive divisions, called maturation divisions. The first maturation division is reductional or meiotic. Hence, the primary spermatocyte divides into two haploid daughter cells called secondary spermatocytes. Both secondary spermatocytes now undergo second maturation division which is an ordinary mitotic division to form four haploid spermatids, by each primary spermatocyte. The transformation of spermatids into spermatozoa is called spermiogenesis or spermateleosis or differentiation phase.

28.(a) : The zona granulosa and theca cells of Graafian follicle remaining in the ovary after ovulation and some surrounding capillaries and connective tissue evolve into the corpus luteum (a temporary endocrine gland). The corpus luteum produces progesterone and in the event of fertilisation, provides the required progesterone until the placenta is formed. In the absence of fertilisation, the life span of the corpus luteum is 14 days. It then degenerates into a corpus albicans, which is mainly a scar tissue.

29.(a) : Sperms remain viable for 48 hours to 72 hours.

30. (b) : Acrosome is the cap-like structure on the front end of a spermatozoan. It breaks down just before fertilisation (the acrosome reaction), releasing a number of hydrolytic enzymes, also called sperm lysins that assist penetration between the follicle cells that still surround the ovum, thus facilitating fertilisation. Failure of the acrosome reaction is a cause of male infertility.

31. (a)

32.(d) : During embryonic development the primordial germ cells migrate to the testis where they become spermatogonia. At puberty the spermatogonia proliferate rapidly by mitosis. Some undergo growth phase to become primary spermatocytes that further undergo through meiotic division I to become secondary spermatocytes. After completion of meiotic division, II the secondary spermatocytes produce spermatids which differentiate to form spermatozoa.

33.(b) : Sertoli cells are present in the germinal epithelium of the seminiferous tubules. These cells nourish the developing sperms. These cells differentiate spermatogonia into sperms. They are under the influence of FSH released by anterior pituitary gland.

34.(b) : The sperm consists of head, neck, middle piece and tail. The middle piece of human sperm contains the mitochondria coiled around the axial filament called mitochondrial spiral. They provide energy for the movement of the sperm.

35.(c) : Spermatogonia are diploid cells which mature into primary spermatocytes (2n) by growth. They then produce two haploid secondary spermatocytes by meiosis I. Each secondary spermatocyte (n) completes the meiosis II and produces two spermatids (n). Each spermatid (n) develops into a spermatozoan or sperm (n). Similarly, in females, oogonia are the diploid cells from which through meiosis, polar bodies (n) and single ovum (n) are produced.

36.(a) : In humans, ovum is released from the ovary in the secondary oocyte stage. The wall of the ovary gets ruptured to release the oocyte. In humans ovulation occurs about 14 days before the onset of the next menstruation. Ovulation is induced by LH.

37.(b) : The first menstruation begins at puberty and is called menarche. Menstrual cycle ceases around 50 years of age in human females, that is called menopause.

38.(a) : FSH, LH and estrogen are at peak during ovulation (release of ovum).

39. (d)

40. (c)

41.(c) : GnRH is secreted by the hypothalamus which stimulates the anterior lobe of pituitary gland to secrete luteinising hormone (LH) and follicle stimulating hormone (FSH). FSH stimulates the growth of the ovarian follicles and stimulates the formation of estrogens. LH stimulates the corpus luteum to secrete progesterone. Rising levels of progesterone and estrogen inhibits the release of GnRH, which in turn, inhibits the production of FSH and LH.

42.(a) : During follicular phase, FSH secretion increases. Follicular phase (proliferative phase) usually includes cycle days 6-13 or 14 in a 28 days cycle. The follicle stimulating hormone (FSH) secreted by the anterior lobe of the pituitary gland stimulates the ovarian follicle to secrete estrogen.

43. (d)

44.(c) : In human females, ovulation is the release of secondary oocyte from the ovary at about 14th day of the menstrual cycle. Both LH and FSH attain a peak level during this period. Rapid secretion of LH induces rupturing of fully developed Graafian follicle and thereby release of ovum. LH surge is actually responsible for ovulation.

45. (b) : Corpus luteum secretes steroid hormones progesterone and estrogen, to make uterus suitable for implantation (in case fertilisation occurs) and its maintenance (mainly endometrium).

46.(c) : The corpus luteum secretes large amount of progesterone which is essential for maintenance of the endometrium necessary for implantation of the fertilized ovum and other events of pregnancy. In the absence of fertilization, the corpus luteum degenerates. This causes disintegration of the endometrium leading to menstruation. The menstrual flow results due to breakdown of endometrial lining of the uterus and its blood vessels which forms liquid that comes out through vagina.

47.(c) : After ovulation which occurs in the middle of menstrual cycle, empty Graafian follicle continues growth under the influence of LH. The follicular cells are converted into lutein cells by deposition of yellowish lipid inclusions. The phenomenon is called luteinization. The ruptured Graafian follicle is now called corpus luteum. It secretes hormones, mainly progesterone and small quantity of estrogen. Both LH and progesterone help in further growth and thickening of endometrium. The major change is that the endometrial glands become secretory. The uterine wall becomes ready for nourishing and anchoring blastocyst if fertilization takes place. Hence, this phase of menstrual cycle is called luteal or secretory phase. The phase lasts for about 13 days, i.e., 15-28 days of 28 days menstrual cycle.

48. (a)

49.(b) : Secretory phase is also called as luteal phase. The luteinising hormone or LH is secreted by the anterior lobe of pituitary gland. LH causes ovulation. LH stimulates cells of ovarian follicles to develop corpus luteum. Corpus luteum secretes large amount of progesterone.

50.(b) : High concentration of sex steroids (estrogen) exerts negative feedback on anterior pituitary, decreasing LH secretion and release thus, lowering LH level in blood. Due to insufficient LH level, no ovulation occurs which causes irregular menstruation.

51.(d) : Menstruation is a process which involves discharge of blood (45–100 mL), serous fluid, cell debris and mucosal fragments from cast off endometrial lining due to reduced titre of both estrogen and progesterone hormone.' Blood clotting does not occur due to presence of fibrinolysin.

52. (d)

53. (b)

54.(a) : The menstrual cycle consists of three phases; proliferative phase, secretory phase and menstrual phase. During menstrual phase the production of LH is considerably reduced. The withdrawal of this hormone causes degeneration of the corpus luteum and, therefore, progesterone production is reduced. The endometrium degenerates and breaks down. Thus, menstruation begins.

55.(d) : Ovulation (the release of secondary oocyte from the Graafian follicle) takes place at the end of proliferative phase of menstrual cycle. During this phase, the follicle stimulating hormone (FSH) secreted by the anterior lobe of the pituitary gland stimulates the ovarian follicle to secrete estrogen.

Estrogen stimulates the proliferation of the endometrium of the uterine wall. The endometrium becomes thicker by rapid cell multiplication and this is accompanied by an increase of uterine glands and blood vessels. This phase ends when the ovarian follicle ruptures and ovulation occurs and at the same time the production of estrogen stops.

56.(a) : A mature ovarian follicle is called Graafian follicle. It contains follicular cells, an antrum and an oocyte. After ovulation, the empty Graafian follicle shows deposition of leutin and forms corpus luteum that ultimately degenerates.

57. (c)

58.(a) : Ovulation is the release of egg by ruptured Graafian follicle. The wall of Graafian follicle is ruptured by sudden increase in the level of luteinising hormone. The length of menstruation cycle is 28 days (average) from the start of one menstruation period to the start of the next. At about 14th day of the cycle, the distended follicle ruptures and the ovum is extruded into the fallopian tube and ovulation takes place.

59.(d) : Progesterone is secreted by the corpus luteum of the ovary. It stimulates further development of the uterine epithelium and mammary glands. It is also required for the formation of the placenta and for the maintenance of pregnancy. Luteotrophic hormone and luteinising hormone are secreted by the anterior lobe of pituitary gland. Estrogen is secreted by the cells of the Graafian follicles.

60. (a)

61.(d) : The corpus luteum secretes large amount of progesterone which is essential for maintenance of the endometrium. This endometrium is necessary for implantation of the fertilised ovum (blastocyst). In the absence of fertilisation the corpus luteum degenerates. This causes disintegration of the endometrium leading to menstruation, marking a new cycle.

62. (a)

63.(b) : Entry of sperm into the secondary oocyte induces the completion of the meiotic division of the secondary oocyte. The second meiotic division is unequal and results in the formation of a second polar body and a haploid ovum (ootid). Soon the haploid nucleus of the sperm and that of the ovum fuse together to form a diploid zygote.

64.(c) : The sperms in the female's genital tract are made capable of fertilising the egg by secretions of the female genital tract. These secretions remove coating substances deposited on the surface of the sperms particularly those on the acrosome. Thus, the receptor sites on the acrosome are exposed and sperm becomes active to penetrate the egg. This phenomenon of sperm activation in mammals is known as capacitation.

65.(d) : The fusion of a haploid male gamete (sperm) and a haploid female gamete (ovum) to form a diploid zygote is called fertilisation. In human beings, it takes place in the ampullaryisthmic junction of the oviduct (fallopian tube).

66.(d) : In human beings, ovum is released from the ovary in the secondary oocyte stage. The maturation of secondary oocyte is completed in the mother's oviduct (fallopian tube) usually after the sperm has entered the secondary oocyte for fertilisation. Entry of the sperm restarts the cell cycle breaking down MPF (M-phase promoting factor) and turning on APC (Anaphase promoting complex). Completion of meiosis II converts the secondary oocyte into a fertilised ovum (egg) or zygote (and also a second polar body).

67. (c)

68.(b) : Establishment of sex through differential development in an individual at an early stage of life is called sex determination. Fusion of male nuclei with that of female nucleus decides the sex of the baby. Chromosome pattern in the human female is XX and that in the male is XY. Therefore, all the haploid gametes produced by the female have the sex chromosome X whereas in the male gametes the sex chromosome could be either X or Y, hence, 50 per cent of sperms carry the X chromosome while the other 50 per cent carry the Y. After fusion of the male and female gametes the zygote would carry either XX or XY depending on whether the sperm carrying X or Y fertilised the ovum. The zygote carrying XX would develop into a female and XY would form a male.

69.(c) : After fertilisation, zygote undergoes rapid mitotic divisions, called cleavage, which is characterised by absence of growth of daughter cells. This leads to the conversion of single celled zygote into a multicellular structure called blastocyst or blastula. Implantation or embedding of zygote into endometrium of uterus occurs in blastocyst stage.

70.(a) : The process of fusion of a sperm with an ovum is called fertilisation. During fertilisation, a sperm comes in contact with the zona pellucida layer of the ovum and induces changes in the membrane that block the entry of additional sperms. Thus, it ensures that only one sperm can fertilise an ovum. The secretions of the acrosome help the sperm enter into the cytoplasm of the ovum through the zona pellucida and the plasma membrane. In contact with the surface of egg covering, the acrosome releases its contained hydrolytic enzymes, also called sperm lysins. It is known as acrosomal reaction. Acrosome reaction results in dissolving of corona cells and degeneration of zona pellucida which helps in sperm penetration.

71.(b) : Oogenesis starts with division of oogonia (gamete mother cells) giving rise to primary oocyte which enters into prophase I of the meiotic division and get temporarily arrested at this stage. The primary oocyte gets surrounded by primary, secondary and tertiary follicles respectively. The tertiary follicle grow in size and completes its first meiotic division to give rise to haploid secondary oocyte. This secondary oocyte forms a new membrane called zona pellucida surrounding it. During fertilisation the sperm enter into the cytoplasm of the ovum through the zona pellucida and the plasma membrane. This induces the completion of the meiotic division (2nd division) of the secondary oocyte. The second meiotic division is also unequal and results in the formation of a second polar body and a haploid ovum (ootid).

72.(a) : A morula is an embryo at an early stage of embryonic development, consisting of cells (called blastomeres) in a solid ball contained within the zona pellucida. The morula is produced by embryonic cleavage, the rapid division of the zygote. The increase in number of cells does not change the size of the original mass. The divisions are rapid because there is no net growth of the embryo-the cell cycle alternates between DNA replication and mitosis. In the absence of growth, the cell number in the embryo increases while the cell size decreases. Thus, it has almost equal quantity of cytoplasm as an uncleaved zygote but much more DNA.

73.(d) : Implantation in endometrial uterine wall takes place at blastocyst stage of embryonic development. Before implantation, the blastomeres of early blastocyst get arranged into an outer layer called trophoblast and an inner group of cells attached to trophoblast called inner cell mass. It is the trophoblast layer through which blastocyst gets attached to the endometrium and the inner cell mass gets differentiated as the embryo.

74.(a) : Cleavage is a series of cell divisions by which a single fertilised egg cell is transformed into a multicellular body, the blastula. Characteristically no growth occurs during cleavage, the shape of the embryo is unchanged except for the formation of central cavity (the blastocoel) and the ratio of nuclear material (DNA) to cytoplasm increases. The mode of cleavage is determined by the amount of yolk and its distribution. On this basis cleavage may be holoblastic or meroblastic.

75.(b) : During cleavage, the zygote divides repeatedly to convert the large cytoplasmic mass into a large number of small blastomeres. It involves cell division without growth in size because cells continue to be retained within the zona pellucida. However, cell size decreases during cleavage.

76.(c) : Mature egg (ovum) secretes a chemical named fertilizin (composed of glycoprotein = monosaccharides + amino acids). Sperm has on its surface a protein substance called antifertilizin (composed of acidic amino acids). The fertilizin of an egg interacts with the antifertilizin of a sperm of the same species. This interaction makes the sperms stick to the egg surface. The adhesion of sperm to the egg of the same species through chemical recognition is known as agglutination.

77.(a) : Cleavage is a series of rapid mitotic divisions of the zygote which convert the single celled zygote into a multicellular structure called blastula (blastocyst). About thirty hours after fertilisation, the newly formed zygote divides into two cells, the blastomeres, in the upper portion of the fallopian tube. This is the first cleavage. The next division occurs within forty hours after fertilisation. The third division occurs about three days after fertilisation. During these early cleavages, the young embryo is slowly moving down the fallopian tube towards the uterus. At the end of fourth day, the embryo reaches the uterus. It has thirty two cells.

78.(b) : During cleavage, the zygote divides repeatedly to convert the large cytoplasmic mass into a large number of small blastomeres. It involves cell division without growth in size because cells continue to be retained within the zona pellucida. However, cell size decreases during cleavage.

79.(b) : The egg released is haploid (has only one X-chromosome and 22 autosomes) as it is formed due to meiotic division of diploid primary oocyte having XX chromosome and 44 autosomes.

80. (d) : The two gametes, i.e., sperm and egg move in opposite direction by an unknown mechanism but most probably by streaming currents of cytoplasm, i.e., due to attraction of their protoplasts. The nucleus of one male gamete fuses with the egg nucleus and the phenomenon is called fertilisation.

81.(a) : Differentiation are the changes from simple to more complex forms undergone by developing tissues and organs so that they become specialised for particular functions. Differentiation occurs during embryonic development and regeneration.

82.(c) : Relaxin is secreted by corpus luteum during the later phase of pregnancy.

83. (d)

84. (c): Placenta is temporary organ that helps in exchange of gases, nutrients and waste materials between mother and fetus. During pregnancy, placenta acts as an endocrine gland and secretes some hormones such as estrogen, progestogens, human chorionic gonadotropin (hCG), human placental lactogen (hPL), chorionic thyrotropin, chorionic corticotropin and relaxin.

85.(a) : Amnion, in reptiles, birds and mammals is a membrane forming a fluid-filled cavity (the amniotic sac) that encloses the embryo. During development, the amnion arises by a folding of a mass of extra-embryonic tissue called the somatopleure. Lined with ectoderm and covered with mesoderm, the amnion contains a thin transparent fluid in which the embryo is suspended, thus providing a cushion against mechanical injury.

86. (b)

87. (b)

88.(d) : Ectopic pregnancy is a complication of pregnancy in which implantation of embryo takes place at site other than uterus. Signs and symptoms include abdominal pain and vaginal bleeding. Most ectopic pregnancies (90%) occur in the fallopian tube, which are known as tubal pregnancies.

89.(c) : The trophoblastic cells secrete human chorionic gonadotropin hormone which has properties similar to those of luteinising hormone (LH) of the pituitary gland. It takes over the job of pituitary LH during pregnancy. The hCG maintains the corpus luteum and stimulates it to secrete progesterone. The latter maintains the endometrium of the uterus and causes it to grow throughout pregnancy. This also prevents menstruation. Progesterone also causes increased secretion of mucus in the cervix of the uterus that forms a protective plug during pregnancy.

90. (b)

91.(b) : In human beings, after one month of pregnancy, the embryo's heart is formed. By the end of the second month of pregnancy, the fetus develops limbs and digits. By the end of 12 weeks (first trimester), most of the major organ systems are formed. The first movements of the fetus and appearance of hair on the head are usually observed during the fifth month. By the end of 24 weeks (second trimester), the body is covered with fine hair, eyelids separate and eyelashes are formed. By the end of nine months of pregnancy, the fetus is fully developed and is ready for delivery.

92.(b) : Amnion is a type of extraembryonic membrane formed by the amniogenic cells inside and splanchnopleuric extraembryonic mesoderm outside. Amnion surrounds the embryo creating the amniotic cavity that is filled with amniotic fluid. The amniotic fluid serves as a shock absorber for the fetus, regulates fetal body temperature and prevents desiccation.

93.(b) : Prolactin is secreted by anterior pituitary gland which stimulates mammary gland development during pregnancy and lactation after child birth.

94.(a) : During embryonic development, the establishment of polarity along anterior/ posterior, dorsal/ventral or medial/ lateral axis is called organiser phenomenon. The organiser is the part of an embryo consisting of undifferentiated cells that follow a specific course of development by identifying the polarity of particular region.

95.(a) : Trophoblast is the layer of cells encircling the blastocoel and the inner cell mass. The latter gives rise to the embryo. The cells of the trophoblast form the placenta and fetal membrane.

96.(a) : Prolactin is secreted by anterior lobe of the pituitary gland during lactation.

97.(b) : Process of parturition is induced by both nervous system and hormones secreted by the endocrine glands of the mother. The signals for child birth (parturition) originate from the fully developed fetus and placenta which induce mild uterine contractions called fetal ejection reflex. This causes quick release of oxytocin from the maternal posterior lobe of pituitary gland which induces labour pains. Prostaglandins, progesterone and estrogen also play a role. Prolactin is the hormone which induces lactation and has no role in parturition.

98. (d)

99. (a)

100. (b)

101. (b)

102. (b): In human adult female, oxytocin is a hormone released by the pituitary gland (neurohypophysis) that causes contraction of the uterus during labour and stimulates milk flow from the breasts by causing contraction of muscle fibres in the milk ducts.

Chapter : 22

REPRODUCTIVE HEALTH

REPRODUCTIVE HEALTH: PROBLEMS AND STRATEGIES

1. Given below are two statements: one is labelled as Assertion (A) : and the other is labelled as Reason (R).

Assertion (A) : Amniocentesis for sex determination is one of the strategies of Reproductive and Child Health Care Programme.

Reason (R) : Ban on amniocentesis checks increasing menace of female foeticide.

In the light of the above statements, choose the correct answer from the options given below: ***(2023)***

(a) (A) is true but (R) is false.
(b) A is false but (R) is true.
(c) Both (A) and (R) are true and (R) is the correct explanation of (A).
(d) Both (A) and (R) are true and (R) is not the correct explanation of (A).

2. In context of amniocentesis, which of the following statements is incorrect? ***(NEET-I 2016)***
(a) It can be used for detection of Down's syndrome.
(b) It can be used for detection of cleft palate.
(c) It is usually done when a woman is between 14-16 weeks pregnant.
(d) It is used for prenatal sex determination.

3. Which of the following cannot be detected in a developing fetus by amniocentesis? ***(2013)***
(a) Down's syndrome
(b) Jaundice
(c) Klinefelter's syndrome
(d) Sex of the fetus

4. The permissible use of the technique amniocentesis is for ***(2010)***
(a) detecting sex of the unborn fetus
(b) artificial insemination
(c) transfer of embryo into the uterus of a surrogate mother
(d) detecting any genetic abnormality.

5. Fetal sex can be determined by examining cells from the amniotic fluid by looking for ***(1997)***
(a) chiasmata (b) kinetochore
(c) barr bodies (d) autosomes.

POPULATION STABILISATION AND BIRTH CONTROL

6. Match List I with List II. ***(2023)***

List I	List II
A. Vasectomy	I. Oral method
B. Coitus interruptus	II. Barrier method
C. Cervical caps	III. Surgical method
D. Saheli	IV. Natural method

Choose the correct answer from the options given below:
(a) A-II, B-III, C-I, D-IV
(b) A-IV, B-II, C-I, D-III
(c) A-III, B-I, C-IV, D-II
(d) A-III, B-IV, C-II, D-I

7. Lippe's loop is a type of contraceptive used as: ***(2022)***
(a) Cervical barrier
(b) Vault barrier
(c) Non-Medicated IUD
(d) Copper releasing IUD.

8. Match list-I with list-II with respect to method of contraception and their respective actions. ***(2022)***

List I	List II
(A) Diaphragms	(i) Inhibit ovulation and implantation
(B) Contraceptive pills	(ii) Increase phagocytosis of sperm within uterus
(C) Intra Uterine devices	(iii) Absence of menstrual cycle and ovulation following parturition
(D) Lactational amenorrhea	(iv) They cover the cervix blocking the entry of sperms

Choose the correct answer from the options given below:

(a) (A)-(iv), (B)-(i),(C)-(iii), (D)-(ii)
(b) (A)-(iv), (B)-(i), (C)-(ii), (D)-(iii)
(c) (A)-(ii), (B)-(iv), (C)-(i), (D)-(iii)
(d) (A)-(iii), (B)-(ii), (C)-(i), (D)-(iv)

9. Match List- I with List- II.

List I	List II
(p) Vaults	(i) Entry of sperm through cervix is blocked
(q) IUDs	(ii) Removal of Vas deferens
(r) Vasectomy	(iii) Phagocytosis of sperms within the uterus
(s) Tubectomy	(iv) Removal of fallopian tube

Choose the correct answer from the options given below. ***(2021)***

	p	q	r	s
(a)	(iii)	(i)	(iv)	(ii)
(b)	(iv)	(ii)	(i)	(iii)
(c)	(i)	(iii)	(ii)	(iv)
(d)	(ii)	(iv)	(iii)	(i)

10. Which one of the following is an example of hormone releasing IUD? ***(2021)***

(a) Multiload 375 (b) CuT
(c) LNG-20 (d) Cu 7

11. Which of the following contraceptive methods involve a role of hormone? ***(2019)***

(a) Pills, Emergency contraceptives, Barrier methods
(b) Lactational amenorrhea, Pills, Emergency contraceptives
(c) Barrier method, Lactational amenorrhea, Pills
(d) CuT, Pills, Emergency contraceptive

12. Select the hormone-releasing Intra-Uterine Devices. ***(2019)***

(a) Lippes Loop, Multiload 375
(b) Vaults, LNG-20
(c) Multiload 375, Progestasert
(d) Progestasert, LNG-20

13. Which of the following is a correct statement? ***(Odisha NEET 2019)***

(a) IUDs once inserted need not be replaced.
(b) IUDs are generally inserted by the user herself.
(c) IUDs increase phagocytosis of sperms in the uterus.
(d) IUDs suppress gametogenesis.

14. The contraceptive 'Saheli' ***(2018)***

(a) blocks estrogen receptors in the uterus, preventing eggs from getting implanted
(b) increases the concentration of estrogen and prevents ovulation in females
(c) is an IUD
(d) is a post-coital contraceptive.

15. The function of copper ions in copper releasing IUDs is ***(2017)***

(a) they inhibit gametogenesis
(b) they make uterus unsuitable for implantation
(c) they inhibit ovulation
(d) they suppress sperm motility and fertilising capacity of sperms.

16. Which of the following is hormone-releasing IUD? ***(NEET-II 2016)***

(a) LNG-20 (b) Multiload 375
(c) Lippes Loop (d) Cu 7

17. Which of the following is incorrect regarding vasectomy? ***(NEET-II 2016)***
(a) No sperm occurs in seminal fluid
(b) No sperm occurs in epididymis
(c) Vasa deferentia is cut and tied
(d) Irreversible sterility

18. Which of the following approaches does not give the defined action of contraceptive?

(a)	Hormonal contraceptives	Prevent/retard entry of sperms, prevent ovulation and fertilisation
(b)	Vasectomy	Prevents spermatogenesis
(c)	Birrier methods.	Prevent fertilisation
(d)	Intra uterine devices	Increase phagocytosis of sperms, suppress sperm motility and fertilising capacity of sperms

19. Tubectomy is a method of sterilisation in which ***(2014)***
(a) small part of the fallopian tube is removed or tied up
(b) ovaries are removed surgically
(c) small part of vas deferens is removed or tied up
(d) uterus is removed surgically.

20. Which of the following is a hormone releasing Intra Uterine Device (IUD)? ***(2014)***
(a) Multiload 375 (b) LNG - 20
(c) Cervical cap (d) Vault

21. One of the following is not a method of contraception. Which one? ***(Karnataka NEET 2013)***
(a) Condoms
(b) Pills of a combination of oxytocin and vasopressin
(c) Lippes Loop
(d) Tubectomy

22. What is the figure given below showing in particular? ***(2012)***

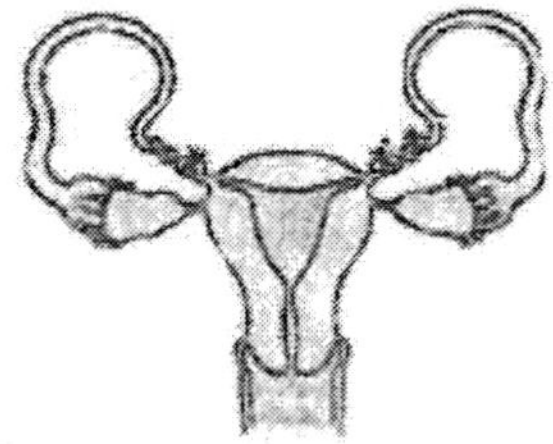

(a) Ovarian cancer (b) Uterine cancer
(c) Tubectomy (d) Vasectomy

23. Which one of the following is the most widely accepted method of contraception in India at present? ***(2011)***
(a) Cervical caps
(b) Tubectomy
(c) Diaphragms
(d) IUDs (Intra uterine devices)

24. Cu ions released from copper-releasing intra uterine devices (IUDs) ***(2010)***
(a) make uterus unsuitable for implantation
(b) increase phagocytosis of sperms
(c) suppress sperm motility
(d) prevent ovulation.

25. Given below are four methods (A-D) and their modes of action (1-iv) in achieving contraception. Select their correct matching from the four options that follow. ***(2008)***

Method	**Mode of Action**
A. The pill	(i) Prevents sperms reaching cervix
B. Condom	(ii) Prevents implantation
C. Vasectomy	(iii) Prevents ovulation
D. Copper T	(iv) Semen contains no sperms

(a) A - (iii), B - (iv), C - (i), D - (ii)
(b) A - (ii), B - (iii), C - (i), D - (iv)
(c) A - (iii), B - (i), C - (iv), D - (ii)
(d) A - (iv), B - (i), C - (ii), D - (iii)

26. What is the work of copper-T? ***(2000)***
(a) To inhibit ovulation
(b) To inhibit fertilisation
(c) To inhibit implantation of blastocyst
(d) To inhibit gametogenesis

27. What is the work of progesterone which is present in oral contraceptive pills? ***(2000)***
(a) To inhibit ovulation
(b) To check oogenesis
(c) To check entry of sperms into cervix and to make them inactive
(d) To check sexual behaviour

28. Tablets to prevent male contraception contain ***(1999)***
(a) progesterone (b) LH
(c) FSH (d) both (b) and (c).

29. The most important component of the oral contraceptive pills is ***(1998)***
(a) thyroxine (b) luteinising hormone
(c) progesterone (d) growth hormone.

MEDICAL TERMINATION OF PREGNANCY (MTP)

30. One of the legal methods of birth control is ***(2013)***
(a) by having coitus at the time of day break
(b) by a premature ejaculation during coitus
(c) abortion by taking an appropriate medicine
(d) by abstaining from coitus from day 10 to 17 of the menstrual cycle.

31. Medical Termination of Pregnancy (MTP) is considered safe up to how many weeks of pregnancy? ***(2011)***
(a) Eight weeks (b) Twelve weeks
(c) Eighteen weeks (d) Six weeks

32. Consider the statements given below regarding contraception and answer as directed *thereafter.* ***(2008)***
(1) Medical termination of pregnancy (MTP) during first trimester is generally safe.
(2) Generally chances of conception are nil until mother breast-feeds the infant upto two years.
(3) Intrauterine devices like copper-T are effective contraceptives.
(4) Contraception pills may be taken upto one week after coitus to prevent conception.

Which two of the above statements are correct?
(a) 1,3 (b) 1,2
(c) 2,3 (d) 3,4

SEXUALLY TRANSMITTED INFECTIONS (STIS)

33. Which one of the following common sexually transmitted diseases is completely curable when detected early and treated properly? **(2023)**
(a) Hepatitis-B (b) HIV Infection
(c) Genital herpes (d) Gonorrhoea

34. Veneral diseases can spread through
(A) using sterile needles
(B) transfusion of blood from infected person
(C) infected mother to fetus
(D) kissing
(E) inheritance
Choose the correct answer from the options given below. ***(2021)***
(a) (A) and (C) only
(b) (A), (B) and (C) only
(c) (B), (C) and (D) only
(d) (B) and (C) only

35. Select the option including all sexually transmitted diseases. ***(2020)***
(a) Gonorrhoea, Syphilis, Genital herpes
(b) Gonorrhoea, Malaria, Genital herpes
(c) AIDS, Malaria, Filaria
(d) Cancer, AIDS, Syphilis

36. Which of the following sexually transmitted diseases is not completely curable? ***(2019)***
(a) Chlamydiasis (b) Gonorrhoea
(c) Genital warts (d) Genital herpes

37. Match the following sexually transmitted diseases (column I) with their causative agent (column II) and select the correct option. ***(2017)***

Column I	Column II
A. Gonorrhoea	(i) HIV
B. Syphilis	(ii) Neisseria
C. Genital warts	(iii) Treponema
D. AIDS	(iv) Human papilloma virus

	A	B	C	D
(a)	(iii)	(iv)	(i)	(ii)
(b)	(iv)	(ii)	(iii)	(i)
(c)	(iv)	(iii)	(ii)	(i)
(d)	(ii)	(iii)	(iv)	(i)

38. Which of the following is not a sexually transmitted disease? (2015 Cancelled)
(a) Trichomoniasis
(b) Encephalitis
(c) Syphilis
(d) Acquired Immuno Deficiency Syndrome (AIDS)

39. Which one of the following statements is correct regarding sexually transmitted diseases (STDs)? ***(Karnataka NEET 2013)***
(a) A person may contract syphilis by sharing milk with one already suffering from the disease.
(b) Haemophilia is one of the STDs.
(c) Genital herpes and sickle-cell anaemia are both STDs.
(d) The chances of a 5-years boy contracting a STD are very little.

40. Which one of the following does correctly match a sexually transmitted disease with its pathogen? ***(1994)***
(a) Syphilis-Treponema pallidum
(b) Gonorrhoea-Entamoeba histolytica
(c) Urethritis-Bacillus anthracis
(d) Softsore-Bacillus brevis

INFERTILITY

41. In which of the following techniques, the embryos are transferred to assist those females who cannot conceive? ***(2020)***
(a) ZIFT and IUT (b) GIFT and ZIFT
(c) ICSI and ZIFT (d) GIFT and ICSI

42. In case of a couple where the male is having a very low sperm count, which technique will be suitable for fertilisation? ***(2017)***
(a) Gamete Intracytoplasmic Fallopian Transfer
(b) Artificial Insemination
(c) Intracytoplasmic sperm injection
(d) Intrauterine transfer

43. Embryo with more than 16 blastomeres formed due to in vitro fertilisation is transferred into ***(NEET-II 2016)***
(a) uterus (b) fallopian tube
(c) fimbriae (d) cervix.

44. A childless couple can be assisted to have a child through a technique called GIFT. The full form of this technique is ***(2015)***
(a) Gamete Internal Fertilisation and Transfer
(b) Germ cell Internal Fallopian Transfer
(c) Gamete Inseminated Fallopian Transfer
(d) Gamete Intra Fallopian Transfer.

45. Assisted reproductive technology, IVF involves transfer of ***(2014)***
(a) ovum into the fallopian tube
(b) zygote into the fallopian tube
(c) zygote into the uterus
(d) embryo with 16 blastomeres into the fallopian tube.

46. Artificial Insemination means ***(2013)***
(a) artificial introduction of sperms of a healthy donor into the vagina
(b) introduction of sperms of a healthy donor directly into the ovary
(c) transfer of sperms of a healthy donor to a test tube containing ova
(d) transfer of sperms of husband to a test tube containing ova.

47. The stage transferred into the uterus after induced fertilisation of ovum in the laboratory is ***(Karnataka NEET 2013)***
(a) embryo at 4 blastomeres stage
(b) embryo at 2 blastomeres stage
(c) morula
(d) zygote.

48. The test-tube baby programme employs which one of the following techniques? ***(2012)***
(a) Intra Cytoplasmic Sperm Injection (ICSI)
(b) Intra Uterine Insemination (IUI)
(c) Gamete Intra Fallopian Transfer (GIFT)
(d) Zygote Intra Fallopian Transfer (ZIFT)

49. The technique called Gamete Intra Fallopian Transfer (GIFT) is recommended for those females ***(Mains 2011)***
(a) who cannot produce an ovum
(b) who cannot retain the fetus inside uterus
(c) whose cervical canal is too narrow to allow passage for the sperms
(d) who cannot provide suitable environment for fertilisation.

50. In vitro fertilisation is a technique that involves transfer of which one of the following into the fallopian tube? ***(2010)***
(a) Embryo only, upto 8 cell stage
(b) Either zygote or early embryo upto 8 cell stage
(c) Embryo of 32 cell stage
(d) Zygote only

51. Test tube baby means a baby born when ***(2003)***
(a) it is developed in a test tube
(b) it is developed through tissue culture method
(c) the ovim is fertilised externally and thereafter implanted in the uterus
(d) it develops from a non-fertilised uterus.

52. The test tube baby means ***(1996)***
(a) fertilisation and development both in uterus
(b) fertilisation in vitro and then transplantation in uterus
(c) a baby grown in test tube
(d) fertilised and developed embryo in test tube.

53. Which of the following statements is correct with reference to a test tube baby? ***(1994)***
(a) Fertilisation of the egg is effected outside the body; the fertilised egg is then placed in the womb of the mother where the gestation is completed.
(b) Fertilisation of the egg is effected in the female genital tract. It is then taken out and grown in a large test tube.
(c) A prematurely born baby is reared in an incubator.
(d) Fertilisation of the egg and growth of the embryo are affected in a large test tube. and embryos with more than 8 blastomeres, into the uterus (IUT - Intra Uterine Transfer), to complete its further development.

ANSWER KEY

1.	(b)	2.	(b)	3.	(b)	4.	(d)	5.	(c)	6.	(d)	7.	(c)
8.	(b)	9.	(c)	10.	(c)	11.	(b)	12.	(d)	13.	(c)	14.	(a)
15.	(d)	16.	(a)	17.	(b)	18.	(b)	19.	(a)	20.	(b)	21.	(b)
22.	(c)	23.	(d)	24.	(c)	25.	(c)	26.	(b, c)	27.	(a)	28.	(d)
29.	(c)	30.	(c)	31.	(b)	32.	(a)	33.	(d)	34.	(d)	35.	(a)
36.	(d)	37.	(d)	38.	(b)	39.	(d)	40.	(a)	41.	(a)	42.	(b,c)
43.	(a)	44.	(d)	45.	(b)	46.	(a)	47.	(c)	48.	(d)	49.	(a)
50.	(b)	51.	(c)	52.	(b)	53.	(a)						

HINTS & EXPLANATIONS

1. (b) : Amniocentesis is one of the reproductive strategies. It is used to determine genetic disorder in fetus and is based on the chromosomal pattern in the amniotic fluid. It has been misused to determine sex of fetus and thus, is legally banned for the determination of sex to avoid female foeticide.

2. (b) : Amniocentesis is fetal sex determination and disorder test based on the chromosomal pattern in the amniotic fluid surrounding the developing embryo. It can be used to determine the sex of the infant, to identify some abnormalities in the number of chromosomes and to detect certain biochemicals and enzymatic abnormalities. It is usually done when woman is 14-16 weeks pregnant. Cleft palate can be detected by ultrasound.

3. (b) : Amniocentesis is a fetal sex determination test in which amniotic fluid containing fetal cells which surrounds the developing embryo is extracted and cells are tested for chromosomal pattern to identify genetic disorders, if any. Jaundice is not a chromosomal disorder thus cannot be tested by amniocentesis.

4. (d) : Amniocentesis is withdrawal of a sample of the fluid (amniotic fluid) surrounding a fetus in the uterus by piercing the amniotic sac through the abdominal wall, under direct ultrasound guidance. As the amniotic fluid contains cells from the fetus, cell cultures enable chromosome patterns to be studied so that prenatal diagnosis of chromosomal abnormalities can be made. Certain metabolic errors and other abnormalities, such as spina bifida, can also be diagnosed prenatally from analysis of the cells or of the fluid.

As this technique also helps in detection of sex of the unborn fetus, it has been banned in order to legally check increasing female feticides.

5. (c) : Barr body is a structure consisting of a condensed X chromosome that is found in non-dividing nuclei of female mammals. Amniotic fluid contains fetal skin cells, that are stained to determine the presence of sex chromatin (barr body). The presence of barr body indicates that the developing fetus is female with two X-chromosome.

6. (d) :

Vasectomy → Surgical method

Coitus interruptus → Natural method

Cervical caps → Barrier method

Saheli → Oral method

7. (c)

8. (b)

9. (c)

10. (c) : LNG-20 is an example of hormone releasing IUD which makes the uterus unsuitable for implantation and the cervix hostile to the sperms.

11. (b) : Lactational amenorrhea method is based on the fact that ovulation and therefore the menstrual cycle do not occur during the period of intense lactation following parturition. This is because breast feeding disrupts the pattern of pulsatile release of GnRH from hypothalamus and hence reduction in gonadotropin releasing hormones. Pills are hormonal preparations (either progestogen or progestogen-estrogen combinations) in the form of tablets which are administrated orally by females. They inhibit ovulation, implantation as well as alter the quality of cervical mucus. Emergency contraceptives are pills that contain levonorgestrel, a type of progestin that helps to prevent pregnancy when taken in few days after sex.

12. (d) : Lippes Loop is non-medicated Intra Uterine Device (IUD) while Multiload 375 is copper releasing IUD. Vault is a barrier method of birth control. It is a hemispheric dome-like rubber or plastic cap with thick rim meant for fitting over the vaginal cervix.

13. (c)

14. (a) : 'Saheli' is a mini pill that contains a non-steroidal preparation called centchroman which is taken once in a week after an initial intake of twice a week dose for 3 months. It blocks estrogen receptors in the uterus hence alters uterine lining and prevents fertilised egg from being implanted.

15. (d) : Copper releasing IUDs (i.e., CuT, LNG-20) are placed in the uterus of the females. They are efficient birth control methods. Copper ions released by them suppress motility and fertilising capacity of the sperms.

16. (a) : LNG-20 is the hormone releasing IUD, Multiload 375 and Cu7 are copper releasing IUDs and Lippes Loop is a non-medicated IUD.

17. (b) : Vasectomy is a surgical contraception method performed in males. In vasectomy, a small part of the vas deferens is removed or tied up through a small cut on the scrotum. This prevents sperm transport. Vasectomy has a poor reversibility. There is no effect on libido and erectile functioning. Seminal vesicles are one pair of sac like structures which join vasa deferentia to form ejaculatory duct. They secrete seminal fluid which contains fructose, prostaglandins and clotting protein, but no sperms. In a male who has undergone vasectomy, the ejaculatory duct will receive seminal fluid but due to cut in vasa deferentia sperms will not be transported from epididymis hence the semen will lack sperms.

18. (b) : Vasectomy is a sterilisation technique for the males in which a small part of the vas deferens is removed or tied up through a small cut on the scrotum to prevent passage of sperms. Spermatogenesis is the series of cell division in the testis that results in the production of spermatozoa or sperms.

19. (a) : Sterilisation provides a permanent and sure birth control. In females, it is called tubectomy. Tubectomy involves the blocking of the fallopian tubes. A small part of the fallopian tube is removed or tied up through a small incision in the abdomen or through vagina.

20. (b) : At present the most widely accepted method of contraception in India is IUDs. Intra uterine devices (IUDs) are plastic or metal objects which are inserted by doctors in the uterus through vagina. These are available as non-medicated IUDs (i.e., Lippes Loop), copper releasing IUDs (CuT, Cu7, Multiload 375) and hormone releasing IUDs (progestasert, LNG-20). Vault cap is hemispheric dome like rubber or plastic cap with a thick rim which is meant for fitting over the vaginal vault over the cervix. Cervical cap is a reusable rubber cup that fits tightly over the cervix.

21. (b) : Oxytocin is a birth hormone and vasopressin (antidiuretic hormone) reabsorbs water from the renal tubules to conserve water in the body. They have no role in contraception.

22. (c) : Tubectomy involves blocking of the fallopian tubes. The fallopian tubes are tied twice and cut between the knot. It prevents the sperms from reaching the ovum and thus prevents fertilisation. It is a permanent method of sterilisation.

23. (d)

24. (c) : Copper releasing IUDs (i.e., CuT, LNG-20) are placed in the uterus of the females. They are efficient birth control methods. Copper ions released by them suppress motility and fertilising capacity of the sperms.

25. (c)

26. (b, c) : Copper-T is an intrauterine device (IUD) used by women as a birth control. An IUD is a small device which is placed inside the uterus. The vertical and horizontal arms of the Copper - T contain copper which is slowly released into the uterine cavity. Copper stops sperm from making their way up through the uterus into the tubes, and it reduces the ability of sperm to fertilise the egg. It also prevents a fertilised egg (blastocyst) from successfully implanting in the lining of the uterus if fertilisation has occurred.

27.(a) : Pills also called contraceptive pills contain small doses of either progestogens or progestogen-estrogen combinations. They inhibit ovulation and implantation.

28.(d) : Male contraceptives work by interfering with sperm production or delivery, that means they inhibit the spermatogenesis as well as the function of male sex hormone testosterone.

LH and FSH (both called gonadotropic hormone are secreted from anterior pituitary) have specific functions in the testis. FSH stimulates male germ cells for spermatogenesis and LH stimulates accessory cells, called Leydig cells to produce sex steroids, especially testosterone. Thus, these two hormones (FSH and LH).prevent male contraception.

29.(c) : The most common type of pill is the so called "combined pill". It contains a combination of synthetic progestins (acting like progesterone) and estrogen. Combined pills inhibit ovulation by inhibiting the normal release of FSH and LH from the pituitary. They mimic the hormones produced by the corpus luteum, causing the uterine walls to thicken, as during normal menstrual cycle and suppressing the release of FSH and LH.

30.(c) : Intentional or voluntary termination of pregnancy by taking an appropriate medicine before full term is called medical termination of pregnancy (MTP) or induced abortion. Nearly

45 to 50 million MTPs are performed in a year all over the world which account to 1 / 5th of the total number of conceived pregnancies in a year. MTP has a significant role in decreasing the population though it is not meant for that purpose. Government of India legalised MTP in 1971 with some strict conditions to avoid its misuse. Such restrictions are all the more important to check indiscriminate and illegal female foeticides.

31.(b) : Medical termination of pregnancy (MTP) or abortion is the termination of pregnancy before the fetus becomes viable. MTP is comparatively safe upto 12 weeks (the first trimester) of pregnancy. It becomes more risky after the first trimester period of pregnancy as the fetus becomes intimately associated with the maternal tissues.

32.(a) : Intrauterine devices like copper-T are effective contraceptives for birth control. It suppresses sperm motility and the fertilising capacity of the sperms. Medical termination of pregnancy or induced abortion is voluntary or intentional termination of pregnancy before full term of fetus. It is comparatively safe upto 12 weeks (the first trimester) of pregnancy.

33.(d) : Except for hepatitis-B, genital herpes and HIV infections, other sexually transmitted diseases are completely curable if detected early and treated properly.

34.(d) : Veneral diseases or STDs can transmitted by sharing of injection needles, surgical instruments etc. with infected person, transfusion of blood or from an infected mother to fetus also.

35.(a) : Malaria, filaria and cancer are not sexually transmitted diseases (STDs).

36.(d) : Antibiotics like tetracycline, erythromycin and rifampicin are effective in chlamydiasis. Gonorrhoea can be treated by antibiotics such as erythromycin, ciprofloxacin, etc. For treating genital warts, cryosurgery is used for removing warts. Genital herpes is an incurable STD.

37. (d)

38. (b)

39.(d) : Syphilis is caused by bacterium Treponema pallidum. It is a sexually transmitted disease (STD) which is transferred through sexual intercourse with infected person. Haemophilia is a X-linked genetic disorder of blood. It is not transmitted via any sexual practice. Genital herpes is an STD while sickle-cell anaemia is an autosomal hereditary disorder. The chances of a 5 year boy contracting an STD are very little since he is unlikely to have sex at this age.

40. (a)

41.(a) : In vitro fertilisation, i.e.,fertilisation outside the body in almost similar conditions as that in the body, followed by embryo transfer (ET) method. In this method, ova from the wife or donor (female) and sperms from husband or donor (male) are collected and are induced to form zygote under simulated conditions in the laboratory. The zygote or early embryos (with upto 8 blastomeres) could then be transferred into the fallopian tube (ZIFT-Zygote Intra Fallopian Transfer) and embryos with more than 8 blastomeres, into the uterus (IUT - Intra Uterine Transfer), to complete its further development.

42. (b,c)

43.(a) : Embryo with more than 16 blastomeres formed due to in-vitro fertilisation is transferred into uterus (intra-uterine transfer, IUT).

44.(d) : Gamete Intra Fallopian Transfer (GIFT) is an assisted reproductive technology in which both the sperm and unfertilised oocytes are transferred into the fallopian tubes. Fertilisation takes place in vivo (inside the body of the female).

45.(b) : Assisted reproductive technologies (ART) include a number of special techniques which assist infertile couples to have children. An important technique of ART is test tube baby programme. The baby produced by conceiving in a culture dish and nursing in the uterus is called a test tube baby. This method involves in vitro fertilisation (IVF), i.e., fertilisation of male and female gamete outside the body in almost similar conditions as that in the body followed by embryo transfer (ET). Zygote or embryo upto 8 blastomeres is transferred into the fallopian tube (ZIFT - Zygote Intra Fallopian Transfer) and mature embryo with more than 8 blastomeres is transferred to uterus to complete its further development.

46.(a) : In Artificial Insemination technique, the semen of a healthy donor male is collected and is introduced artificially through a flexible polyethylene catheter into the vagina or into uterus called intra-uterine insemination (IUI). Best results are obtained when the motile sperm count is more than 10 million. The fertilising capacity of spermatozoa (sperms) is for 24- 48 hours. The procedure may be repeated 2-3 times over a period of 2–3 days.

47. (c) : Cleavage divisions produce a solid ball of cells called morula. It has 8–16 cells, occasionally 32 cells. It is transferred into uterus (IUT-Intra-uterine transfer) for further development.

48. (d)

49.(a) : Gamete Intra Fallopian Transfer (GIFT) is transfer of an ovum collected from a donor into the fallopian tube of another female who cannot produce ova but can provide proper environment for fertilisation and further development.

50. (b)

51.(c) : By in vitro fertilisation, the ovum is fertilised with sperm outside the body of a woman, providing the ovum with the same environmental conditions as it would have got inside the uterus. The zygote is grown inside a culture and when embryo is formed, it is then implanted into uterus where it develops into fetus and then into a child. This is called test tube baby.

52. (b)

53. (a)

Chapter : 23 PRINCIPLES OF INHERITANCE AND VARIATION

MENDEL'S LAWS OF INHERITANCE

1. Given below are two statements : ***(2022)***

Statement I : Mendel studied seven pairs of contrasting traits in pea plants and proposed the laws of inheritance.

Statement II: Seven characters examined by Mendel in his experiment on pea plants were seed shape and colour, flower colour, pod shape and colour, flower position and stem height.

In the light of the above statements, choose the correct answer from the options given below :

(a) Both Statement I and Statement II are correct
(b) Both Statement I and Statement II are incorrect
(c) Statement I is correct but Statement II is incorrect
(d) Statement I is incorrect but Statement II is correct

2. How many true breeding pea plant varieties did Mendel select as pairs, which were similar except in one character with contrasting traits? ***(2020)***

(a) 4 (b) 2
(c) 14 (d) 8

3. Among the following characters, which one was not considered by Mendel in his experiments on pea? ***(2017)***

(a) Trichomes-Glandular or non-glandular
(b) Seed-Green or yellow
(c) Pod-Inflated or constricted
(d) Stem-Tall or dwarf

4. Which one from those given below is the period for Mendel's hybridisation experiments? ***(2017)***

(a) 1840-1850 (b) 1857-1869
(c) 1870-1877 (d) 1856-1863

5. In his classic experiments on pea plants, Mendel did not use ***(2015)***

(a) seed shape (b) flower position
(c) seed colour (d) pod length.

6. How many pairs of contrasting characters in pea plants were studied by Mendel in his experiments? ***(2015 Cancelled)***

(a) Eight (b) Seven
(c) Five (d) Six

7. Which one of the following traits of garden pea studied by Mendel was a recessive feature? ***(2003)***

(a) Axial flower position
(b) Green seed colour
(c) Green pod colour
(d) Round seed shape

8. The genes controlling the seven pea characters studied by Mendel are now known to be located on how many different chromosomes? ***(2003)***

(a) Seven (b) Six
(c) Five (d) Four

9. According to Mendelism, which character shows dominance? ***(2000)***

(a) Terminal position of flower
(b) Green colour in seed coat
(c) Wrinkled seeds
(d) Green pod colour

10. First geneticist/father of genetics was ***(1991)***

(a) De Vries (b) Mendel
(c) Darwin (d) Morgan.

11. Which contribute to the success of Mendel? ***(1988)***

(a) Qualitative analysis of data
(b) Observation of distinct inherited traits
(c) His knowledge of biology
(d) Consideration of one character at one time

INHERITANCE OF ONE GENE

12. The production of gametes by the parents, formation of zygotes, the F1 and F2 plants, can be understood from a diagram called ***(2021)***

(a) net square (b) bullet square
(c) punch square (d) Punnett square

13. In a cross between a male and female, both heterozygous for sickle cell anaemia gene, what percentage of the progeny will be diseased? ***(2021)***

(a) 100% (b) 50%
(c) 75% (d) 25%

14. Identify the wrong statement with reference to the gene ' I that controls ABO blood groups. ***(2020)***

(a) The gene (I) has three alleles.
(b) A person will have only two of the three alleles.
(c) When IA and IB are present together, they express same type of sugar.
(d) Allele i does not produce any sugar.

15. In Antirrhinum (Snapdragon), a red flower was crossed with a white flower and in F1 generation all pink flowers were obtained. When pink flowers were selfed, the F2 generation showed white, red and pink flowers. Choose the incorrect statements from the following. ***(2019)***

(a) Law of segregation does not apply in this experiment.
(b) This experiment does not follow the Principle of Dominance.
(c) Pink colour in F1 is due to incomplete dominance.
(d) Ratio of F2 is 1/4 (red) : 2/4 (pink) : 1/4 (white).

16. The genotypes of a husband and wife are IA IB and IA i. Among the blood types of their children, how many different genotypes and phenotypes are possible? ***(2017)***

(a) 3 genotypes; 4 phenotypes
(b) 4 genotypes; 3 phenotypes
(c) 4 genotypes; 4 phenotypes
(d) 3 genotypes; 3 phenotypes

17. A tall true breeding garden pea plant is crossed with a dwarf true breeding garden pea plant. When the F1 plants were selfed the resulting genotypes were in the ratio of ***(NEET-I 2016)***

(a) 3 : 1 : : Tall : Dwarf
(b) 3 : 1 : : Dwarf : Tall
(c) 1 : 2 : 1 : : Tall homozygous : Tall heterozygous : Dwarf
(d) 1 : 2 : 1 : : Tall heterozygous : Tall homozygous : Dwarf.

18. A gene showing co-dominance has ***(2015)***

(a) alleles that are recessive to each other
(b) both alleles independently expressed in the heterozygote
(c) one allele dominant on the other
(d) alleles tightly linked on the same chromosome.

19. Alleles are ***(2015 Cancelled)***

(a) different molecular forms of a gene
(b) heterozygotes
(c) different phenotype
(d) true breeding homozygotes.

20. Multiple alleles are present ***(2015 Cancelled)***

(a) at the same locus of the chromosome
(b) on non-sister chromatids
(c) on different chromosomes
(d) at different loci on the same chromosome.

21. A man with blood group 'A' marries a woman with blood group 'B'. What are all the possible blood groups of their offspring? ***(2015 Cancelled)***

(a) A, B, AB and O (b) O only
(c) A and B only (d) A, B and AB only

22. If two persons with 'AB' blood group marry and have sufficiently large number of children, these children could be classified as 'A' blood group:

'AB' blood group: 'B' blood group in 1 : 2 : 1 ratio. Modern technique of protein electrophoresis

reveals presence of both 'A' and 'B' type proteins in 'AB' blood group individuals. This in an example of ***(2013)***
(a) partial dominance
(b) complete dominance
(c) co-dominance
(d) incomplete dominance.

23. Which idea is depicted by a cross in which the F1 generation resembles both the parents? ***(2013)***
(a) Inheritance of one gene
(b) Co-dominance
(c) Incomplete dominance
(d) Complete dominance

24. F2 generation in a Mendelian cross showed that both genotypic and phenotypic ratios are same as 1:2:1. It represents a case of ***(2012)***
(a) co-dominance
(b) dihybrid cross
(c) monohybrid cross with complete dominance
(d) monohybrid cross with incomplete dominance.

25. A test cross is carried out to ***(Mains 2012)***
(a) determine the genotype of a plant at F2
(b) predict whether two traits are linked
(c) assess the number of alleles of a gene
(d) determine whether two species or varieties will breed successfully.

26. Test cross in plants or in Drosophila involves crossing ***(Mains 2011)***
(a) between two genotypes with recessive trait
(b) between two F1 hybrids
(c) the F1 hybrid with a double recessive genotype
(d) between two genotypes with dominant trait.

27. ABO blood groups in humans are controlled by the gene I. It has three alleles - IA,IB and i. Since there are three different alleles, six different genotypes are possible. How many phenotypes can occur? ***(2010)***
(a) Three (b) One
(c) Four (d) Two

28. The genotype of a plant showing the dominant phenotype can be determined by ***(2010)***
(a) test cross (b) dihybrid cross
(c) pedigree analysis (d) back cross.

29. Which one of the following cannot be explained on the basis of Mendel's law of dominance? ***(2010)***
(a) The discrete unit controlling a particular character is called a factor.
(b) Out of one pair of factors one is dominant, and the other recessive.
(c) Alleles do not show any blending and both the characters recover as such in F2 generation.
(d) Factors occur in pairs.

30. ABO blood grouping is controlled by gene I which has three alleles and show co-dominance. There are six genotypes. How many phenotypes in all are possible? ***(Mains 2010)***
(a) Six (b) Three
(c) Four (d) Five

31. A cross in which an organism showing a dominant phenotype is crossed with the recessive parent in order to know its genotype is called ***(Mains 2010)***
(a) monohybrid cross (b) back cross
(c) test cross (d) dihybrid cross.

32. In Antirrhinum two plants with pink flowers were hybridized. The F1 plants produced red, pink and white flowers in the proportion of 1 red, 2 pink and 1 white. What could be the genotype of the two plants used for hybridisation? Red flower colour is determined by RR and white by rr genes. ***(Mains 2010)***
(a) rrrr (b) RR
(c) Rr (d) rr

33. In pea plants, yellow seeds are dominant to green. If a heterozygous yellow seeded plant is crossed with a green seeded plant, what ratio of yellow and green seeded plants would you expect in F1 generation? ***(2007)***

(a) 9:1 (b) 1:3
(c) 3:1 (d) 50:50

34. A common test to find the genotype of a hybrid is by ***(2007)***

(a) crossing of one F2 progeny with female parent
(b) studying the sexual behaviour of F1 progenies
(c) crossing of one F1 progeny with male parent
(d) crossing of one F2 progeny with male parent.

35. Test cross involves ***(2006)***

(a) crossing between two genotypes with dominant trait
(b) crossing between two genotypes with recessive trait
(c) crossing between two F1 hybrids
(d) crossing the F1 hybrid with a double recessive genotype.

36. Phenotype of an organism is the result of ***(2006)***

(a) genotype and environment interactions
(b) mutations and linkages
(c) cytoplasmic effects and nutrition
(d) environmental changes and sexual dimorphism.

37. A gene is said to be dominant if ***(2002)***

(a) it expresses its effect only in homozygous state
(b) it expresses its effect only in heterozygous condition
(c) it expresses its effect both in homozygous and heterozygous condition
(d) it never expresses its effect in any condition.

38. When dominant and recessive alleles express itself together it is called ***(2001)***

(a) co-dominance (b) dominance
(c) amphidominance (d) pseudodominance.

39. In hybridisation, Tt × tt gives rise to the progeny of ratio ***(1999)***

(a) 2:1 (b) 1:2:1
(c) 1:1 (d) 1:2.

40. A child's blood group is 'O'. The parent's blood groups cannot be ***(1994)***

(a) A and B (b) A and A
(c) AB and O (d) B and O.

41. A child of O-group has B-group father. The genotype of father will be ***(1992)***

(a) IO IO (c) IA IB
(b) IB IB (d) IB IO

42. An allele is dominant if it is expressed in ***(1992)***

(a) both homozygous and heterozygous states
(b) second generation
(c) heterozygous combination
(d) homozygous combination.

43. An organism with two identical alleles is (1992)

(a) dominant (b) hybrid
(c) heterozygous (d) homozygous.

44. A man of A-blood group marries a woman of AB blood group. Which type of progeny would indicate that man is heterozygous A ? ***(1991)***

(a) AB (b) A
(c) O (d) B

45. Multiple alleles control inheritance of ***(1991)***

(a) phenylketonuria (b) colour blindness
(c) sickle cell anaemia (d) blood groups.

46. The contrasting pairs of factors in Mendelian crosses are called ***(1991)***

(a) multiple alleles (b) allelomorphs
(c) alloloci (d) paramorphs.

47. Mendel's last law is ***(1991)***

(a) segregation
(b) dominance
(c) independent assortment
(d) polygenic inheritance.

48. Blue eye colour is recessive to brown eye colour. A brown eyed man whose mother was blue eyed marries a blue-eyed woman. The children will be ***(1991)***
(a) both blue eyed and brown eyed 1:1
(b) all brown eyed
(c) all blue eyed
(d) blue eyed and brown eyed 3:1.

49. RR (Red) Antirrhinum is crossed with white (rr) one. Offspring Rr are pink. This is an example of ***(1991)***
(a) dominant-recessive
(b) incomplete dominance
(c) hybrid
(d) supplementary genes.

50. ABO blood group system is due to ***(1990)***
(a) multifactor inheritance
(b) incomplete dominance
(c) multiple allelism
(d) epistasis.

51. tt mates with Tt. What will be characteristic of offspring? ***(1990)***
(a) 75% recessive (b) 50% recessive
(c) 25% recessive (d) All dominant

52. Haploids are able to express both recessive and dominant alleles/mutations because there are ***(1988)***
(a) many alleles for each gene
(b) two alleles for each gene
(c) only one allele for each gene in the individual
(d) only one allele in a gene.

INHERITANCE OF TWO GENES

53. Frequency of recombination between gene pairs on same chromosome as a measure of the distance between genes to map their position on chromosome, was used for the first time by ***(2023)***
(a) Alfred Sturtevant
(b) Henking
(c) Thomas Hunt Morgan
(d) Sutton and Boveri.

54. Given below are two statements : one is labelled as Assertion (A) and the other is labelled as Reason (R).

Assertion (A) : Mendel's law of independent assortment does not hold good for the genes that are located closely on the same chromosome.

Reason (R) : Closely located genes assort independently.

In the light of the above statements, choose the correct answer from the options given below : ***(2022)***
(a) Both (A) and (R) are correct and (R) is the correct explanation of (A)
(b) Both (A) and (R) are correct but (R) is not the correct explanation of (A)
(c) (A) is correct but (R) is not correct.
(d) (A) is not correct but (R) is correct.

55. The recombination frequency between the genes a & c is 5%, b & c is 15%, b & d is 9%, a & b is 20%, c & d is 24% and a & d is 29%. What will be the sequence of these genes on a linear chromosome? ***(2022)***
(a) a,d,b,c (c) a,b,c,d
(b) d,b,a,c (d) a,c,b,d

56. Experimental verification of the chromosomal theory of inheritance was done by ***(2020)***
(a) Mendel (b) Sutton
(c) Boveri (d) Morgan.

57. What map unit (centimorgan) is adopted in the construction of genetic maps? ***(2019)***
(a) A unit of distance between genes on chromosomes, representing 50% cross over.
(b) A unit of distance between two expressed genes, representing 10% cross over.
(c) A unit of distance between two expressed genes, representing 100% cross over.
(d) A unit of distance between genes on chromosomes, representing 1% cross over.

58. The frequency of recombination between gene present on the same chromosome as a measure of the distance between genes was explained by ***(2019)***

(a) Sutton Boveri (b) T.H. Morgan
(c) Gregor J.Mendel (d) Alfred Sturtevant.

59. The mechanism that causes a gene to move from one linkage group to another is called ***(NEET-II 2016)***

(a) inversion (b) duplication
(c) translocation (d) crossing-over.

60. In a test cross involving F1 dihybrid flies, more parental-type offspring were produced than the recombinant-type offspring. This indicates ***(NEET-I 2016)***

(a) the two genes are linked and present on the same chromosome
(b) both of the characters are controlled by more than one gene
(c) the two genes are located on two different chromosomes
(d) chromosomes failed to separate during meiosis.

61. The term "linkage" was coined by ***(2015)***

(a) G. Mendel (b) W. Sutton
(c) T.H. Morgan (d) T. Boveri.

62. The movement of a gene from one linkage group to another is called ***(2015 Cancelled)***

(a) translocation (b) crossing over
(c) inversion (d) duplication.

63. Fruit colour in squash is an example of ***(2014)***

(a) recessive epistasis
(b) dominant epistasis
(c) complementary genes
(d) inhibitory genes

64. Which of the following statements is not true of two genes that show 50% recombination frequency? ***(2013)***

(a) The gene show independent assortment.
(b) If the genes are present on the same chromosome, they undergo more than one cross-overs in every meiosis.
(c) The genes may be on different chromosomes.
(d) The genes are tightly linked.

65. When two unrelated individuals or lines are crossed, the performance of F1 hybrid is often superior to both its parents. This phenomenon is called ***(2011)***

(a) heterosis (b) transformation
(c) splicing (d) metamorphosis.

66. Select the correct statement from the ones given below with respect to dihybrid cross. ***(2010)***

(a) Tightly linked genes on the same chromosomes show higher recombinations.
(b) Genes far apart on the same chromosome show very few recombinations.
(c) Genes loosely linked on the same chromosome show similar recombinations.
(d) Tightly linked genes on the same chromosome show very few recombinations.

67. A human male produces sperms with the genotypes AB, Ab, aB and ab pertaining to two diallelic characters in equal proportions. What is the corresponding genotype of this person? ***(2007)***

(a) AaBB (b) AABb
(c) AABB (d) AaBb

68. In Mendel's experiments with garden pea, round seed shape (RR) was dominant over wrinkled seeds (rr), yellow cotyledon (YY) was dominant over green cotyledon (yy). What are the expected phenotypes in the F2 generation of the cross RRYY × rryy? ***(2006)***

(a) Round seeds with yellow cotyledons, and wrinkled seeds with yellow cotyledons
(b) Only round seeds with green cotyledons
(c) Only wrinkled seeds with yellow cotyledons
(d) Only wrinkled seeds with green cotyledons

69. In order to find out the different types of gametes produced by a pea plant having the genotype AaBb it should be crossed to a plant with the genotype ***(2005)***
(a) AABB (b) AaBb
(c) aabb (d) aaBB.

70. In a plant, red fruit (R) is dominant over yellow fruit (r) and tallness (T) is dominant over shortness (t). If a plant with RRTt genotype is crossed with a plant that is rrtt, ***(2004)***
(a) 25% will be tall with red fruit
(b) 50% will be tall with red fruit
(c) 75% will be tall with red fruit
(d) all the offspring will be tall with red fruit.

71. Lack of independent assortment of two genes A and B in fruit fly Drosophila is due to ***(2004)***
(a) repulsion (b) recombination
(c) linkage (d) crossing over.

72. There are three genes a,b,c. Percentage of crossing over between a and b is 20%,b and c is 28% and a and c is 8%. What is the sequence of genes on chromosome? ***(2002)***
(a) b,a,c (b) a,b,c
(c) a,c,b (d) None of these

73. A and B genes are linked. What shall be genotype of progeny in a cross between AB/ab and ab/ab ? ***(2001)***
(a) AAbb and aabb (b) AaBb and aabb
(c) AABB and aabb (d) None of these

74. Independent assortment of genes does not take place when ***(2001)***
(a) genes are located on homologous chromosomes
(b) genes are linked and located on same chromosome
(c) genes are located on non-homogenous chromosome
(d) all of these.

75. Due to the cross between TTRr × ttrr the resultant progenies show what percent of tall, red flowered plants? ***(2000)***
(a) 50% (b) 75%
(c) 25% (d) 100%

76. If Mendel had studied the seven traits using a plant with 12 chromosomes instead of 14 , in what way would his interpretation have been different? ***(1998)***
(a) He would not have discovered the law of independent assortment.
(b) He would have discovered sex linkage.
(c) He could have mapped the chromosome.
(d) He would have discovered blending or incomplete dominance.

77. Crossing over in diploid organism is responsible for ***(1998)***
(a) segregation of alleles
(b) recombination of linked alleles
(c) dominance of genes
(d) linkage between genes.

78. In a cross between AABB× aabb, the ratio of F2 genotypes between AABB, AaBB,Aabb and aabb would be ***(1992)***
(a) 9 : 3 : 3 : 1 (b) 2 : 1 : 1 : 2
(c) 1 : 2 : 2 : 1 (d) 7 : 5 : 3 : 1

79. Segregation of Mendelian factors (no linkage, no crossing over) occurs during ***(1992)***
(a) anaphase I (b) anaphase II
(c) diplotene (d) metaphase I.

80. The allele which is unable to express its effect in the presence of another is called ***(1991)***
(a) codominant (b) supplementary
(c) complementary (d) recessive.

81. Cross between AaBB and aaBB will form ***(1990)***
(a) 1AaBB : 1aaBB (b) all AaBB
(c) 3AaBB : 1aaBB (d) 1AaBB : 3aaBB

82. Segregation of Mendelian factor (Aa) occurs during ***(1990)***
(a) diplotene
(b) anaphase I
(c) zygotene/pachytene
(d) anaphase II.

POLYGENIC INHERITANCE

83. Which of the following characteristics represent 'inheritance of blood groups' in humans? ***(2018)***

(i) Dominance

(ii) Co-dominance

(iii) Multiple allele

(iv) Incomplete dominance

(v) Polygenic inheritance

(a) (ii), (iii) and (v) (b) (i), (ii) and (iii)
(c) (ii), (iv) and (v) (d) (i), (iii) and (v)

84. Inheritance of skin colour in humans is an example of ***(2007)***
(a) point mutation
(b) polygenic inheritance
(c) codominance
(d) chromosomal aberration.

85. How many different kinds of gametes will be produced by a plant having the genotype AABbCC ? ***(2006)***
(a) Two (b) Three
(c) Four (d) Nine

86. Which one of the following is an example of polygenic inheritance? ***(2006)***
(a) Skin colour in humans
(b) Flower colour in Mirabilis jalapa
(c) Production of male honeybee
(d) Pod shape in garden pea

87. On selfing a plant of F1-generation with genotype "AABbCC", the genotypic ratio in F2-generation will be ***(2002)***
(a) 3 : 1 (b) 1 : 1
(c) 9 : 3 : 3 : 1 (d) 27 : 9 : 9 : 9 : 3 : 3 : 3 : 1.

88. In human beings, multiple genes are involved in the inheritance of ***(1999)***
(a) sickle-cell anaemia (b) skin colour
(c) colour blindness (d) phenylketonuria.

89. How many different types of genetically different gametes will be produced by a heterozygous plant having the genotype AABbCc ? ***(1998)***
(a) Six (b) Nine
(c) Two (d) Four

90. The polygenic genes show ***(1996)***
(a) different karyotypes
(b) different genotypes
(c) different phenotypes
(d) none of these.

91. A polygenic inheritance in human beings is ***(1993)***
(a) skin colour (b) phenylketonuria
(c) colour blindness (d) sickle cell anaemia.

PLEIOTROPY

92. The phenomenon of pleiotropism refers to ***(2023)***
(a) a single gene affecting multiple phenotypic expression
(b) more than two genes affecting a single character
(c) presence of several alleles of a single gene controlling a single crossover
(d) presence of two alleles, each of the two genes controlling a single trait.

93. Match the terms in column I with their description in column II and choose the correct option. ***(NEET-I 2016)***

Column I	Column II
A. Dominance	(i) Many genes govern a single character
B. Co-dominance	(ii) In a heterozygous organism only one allele expresses itself
C. Pleiotropy	(iii) In a heterozygous organism both alleles express themselves fully
D. Polygenic	(iv) A single gene inheritance influences many characters

	A	B	C	D
(a)	(iv)	(i)	(ii)	(iii)
(b)	(iv)	(iii)	(i)	(ii)
(c)	(ii)	(i)	(iv)	(iii)
(d)	(ii)	(iii)	(iv)	(i)

94. A pleiotropic gene ***(2015)***
(a) controls a trait only in combination with another gene
(b) controls multiple traits in an individual
(c) is expressed only in primitive plants
(d) is a gene evolved during Pliocene.

95. Which of the following is an example of pleiotropy? ***(2002)***
(a) Haemophilia (b) Thalassemia
(c) Sickle cell anaemia (d) Colour blindness

96. When a single gene influences more than one trait it is called ***(1998)***
(a) pseudodominance (b) pleiotropy
(c) epistasis (d) none of these.

SEX DETERMINATION

97. XO type of sex determination can be found in : ***2022)***
(a) Drosophila (b) Birds
(c) Grasshoppers (d) Monkeys

98. Select the incorrect statement. ***(2019)***
(a) Human males have one of their sex-chromosome much shorter than other.
(b) Male fruit fly is heterogametic.
(c) In male grasshoppers, 50% of sperms have no sex-chromosome.
(d) In domesticated fowls, sex of progeny depends on the type of sperm rather than egg.

99. Which of the following pairs is wrongly matched? ***(2018)***
(a) Starch synthesis in pea : Multiple alleles
(b) ABO blood grouping : Co-dominance
(c) XO type sex determination: Grasshopper
(d) T.H. Morgan : Linkage

100. Which one of the following conditions of the zygotic cell would lead to the birth of a normal human female child? ***(Mains 2011)***
(a) Two X chromosomes
(b) Only one Y chromosome
(c) Only one X chromosome
(d) One X and one Y chromosome

101. In Drosophila, the sex is determined by ***(2003)***
(a) the ratio of number of X-chromosome to the sets of autosomes
(b) X and Y chromosomes
(c) the ratio of pairs of X-chromosomes to the pairs of autosomes
(d) whether the egg is fertilized or develops parthenogenetically.

102. Number of Barr bodies in XXXX female is ***(2001)***
(a) 1 (b) 2
(c) 3 (d) 4

103. Male XX and female XY sometime occur due to ***(2001)***
(a) deletion
(b) transfer of segments in X and Y chromosome
(c) aneuploidy
(d) hormonal imbalance.

104. Probability of four sons to a couple is (2001)
(a) 1/4 (b) 1/8
(c) 1/16 (d) 1/32.

105. Genetic identity of a human male is determined by ***(1997)***
(a) sex-chromosome
(b) cell organelles
(c) autosome
(d) nucleolus.

106. Sex is determined in human beings ***(1993)***
(a) by ovum
(b) at time of fertilisation
(c) 40 days after fertilisation
(d) seventh to eight week when genitals differentiate in fetus.

107. A family of five daughter only is expecting sixth issue. The chance of its being a son is ***(1988)***

(a) zero (b) 25%
(c) 50% (d) 100%.

MUTATION

108. Which of the following occurs due to the presence of autosome linked dominant trait? ***(2022)***

(a) Sickle cell anaemia (b) Myotonic dystrophy
(c) Haemophilia (d) Thalessemia

109. If a colourblind female marries a man whose mother was also colourblind, what are the chances of her progeny having colour blindness ? **(2022)**

(a) 25% (b) 50% (c) 75% (d) 100%

110. One of the parents of a cross has a mutation in its mitochondria. In that cross, that parent is taken as a male. During segregation of F2 progenies that mutation is found in ***(2004)***

(a) one-third of the progenies
(b) none of the progenies
(c) all the progenies
(d) fifty percent of the progenies.

111. The most striking example of point mutation is found in a disease called ***(1995)***

(a) Down's syndrome
(b) sickle cell anaemia
(c) thalassaemia
(d) night blindness.

GENETIC DISORDERS

112. Which one of the following symbols represents mating between relatives in human pedigree analysis? ***(2023)***

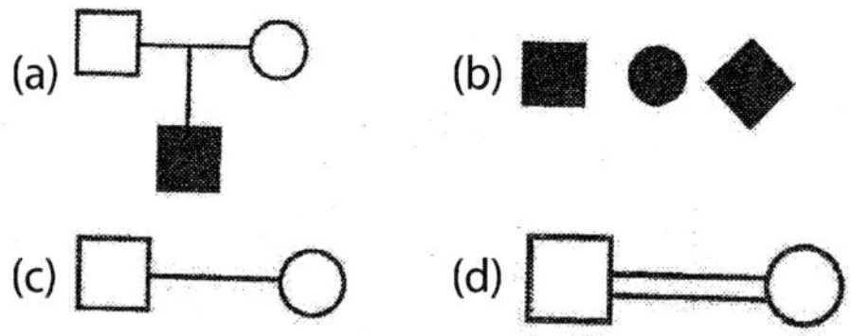

113. Which of the following statements are correct about Klinefelter's Syndrome? ***(2023)***

A. This disorder was first described by Langdon Down (1866).

B. Such an individual has overall masculine development. However, the feminine development is also expressed.

C. The affected individual is short statured.

D. Physical, psychomotor and mental development is retarded.

E. Such individuals are sterile.

Choose the correct answer from the options given below:

(a) B and E only (b) A and E only
(c) A and B only (d) C and D only

114. Broad palm with single palm crease in a person suffering from ***(2023)***

(a) Klinefelter's syndrome
(b) Thalassemia
(c) Down's syndrome
(d) Turner's syndrome

115. Select the correct match. ***(2020)***

(a) Haemophilia -Y linked
(b) Phenylketonuria - Autosomal dominant trait
(c) Sickle cell anaemia - Autosomal recessive trait, chromosome -11
(d) Thalassemia – X linked

116. What is the genetic disorder in which an individual has an overall masculine development, genetic disorder in which an individual has an overall masculine development, gynaecomastia and is sterile? ***(2019)***

(a) Down's syndrome
(b) Turner's syndrome
(c) Klinefelter's syndrome
(d) Edward syndrome

117. A woman has an X-linked condition on one of her X chromosomes. This chromosome can be inherited by ***(2018)***
(a) only daughters
(b) only sons
(c) only grandchildren
(d) both sons and daughters.

118. Thalassemia and sickle cell anaemia are caused due to a problem in globin molecule synthesis. Select the correct statement ***(2017)***
(a) Both are due to a quantitative defect in globin chain synthesis.
(b) Thalassemia is due to less synthesis of globin molecules.
(c) Sickle cell anaemia is due to a quantitative problem of globin molecules.
(d) Both are due to a qualitative defect in globin chain synthesis.

119. A disease caused by an autosomal primary non disjunction is ***(2017)***
(a) Klinefelter's syndrome
(b) Turner's syndrome
(c) Sickle cell anaemia
(d) Down's syndrome.

120. If a colour-blind man marries a woman who is homozygous for normal colour vision, the probability of their son being colour-blind is ***(NEET-II 2016)***
(a) 0 (b) 0.5 (c) 0.75 (d) 1

121. Pick out the correct statements. (NEET-I 2016)
(1) Haemophilia is a sex-linked recessive disease
(2) Down's syndrome is due to aneuploidy.
(3) Phenylketonuria is an autosomal recessive gene disorder.
(4) Sickle cell anaemia is an X-linked recessive gene disorder.
(a) (1), (3) and (4) are correct.
(b) (1), (2) and (3) are correct.
(c) (1) and (4) are correct.
(d) (2) and (4) are correct.

122. Which of the following most appropriately describes haemophilia? ***(NEET-I 2016)***
(a) Chromosomal disorder
(b) Dominant gene disorder
(c) Recessive gene disorder
(d) X-linked recessive gene disorder

123. A colour blind man marries a woman with normal sight who has no history of colour blindness in her family. What is the probability of their grandson being colour blind ? ***(2015)***
(a) Nil (b) 0.25 (c) 0.5 (d) 1

124. In the following human pedigree, the filled symbols represent the affected individuals. Identify the type of given pedigree. ***(2015)***

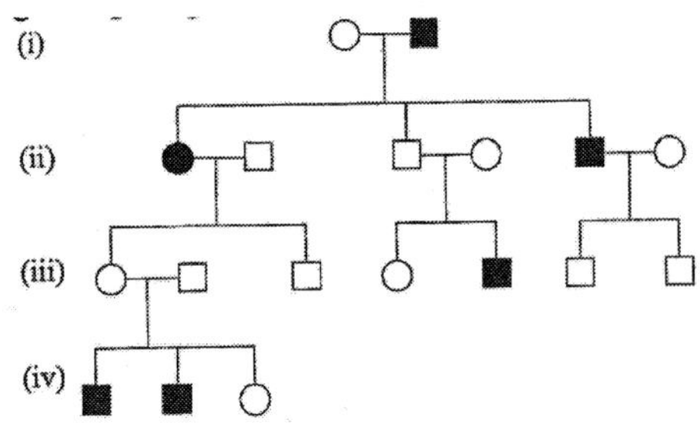

(a) Autosomal recessive
(b) X-linked dominant
(c) Autosomal dominant
(d) X-linked recessive

125. An abnormal human baby with 'XXX' sex chromosomes was born due to ***(2015 Cancelled)***
(a) fusion of two ova and one sperm
(b) fusion of two sperms and one ovum
(c) formation of abnormal sperms in the father
(d) formation of abnormal ova in the mother.

126. A man whose father was colour blind marries a woman who had a colour blind mother and normal father. What percentage of male children of this couple will be colour blind? (2014)
(a) 25% (b) 0% (c) 50% (d) 75%

127. A human female with Turner's syndrome **(2014)**

(a) has 45 chromosomes with XO
(b) has one additional X chromosome
(c) exhibits male characters
(d) is able to produce children with normal husband.

128. Select the incorrect statement with regard to haemophilia. **(2013)**

(a) It is a dominant disease.
(b) A single protein involved in the clotting of blood is affected.
(c) It is a sex-linked disease.
(d) It is a recessive disease.

129. If both parents are carriers for thalassaemia, which is an autosomal recessive disorder, what are the chances of pregnancy resulting in an affected child? **(2013)**

(a) 25% (b) 100%
(c) No chance (d) 50%

130. Which one is the incorrect statement with regard to the importance of pedigree analysis? ***(Karnataka NEET 2013)***

(a) It confirms that DNA is the carrier of genetic information.
(b) It helps to understand whether the trait in question is dominant or recessive.
(c) It confirms that the trait is linked to one of the autosome.
(d) It helps to trace the inheritance of a specific trait.

131. Down's syndrome in humans is due to ***(Karnataka NEET 2013)***

(a) three 'X' chromosomes
(b) three copies of chromosome 21
(c) monosomy
(d) two 'Y' chromosomes.

132. A normal-visioned man whose father was colourblind, marries a woman whose father was also colour-blind. They have their first child as a daughter. What are the chances that this child would be colour-blind? **(2012)**

(a) 100% (b) Zero percent
(c) 25% (d) 50%

133. Represented here is the inheritance pattern of a certain type of trait in humans. Which one of the following conditions could be an example of this pattern? ***(Mains 2012)***

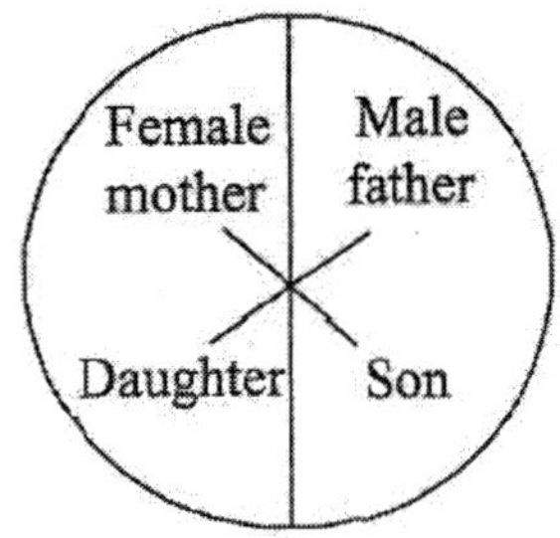

(a) Phenylketonuria
(b) Sickle cell anaemia
(c) Haemophilia
(d) Thalassemia

134. Which one of the following conditions correctly describes the manner of determining the sex? **(2011)**

(a) Homozygous sex chromosomes (ZZ) determine female sex in birds.
(b) XO type of sex chromosomes determine male sex in grasshopper.
(c) XO condition in humans as found in Turner's syndrome, determines female sex.
(d) Homozygous sex chromosomes (XX) produce male in Drosophila.

135. Which one of the following symbols and its representation, used in human pedigree analysis is correct? **(2010)**

(a) 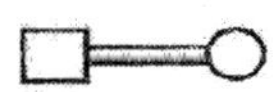 – Mating between relatives

(b) 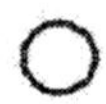 = Unaffected male

(c) 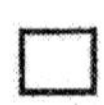 = Unaffected female

(d)  = Male affected

136. Study the pedigree chart of a certain family given below and select the correct conclusion which can be drawn for the character. ***(Mains 2010)***

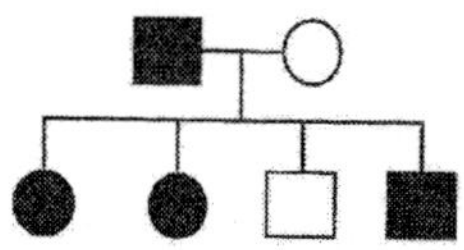

(a) The female parent is heterozygous.
(b) The parents could not have had a normal daughter for this character.
(c) The trait under study could not be colour blindness.
(d) The male parent is homozygous dominant.

137. Sickle-cell anaemia is ***(2009)***
(a) caused by substitution of valine by glutamic acid in the beta globin chain of haemoglobin
(b) caused by a change in a single base pair of DNA
(c) characterized by elongated sickle like RBCs with a nucleus
(d) an autosomal linked dominant trait.

138. Study the pedigree chart given below. What does it show? ***(2009)***

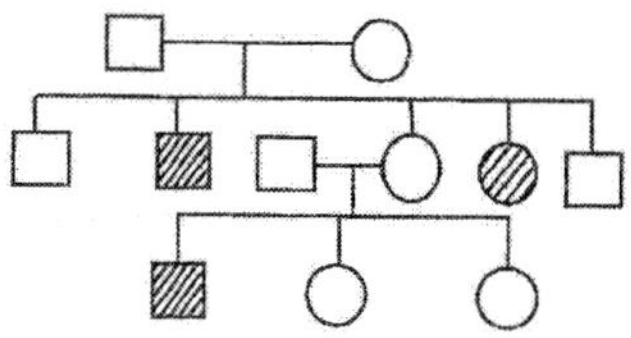

(a) Inheritance of a condition like phenylketonuria as an autosomal recessive trait.
(b) The pedigree chart is wrong as this is not possible.
(c) Inheritance of a recessive sex-linked disease like haemophilia.
(d) Inheritance of a sex-linked inborn error of metabolism like phenylketonuria.

139. Which one of the following conditions in humans is correctly matched with its chromosomal abnormality/linkage? ***(2008)***
(a) Erythroblastosis fetalis - X-linked
(b) Down's syndrome - 44 autosomes +XO
(c) Klinefelter's syndrome - 44 autosomes + XXY
(d) Colour blindness - Y-linked

140. Both sickle cell anaemia and Huntington's chorea are ***(2006)***
(a) virus-related diseases
(b) bacteria-related diseases
(c) congenital disorders
(d) pollutant-induced disorders.

141. If a colour blind woman marries a normal visioned man, their sons will be ***(2006)***
(a) all colour blind
(b) all normal visioned
(c) one-half colour blind and one-half normal
(d) three-fourths colour blind and one-fourth normal.

142. Cri-du-chat syndrome in humans is caused by the ***(2006)***
(a) trisomy of 21st chromosome
(b) fertilisation of an XX egg by a normal Y-bearing sperm
(c) loss of half of the short arm of chromosome 5
(d) loss of half of the long arm of chromosome 5.

143. Sickle cell anaemia has not been eliminated from the African population because ***(2006)***
(a) it is controlled by dominant genes
(b) it is controlled by recessive genes
(c) it is not a fatal disease
(d) it provides immunity against malaria.

144. A man and a woman, who do not show any apparent signs of a certain inherited disease, have seven children (2 daughters and 5 sons). Three of the sons suffer from the given disease but none of the daughters affected. Which of the following mode of inheritance do you suggest for this disease? ***(2005)***
(a) Sex-linked dominant
(b) Sex-linked recessive
(c) Sex-limited recessive
(d) Autosomal dominant

145. A woman with 47 chromosomes due to three copies of chromosome 21 is characterised by ***(2005)***
(a) superfemaleness
(b) triploidy
(c) Turner's syndrome
(d) Down's syndrome.

146. Haemophilia is more commonly seen in human males than in human females because ***(2005)***
(a) a greater proportion of girls die in infancy
(b) this disease is due to a Y-linked recessive mutation
(c) this disease is due to an X-linked recessive mutation
(d) this disease is due to an X-linked dominant mutation.

147. Which of the following is not a hereditary disease? ***(2005)***
(a) Cystic fibrosis (b) Thalassaemia
(c) Haemophilia (d) Cretinism

148. A woman with normal vision, but whose father was colour blind, marries a colour blind man. Suppose that the fourth child of this couple was a boy. This boy ***(2005)***
(a) may be colour blind or may be of normal vision
(b) must be colour blind
(c) must have normal colour vision
(d) will be partially colour blind since he is heterozygous for the colour blind mutant allele.

149. A normal woman, whose father was colour-blind is married to a normal man. The sons would be ***(2004)***
(a) 75% colour-blind (b) 50% colour-blind
(c) all normal (d) all colour-blind.

150. The recessive genes located on X-chromosome humans are always ***(2004)***
(a) lethal (b) sub-lethal
(c) expressed in males
(d) expressed in females.

151. Which one of the following conditions though harmful in itself, is also potential saviour from a mosquito borne infectious disease? ***(2003)***
(a) Thalassaemia
(b) Sickle cell anaemia
(c) Pernicious anaemia
(d) Leukaemia

152. Down's syndrome is caused by an extra copy of chromosome number 21. What percentage of offspring produced by an affected mother and a normal father would be affected by this disorder? ***(2003)***
(a) 100% (b) 75%
(c) 50% (d) 25%

153. Christmas disease is another name for ***(2003)***
(a) haemophilia B (b) hepatitis B
(c) Down's syndrome (d) sleeping sickness.

154. A diseased man marries a normal woman. They get three daughters and five sons. All the daughters were diseased and sons were normal. The gene of this disease is (2002)
(a) sex linked dominant
(b) sex linked recessive
(c) sex limited character
(d) autosomal dominant.

155. Which of the following is a correct match? ***(2002)***
(a) Down's syndrome -21st chromosome
(b) Sickle cell anaemia - X-chromosome
(c) Haemophilia - Y-chromosome
(d) Parkinson's disease - X and Y chromosome

156. Sickle cell anaemia induce to ***(2001)***
(a) change of amino acid in α-chain of haemoglobin
(b) change of amino acid in β-chain of haemoglobin
(c) change of amino acid in both α and β chains of haemoglobin
(d) change of amino acid either α or β chains of haemoglobin.

157. Mongolian Idiocy due to trisomy in 21st" chromsome is called ***(2000)***
(a) Down's syndrome
(b) Turner's syndrome
(c) Klinefelter's syndrome
(d) Triple X syndrome.

158. In Drosophila, the XXY condition leads to femaleness whereas in human beings the same condition leads to Klinefelter's syndrome in male. It proves ***(2000)***
(a) in human beings Y chromosome is active in sex determination
(b) Y chromosome is active in sex determination in both human beings and Drosophila
(c) in Drosophila Y chromosome decides femaleness
(d) Y chromosome of man have genes for syndrome.

159. A marriage between normal visioned man and colour blind woman will produce offspring ***(1999)***
(a) colour blind sons and 50% carrier daughter
(b) 50% colourblind sons and 50% carrier daughter
(c) normal males and carrier daughters
(d) colour blind sons and carrier daughters.

160. Haemophilic man marries a normal woman. Their offspring will be ***(1999)***
(a) all haemophilic
(b) all boys haemophilic
(c) all girls haemophilic
(d) all normal.

161. A woman with two genes for haemophilia and one gene for colour blindness on one of the ' X ' chromosomes marries a normal man. How will the progeny be? ***(1998)***
(a) 50% haemophilic colour-blind sons and 50% haemophilic sons.
(b) 50% haemophilic daughters (carrier) and 50% colour blind daughters (carrier).
(c) All sons and daughters haemophilic and colourblind.
(d) Haemophilic and colour-blind daughters.

162. Mental retardation in man, associated with sex chromosomal abnormality is usually due to ***(1998)***
(a) moderate increase in Y complement
(b) large increase in Y complement
(c) reduction in X complement
(d) increase in X complement.

163. A person with the sex chromosomes XXY suffers from ***(1997)***
(a) gynandromorphism
(b) Klinefelter's syndrome
(c) Down's syndrome
(d) Turner's syndrome.

164. In which of the following diseases, the man has an extra X-chromosome? ***(1996)***
(a) Turner's syndrome
(b) Klinefelter's syndrome
(c) Down's syndrome
(d) Haemophilia

165. A person whose father is colour blind marries a lady whose mother is daughter of a colour blind man. Their children will be ***(1996)***
(a) all sons colour blind
(b) some sons normal and some colour blind
(c) all colour blind
(d) all daughters normal.

166. A genetically diseased father (male) marries with a normal female and gives birth to 3 carrier girls and 5 normal sons. It may be which type of genetic disease? ***(1996)***
(a) Sex-influenced disease
(b) Blood group inheritance disease
(c) Sex-linked disease
(d) Sex-recessive disease

167. An abnormal human male phenotype involving an extra X-chromosome (XXY) is a case of ***(1995)***
(a) Edward's syndrome
(b) Klinefelter's syndrome
(c) intersex
(d) Down's syndrome.

168. The colour blindness is more likely to occur in males than in females because ***(1994)***
(a) the Y-chromosome of males have the genes for distinguishing colours
(b) genes for characters are located on the sex chromosomes
(c) the trait is dominant in males and recessive in females
(d) none of these.

169. Of both normal parents, the chances of a male child becoming colour blind are ***(1993)***
(a) none
(b) possible only when all the four grand parents had normal vision
(c) possible only when father's mother was colour blind
(d) possible only when mother's father was colour blind.

170. Of a normal couple, half the sons are haemophiliac while half the daughters are carriers. The gene is located on ***(1993)***
(a) X-chromosome of father
(b) Y-chromosome of father
(c) one X-chromosome of mother
(d) both the X-chromosomes of mother.

171. A colour blind mother and normal father would have ***(1992)***
(a) colour blind sons and normal/carrier daughters
(b) colour blind sons and daughters
(c) all colour blind
(d) all normal.

172. Down's syndrome is due to ***(1992)***
(a) crossing over
(b) linkage
(c) sex-linked inheritance
(d) non-disjunction of chromosomes.

173. In human beings 45 chromosomes/single X/XO abnormality causes ***(1992)***
(a) Down's syndrome
(b) Kinefelter's syndrome
(c) Turner's syndrome
(d) Edward's syndrome

174. A colour blind girl is rare because she will be born only when ***(1991)***
(a) her mother and maternal grand father were colour blind
(b) her father and maternal grand father were colour blind
(c) her mother is colour blind and father has normal vision
(d) parents have normal vision but grand parents were colour blind.

175. In Down's syndrome of a male child, the sex complement is ***(1990)***
(a) XO (b) XY (c) XX (d) XXY.

176. Haemophilia is more common in males because it is a ***(1990)***
(a) recessive character carried by Y-chromosome
(b) dominant character carried by Y-chromosome
(c) dominant trait carried by X-chromosome
(d) recessive trait carried by X-chromosome.

177. Which one is a hereditary disease? ***(1990)***
(a) Cataract (b) Leprosy
(c) Blindness (d) Phenylketonuria

178. Both husband and wife have normal vision though their fathers were colour blind. The probability of their daughter becoming colour blind is ***(1990)***
(a) 0% (b) 25%
(c) 50% (d) 75%.

ANSWER KEY

1.	(a)	2.	(c)	3.	(a)	4.	(d)	5.	(d)	6.	(b)	7.	(b)
8.	(d)	9.	(d)	10.	(b)	11.	(d)	12.	(d)	13.	(d)	14.	(c)
15.	(a)	16.	(b)	17.	(c)	18.	(b)	19.	(a)	20.	(a)	21.	(a)
22.	(c)	23.	(b)	24.	(d)	25.	(a)	26.	(c)	27.	(c)	28.	(a)
29.	(c)	30.	(c)	31.	(c)	32.	(c)	33.	(d)	34.	(c)	35.	(d)
36.	(a)	37.	(c)	38.	(a)	39.	(c)	40.	(c)	41.	(d)	42.	(a)
43.	(d)	44.	(d)	45.	(d)	46.	(b)	47.	(c)	48.	(a)	49.	(b)
50.	(c)	51.	(b)	52.	(c)	53.	(a)	54.	(c)	55.	(d)	56.	(d)
57.	(d)	58.	(d)	59.	(c)	60.	(a)	61.	(c)	62.	(a)	63.	(b)
64.	(d)	65.	(a)	66.	(d)	67.	(d)	68.	(a)	69.	(c)	70.	(b)
71.	(c)	72.	(a)	73.	(b)	74.	(b)	75.	(a)	76.	(a)	77.	(b)
78.	(c)	79.	(a)	80.	(d)	81.	(a)	82.	(b)	83.	(b)	84.	(b)
85.	(a)	86.	(a)	87.	(a)	88.	(b)	89.	(d)	90.	(c)	91.	(a)
92.	(a)	93.	(d)	94.	(b)	95.	(c)	96.	(b)	97.	(c)	98.	(d)
99.	(a)	100.	(a)	101.	(c)	102.	(c)	103.	(b)	104.	(c)	105.	(a)
106.	(b)	107.	(c)	108.	(b)	109.	(d)	110.	(b)	111.	(b)	112.	(d)
113.	(a)	114.	(c)	115.	(c)	116.	(c)	117.	(d)	118.	(b)	119.	(d)
120.	(a)	121.	(b)	122.	(d)	123.	(b)	124.	(a)	125.	(d)	126.	(c)
127.	(a)	128.	(a)	129.	(a)	130.	(a)	131.	(b)	132.	(b)	133.	(c)
134.	(b)	135.	(a)	136.	(a)	137.	(b)	138.	(a)	139.	(c)	140.	(c)
141.	(a)	142.	(c)	143.	(d)	144.	(b)	145.	(d)	146.	(c)	147.	(d)
148.	(a)	149.	(b)	150.	(c)	151.	(b)	152.	(c)	153.	(a)	154.	(a)
155.	(a)	156.	(b)	157.	(a)	158.	(a)	159.	(d)	160.	(d)	161.	(a)
162.	(d)	163.	(b)	164.	(b)	165.	(d)	166.	(c)	167.	(b)	168.	(b)
169.	(d)	170.	(c)	171.	(a)	172.	(d)	173.	(c)	174.	(b)	175.	(b)
176.	(d)	177.	(d)	178.	(a)								

HINTS & EXPLANATIONS

1. (a)

2.(c) : Mendel conducted artificial pollination or cross pollination experiments using several true-breeding pea lines. He selected 14 true-breeding pea plant varieties, as pairs which were similar except for one character with contrasting traits. Some of the contrasting traits selected were smooth or wrinkled seeds, yellow or green seeds, inflated (full) or constricted green or yellow pods and tall or dwarf plants.

3.(a) : Mendel considered the following characters of pea in his experiments:

	Character	Dominant	Recessive
(i)	Seed shape	Round (R)	Wrinkled (r)
(ii)	Seed cotyledon colour	Yellow (Y)	Green (y)
(iii)	Flower colour	Violet (V)	White (v)
(iv)	Pod shape	Inflated (I)	Constricted (i)

4.(d) : Mendel carried out hybridisation experiments on garden pea for 7 years from 1856-1863.

5.(d)

6. (b)

7. (b)

8. (d) : Mendel worked on seven characters. These characters showed complete independent assortment despite the seven characters chosen by him were present on four chromosomes – 1, 4, 5 and 7 .

9. (d)

10.(b) : An Austrian monk, Gregor Mendel, developed his theory of inheritance. He formulated the Law of Heredity. Therefore, he is called the 'father of genetics'.

11.(d) : Consideration of one character at one time contribute to the success of Mendel. Mendel's contribution was unique because of his methodological approach to a definite problem, use of clear cut variables and application of mathematics (statistics) to the problem. Using pea plants and statistical methods, Mendel was able to demonstrate that traits were passed from each parent inheritance of genes.

12.(d) : The prodcuction of gametes by the parents, formation of the zygotes, the F1 and F2 plants can be understood from a diagram called Punnett square developed by a British geneticist, Reginald C. Punnett.

13.(d) : Sickle cell anaemia is an autosomal recessive disorder

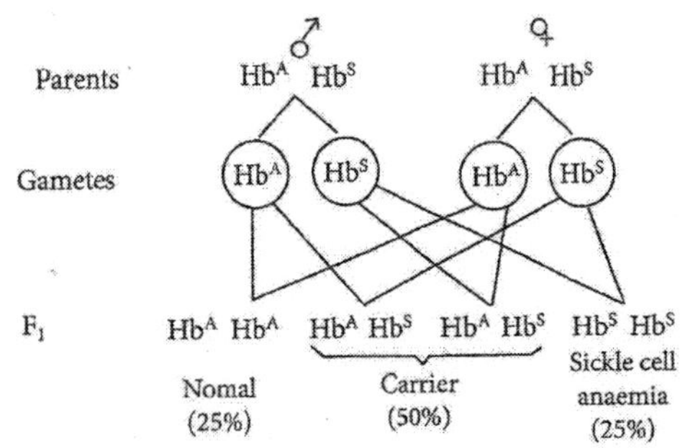

14.(c) : ABO blood groups are controlled by the gene I. The gene (I) has three alleles IA,IB and i. The alleles IA and IB produce a slightly different form of the sugar while allele i does not produce any sugar. Because humans are diploid organisms, each person possesses any two of the three I gene alleles. When IA and IB are present together they both express their own types of sugars, because of co-dominance.

15.(a) : Law of segregation applies in this case as when pink flowers obtained in F1 are selfed then red and white flowers are obtained in F2 which indicates that there is no mixing of gametes.

16.(b) : If the genotypes of husband and wife are IA IB and IA i respectively, then the probabilities of genotypes and phenotypes among their children can be worked out as:

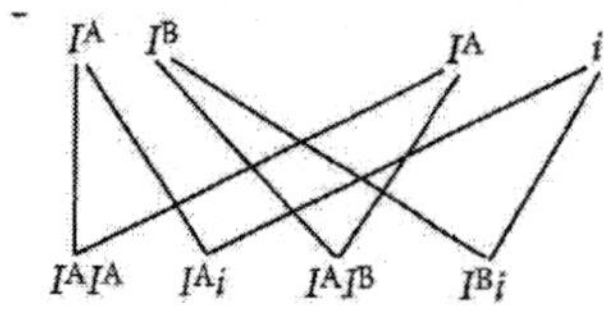

Genotype:	$I^A I^A$	I^Ai	I^AI^B	I^Bi
Phenotype:	A	A	AB	B

Thus, there are four possible genotypes, viz., $I^A I^A$ $I^A i$, $I^A I^B$ and $I^B i$ and three possible phenotypes, viz., A, AB and B among the children.

17.(c) : When a tall true breeding garden pea plant is crossed with a dwarf true breeding garden pea plant and the F1 plants were selfed the resulting genotypes were in the ratio of 1 : 2 : 1, i.e., Tall homozygous : Tall heterozygous : Dwarf It can be illustrated as given below:

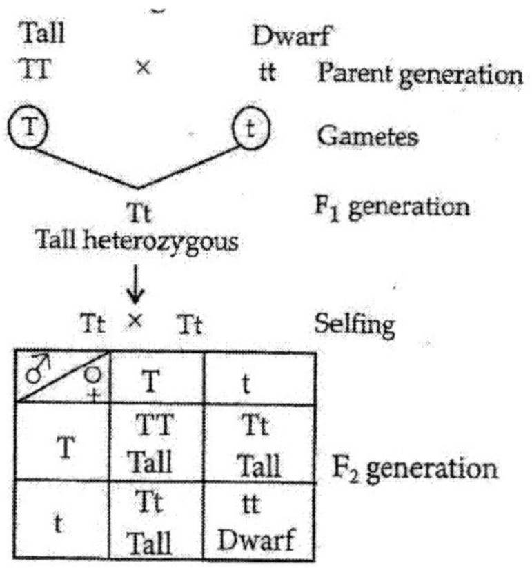

Phenotypic ratio :3 : 1 : : Tall : Dwarf

Genotypic ratio -1 : 2 : 1 : : TT : Tt : tt

18.(b) : The phenomenon of expression of both the alleles in a heterozygote is called co-dominance. The alleles which do not show dominance-recessive relationship and are able to express themselves independently when present together are called codominant alleles. As a result the heterozygous condition has a phenotype different from either of homozygous genotypes, e.g., alleles for biood group A(IA) and for blood group B(IB) are codominant so that when they come together in an individual, they produce blood group AB.

19.(a) : Genes are the units of inheritance and contain the information that is required to express a particular trait in an organism. Alternating forms of a single gene which code for a pair of contrasting traits are known as alleles. For example, two alleles determine the height of pea plant (tall and dwarf).

20. (a)

21.(a) : The man has blood group A, thus its genotype can either be IA IA or IA IO. Similarly, woman can either have IB IB, or IB IO genotype. Thus, their offspring can have any of the blood groups A(IA IA or IA IO), B(IB IB or IB IO), AB(IA IB) or O (IO IO).

22. (c)

23.(b) : In co-dominance, both the alleles are able to express themselves independently when present together resulting in a phenotype that is intermediate between both the parental homozygous phenotypes, thereby resembling both of them. E.g., roan coat colour in cattle is a result of co-dominance of alleles for white and red coat colour.

24.(d) : The inheritance of flower colour in the dog flower (snapdragon or Antirrhinum sp.) is a an example of incomplete dominance. In a cross between true-breeding red-flowered (RR) and true-breeding white-flowered plants (rr), the F1 (Rr) was pink. When the F1 was self-pollinated the F2 resulted in the following ratio, 1 (RR) Red : 2 (Rr) Pink: 1 (rr) White. Here, the genotype ratios were 1 : 2 : 1 as in any Mendelian monohybrid cross, but the phenotype ratios had changed from the 3:1 dominant : recessive ratio to 1 : 2 : 1.

25.(a) : Test cross is performed to determine the genotype of F2 plant. In a typical test cross, an organism showing dominant phenotype and whose genotype is to be determined is crossed with one that is homozygous recessive for the allele being investigated, instead of self-crossing. The progenies of such a cross can easily be analysed to predict the genotype of the test organism. Given below is an illustration of test cross:

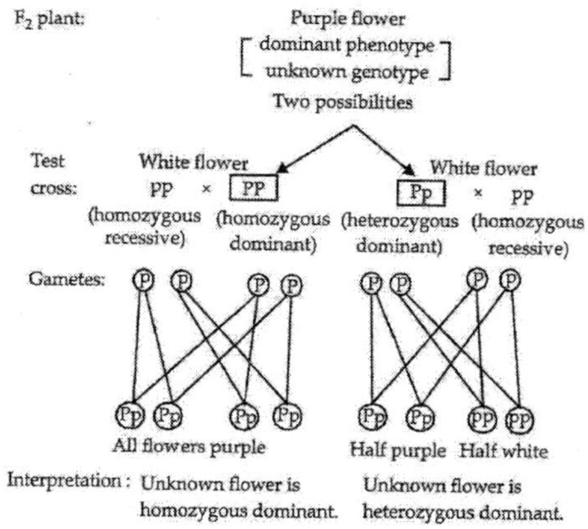

26. (c)

27.(c) : The three alleles IA,IB and i of gene I in ABO blood group system can produce six different genotypes and four different phenotypes as shown below :

Genotypes		Phenotypes
I^AI^A, I^Ai		Blood group A
I^BI^B, I^Bi		Blood group B
I^AI^B	–	Blood group AB
ii	–	Blood group O

28. (a)

29.(c) : According to Mendel's law of dominance, in heterozygous individuals a character is represented by two contrasting factors called alleles or allelomorphs which occur in pairs. Out of the two contrasting alleles, only one is able to express its effect in the individual. It is called dominant factor or dominant allele. The other allele which does not show its effect in the heterozygous individual is called recessive factor or recessive allele. The option (c) in the given question cannot be explained on the basis of law of dominance. It can only be explained on the basis of Mendel's law of independent assortment, according to which in a dihybrid cross, the two alleles of each character assort independently (do not show any blending) of the alleles of other character and separate at the time of gamete formation. Both the characters are recovered as such in F2 generation producing both parental and new combinations of traits.

30. (c)

31. (c)

32.(c) : The given situation is an example of incomplete dominance where phenotype found in F1 generation do not resemble either of the two parents. The genotype of the two plants used for cross will be:

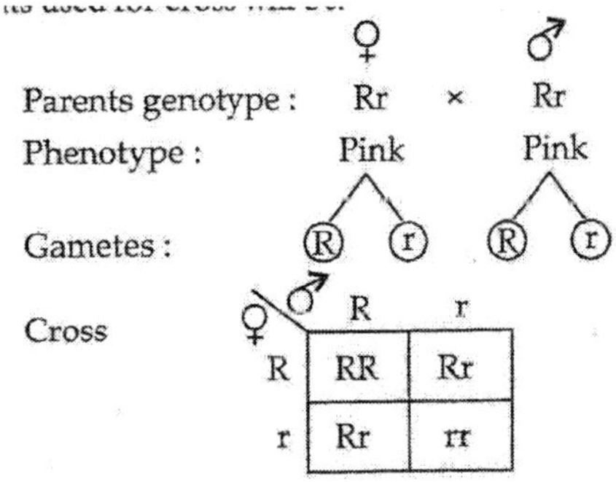

Genotypic ratio : RR : Rr : rr

1 : 2 : 1

Phenotype: Red : Pink : White

The incomplete dominance of dominant allele (here ' R ') over recessive allele (here ' r ') could be due to mutations (insertion, deletion, substitution or inversion of nucleotides). The mutant allele generally produces a faulty or no product. This modification in the product may lead to incomplete dominance of the (unmodified) wild type dominant allele.

33.(d) : Yellow (Y) seeds are dominant to green (y). So, a heterozygous yellow seeded plant will have the genotype of (Yy) and a green seeded plant will have genotype of (yy). When these two plants are crossed, the F1 generation will have the ratio of yellow : green as 50:50. It is shown as:

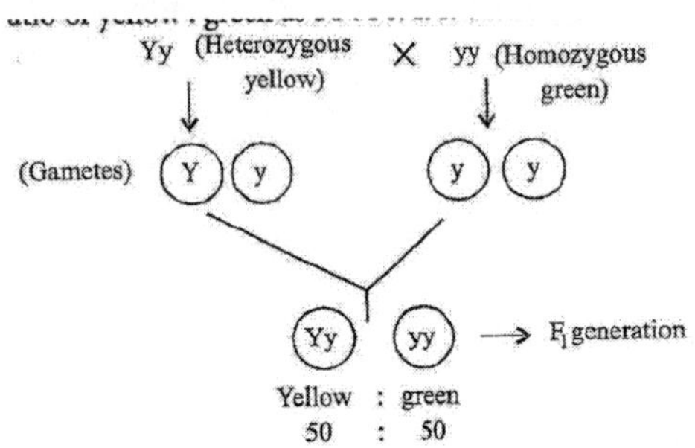

34.(c) : A common test to find the genotypes of a hybrid is by crossing of one F1 progeny with male parent.

35. (d)

36.(a) : The external manifestation, morphological or physiological expression of an individual with regard to one or more characters is called phenotype. For recessive genes, phenotype and genotype are similar. For dominant genes, the phenotype is same for both homozygous states. Phenotype is influenced by environment as well as age. A child definitely differs from adolescent, the latter from adult and an adult from aged one. Many phenotypes are determined by multiple genes. Thus, the identity of phenotype is determined by genotype and environment.

37.(c) : Dominant factor is an allele or Mendelian factor which expressess itself in the hybrid (heterozygous) as well as in homozygous state. It is denoted by capital letter.

38. (a)

39.(c) : Crossing of individuals having dominant phenotype with its homozygous recessive is a test cross, which can be represented as:

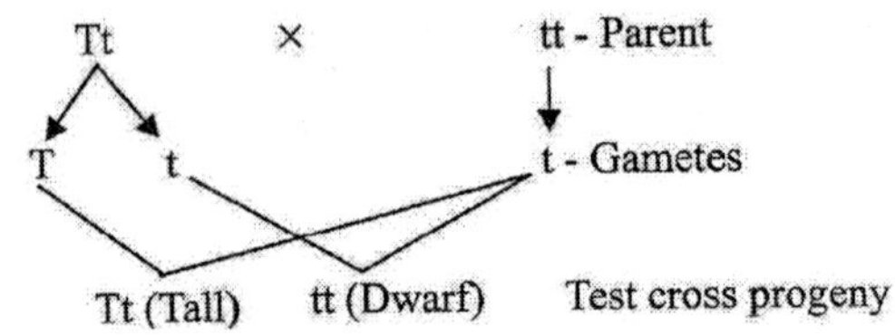

Thus, ratio of progeny is = 1 : 1

40.(c) : O blood group of a child cannot be obtained from the parents having blood group O × AB. The parents blood groups may be A × O, A × B, B × O, B ×A , O × A and O × B.

41.(d) : The genotype of the child would be IO IO (recessive). Hence, the genotype of the father can only be IB IO.

42. (a)

43.(d) : An organism with two identical alleles is homozygous. Homozygous have identical genes at the same locus on each member of a pair of homologous/chromosomes.

44.(d) : $I^A I^O \times I^A I^B$ gives us the following genotypes $I^A I^A$, $I^O I^B$,$I^A I^B$. Hence, when a man of blood group A marries a woman of AB blood group, B progeny would indicate that man is heterozygous A.

45.(d) : ABO blood group system is due to multiple allelism. A gene can have more than two alleles or allelomorphs, which can be expressed by mutation in wild form in more than one ways. These alleles or allelomorphs make a series of multiple alleles. The mode of inheritance in case of multiple alleles is called multiple allelism. A well known and simplest example of multiple allelism is the inheritance of ABO blood groups in human beings. In human population, 3 different alleles for this character are found -IA IB and IO. A person is having only two of these three alleles and blood type can be determined.

46.(b) : The contrasting pairs of factors in Mendelian crosses are called allelomorphs. Alleles or allelomorphs are the different forms of a gene, having the same locus on homologous chromosomes and are subject to Mendelian (alternative) inheritance.

47.(c) : Mendel's last law is independent assortment. The principle of independent assortment states that when two individuals differ from each other in two or more pairs of factors, the inheritance of one pair is quite independent of the inheritance of other.

48.(a) : The brown eyed man will have the genotype Bb and his wife bb. Hence, Bb × bb = Bb : bb. Therefore, the children shall be both blue eyed and brown eyed the ratio is 1:1.

49.(b) : The inheritance of flower colour in the dog flower (snapdragon or Antirrhinum sp.) is a an example of incomplete dominance. In a cross between true-breeding red-flowered (RR) and true-breeding white-flowered plants (rr), the F1 (Rr) was pink. When the F1 was self-pollinated the F2 resulted in the following ratio, 1(RR) Red : 2 (Rr) Pink : 1 (rr) White. Here, the genotype ratios were 1 : 2 : 1 as in any Mendelian monohybrid cross, but the phenotype ratios had changed from the 3 : 1 dominant : recessive ratio to 1 : 2 : 1.

50. (c)

51. (b)

52.(c) : Haploids are able to express both recessive and dominant alleles/ mutations because there are only one allele for each gene in the individual. Diploid is an organism containing two different alleles or individual containing both dominant and recessive genes of an allelic pairs.

53.(a) : Alfred Sturtevant used the frequency of recombination between gene pairs on the same chromosomes as a measure of the distance between genes and 'mapped' their position on the chromosome.

54.(c) : The law of independent assortment is applicable to only those factors or genes which are either located distantly on the same chromosome or occur on different chromosomes.

55. (d)

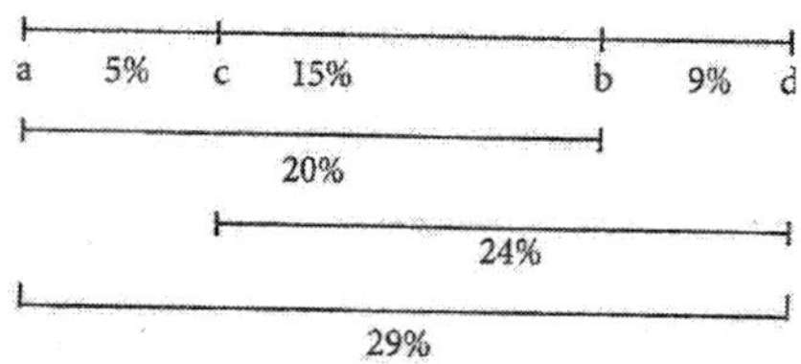

56.(d) : Sutton and Boveri proposed the chromosomal theory of inheritance but its experimental verification was done by Thomas Hunt Morgan

57.(d) : Genetic map is a linear graphic representation of the sequence and relative distance of various genes present in a chromosome. 1% crossing over between two linked genes is known as 1 map unit or centiMorgan (cM).

58.(d) : T.H. Morgan coined the term linkage to describe the physical association of genes on chromosome and term recombination to describe the generation of non-parental gene combinations. Alfred Sturtevant used the frequency of recombination between gene pairs on the same chromosome as a measure of the distance between genes.

59.(c) : Translocation is a chromosomal abnormality caused by rearrangement of parts between non-homologous chromosomes. It may cause a gene to move from one linkage group to another.

60.(a) : If in a dihybrid test cross more parental combinations appear as compared to the recombinants in F2 generation, then it is indicative of involvement of linkage. Linkage is the tendency of two different genes on the same chromosome to remain together during the separation of homologous chromosomes at meiosis. During complete linkage no recombinants are formed whereas in incomplete linkage few recombinants are produced along with parental combinations.

61.(c) : Linkage is the phenomenon of certain genes staying together during inheritance through generations without any change or separation due to their being present on the same chromosome. Linkage was first suggested by Sutton and Boveri (1902-1903) when they propounded the famous "chromosomal theory of inheritance." Bateson and Punnett (1906) while working on sweet pea found that the factors for certain characters do not show independent assortment. However, it was Morgan (1910) who clearly proved and defined linkage on the basis of his breeding experiments in fruit fly (Drosophila melanogaster).

62. (a)

63.(b) : A dominant epistatic allele suppresses the expression of a non-allelic gene whether the latter is dominant or recessive. The gene which suppresses the expression of a nonallelic gene is known as epistatic gene. The gene or locus which is suppressed by the presence of non-allelic gene is termed as hypostatic gene. In summer squash or Cucurbita pepo, there are three types of fruit colour-yellow, green and white. White colour is dominant over other colours while yellow is dominant over green. Yellow colour is formed only when the dominant epistatic gene is represented by its recessive allele (w). When the hypostatic gene is also recessive (y), the colour of the fruit is green, i.e.

$W\_\,Yy, W\_\,yy \rightarrow$ White

$wwY\_ \rightarrow$ Yellow

$wwyy \rightarrow$ Green

64. (d)

65.(a) : The increased vigour displayed by the offspring from a cross between genetically different parents is called heterosis. Hybrids from crosses between different crop varieties (F1 hybrids) are often stronger and produce better yields than the original varieties.

66.(d) : Linkage is the phenomenon of certain genes staying together during inheritance through generations without any change or separation due to their being present on the same chromosome. Linked genes occur in the same chromosome. Strength of the linkage between two genes is inversely proportional to the distance between the two, i.e., two linked genes show higher frequency of crossing over (recombination) if the distance between them is higher and lower frequency if the distance is small.

67.(d) : As sperms produced are with genotypes AB,Ab,aB, ab (two diallelic character) the person must be heterozygous for both genes. So, his genotype will be AaBb.

68.(a) : Since round seed shape is dominant over wrinkled seed shape and yellow cotyledon is dominant over green cotyledon so RRYY individuals is round yellow and rryy is wrinkled green.

Round yellow seeds × Wrinkled green seeds
RRYY rryy
↓
F_1 generation RrYy
F_2 generation is obtained by selfing F_1.

♀ \ ♂	RY	Ry	rY	ry
RY	RRYY	RRYy	RrYY	RrYy
Ry	RRYy	RRyy	RrYy	Rryy
rY	RrYY	RrYy	rrYY	rrYy
ry	RrYy	Rryy	rrYy	rryy

Expected phenotypes in F_2 generation

Round yellow seed 9 — Wrinkled yellow seed 3

Round green seed 3 — Wrinkled green seed 1

69.(c) : A test cross involving the crossing of F1 individual with the homozygous recessive parent. It is done to find out homozygous and heterozygous individuals. So, AaBb should be crossed with aabb.

70.(b) : Since red fruit colour is dominant over yellow fruit colour and tallness is dominant over shortness.

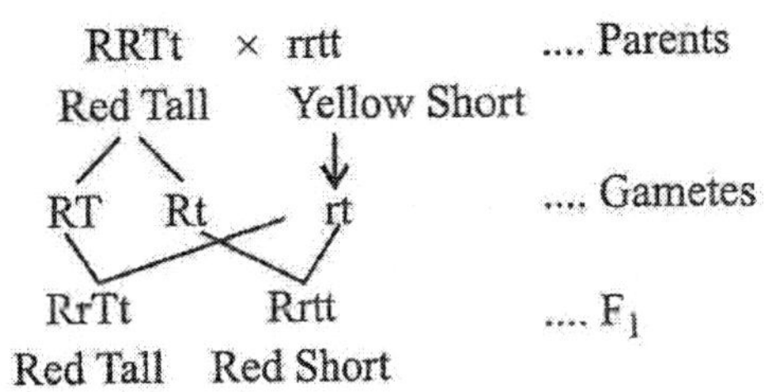

These are produced in 1:1 ratio.

71.(c) : Mendel's law of independent assortment states that when the parent differs from each other in two or more pairs of contrasting characters, the inheritance of one pair of factor is independent of the other. For the character to assort independently they should be located on separate non-homologous chromosomes. Genes present on the same chromosome show linkage. It means that these characters remain together and thus low numbers of combinations are formed. This phenomenon is called linkage and such genes are called linked genes. So, A and B are linked genes.

72.(a) : Linkage/ Cross over/Chromosome map is a graphic representation of relative positions/ order and relative distances of genes in a chromosome in the form of line like a linear road map depicting different places and their relative distances without giving exact mileage. It is based on Morgan's hypothesis (1911) that frequency of crossing over/ recombination between two linked genes is directly proportional to the physical distance between the two. 1 map unit or centrimorgan is equivalent to 1% recombination between two genes. Percentage of crossing over between a and b is 20% so they are 20 map distance apart and b and c are 28 map distance apart. So, that correct sequence of genes on chromosomes will be as

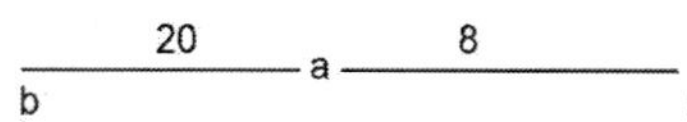

73.(b) : The tendency of potential combinations to remain together, which is expressed in terms of low frequency of recombinations (new combinations) is called linkage. Genes present on same chromosomes show linkage. These genes are called linked genes. Since A and B genes are linked they will be passed on together in the progeny.

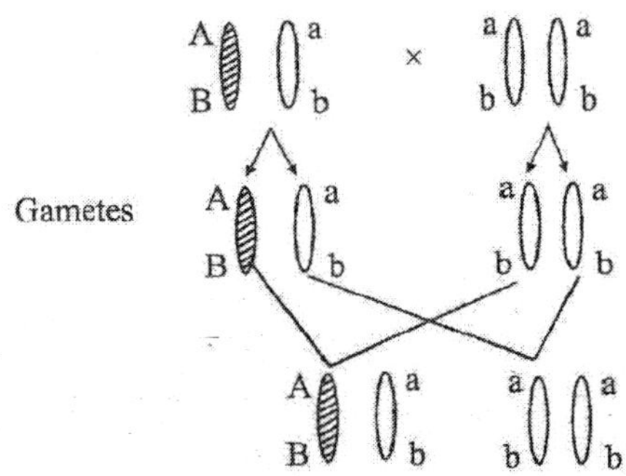

74.(b) : According to law of independent assortment, the two factors of each trait assort at random and independent of the factors of other traits at the time of meiosis and get randomly as well as independently rearranged in the offspring. Principle of law of independent assortment is applicable to only those factors or genes which are present on different chromosomes.

75.(a) : The cross can be represented as:

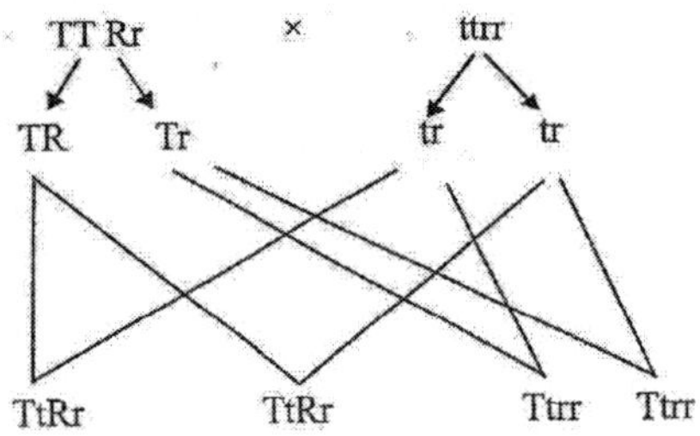

Tall Red TtRr – 50%

Tall White Ttrr – 50%

76.(a) : According to principle of independent assortment, the two factors of each trait assort at random and independent of the factors of other traits at the time of meiosis and get randomly as well as independently rearranged in the offspring. Principle of independent assortment is applicable to only those factors or genes which are present on different chromosomes. Chromosome have hundreds of genes which show linked inheritance or linkage. Linkage is the phenomenon of certain genes (present on the same chromosome) to remain together and get inherited through generations. The seven characters that Mendel chose were present on 14 chromosomes and so they did not show linkage but if present on 12 chromosomes they would have shown linkage and the principle of independent assortment would not have been discovered.

77.(b) : Crossing over is the reciprocal exchange of segments between non-sister chromatids of a pair of homologous chromosomes. It results in recombination of genes.

78.(c) : In a cross between AABB × aabb, the ratio of F2 genotypes between AABB, AaBB, Aabb and aabb would be 1 : 2 : 2 : 1.

79.(a) : Segregation of Mendelian factors (no linkage, no crossing over) occurs during anaphase I. At anaphase I, actual segregation occurs, but two similar alleles occurs in the dyad chromosome which separate at anaphase II.

80.(d) : The allele which is unable to express its effect in the presence of another is called recessive. A member of a pair of alleles that does not show its effect in the phenotype in the presence of any other allele. It is denoted by small letter.

81.(a) : Cross between AaBB and aaBB will form 1AaBB:1 aaBB. On crossing, AaBB× aaBB gives 50% individuals having genotype AaBB and 50% individuals having genotype aaBB.

82.(b) : Segregation of Mendelian factor (Aa) occurs during anaphase I. The paired homologous chromosomes separate in meiosis I so that each gamete receives one chromosomes of each homologous pair. During anaphase I chromosome divides at the point of centromere or kinetochore and thus two sister chromatids are formed, which are called as chromosomes.

83.(b) : ABO blood group system in human beings is an example of dominance, co-dominance and multiple allelism. I^A I^O,I^B I^O or i - Alleles shows dominant-recessive relationship. IA IB – Co-dominance is a phenomenon in which alleles of a gene do not show dominant recessive relationship and express themselves independently when present together.

I^A,I^B I^O or *i* - More than two alternate forms of a gene present on the same locus are called as multiple alleles and the mode of inheritance in the alleles is called multiple allelism.

84.(b) : Polygenic (or Quantitative) inheritance is that type of inheritance in which the complete expression of a trait is controlled by two or more genes in which a dominant allele of each gene contributes only a unit fraction of the trait and total phenotypic expression is the sum total of a additive or cumulative effect of all the dominant alleles of genes/ polygenes. Human skin colour is an example of such polygenic inheritance which is controlled by three pairs of polygenes A, B and C. Negro/black colour is due to presence of all the six dominant contributing alleles AABBCC. Very light colour or white colour is due to presence of all six recessive non contributing alleles aabbcc.

85.(a) : The plant having genotype AABbCC is heterozygous for only one character B. Number of gametes = 2n, where n is the heterozygosity.

Since n = 1 so 2 gametes will be formed. Those are ABC and AbC.

86. (a)

87.(a) : Selfing is the process of fertilisation with polar or male gametes of the same individual. AABbCC will produce two type of gametes ABC and AbC. Thus, in F2 generation three genotypes will be obtained. These are AABBCC, AABBCC and AABbCC in the ratio of 1:2:1. Phenotypically AABBCC and AABbCC are same. So, the phenotypic ratio in F2 generation will be 3:1.

88. (b)

89.(d) : Number of gametes = 2n = 22 = 4. where n is the number of gene in heterozygous form.

The four gametes formed will be → ABc, AbC, Abc and ABC.

90. (c)

91. (a)

92.(a) : Pleiotropy is a phenomena where a single gene can exhibit multiple phenotypic expression. Such a gene is called a pleiotropic gene.

93. (d)

94.(b) : The ability of a gene to have multiple phenotypic effects because it influences a number of characters simultaneously is known as pleiotropy. The gene having a multiple phenotypic effect because of its ability to control expression of two or more characters is called pleiotropic gene. In human beings pleiotropy is exhibited by syndromes called sickle cell anaemia and phenylketonuria.

95.(c) : Pleiotropic gene is such a gene which has a wider effect on phenotype, i.e., it controls several phenotypic traits. Sickle cell anaemia is considered to be caused by one such pleiotropic gene. It is caused due to mutation in β-globin gene of haemoglobin.

96.(b) : The ability of a gene to have multiple phenotypic effect because it influences a number of characters simultaneously is known as pleiotropy.

97.(c) : Grasshopper is an example of XO type of sex determination in which the males have only X chromosome besides the autosomes, whereas females have a pair of X-chromosomes.

98.(d) : In birds, e.g., fowls, males have homomorphic sex chromosomes (AA + ZZ) and females have heteromorphic sex chromosomes (AA+ZW). So, males produce only one type of sperms containing (A+Z) whereas females produce two types of eggs (A+Z and A+W). Therefore, the sex of the progeny depends on the type of the egg which is fertilised by the sperm.

99.(a) : The gene for starch synthesis in pea seeds can produce more than one effect which implies it is a pleiotropic gene.

100. (a) : In humans, the female has a pair of X chromosome (homogametic composition) and the male has XY chromosomes (heterogametic composition). Therefore, two normal X chromosomes in zygotic cell lead to the birth of a normal human female child.

101.(c) : According to genic balance theory of sex determination the ratio between the number of X-chromosomes and number of complete sets of autosomes will determine the sex. The X-chromosome is believed to carry female tendency genes, while autosomes carry male tendency genes. Both these sets of genes start functioning and there has to be a balance between them for an individual to become male or female. If the ratio between X and A is 1.0 it will be a female individual and when it is 0.5 , it would be male.

102.(c) : Barr body is a mass of condensed sex chromatin in the nuclei of normal female somatic cells due to inactive X chromosome. Whenever the number of X-chromosomes is two or more than two, the number of Barr bodies is one less than the number of X-chromosomes. Therefore, the number of Barr bodies in XXXX female is three.

103.(b) : Male XX and female XY sometimes occur due to transfer of segments in X and Y chromosomes. Deletion is the loss of an intercalary segment of a chromosome which is produced by a double break in the chromosomes followed by the union of remaining parts. Aneuploidy is a condition of having fewer or extra chromosomes than the normal genome number of the species.

104. (c)

105.(a) : Sex-chromosomes are those chromosomes whose presence, absence or particular form determines the sex of the individual in unisexual or dioecious organisms, e.g., XX denotes female and XY denotes male.

106. (b): Sex is determined in human beings at the time of fertilisation. Sex of the baby depends upon the sperm which fertilises the ovum.

107.(c) : A family of five daughter only is expecting sixth issue. The chance of its beings a son is 50%. Human have 22 pairs chromosomes which are XX in females and XY in males So if we cross the parents there is 1 : 1 chance for boy and girl.

108.(b) : Sickle cell anaemia and thalassemia are autosomal linked recessive disease while haemophilia is a sex linked recessive disease.

109.(d) : If a colourblind female (Xc Xc) marries a man whose mother is colourblind, (XcY) then

♀ \ ♂	X^c	Y
X^c	X^cX^c	X^cY
X^c	X^cX^c	X^cY

110.(b) : Mutation is a sudden alteration of the chemical structure of a gene or the alteration of its position on the chromosome by breaking and rejoining of the chromosome. It has occurred in male parent. But organelles like mitochondria, chloroplast etc., are a part of cytoplasmic inheritance.

Cytoplasmic inheritance is the passage of traits from parents to offspring through structures present inside the cytoplasm of contributing gametes. Plasma genes occur in plastids, mitochondria, plasmids and some special particles like kappa particles, sigma particles, etc. In higher organisms cytoplasmic inheritance is called maternal inheritance because the zygote receives most of its cytoplasm from the ovum. Therefore, cytoplasmic inheritance is usually uniparental. So, none of the progeny will show mutation.

111. (b): Point mutation involves only the replacement of one nucleotide with another. One type of point mutation is missense mutation. These are base changes that alter the codon for an amino acid resulting in its substitution with a different amino acid. For example, mutation of the codon CTT to ATT would result in the replacement of the hydrophobic amino acid leucine with isoleucine, another hydrophobic amino acid. Many other missense mutations have been described which do affect the encoded protein and result in genetic diseases. These include an A to T mutation in the gene for β-globin, one of the polypeptides of haemoglobin. This mutation changes codon six of the gene from GAG which encodes glutamic acid to GTG which encodes valine. The mutation results in a condition called sickle cell anaemia.

112.(d) : In pedigree analysis, 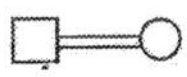 symbol shows consanguineous mating, i.e., mating between relatives.

113. (a) : Klinefelter's syndrome is a genetic disorder caused due to the presence of an additional copy of X-chromosome resulting into a karyotype of 47 , XXY. Such an individual has overall masculine development, however the feminine development (development of breast i.e., gynaecomastia) is also expressed. Such individuals are sterile.

114. (c) : Broad palm with characteristic palm crease small round head, furrowed tongue and retarded mental development are characteristics of Down's syndrome. It is a genetic disorder due to the presence of an additional copy of chromosome number 21 (trisomy of 21).

115. (c)

116.(c) : Klinefelter's syndrome occurs by the union of an abnormal XX egg and a normal Y sperm or a normal X egg and abnormal XY sperm. The individual has 47 chromosomes (44+XXY). Such persons are sterile males with undeveloped testes, mental retardation, sparse body hair, long limbs and with some female characteristics such as enlarged breast, i.e., gynaecomastia.

117.(d) : Woman acts as a carrier when she has the X-linked condition on one of her X-chromosomes. Both son and daughter inherit X-chromosome from mother. Hence, one of the two daughters will be carrier and one of the two sons will be diseased. It can be explained by the given cross :

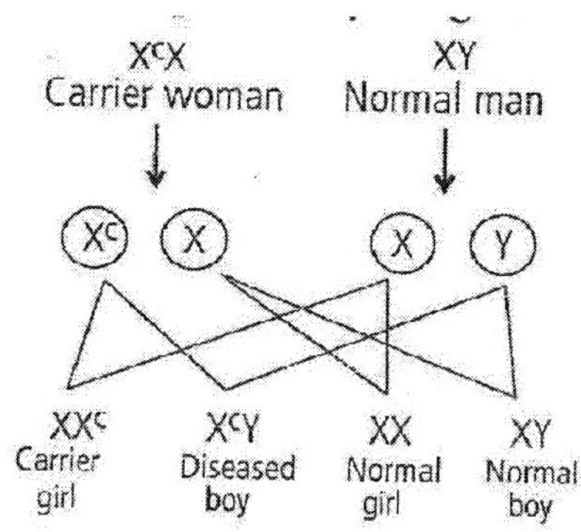

where X^c is the X-chromosome carrying the gene for the condition.

118.(b) : Sickle cell anaemia is caused due to point mutation in which at the 6th position of beta globin chain, glutamic acid is replaced by valine. Thus, it is a qualitative defect in functioning of globin molecules.

Thalassemia is caused due to either mutation or deletion which ultimately results in reduced rate of synthesis of one of the globin chains that make up haemoglobin. Hence, it is a quantitative defect in functioning of globin molecules.

119.(d) : Down's syndrome is an autosomal aneuploidy, caused by the presence of an extra-chromosome number 21 . Both the chromosomes of the pair 21 pass into a single egg due to non disjunction during oogenesis.

120.(a) : Genotype of colour blind man - XC Y

Genotype of woman homozygous - XX

for normal woman

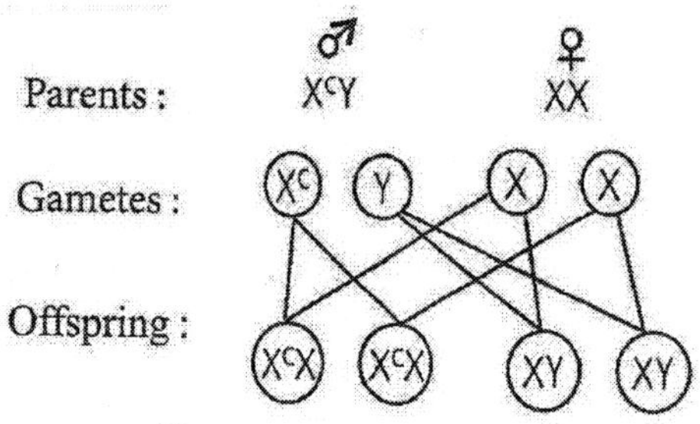

All carrier daughters All normal sons

Hence, there is zero (0) probability of their son to be colour-blind.

121.(b): Sickle-cell anaemia is an autosomal recessive genetic disorder. It can be transmitted from parents to the offspring when both the partners are carriers of the gene (or heterozygous),

122.(d): Haemophilia is a sex-linked disease. It occurs due to the presence of a recessive sex linked gene h, which is carried by X-chromosome.

123.(b) : When a colour blind man (XC Y) marries a normal woman (XX), all of their daughters are carriers and all of their sons are normal, as shown in following figure:

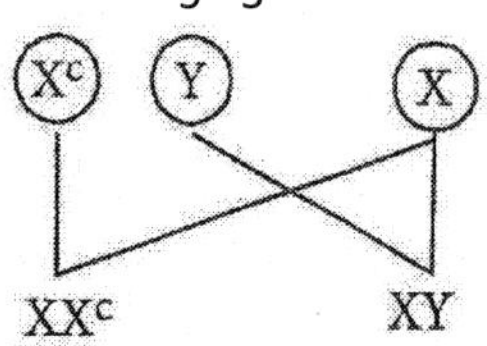

Carrier daughter   Normal son

When the carrier daughter (XX^C) is married to a normal man, the probability of their son being colour blind is 0.25 , as shown in following figure:

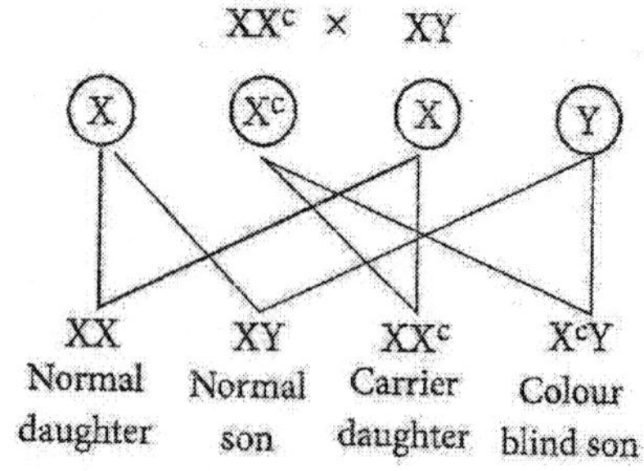

From above crosses, it is clear that the probability of occurrence of colour blindness in the grandson of a colour blind man and a normal woman is 0.25.

124.(a) : Autosomal recessive traits are the traits which are caused by recessive autosomal genes when present in homozygous condition. The given pedigree can be explained as:

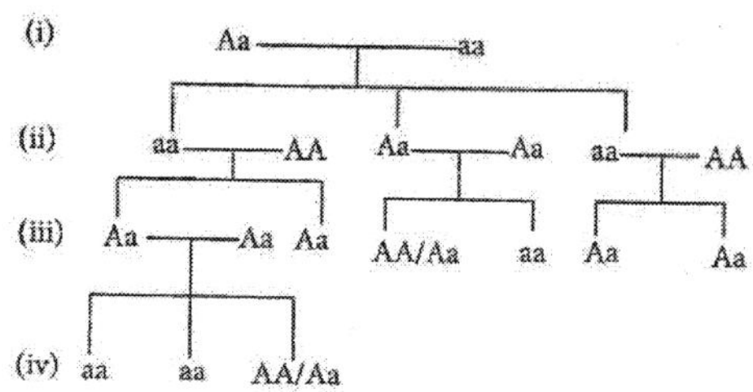

As the trait appears only in homozygous recessive individuals (aa), therefore it is an autosomal recessive trait.

125.(d) : The abnormal baby has an extra X chromosome, thus it must have been produced by fusion of abnormal XX ovum with a normal X sperm. Abnormal XX sperm is not possible because, males have XY genotype, and if produce abnormal sperms, then XY sperms and O sperms will be produced. If fusion of multiple gametes have occurred (either two ova with one sperm or two sperms with one ovum), then the human baby will have triploid genotype not the trisomy of sex chromosomes.

126.(c) : It is given that the man had colour blind father, i.e., man's genotype would be XY.

Now, the woman had a colourblind mother and normal father, thus her genotype would be X^C X. A cross between them can be represented as below.

Parents: X^cX × X Y
Gametes : X^c X X Y

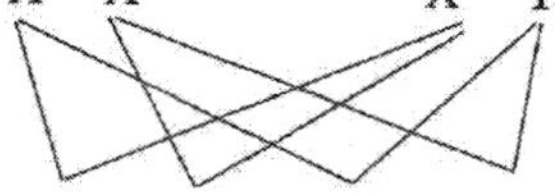

Progeny : X^cX XX X^cY XY
Carrier female, Normal female, Colour blind male, Normal male

Therefore, 50% of male children of this couple will be colour blind.

127.(a) : A human female with Turner's syndrome has single sex chromosome i.e., 44 + X0 (45). Such females are called sterile females with rudimentary ovaries. Other associated phenotypes of this condition are short stature, webbedneck, broad chest, lack of secondary sexual characteristics and sterility. Thus, any imbalance in the copies of the sex chromosomes may disrupt the genetic information necessary for normal sexual development.

128.(a) : Haemophilia is sex-linked disease which is also known as bleeder's disease as the patient will continue to bleed even from a minor cut since he or she does not possess the natural phenomenon of blood clotting due to absence of antihaemophiliac globulin or factor VIII (haemophilia A) and plasma thromboplastin factor IX (haemophilia-B, Christmas disease) essential for it. As a result of continuous bleeding, the patient may die of blood loss. It is genetically due to the presence of a recessive sex linked gene h, carried by X-chromosome. A female becomes haemophiliac only when both of her X-chromosomes carry the gene (Xh Xh). However, such females generally die before birth because the combination of these two recessive alleles is lethal. A female having only one allele for haemophilia (XXh) appears normal because the allele for normal blood clotting present on the other X-chromosome is dominant. Such females are known as carriers. In case of males, a single gene for the defect is able to express itself as the Y-chromosome is devoid of any corresponding allele (XhY).

129. (a) : Thalassaemia is an autosomal recessive blood disorder. In the given case, both the partners are unaffected carriers for the gene, i.e., have heterozygous genotype Tt. Persons homozygous for the autosomal recessive gene of β-thalassaemia suffer from severe haemolytic anaemia. Heterozygous persons are also not normal, but show the defect in a less severe form (thalassaemia minor).

Parents genotype: Tt × Tt
↓
Offspring genotype: TT : Tt : tt
1 : 2 : 1
Normal Carriers Affected
25% 50% 25%

130.(a) : Pedigree analysis is a system of analysis by following the movement and distribution of certain genetic traits in many generations of a family. Pedigree analysis cannot confirm that DNA Is the carrier of genetic information because it is an analysis system. For DNA based experiments, molecular biology techniques are used.

131.(b) : Down's syndrome is the trisomy of 21st chromosome in man. Down's syndrome is characterised by short stature, warty skin, protruding tongue, slanting eyes, with folded eyelids. The affected person's face presents a typical mongoloid look. Hence, it is also called as mongoloid idiocy. It occurs due to the phenomenon of non-disjunction. Non-disjunction occurs when a pair of homologous chromosomes do not separate in meiosis but migrate to the same pole of the cell resulting in an uneven number of chromosomes in the daughter cells (45 in one and 47 in other). This numerical abnormality results in trisomy (2n + 1) and monosomy (2n – 1). Non-disjunction is more common in sex chromosomes.

132.(b) : In the given condition the chances of child to be colour-blind is zero percent. It can be understood by the given cross :

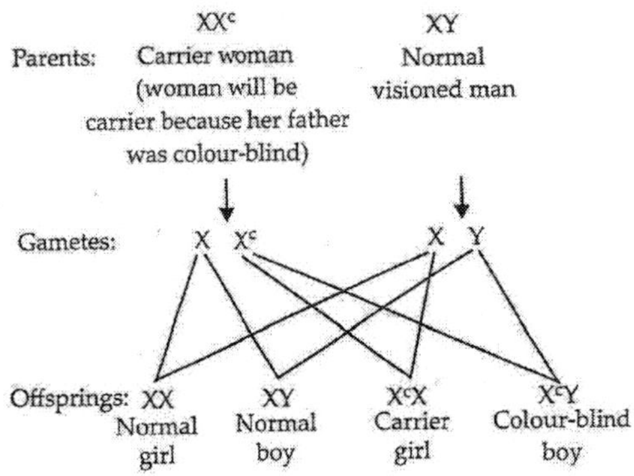

133. (c)

134.(b) : XO type of sex chromosomes determine male sex in grasshoppers. This type of sex-determination comes under XX–XO type. Its common examples are cockroaches, grasshoppers and bugs. The female has two homomorphic sex chromosomes XX and is homogametic. It produces similar eggs, each with X-chromosome. The male has one chromosome only and is heterogametic. It produces 2 types of sperms : gynosperms with X and androsperms without X. Fertilisation of an egg by X-bearing sperm yields female offspring and by no X bearing sperm yields male offspring

		Male	Female
Parents	Phenotypes	Male	Female
	Genotypes	AA + XO	AA + XX
Gametes		A + X, A + O	A + X, A + X

F_1 Generation

♂ \ ♀	A + X	A + X	
A + X	AA + XX	AA + XX	Females
A + O	AA + XO	AA + XO	Males
	Genotypes		Phenotypes

135.(a) : A record of inheritance of certain genetic traits for two or more generations presented in the form of a diagram or family tree is called pedigree. In a pedigree, a square represents the male, a circle the female, solid (blackened) symbol shows the trait under study or affected individual; unaffected or normal individual by an open or clear symbol and a cross or shade (of any type) in the symbol signifies the carrier of a recessive allele Words can also be used in place of symbols. Parents are shown by horizontal line while their offspring are connected to it by a vertical line. The offspring are then shown in the form of horizontal line below the parents and numbered with arabic numerals.

136. (a)

137.(b) : Sickle-cell anaemia is an autosomal hereditary disorder in which erythrocytes become sickle shaped. It is caused by the formation of abnormal haemoglobin called haemoglobin-S. Haemoglobin-S is formed when 6th amino acid of β-chain, i.e., glutamic acid is replaced by valine due to substitution. It occurs due to a single nucleotide change (A→T) in the β-globin gene of coding strand. In the normal β-globin gene the DNA sequence is CCTGAGGAG, while in sickle-cell anaemia, the sequence is CCTGTGGAG.

138.(a) : This chart shows inheritance of an autosomal recessive trait like phenylketonuria. An autosomal recessive trait may skip a generation. It appears in case of marriage between two heterozygous individuals (Aa × Aa = 3Aa + 1aa), a recessive individual with hybrid (Aa × aa = 2Aa + 2aa) and two recessive (aa × aa = all aa). Phenylketonuria is an inborn, autosomal, recessive metabolic disorder in which homozygous recessive individual lacks the enzyme phenylalanine hydroxylase. The heterozygous individuals are normal but carriers.

139.(c) : Klinefelter's syndrome is a genetic disorder in which there are three sex chromosomes, XXY, rather than the normal XX or XY. The number of autosomes are normal, i.e., 44. Affected individuals are apparently male but are tall and thin, with small testes, failure of normal sperm production (azoospermia), enlargement of the breasts (gynaecomastia) and absence of facial and body hairs.

140.(c) : A congenital disorder is a medical condition that is present at birth. Congenital disorders can be a result of genetic abnormalities, the intrauterine environment, or unknown factors. Sickle cell disease (a group of genetic disorders caused by sickle haemoglobin (HbS). HbS molecules tend to clump together, making red blood cells sticky, stiff and more fragile and causing them to form into a curved, sickle shape) and Huntington's chorea (an inherited disorder characterised by degenerative changes in the basal ganglia structures, which ultimately result in a severely shrunken brain and enlarged ventricles, abnormal body movements called chorea and loss of memory) are congenital disorders.

141.(a) : Colour blindness is a recessive sex-linked trait.

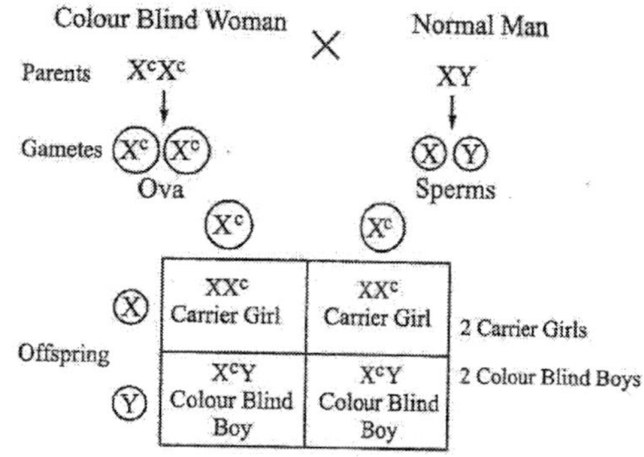

All sons will be colour blind and all daughters will be carriers.

142.(c) : Cri-du-chat syndrome, also called deletion 5p syndrome, (or 5p minus), is a rare genetic disorder. Cri-duchat syndrome is due to a partial deletion of the short arm of chromosome number 5. The name of this syndrome is French for "cry of the cat," referring to the distinctive cry of children with this disorder. The cry is caused by abnormal larynx development, which becomes normal within a few weeks of birth. Infants with cri-du-chat have low birth weight and may have respiratory problems. Some people with this disorder have a shortened lifespan, but most have a normal life expectancy.

143.(d) : Sickle cell anaemia is an autosomal hereditary disorder in which the erythrocytes become sickle shaped. The disorder or disease is caused by the formation of an abnormal haemoglobin called haemoglobin-S. Carriers of the sickle cell anaemia gene are protected against malaria because of their particular haemoglobin mutation; this explains why sickle cell anaemia is particularly common among people of African origin. The malarial parasite has a complex life cycle and spends part of it in red blood cells and feeds on haemoglobin. Both sickle-cell anaemia and thalassemia are more common in malaria areas, because these mutations convey some protection against the parasite. In a carrier, the presence of the malaria parasite causes the red blood cell to rupture, making the Plasmodium unable to reproduce. Further, the polymerisation of Hb affects the ability of the parasite to digest Hb in the first place. Therefore, in areas where malaria is a problem, people's chances of survival actually increase if they carry sickle cell anaemia. Thus, sickle-cell anaemia is a potential saviour from malaria.

144.(b) : Traits governed by sex-linked recessive genes : (a) produce disorders in males more often than in females, (b) express themselves in males even when represented by a single allele because Y-chromosome does not carry any corresponding alleles, (c) seldom appear in both father and son, (d) fail to appear in females unless their father also possesses the same and the mother is a carrier, (e) female heterozygous for the trait function as carrier and (f) female homozygous for the recessive trait transfer the trait to all the sons.

Take the example of colour blindness which is a recessive sexlinked trait. In the question, as man and woman do not show any signs of disease, so man must be normal and woman must be carrier.

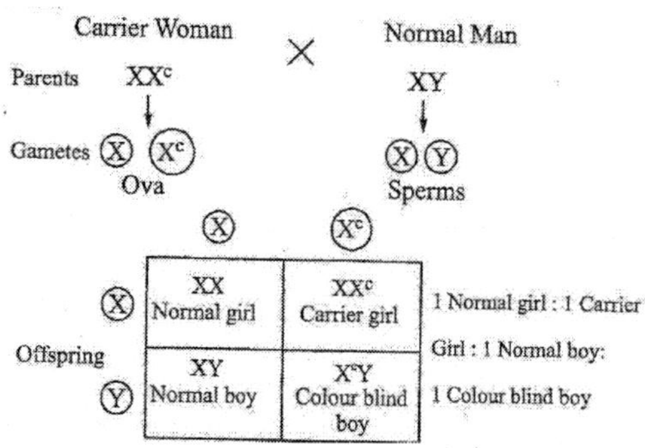

145.(d) : Down's syndrome is caused by the presence of an extra chromosome number 21. Both the chromosomes of the pair 21 pass into a single egg. Thus, the egg possesses 24 chromosomes instead of 23 and offspring has 47 chromosomes (45+XY in males, 45+XX in males) instead of 46 . Turner's syndrome is formed by the union of an abnormal 0 egg and a normal X sperm or a normal egg and an abnormal 0 sperm. The individual has 45 chromosomes (44+X) instead of 46 .

Female with more than two X chromosomes is called superfemale. Triploidy is a condition in which an organism has three times (3n) the haploid number (n) of chromosomes.

146. (c)

147.(d) : Cretinism occurs due to hyposecretion of thyroid hormones. Haemophilia is a sex linked recessive trait. Cystic fibrosis is also a recessive autosomal disorder resulting in mucus clogging in lungs. Thalassemia involves a gene mutation in the polypeptide chains of haemoglobin.

148.(a) : Colour blindness is a recessive sex-linked trait. Since the woman's father was colour blind, she should be carrier of the colour blind gene (X^C X). When she marries to colour blind man their progeny could be

Parent:	X^cX Carrier woman	×	X^cY Colourblind man	
Progeny:	X^cX^c Colour blind girl	X^cX Carrier girl	X^cY Colour blind son	XY Normal son

149.(b) : In question, where the genotype of the other parent is not mentioned then that should be considered normal. Colour blindness is a recessive sex-linked trait

(i) To find out the genotype of a woman.

Her father is colour-blind so his genotype is X^c Y and her mother is normal so her genotype is XX.

∴

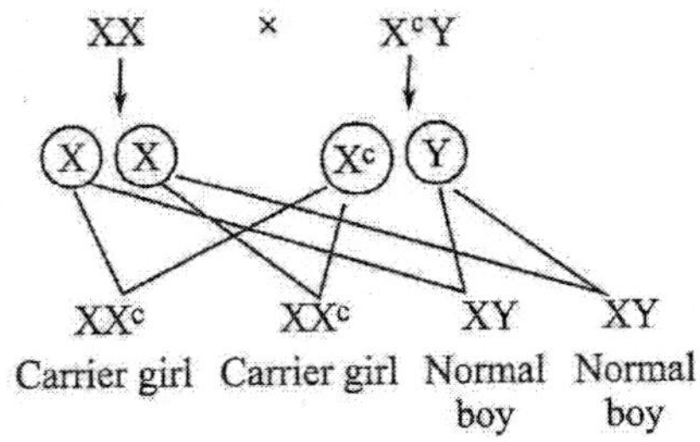

So, woman is carrier.

(ii) When this woman marries normal man

∴ 50% of the sons would be colour blind.

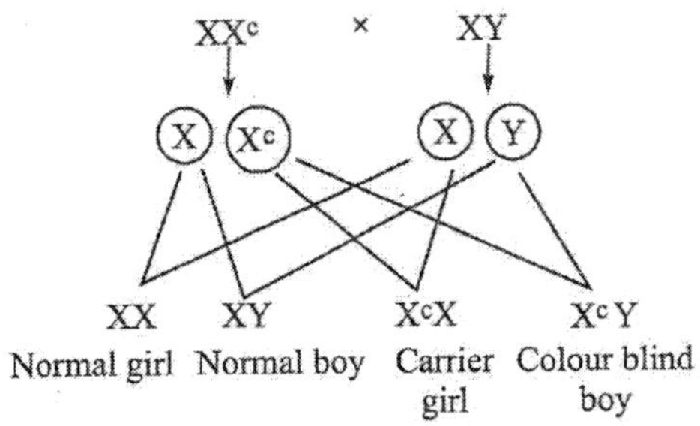

150.(c) : The recessive genes located on X-chromosome of humans are always expressed in males, e.g., colour blindness is a recessive sex-linked trait in which the eye fails to distinguish red and green colours. The gene for the normal vision is dominant. The normal gene and its recessive allele are carried by X-chromosomes. In females colour blindness appears only when both the sex chromosomes carry the recessive gene (Xc Xc). The females have normal vision but function as carrier if a single recessive gene for colour blindness is present (XXc). However, in human males the defect appears in the presence of a single recessive gene (XC Y) because Y-chromosome of male does not carry any gene for colour vision.

151.(b) :

152.(c) : Down's syndrome is the example of autosomal aneuploidy. Here, an extra copy of chromosome 21 occurs. As it is an autosomal disease, the offspring produced from affected mother and normal father should be 50%.

153.(a) : Haemophilia B, a type of haemophilia is also known as christmas disease. It is due to deficiency of a blood coagulation factor, the christmas factor (factor IX). Christmas was the person (20th century) in whom the factor was first identified. Haemophilia B is a defect of the blood which prevents its clotting.

154.(a) : In the inheritance pattern of sex chromosomes, X-chromosome of father always passes to daughter and X-chromosome of mother passes to son. As the father is diseased and all the girls inherit it, it is obvious the disease is sex-linked. The mother is not a carrier (as evident from the fact that no son is diseased). Thus, the gene is dominant and expresses even in heterozygous condition.

155.(a) : Down's syndrome (Mongolian Idiocy, Mongolism) is caused by the presence of an extra chromosome number 21. Sickle cell anaemia is not a sex linked (i.e., X linked) disease but an autosomally inherited recessive trait.

Haemophilia is X-linked but not holandric/Y-linked.

Parkinson's disease is a degenerative disease. It is not at all hereditary.

156.(b)

157. (a)

158. (a): Y-chromosome does not play any role in determination of sex in Drosophila. In human being, XXY is phenotypically male with underdeveloped testes, gynaecomastia and often mental retardation. It is caused by the union of a non-disjunct XX egg and sperm and a normal X egg and abnormal XY sperm. This indicates that in human being Y chromosome is active in sex determination.

159.(d) : Colour blindness is produced by a recessive gene which lies on X chromosome. A marriage between normal visioned man (XY) and colour blind woman (XC XC), results in colour blind sons (XC YC) and carrier daughters (XXC).

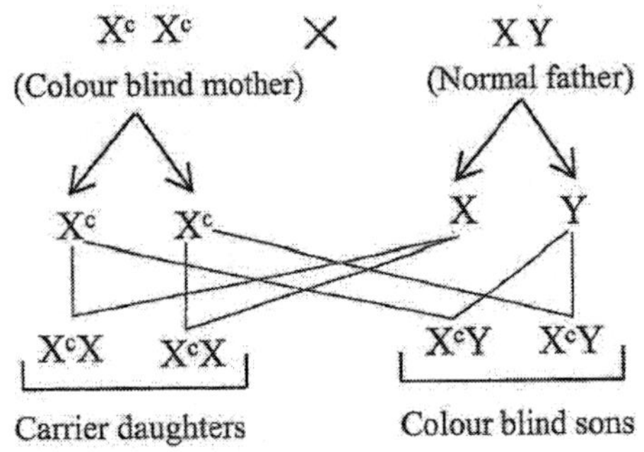

160.(d) : Haemophilia is caused by a recessive gene located in the X-chromosome. When a haemophilic man (Xh Y) marries a normal woman (XX), produces carrier girls (XXh) and normal boys (XY), i.e. all their offspring will be normal.

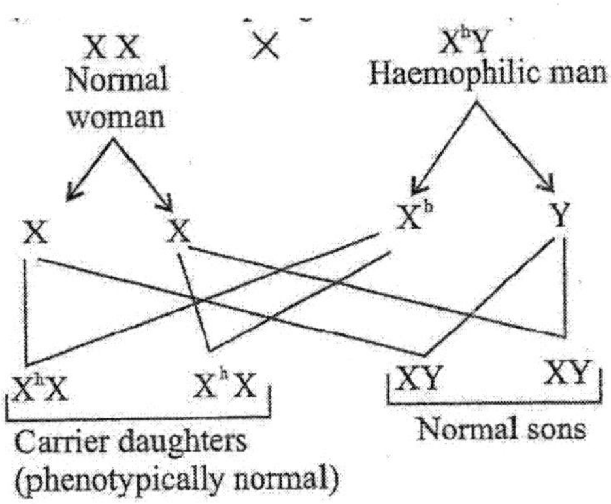

161.(a) : Both diseases are produced by a recessive genes which lies on the X-chromosomes. A woman with both gene for haemophilia and one gene for colour blindness on one of the X-chromosome will have genotype Xhc Xh.

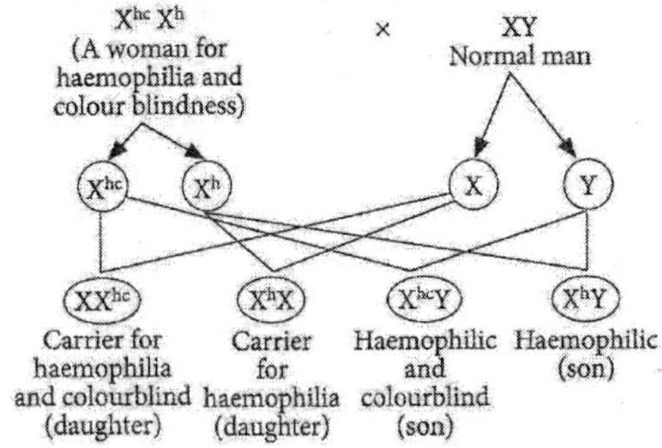

Thus, progeny includes 50% haemophilic colourblind sons and 50% haemophilic sons.

162.(d) : In humans, sex chromosomal abnormality is due to gene carried on X-chromosome. Increase in X-complement leads to Klinefelter's syndrome. The individiuals of Klinefelter's syndrome has 47 chromosomes (44 + XXY), this condition caused by a chromosome aneuploidy. Affected males have an extra X sex chromosome. It is formed by the union of an XX egg and normal Y sperm or normal X egg and abnormal XY sperm. Affected males are almost always effectively sterile, although advanced reproductive assistance is sometimes possible and some degree of language learning impairment and mental retardation may be present. In adults, possible characteristics vary widely and include little to no signs of affectedness, a lanky, youthful build and facial appearance, or a rounded body type with some degree of gynecomastia (increased breast tissue).

163. (b)

164. (b)

165.(d) : In question where the genotype of the other parent is not mentioned then that should be considered as normal.

(i) To find out the genotype of person.

His father is colour blind.

∴ genotype $=X^cY$ ...(i)

His mother is normal XX ...(ii)

Offspring X^cX, X^cX, XY, XY

As all sons will be normal therefore the genotype of the person will be XY.

(ii) To find out the genotype of lady ...(iii)

Father's genotype - XY ...(iv)

Her mother is a daughter of colourblind father and normal mother.

$X^cY \times XX$
X^cX, X^cX, XY, XY

So the mother of lady would be carrier having genotype X^cX ...(v)

Performing cross between (iv) and (v) to find out lady's genotype.

$XY \times X^cX$
X^cX, XX, X^cY, XY

As 50% daughter are carrier and 50% daughter are normal. So the lady can be normal or carrier having genotype XX, X'X respectively.

Now considering both the genotype of the lady and the genotype of the person, the result would be as follows.

$XY \times X^cX$ $\quad$ $XY \times XX$
X^cX, XY, XX, X^cY $\quad$ XX, XX, XY, XY

About cases show that if mother (lady) is carrier then options (a) and (c) are not true. Option (b) is true and option (d) all daughters normal (though phenotypically) is also true. If mother is normal then options (a), (b) and (c) are not true and option (d) is true so from the cases, it is concluded that option (d) is true.

166. (c)

167. (b)

168. (b)

169.(d) : The chance of a male child becoming colour blind are possible only when mother's father was colour blind. It is an example of criss cross inheritance. If a cross is made between two sexes differing in certain characters, in such a way that character of one sex remains hidden in the opposite sex of F1 generation, but it is passed on to the same sex in the F2 generation, it is said to exhibit criss cross inheritance.

170.(c) : The gene is located on one X-chromosomes of mother. Cross between a haemophilic carrier female Xh X and normal male would yield 50% of the sons being haemophilic and 50% of the daughter are carriers.

171. (a)

172. (d)

173.(c) : In human beings, 45 chromosomes/single X/XO abnormality causes Turner's syndrome. Individuals having a single X chromosome 2 A + XO (45) have female sexual differentiation but ovaries are rudimentary. Other associated phenotypes of this condition are short stature, webbed neck, broad chest, lack of secondary sexual characteristics and sterility. Thus, any unbalance in the copies of the sex chromosomes may disrupt the genetic information necessary for normal sexual development.

174.(b) : A colour blind girl is rare because she will be born only when her father and maternal grand-father were colour blind. The genotype of the mother was to be either XC XC or XCX and that of father XCY so that the daughter becomes colour blind.

175.(b) : In Down's syndrome of a male child, the sex complement is XY. Down syndrome is an autosomal birth defect caused by the presence of an extra chromosome number 21 (three instead of two number 21 chromosomes or trisomy 21).

176.(d) : Haemophilia is more common in males because it is a recessive trait carried by X-chromosome. Haemophilia A is the most common X-linked genetic disease that prevents normal blood clotting when blood vessels are ruptured.

177.(d) : Phenylketonuria is a hereditary disease. Phenylketonuria is an inherited error of metabolism caused by a deficiency in the enzyme phenylalanine hydroxylase. It results in mental retardation and is inherited as an autosomal recessive trait. It is a hereditary human condition resulting from the inability to convert phenylalanine into tyrosine. This change can be traced to a tiny mutation in a single gene on chromosome 12.

178.(a) : Both husband and wife have normal vision through their fathers were colour blind, the probability of their daughter becoming colour blind is 0%. The chances of daughter becoming colour blind arises only when the father is also colour blind.

Chapter : 24 MOLECULAR BASIS OF INHERITANCE

THE DNA

1. Given below are two statements: ***(2023)***

Statement I: In prokaryotes, the positively charged DNA is held with some negatively charged proteins in a region called nucleoid.

Statement II: In eukaryotes, the negatively charged DNA is wrapped around the positively charged histone octamer to form nucleosome.

In the light of the above statements, choose the correct answer from the options given below:

(a) Statement I is correct but Statement II is false.
(b) Statement I incorrect but Statement II is true
(c) Both Statement I and Statement II are true.
(d) Both Statement I and Statement II are false.

2. Read the following statements and choose correct statements : ***(2022)***

(A) Euchromatin is loosely packed chromatin.
(B) Heterochromatin is transcriptionally active.
(C) Histone octamer is wrapped by negatively charged DNA in nucleosome
(D) Histones are rich in lysine and arginine
(E) A typical nucleosome contains 400bp of DNA helix.

Choose the correct answer from the option below :

(a) (B), (D), (E) only (b) (A), (C), (D) only
(c) (B), (E) only (d) (A), (C), (E) only

3. If the length of a DNA molecule is 1.11 metres, what will be the approximate number of base pairs? ***(2022)***

(a) 3.3×10^9 bp (b) 6.6×10^9 bp
(c) 3.3×10^6 bp (d) 6.6×10^6 bp

4. Complete the flow chart on central dogma. ***(2021)***

$$P \circlearrowleft DNA \xrightarrow{Q} mRNA \xrightarrow{R} S$$

(a) (P)-Transduction; (Q)Translation; (R)-Replication; (S)-Protein
(b) (P)-Replication; (Q)-Transcription; (R)-Transduction; (S)-Protein
(c) (P)-Translation; (Q)-Replication; (R)-Transcription; (S)-Transduction
(d) (P)-Replication; (Q)-Transcription; (R)-Translation; (S)-Protein

5. If adenine makes 30% of the DNA molecule, what will be the percentage of thymine, guanine and cytosine in it? ***(2021)***

(a) T:20;G:25;C:25 (b) T:20;G:30;C:20
(c) T:20;G:20;C:30 (d) T:30;G:20;C:20

6. Which one of the following statements about histones is wrong? ***(2021)***

(a) Histones carry positive charge in the side chain.
(b) Histones are organized to form a unit of 8 molecules.
(c) The pH of histones is slightly acidic.
(d) Histones are rich in amino acids - Lysine and Arginine.

7. Which of the following statements is correct? ***(2020)***

(a) Adenine pairs with thymine through two H-bonds.
(b) Adenine pairs with thymine through one H-bond.
(c) Adenine pairs with thymine through three H-bonds.
(d) Adenine does not pair with thymine.

8. If the distance between two consecutive base pairs is 0.34 nm and the total number of base pairs of a DNA double helix in a typical mammalian cell is 6.6×10^9 bp, then the length of the DNA is approximately ***(2020)***

(a) 2.0 meters (b) 2.5 meters
(c) 2.2 meters (d) 2.7 meters.

9. Purines found both in DNA and RNA are ***(2019)***
(a) cytosine and thymine
(b) adenine and thymine
(c) adenine and guanine
(d) guanine and cytosine.

10. The association of histone H1 with a nucleosome indicates that ***(2017)***
(a) DNA replication is occurring
(b) the DNA is condensed into a chromatin fibre
(c) the DNA double helix is exposed
(d) transcription is occurring.

11. In sea urchin DNA, which is double stranded, 17% of the bases were shown to be cytosine. The percentages of the other three bases expected to be present in this DNA are ***(2015 Cancelled)***
(a) G 17%, A33%, T 33%
(b) G 8.5%, A 50%, T 24.5%
(c) G 34%, A 24.5%, T 24.5%
(d) G 17%, A 16.5%, T 32.5%.

12. The diagram shows an important concept in the genetic implication of DNA. Fill in the blanks A to C. ***(2013)***

$$\text{DNA} \xrightarrow{A} m\text{RNA} \xrightarrow{B} \text{Protein} \xrightarrow{\text{Proposed by}} C$$

(a) A - Transcription, B -Translation, C - Francis Crick
(b) A - Translation, B - Extension, C - Rosalind Franklin
(c) A - Transcription, B - Replication, C - James Watson
(d) A - Translation, B - Transcription, C - Ervin Chargaff

13. $$\text{DNA} \xrightarrow{C} m\text{RNA} \xrightarrow{B} \text{Protein} \xrightarrow{\text{Proposed by}} A$$

The figure gives an important concept in the genetic implication of DNA. Fill the blanks A, B and C. ***(Karnataka NEET 2013)***
(a) A-Maurice Wilkins, B-Transcription, C-Translation
(b) A-James Watson, B-Replication, C-Extension
(c) A-Erwin Chargaff, B-Translation, C-Replication
(d) A-Francis Crick, B-Translation, C-Transcription

14. What are the structures called that give an appearance as 'beads-on-string' in the chromosomes when viewed under electron microscope? ***(2011)***
(a) Genes (b) Nucleotides
(c) Nucleosomes (d) Base pairs

15. Which one of the following does not follow the central dogma of molecular biology? ***(2010)***
(a) Pea (b) Mucor
(c) Chlamydomonas (d) HIV

16. The 3–5 phosphodiester linkages inside a polynucleotide chain serve to join (Mains 2010)
(a) one DNA strand with the other DNA strand
(b) one nucleoside with another nucleoside
(c) one nucleotide with another nucleotide
(d) one nitrogenous base with pentose sugar.

17. Which one of the following statements about the particular entity is true? ***(Mains 2010)***
(a) Centromere is found in animal cells, which produces aster during cell division.
(b) The gene for producing insulin is present in every body cell.
(c) Nucleosome is formed of nucleotides.
(d) DNA consists of core of eight histones.

18. In the DNA molecule, ***(2008)***
(a) the proportion of adenine in relation to thymine varies with the organism
(b) there are two strands which run antiparallel- one in 5→3 direction and other in 3→5
(c) the total amount of purine nucleotides and pyrimidine nucleotides is not always equal
(d) there are two strands which run parallel in the 5→3 direction.

19. Which one of the following pairs of nitrogenous bases of nucleic acids, is wrongly matched with the category mentioned against it? ***(2008)***
(a) Guanine, Adenine - Purines
(b) Adenine, Thymine - Purines
(c) Thymine, Uracil - Pyrimidines
(d) Uracil, Cytosine - Pyrimidines

20. One turn of the helix in a B-form DNA is approximately ***(2006)***
(a) 2 nm (b) 20 nm
(c) 0.34 nm (d) 3.4 nm.

21. Antiparallel strands of a DNA molecule means that ***(2006)***
(a) one strand turns clockwise
(b) one strand turns anti-clockwise
(c) the phosphate groups of two DNA strands, at their ends, share the same position
(d) the phosphate groups at the start of two DNA strands are in opposite position (pole).

22. Which one of the following makes use of RNA template to synthesise DNA? ***(2005)***
(a) DNA polymerase
(b) RNA polymerase
(c) Reverse transcriptase
(d) DNA dependant RNA polymerase

23. Which one of the following hydrolyses internal phosphodiester bonds in a polynucleotide chain? ***(2005)***
(a) Lipase (b) Protease
(c) Endonuclease (d) Exonuclease

24. The following ratio is generally constant for a given species: ***(2004)***
(a) A+G/C+T (b) T+C/G+A
(c) G+C/A+T (d) A+C/T+G.

25. In a DNA percentage of thymine is 20% then what will be percentage of guanine? (2002)
(a) 20% (b) 40% (c) 30% (d) 60%

26. Length of one loop of B-DNA ***(2000)***
(a) 3.4nm (c) 20 nm
(b) 0.34 nm (d) 10 nm.

27. DNA is mainly found in ***(1999)***
(a) nucleolus (c) cytoplasm only
(b) nucleus only (d) none of these

28. In prokaryotes, the genetic material is ***(1999)***
(a) linear DNA without histones
(b) circular DNA without histones
(c) linear DNA with histones
(d) circular DNA with histones.

29. In DNA, when AGCT occurs, their association is as per which of the following pair? ***(1999)***
(a) AT-GC (b) AG-CT
(c) AC-GT (d) All of these

30. The eukaryotic genome differs from the prokaryotic genome because ***(1999)***
(a) the DNA is complexed with histone in prokaryotes
(b) the DNA is circular and single stranded in prokaryotes
(c) repetitive sequences are present in eukaryotes
(d) genes in the former case are organised into operons.

31. Genes are packaged into a bacterial chromosome by ***(1997)***
(a) acidic protein (b) actin
(c) histones (d) basic protein.

32. Radiotracer technique shows that DNA is in ***(1996)***
(a) multi-helix stage (b) single-helix stage
(c) double-helix stage (d) none of these.

33. Nucleosome core is made of ***(1993)***
(a) H_0, H_2 A, H_2B and H_3
(b) H_1, H_2A, H_2B, H_4
(c) H_1, H_2A, H_2B, H_3 and H_4
(d) H_2A, H_2B, H_3 and H_4.

34. A DNA with unequal nitrogen bases would most probably be ***(1993)***
(a) single stranded (b) double stranded
(c) triple stranded (d) four stranded.

35. Nucleotide arrangement in DNA can be seen by (1993)
(a) X-ray crystallography
(b) electron microscope
(c) ultracentrifuge
(d) light microscope.

36. An octamer of 4 histones complexed with DNA forms ***(1990)***
(a) endosome (b) nucleosome
(c) mesosome (d) centromere.

THE SEARCH FOR GENETIC MATERIAL

37. Given below are two statements: ***(2023)***

Statement I: RNA mutates at a faster rate.

Statement II: Viruses having RNA genome and shorter life span mutate and evolve faster.

In the light of the above statements, choose the correct answer from the options given below:
(a) Statement I is true but Statement II is false.
(b) Statement I false but Statement II is true.
(c) Both Statement I and Statement II are true.
(d) Both Statement I and Statement II are false.

38. Unequivocal proof that DNA is the genetic material was first proposed by ***(2023)***
(a) Avery, Macleoid and McCarthy
(b) Wilkins and Franklin
(c) Frederick Griffith
(d) Alfred Hershey and Martha Chase

39. The experimental proof for semi-conservative replication of DNA was first shown in a ***(2018)***
(a) fungus (b) bacterium
(c) plant (d) virus.

40. Select the correct match. ***(2018)***
(a) Ribozyme – Nucleic acid
(b) $F_2 \times$ Recessive parent – Dihybrid cross
(c) T.H. Morgan – Transduction
(d) G. Mendel – Transformation

41. The final proof for DNA as the genetic material came from the experiments of ***(2017)***
(a) Hershey and Chase
(b) Avery, MacLeod and McCarty
(c) Hargobind Khorana
(d) Griffith.

42. Taylor conducted the experiments to prove semiconservative mode of chromosome replication on ***(NEET-II 2016)***
(a) Vinca rosea
(b) Vicia faba
(c) Drosophila melanogaster
(d) E. coli.

43. A molecule that can act as a genetic material must fulfill the traits given below, except ***(NEET-II 2016)***
(a) it should be able to express itself in the form of 'Mendelian characters'
(b) it should be able to generate its replica
(c) it should be unstable structurally and chemically
(d) it should provide the scope for slow changes that are required for evolution.

44. Transformation was discovered by ***(2014)***
(a) Meselson and Stahl
(b) Hershey and Chase
(c) Griffith
(d) Watson and Crick.

45. The unequivocal proof of DNA as the genetic material came from the studies on a ***(Mains 2011)***
(a) bacterium (b) fungus
(c) viroid (d) bacterial virus.

46. Semi-conservative replication of DNA was first demonstrated in ***(2009)***
(a) Escherichia coli
(b) Streptococcus pneumoniae
(c) Salmonella typhimurium
(d) Drosophila melanogaster.

47. Transformation experiment was first performed on which bacteria? ***(2002)***
(a) E. coli
(b) Diplococcus pneumoniae
(c) Salmonella
(d) Pasteurella pestis

48. The Pneumococcus experiment proves that ***(1999)***
(a) bacteria do not reproduce sexually
(b) RNA sometime controls the production of DNA and proteins
(c) DNA is the genetic material
(d) bacteria undergo binary fission.

49. DNA synthesis can be specifically measured by estimating the incorporation of radio-labelled ***(1997)***
(a) thymidine (b) deoxyribose sugar
(c) uracil (d) adenine.

50. The transforming principle of Pneumococcus as found out by Avery, MacLeod and McCarty was ***(1993)***
(a) mRNA (b) DNA
(c) protein (d) polysaccharide.

51. Who proved that DNA is basic genetic material? ***(1993)***
(a) Griffith (b) Watson
(c) Boveri and Sutton (d) Hershey and Chase

52. Escherichia coli fully labelled with 15N is allowed to grow in 14N medium. The two strands of DNA molecule of the first generation bacteria have ***(1992)***
(a) different density and do not resemble parent DNA
(b) different density but resemble parent DNA
(c) same density and resemble parent DNA
(d) same density but do not resemble parent DNA.

RNA WORLD

53. Which one of the following is not applicable to RNA? ***(2015)***
(a) Heterocyclic nitrogenous bases
(b) Chargaff's rule
(c) Complementary base pairing
(d) 5′ phosphoryl and 3′ hydroxyl ends

54. Similarity in DNA and RNA is that ***(2000)***
(a) both are polymer of nucleotides
(b) both have similar pyrimidine
(c) both have similar sugar
(d) both are genetic material.

REPLICATION

55. Ten E.coli cells with 15N-dsDNA are incubated in medium containing 14N nucleotide. After 60 minutes, how many E.coli cells will have DNA totally free from 15N ? ***(2005)***
(a) 20 cells (b) 40 cells
(c) 60 cells (d) 80 cells

56. During DNA replication, Okazaki fragments are used to elongate ***(2017)***
(a) the lagging strand towards replication fork
(b) the leading strand away from replication fork
(c) the lagging strand away from the replication fork
(d) the leading strand towards replication fork.

57. During replication of a bacterial chromosome DNA synthesis starts from a replication origin site and ***(2004)***
(a) RNA primers are involved
(b) is facilitated by telomerase
(c) moves in one direction of the site
(d) moves in bidirectional way.

58. Method of DNA replication in which two strands of DNA separate and synthesise new strands is called ***(2000)***
(a) dispersive (b) conservative
(c) semi-conservative (d) non conservative.

59. There are special proteins that help to open up DNA double helix in front of the replication fork. These proteins are ***(1994)***
(a) DNA ligase (b) DNA topoisomerase I
(c) DNA gyrase (d) DNA polymerase I.

60. During DNA replication, the strands separate by ***(1993)***
(a) DNA polymerase (b) topoisomerase
(c) unwindase/helicase (d) gyrase,

61. Experimental material in the study of DNA replication has been ***(1992)***
(a) Escherichia coli (b) Neurospora crassa
(c) Pneuтococcus
(d) Drosophila melanogaster.

62. DNA replication is ***(1989)***
(a) conservative and discontinuous
(b) semi-conservative and semi-discontinuous
(c) semi-conservative and discontinuous
(d) conservative.

TRANSCRIPTION

63. What is the role of RNA polymerase III in the process of transcription in Eukaryotes? ***(2023)***
(a) Transcription of precursor of mRNA
(b) Transcription of only snRNAs
(c) Transcription of rRNAs (28S, 18S and 5.8S)
(d) Transcription of tRNA, 5 SrRNA and snRNA

64. Which one of the following is the sequence on corresponding coding strand, if the sequence on mRNA formed is as follows. ***(2023)***

5′ AUCGAUCGAUCGAUCGAUCGAUCGAUCG 3′?
(a) 5′ ATCGATCGATCGATCGATCGATCGATCG 3′
(b) 3′ ATCGATCGATCGATCGATCGATCGATCG 5
(c) 5′ UAGCUAGCUAGCUAGCUAGCUAGC UAGC 3′
(d) 3′ UAGCUAGCUAGCUAGCUAGCUAGCUAGC 5′

65. What is the role of RNA polymerase III in the process of transcription in eukaryotes? ***(2021)***
(a) Transcribes only snRNAs
(b) Transcribes r RNAs (28S, 18S and 5.8S)
(c) Transcribes t RNA, 5S rRNA and snRNA
(d) Transcribes precursor of mRNA

66. Identify the correct statement. ***(2021)***
(a) Split gene arrangement is characteristic of prokaryotes.
(b) In capping, methyl guanosine triphosphate is added to the 3′ end of hnRNA.
(c) RNA polymerase binds with Rho factor to terminate the process of transcription in bacteria.
(d) The coding strand in a transcription unit is copied to an mRNA.

67. Which is the "only enzyme" that has "capability" to catalyse initiation, elongation and termination in the process of transcription in prokaryotes? ***(2021)***
(a) DNase
(b) DNA dependent DNA polymerase
(c) DNA dependent RNA polymerase
(d) DNA Ligase

68. Name the enzyme that facilitates opening of DNA helix during transcription. ***(2020)***
(a) DNA ligase (b) DNA helicase
(c) DNA polymerase (d) RNA polymerase

69. What will be the sequence of m RNA produced by the following stretch of DNA? ***(Odisha NEET 2019)***

3′ ATGCATGCATGCATG5′TEMPLATE STRAND
5′TACGTACGTACGTAC3′ CODING STRAND
(a) 3′AUGCAUGCAUGCAUG5′
(b) 5′UACGUACGUACGUAC 3′
(c) 3′ UACGUACGUACGUAC 5′
(d) 5′ AUGCAUGCAUGCAUG 3′

70. Match the following RNA polymerase with their transcribed products : ***(Odisha NEET 2019)***

1. RNA polymerase I	(i) tRNA
2. RNA polymerase II	(ii) rRNA
3. RNA polymerase III	(iii) hnRNA

Select the correct option from the following :
(a) 1-i, 2-iii, 3-ii (b) 1-i, 2-ii, 3-iii
(c) 1-ii, 2-iii, 3-i (d) 1-iii, 2-ii, 3-i

71. Select the correct statement. ***(2018)***
(a) Franklin Stahl coined the term "linkage".
(b) Punnett square was developed by a British scientist.
(c) Spliceosomes take part in translation.
(d) Transduction was discovered by S. Altman.

72. AGGTATCGCAT is a sequence from the coding strand of a gene. What will be the corresponding sequence of the transcribed m RNA? ***(2018)***
(a) AGGUAUCGCAU (b) UGGTUTCGCAT
(c) ACCUAUGCGAU (d) UCCAUAGCGUA

73. Which of the following RNAs should be most abundant in animal cell? ***(2017)***
(a) tRNA (b) mRNA
(c) miRNA (d) r RNA

74. Spliceosomes are not found in cells of ***2017)***
(a) fungi (b) animals
(c) bacteria (d) plants

75. The equivalent of a structural gene is ***(NEET-II 2016)***
(a) muton (b) cistron
(c) operon (d) recon

76. Which of the following rRNAs acts as structural RNA as well as ribozyme in bacteria? ***(NEET-II 2016)***
(a) 5S rRNA (b) 18S rRNA
(c) 23S rRNA (d) 5.8S rRNA

77. DNA-dependent RNA polymerase catalyses transcription on one strand of the DNA which is called the ***(NEET-II 2016)***
(a) template strand (b) coding strand
(c) alpha strand (d) antistrand.

78. Select the correct option. ***(2014)***

	Direction of RNA synthesis	**Direction of reading of the template DNA strand**
(a)	5′-3′	3′–5′
(b)	3′-5′	5′–3′
(c)	5′–3′	5′–3′
(d)	3′–5′	3′–5′

79. Removal of introns and joining of exons in a defined order during transcription is called ***(2012,2009)***
(a) looping (b) inducing
(c) slicing (d) splicing.

80. If one strand of DNA has the nitrogenous base sequence as ATCTG, what would be the complementary RNA strand sequence? ***(2012)***
(a) TTAGU (b) UAGAC
(c) AACTG (d) ATCGU

81. Ribosomal RNA is actively synthesised in ***(2012)***
(a) lysosomes (b) nucleolus
(c) nucleoplasm (d) ribosomes.

82. Which one of the following is not a part of a transcription unit in DNA? ***(2012)***
(a) The inducer (b) A terminator
(c) A promoter (d) The structural gene

83. Removal of RNA polymerase III from nucleoplasm will affect the synthesis of ***(2012)***
(a) tRNA (b) hnRNA
(c) mRNA (d) r RNA.

84. Which one of the following also acts as a catalyst in a bacterial cell? ***(2011)***
(a) 5S rRNA (b) snRNA
(c) hnRNA (d) 23S rRNA

85. In eukaryotic cell transcription, RNA splicing and RNA capping take place inside the ***(Main 2010)***
(a) ribosomes (b) nucleus
(c) dictyosomes (d) ER.

86. Which form of RNA has a structure resembling clover leaf? ***(2004)***
(a) rRNA (b) hnRNA
(c) mRNA (d) t RNA

87. During transcription, if the nucleotide sequence of the DNA strand that is being coded is ATACG then the nucleotide sequence in the m RNA would be ***(2004)***
(a) TATGC (b) TCTGG
(c) UAUGC (d) UATGC.

88. During transcription, the DNA site at which RNA polymerase binds is called ***(2003)***
(a) promoter (b) regulator
(c) receptor (d) enhancer.

89. Which of the following reunites the exon segments after RNA splicing? ***(2002)***
(a) RNA polymerase (b) RNA primase
(c) RNA ligase(d) RNA proteoses

90. Exon part of mRNAs have code for ***(2002)***
(a) protein (b) lipid
(c) carbohydrate (d) phospholipid.

91. mRNA is synthesised on DNA template in which direction? ***(2001)***
(a) $5 \rightarrow 3$ (b) $3 \rightarrow 5$
(c) Both (a) and (b) (d) Any

92. Gene and cistron words are sometimes used synonymously because ***(2001)***
(a) one cistron contains many genes
(b) one gene contains many cistrons
(c) one gene contains one cistron
(d) one gene contains no cistron.

93. Types of RNA polymerase required in nucleus of eukaryotes for RNA synthesis (2001)
(a) 1 (b) 2 (c) 3 (d) 4

94. Anticodon occurs in ***(2000)***
(a) tRNA (c) rRNA
(b) mRNA (d) DNA.

95. In three dimensional view the molecule of t RNA is ***(2000)***
(a) L-shaped (b) S-shaped
(c) Y-shaped (d) E-shaped.

96. Genes that are involved in turning on or off the transcription of a set of structural genes are called ***(1998)***
(a) redundant genes
(b) regulatory genes
(c) polymorphic genes
(d) operator genes.

97. DNA elements, which can switch their position, are called ***(1998)***
(a) cistrons (b) transposons
(c) exons (d) introns.

GENETIC CODE

98. Statement I : The codon 'AUG' codes for methionine and phenylalanine. ***(2021)***

Statement II: 'AAA' and 'AAG' both codons code for the amino acid lysine.

In the light of the above statements, choose the correct answer from the options given below.
(a) Statement I is incorrect but Statement II is true.
(b) Both Statement I and Statement II are true.
(c) Both Statement I and Statement II are false.
(d) Statement I is correct but Statement II is false.

99. Under which of the following conditions there will be no change in the reading frame of following m RNA? ***(2019)***

5 AACAGCGGUGCUAUU 3
(a) Deletion of GGU from 7th, 8th and 9th positions
(b) Insertion of G at 5th position
(c) Deletion of G from 5th position
(d) Insertion of A and G at 4th and 5th position respectively

100. Which of the following features of genetic code does allow bacteria to produce human insulin by recombinant DNA technology? ***(2019)***
(a) Genetic code is specific.
(b) Genetic code is not ambiguous.
(c) Genetic code is redundant.
(d) Genetic code is nearly universal.

101. If there are 999 bases in an RNA that code for a protein with 333 amino acids; and the base at position 901 is deleted such that the length of the RNA becomes 998 bases, how many codons will be altered? ***(2017)***
(a) 11 (b) 33
(c) 333 (d) 1

102. Which one of the following is the starter codon? ***(NEET-I 2016)***
(a) UAA (b) UAG
(c) AUG (d) UGA

103. Which of the following is not a property of the genetic code? ***(Karnataka NEET 2013)***
(a) Non-overlapping (b) Ambiguous
(c) Degeneracy (d) Universal

104. The one aspect which is not a salient feature of genetic code, is its being (2010)
(a) degenerate (b) ambiguous
(c) universal (d) specific.

105. Whose experiments cracked the DNA and discovered unequivocally that a genetic code is a "triplet"? ***(2009)***
(a) Hershey and Chase
(b) Morgan and Sturtevant
(c) Beadle and Tatum
(d) Nirenberg and Mathaei

106. What is not true for genetic code? ***(2009)***
(a) It is nearly universal.
(b) It is degenerate.
(c) It is unambiguous.
(d) A codon in mRNA is read in a non-contiguous fashion.

107. Which one of the following pairs of codons is correctly matched with their function or the signal for the particular amino acid? (2008)
(a) AUG, ACG - Start/methionine
(b) UUA, UCA - Leucine
(c) GUU, GCU - Alanine
(d) UAG, UGA - Stop

108. After a mutation at a genetic locus the character of an organism changes due to change in ***(2004)***
(a) protein structure
(b) DNA replication
(c) protein synthesis pattern
(d) RNA transcription pattern.

109. In mutational event, when adenine is replaced by guanine, it is a case of ***(2004)***
(a) frame shift mutation
(b) transcription
(c) transition
(d) transversion.

110. What would happen if in a gene encoding a polypeptide of 50amino acids, 25th codon (UAU) is mutated to UAA? ***(2003)***
(a) A polypeptide of 24 amino acids will be formed.
(b) Two polypeptides of 24 and 25 amino acids will be formed.
(c) A polypeptide of 49 amino acids will be formed.
(d) A polypeptide of 25 amino acids will be formed.

111. Which one of the following triplet codes, is correctly matched with its specificity for an amino acid in protein synthesis or as 'start' or 'stop' codon? ***(2003)***
(a) UCG - Start (b) UUU - Stop
(c) UGU - Leucine (d) UAC - Tyrosine

112. Degeneration of a genetic code is attributed to the ***(2003)***
(a) first member of a codon
(b) second member of codon
(c) entire codon
(d) third member of a codon.

113. In the genetic code dictionary, how many codons are used to code for all the 20 essential amino acids? ***(2003)***
(a) 20 (b) 64
(c) 61 (d) 60

114. Out of 64 codons, 61 codons code for 20 types of amino acid. It is called ***(2002)***
(a) degeneracy of genetic code
(b) overlapping of gene
(c) wobbling of codon
(d) universility of codons.

115. Change in sequence of nucleotide in DNA is called ***(2002)***
(a) mutagen (b) mutation
(c) recombination (d) translation.

116. Which of the following is initiation codon? ***(2000)***
(a) UAG (b) AUC (c) AUG (d) CCU

117. Initiation codon in eukaryotes is ***(1999, 1994)***
(a) GAU (b) AGU
(c) AUG (d) UAG.

118. The codons causing chain termination are ***(1997)***
(a) AGT, TAG, UGA (b) UAG, UGA, UAA
(c) TAG, TAA, TGA (d) GAT, AAT, AGT.

119. Which of the following serves as a terminal codon? ***(1996)***
(a) UAG (b) AGA
(c) AUG (d) GCG

120. If the DNA codons are ATG ATG ATG and a cytosine base is inserted at the beginning, then which of the following will result? ***(1995)***
(a) CAT GAT GAT G
(b) A non-sense mutation
(c) C ATG ATG ATG
(d) CA TGA TGA TG

121. Anticodon is an unpaired triplet of bases in an exposed position of ***(1995)***
(a) tRNA (b) mRNA
(c) rRNA(d) both (b) and (c)

122. Initiation codon of protein synthesis (in eukaryotes) is ***(1993)***
(a) GUA (b) GCA
(c) CCA (d) AUG.

123. In the genetic dictionary, there are 64 codons as ***(1990)***
(a) 64 amino acids are to be coded
(b) 64 types of tRNAs are present
(c) there are 44 nonsense codons and 20 sense codons
(d) genetic code is triplet.

124. Genetic code consists of ***(1988)***
(a) adenine and guanine
(b) cytosine and uracil
(c) cytosine and guanine
(d) all of these.

TRANSLATION

125. The process of translation of mRNA to proteins begins as soon as ***(2022)***
(a) the small subunit of ribosome encounter mRNA
(b) the larger subunit of ribosome encounters m RNA
(c) both the subunits join together to bind with m RNA
(d) the tRNA is activated and the larger subunit of ribosome encounters m RNA.

126. Which of the following RNAs is not required for the synthesis of protein? ***(2021)***
(a) siRNA (b) mRNA
(c) tRNA (d) rRNA

127. The first phase of translation is ***(2020)***
(a) binding of mRNA to ribosome
(b) recognition of DNA molecule
(c) aminoacylation of t RNA
(d) recognition of an anti-codon.

128. Many ribosomes may associate with a single mRNA to form multiple copies of a polypeptide simultaneously. Such strings of ribosomes are termed as ***(2018)***
(a) polysome (b) polyhedral bodies
(c) plastidome (d) nucleosome.

129. A complex of ribosomes attached to a single strand of RNA is known as ***(NEET-I 2016)***
(a) polypeptide (b) Okazaki fragment
(c) polysome (d) polymer.

130. Polysome is formed by ***(2008)***
(a) a ribosome with several subunits
(b) ribosomes attached to each other in a linear arrangement
(c) several ribosomes attached to a single mRNA
(d) many ribosomes attached to a strand of endoplasmic reticulum.

131. The two sub-units of ribosome remain united at a critical ion level of ***(2008)***
(a) magnesium (b) calcium
(c) copper (d) manganese.

132. Which antibiotic inhibits interaction between t RNA and m RNA during bacterial protein synthesis? ***(2006)***
(a) Tetracycline (b) Erythromycin
(c) Neomycin (d) Streptomycin

133. Amino acid sequence, in protein synthesis is decided by the sequence of ***(2006)***
(a) rRNA (b) t RNA
(c) mRNA (d) cDNA.

134. Using imprints from a plate with complete medium and carrying bacterial colonies, you can select streptomycin resistant mutants and prove that such mutations do not originate as adaptation. These imprints need to be used ***(2005)***
(a) on plates with and without streptomycin
(b) on plates with minimal medium
(c) only on plates with streptomycin
(d) only on plates without streptomycin.

135. Protein synthesis in an animal cell occurs ***(2005)***
(a) only on the ribosomes present in cytosol
(b) only on ribosome attached to the nuclear envelope and endoplasmic reticulum
(c) on ribosome present in the nucleolus as well as in cytoplasm
(d) on ribosomes present in cytoplasm as well as in mitochondria.

136. During translation initiation in prokaryotes, a GTP molecule is needed in ***(2003)***
(a) formation of formyl-met- tRNA
(b) binding of 30S subunit of ribosome with mRNA
(c) association of 30S mRNA with formyl-mettRNA
(d) association of 50S subunit of ribosome with initiation complex.

137. The RNA that pick up specific amino acid from amino acid pool in the cytoplasm to ribosome during protein synthesis is called ***(1997)***
(a) rRNA (b) RNA
(c) mRNA (d) t RNA.

138. Protein synthesis in an animal cell, takes place ***(1997)***
(a) in the cytoplasm as well as endoplasmic reticulum
(b) only on ribose attached to nucleon
(c) only in the cytoplasm
(d) in the nucleolus as well as in the cytoplasm.

139. In protein synthesis, the polymerisation of amino acids involves three steps. Which one of the following is not involved in the polymerisation of protein? ***(1994)***
(a) Termination (b) Initiation
(c) Elongation (d) Transcription

140. Because most of the amino acids are represented by more than one codon, the genetic code is ***(1993)***
(a) overlapping (b) wobbling
(c) degenerate (d) generate.

141. The process of translation is ***(1993)***
(a) ribosome synthesis
(b) protein synthesis
(c) DNA synthesis
(d) RNA synthesis.

REGULATION OF GENE EXPRESSION

142. Match List I with List II. ***(2023)***

List I	List II
A. Gene 'a'	I. β-galactosidae
B. Gene 'y'	II. Transacetylase
C. Gene 'i'	III. Permease
D. Gene 'z'	IV. Repressor protein

Choose the correct answer from the options given below:
(a) A-III, B-IV, C-I, D-II (b) A-III, B-I, C-IV, D-II
(c) A-II, B-I, C-IV, D-III (d) A-II, B-III, C-IV, D-I

143. In an E.coli strain i gene gets mutated and its product cannot bind the inducer molecule. If growth medium is provided with lactose, what will be the outcome? ***(2022)***

(a) Only z gene will get transcribed
(b) z,y, a genes will be transcribed
(c) z,y, a genes will not be translated
(d) RNA polymerase will bind the promoter region

144. Match the following genes of the Lac operon with their respective products. ***(2019)***

(A) *i* gene	(i) β-galactosidase
(B) *z* gene	(ii) Permease
(C) *a* gene	(iii) Repressor
(D) *y* gene	(iv) Transacetylase

Select the correct option.

	A	B	C	D
(a)	(iii)	(iv)	(i)	(ii)
(b)	(i)	(iii)	(ii)	(iv)
(c)	(iii)	(i)	(ii)	(iv)
(d)	(iii)	(i)	(iv)	(ii)

145. Select the correct match. ***(2018)***

(a) Alec Jeffreys – Streptococcus pneumoniae
(b) Alfred Hershey and Martha Chase – TMV
(c) Matthew Meselson and F. Stahl – Pisum sativum
(d) Francois Jacob and Jacques Monod – Lac operon

146. All of the following are part of an operon except ***(2018)***

(a) an operator (b) structural genes
(c) an enhancer (d) a promoter.

147. Which of the following is required as inducer(s) for the expression of Lac operon? ***(NEET-I 2016)***

(a) Lactose
(b) Lactose and galactose
(c) Glucose
(d) Galactose

148. Gene regulation governing lactose operon of E.coli that involves the lac I gene product is ***(2015 Cancelled)***

(a) negative and repressible because repressor protein prevents transcription
(b) feedback inhibition because excess of β-galactosidase can switch off transcription
(c) positive and inducible because it can be induced by lactose
(d) negative and inducible because repressor protein prevents transcription.

149. Which one of the following is wrongly matched? ***(2014)***

(a) Transcription - Writing information from DNA to t RNA.
(b) Translation - Using information in mRNA to make protein.
(c) Repressor protein - Binds to operator to stop enzyme synthesis.
(d) Operon - Structural genes, operator and promoter.

150. Which enzyme will be produced in a cell if there is a nonsense mutation in the lac Y gene? ***(2013)***

(a) Transacetylase
(b) Lactose permease and transacetylase
(c) β-galactosidase
(d) Lactose permease

151. In an inducible operon, the genes are ***(Karnataka NEET 2013)***

(a) usually not expressed unless a signal turns them "on".
(b) usually expressed unless a signal turns them "off".
(c) never expressed
(d) always expresser.

152. Select the two correct statements out of the four (i - iv) statements given below about lac operon. ***(2010)***

(i) Glucose or galactose may bind with the repressor and inactivate it.

(ii) In the absence of lactose, the repressor binds with the operator region.
(iii) The z-gene codes for permease.
(iv) This was elucidated by Francois Jacob and Jacques Monod.

The correct statements are
(a) (ii) and (iii)
(b) (i) and (iii)
(c) (ii) and (iv)
(d) (i) and (ii).

153. The lac operon consists of *(Mains 2010)*
(a) four regulatory genes only
(b) one regulatory gene and three structural genes
(c) two regulatory genes and two structural genes
(d) three regulatory genes and three structural genes.

154. E.coli cells with a mutated z gene of the lac operon cannot grow in medium containing only lactose as the source of energy because *(2005)*
(a) the lac operon is constitutively active in these cells
(b) they cannot synthesise functional beta galactosidase
(c) in the presence of glucose, E.coli cells do not utilise lactose
(d) they cannot transport lactose from the medium into the cell.

155. What does "lac" refer to in what we call the lac operon? *(2003)*
(a) Lactose
(b) Lactase
(c) Lac insect
(d) The number 1,00,000

156. Jacob and Monod studied lactose metabolism in E. coli and proposed operon concept. Operon concept is applicable for *(2002)*
(a) all prokaryotes
(b) all prokaryotes and some eukaryotes
(c) all prokaryotes and all eukaryotes
(d) all prokaryotes and some protozoans.

157. In E.coli, during lactose metabolism repressor binds to *(2002)*
(a) regulator gene
(b) operator gene
(c) structural gene
(d) promoter gene.

158. In negative operon, *(2001)*
(a) co-repressor binds with repressor
(b) co-repressor does not bind with repressor
(c) co-repressor binds with inducer
(d) CAMP have negative effect on lac operon.

159. The wild type E.coli cells are growing in normal medium with glucose. They are transferred to a medium containing only lactose as sugar. Which of the following changes take place? *(1995)*
(a) The lac operon is induced.
(b) E.coli cells stop dividing.
(c) The lac operon is repressed.
(d) All operons are induced.

160. The lac operon is an example of *(1995)*
(a) repressible operon
(b) overlapping genes
(c) arabinose operon
(d) inducible operon.

HUMAN GENOME PROJECT

161. Expressed Sequence Tags (EST's) refers to *(2023)*
(a) all genes whether expressed or unexpressed
(b) certain important expressed genes
(c) all genes that are expressed as RNA
(d) all genes that are expressed as proteins

162. If a geneticist uses the blind approach for sequencing the whole genome of an organism, followed by assignment of function to different segments, the methodology adopted by him is called as: *(2022)*
(a) Sequence annotation
(b) Gene mapping
(c) Expressed sequence tags
(d) Bioinformatics

163. Expressed Sequence Tags (ESTs) refers to ***(2019)***

(a) novel DNA sequences
(b) genes expressed as RNA
(c) polypeptide expression
(d) DNA polymorphism.

164. Identify the correct order of organisation of genetic material from largest to smallest. (2015)

(a) Genome, chromosome, gene, nucleotide
(b) Chromosome, genome, nucleotide, gene
(c) Chromosome, gene, genome, nucleotide
(d) Genome, chromosome, nucleotide, gene

165. Satellite DNA is important because it ***(2015)***

(a) does not code for proteins and is same in all members of the population
(b) codes for enzymes needed for DNA replication
(c) codes for proteins needed in cell cycle
(d) showshigh degree of polymorphism in population and also the same degree of polymorphism in an individual, which is heritable from parents to children.

DNA FINGERPRINTING

166. DNA polymorphism forms the basis of ***(2022)***

(a) genetic mapping
(b) DNA finger printing
(c)both genetic mapping and DNA fingerprinting
(d) translation.

167. DNA fingerprinting involves identifying differences in some specific regions in DNA sequence, called as ***(2021)***

(a) polymorphic DNA (b) satellite DNA
(c) repetitive DNA (d) single nucleotides.

168. Which of the following is not required for any of the techniques of DNA fingerprinting available at present? ***(NEET-I 2016)***

(a) Restriction enzymes
(b) DNA-DNA hybridisation
(c) Polymerase chain reaction
(d) Zinc finger analysis

169. One of the most frequently used techniques in DNA fingerprinting is ***(Karnataka NEET 2013)***

(a) VNTR (b) SSCP
(c) SCAR (d) AFLP.

170. What is it that forms the basis of DNA fingerprinting? ***(Mains 2012)***

(a) The relative proportions of purines and pyrimidines in DNA.
(b) The relative difference in the DNA occurrence in blood, skin and saliva.
(c) The relative amount of DNA in the ridges and grooves of the fingerprints.
(d) Satellite DNA occurring as highly repeated short DNA segments.

171. DNA fingerprinting refer to ***(2004)***

(a) molecular analysis of profiles of DNA samples
(b) analysis of DNA samples using imprinting devices
(c) techniques used for molecular analysis of different specimens of DNA
(d) techniques used for identification of fingerprints of individuals.

ANSWER KEY

1.	(b)	2.	(b)	3.	(a)	4.	(d)	5.	(d)	6.	(c)	7.	(a)
8.	(c)	9.	(c)	10.	(b)	11.	(a)	12.	(a)	13.	(d)	14.	(c)
15.	(d)	16.	(c)	17.	(b)	18.	(b)	19.	(b)	20.	(d)	21.	(d)
22.	(c)	23.	(c)	24.	(c)	25.	(c)	26.	(a)	27.	(b)	28.	(b)
29.	(a)	30.	(b)	31.	(d)	32.	(c)	33.	(d)	34.	(a)	35.	(a)
36.	(b)	37.	(c)	38.	(d)	39.	(b)	40.	(a)	41.	(a)	42.	(b)
43.	(c)	44.	(c)	45.	(d)	46.	(a)	47.	(b)	48.	(c)	49.	(a)
50.	(b)	51.	(d)	52.	(a)	53.	(b)	54.	(a)	55.	(c)	56.	(c)
57.	(d)	58.	(c)	59.	(b)	60.	(c)	61.	(a)	62.	(c)	63.	(d)
64.	(a)	65.	(a)	66.	(c)	67.	(c)	68.	(d)	69.	(b)	70.	(c)
71.	(b)	72.	(a)	73.	(d)	74.	(c)	75.	(b)	76.	(c)	77.	(a)
78.	(a)	79.	(d)	80.	(b)	81.	(b)	82.	(a)	83.	(a)	84.	(d)
85.	(b)	86.	(d)	87.	(c)	88.	(a)	89.	(c)	90.	(a)	91.	(a)
92.	(c)	93.	(c)	94.	(a)	95.	(a)	96.	(d)	97.	(b)	98.	(a)
99.	(a)	100.	(d)	101.	(b)	102.	(c)	103.	(b)	104.	(b)	105.	(d)
106.	(d)	107.	(d)	108.	(a)	109.	(c)	110.	(a)	111.	(d)	112.	(d)
113.	(c)	114.	(a)	115.	(b)	116.	(c)	117.	(c)	118.	(b)	119.	(a)
120.	(a)	121.	(a)	122.	(d)	123.	(d)	124.	(d)	125.	(a)	126.	(a)
127.	(c)	128.	(a)	129.	(c)	130.	(c)	131.	(a)	132.	(c)	133.	(c)
134.	(c)	135.	(d)	136.	(c)	137.	(d)	138.	(d)	139.	(d)	140.	(c)
141.	(b)	142.	(d)	143.	(c)	144.	(d)	145.	(d)	146.	(c)	147.	(a)
148.	(d)	149.	(a,d)	150.	(c)	151.	(a)	152.	(c)	153.	(b)	154.	(b)
155.	(a)	156.	(b)	157.	(b)	158.	(a)	159.	(a)	160.	(d)	161.	(c)
162.	(a)	163.	(b)	164.	(a)	165.	(d)	166.	(c)	167.	(c)	168.	(d)
169.	(a)	170.	(d)	171.	(a)								

HINTS & EXPLANATIONS

1.(b) : In prokaryotes, DNA being negatively charged is held with positively charged proteins in region termed as 'nucleoid'.

2.(b) : In a typical nucleus, some region of chromatin are loosely packed (and stains light) and are referred to as euchromatin. Euchromatin is transcriptionally active chromatin whereas heterochromatin is inactive. Histone octamer is wrapped by negatively charged DNA to form nucleosome. Histones are rich in basic amino acid residues lysine and arginine. A typical nucleosome contains 200bp of DNA helix.

3.(a) : Length of DNA double helix = Total number of bp × Distance between two consecutive bp.

So, total number of bp

$$= \frac{\text{length of DNA double helix}}{\text{Distance between two consecutive bp}}$$

$$= \frac{1.11 \text{ metres}}{0.34 \times 10^{-9} \text{ m/bp}} = 3.26 \times 10^9 \text{ bp}$$

Therefore, approximate number of base pair will be 3.3×10^9 bp.

4.(d)

5.(d) : According to the Chargaff's rule,

$A = T$ and $G = C$

$A + G = T + C$

$\therefore$ If $A = 30\%$, then $T = 30\%$

$\Rightarrow A + T = 60\%$

$G + C = 100 - 60 = 40\%$

$G = C = 20\%$

$T = 30\%$, $G = 20\%$, $C = 20\%$

6.(c) : Histones are positively charged basic proteins, thus, pH is alkaline.

7.(a) : Adenine pairs with thymine by forming two hydrogen bonds, A = T.

8.(c) : If the distance between two consecutive base pairs is 0.34 nm i.e., 0.3×10^{-9} m and the total number of base pairs of a DNA double helix in a typical mammalian cells is 6.6×10^9 bp the length of DNA is calculated by multiplying the total number of base pairs with distance between two consecutive base pair i.e.,

6.6×10^9 bp × 0.34 nm = 2.2"" m (approx.)

9. (c)

10.(b) : Histones help in packaging of DNA. In eukaryotes, DNA packaging is carried out with the help of positively charged basic proteins called histones. Histones are of five types -H_1,H_2 " " A,H_2 B,H_3 and H4. The association of H1 histone with nucleosome indicates that DNA remains in its condensed form. Nucleosome is the unit of compaction. H1 is attached over the linker DNA. The linker DNA, consisting of H_1 histone connects two adjacent nucleosomes. They together consititute chromatosome. It gives rise to a chromatin fibre after further condensation.

11.(a) :According to Chargaff's rule, the amount of adenine is always equal to that of thymine and the amount of guanine is always equal to that of cytosine, i.e., A = T and G = C. Also, the purines and pyrimidines are always in equal amounts, i.e., A + G = T + C. Now, given dsDNA has 17% cytosine and hence guanine will be also 17%. So, A + T must be 66%, therefore, percentage of adenine or thymine would be 66/2 = 33%.

12.(a) : The expression of the genetic material occurs normally through the production of proteins. This involves two consecutive steps. These are transcription and translation. The DNA codes for the production of messenger RNA (mRNA) during transcription. Messenger RNA carries coded information to ribosomes. The ribosomes read this information and use it for protein synthesis. This process is called translation. F.H.C. Crick described this unidirectional flow of information in 1958 as the 'central dogma of molecular biology'.

13. (d)

14.(c) : Nucleosomes appear as 'beads-on-string' in the chromosome when viewed under electron microscope. The beads in 'beads-on-string' arrangement are complexes of histones and DNA. The bead plus the connecting DNA leads to the next bead from the nucleosome. Nucleosome is the fundamental unit of organisation on which the higher-order packaging of chromatin is built. The bead of each nucleosome contains eight histone molecules in which two copies each of H_2A, H_2B, H3 and H4 are found.

15.(d) : $\text{DNA} \xrightarrow{\text{Transcription}} \text{mRNA} \xrightarrow{\text{Transcription}} \text{Protein}$

This one-way flow of information from DNA to m RNA and then to protein is called the central dogma of molecular biology by F.H.C. Crick (1958). But later on two American workers H. Temin and D. Baltimore reported that DNA is also formed from RNA in retroviruses, e.g., HIV. This is called reverse transcription or teminism, i.e.,

$$\text{DNA} \underset{\text{Reverse transcription}}{\overset{\text{Transcription}}{\rightleftarrows}} \text{mRNA} \xrightarrow{\text{Transcription}} \text{Protein}$$

This reverse transcription occurs under the influence of reverse transcriptase enzyme. So, HIV viruses does not follow central dogma.

16.(c) : The phosphodiester bonds is formed between the phosphate group, which is connected to carbon 5′ of the sugar residue of one nucleotide and carbon 3′ of the sugar residue of the next nucleotide.

17.(b) : Insulin gene is found in every body cell but is not expressed in all cells. It is nucleosome which consists of a core of eight histones. DNA is composed of nucleotides. Centriole is found in animal cells, which produces aster during cell division.

18.(b) : A DNA molecule has two unbranched complementary strands which are spirally coiled. The two chains are antiparallel, i.e., they run parallel but in opposite direction. One chain has the polarity $5 \rightarrow 3$ whereas, other has $3 \rightarrow 5$. Both are held together by hydrogen bonds between their bases, i.e., $A = T$ and $G \equiv C$ and the amount of adenine is equal to thymine and guanine equals to cytosine. The base ratio $A + T/G + C$ may vary from one species to another but is constant for a given species. The purine and pyrimidines are always in equal amount $(A + G = T + C)$ but $A + T$ is not necessarily equal to $G + C$.

19.(b) : The two DNA chains are held together by hydrogen bonds between their nitrogenous bases. Adenine (A), a purine of one chain lies exactly opposite thymine (T), a pyrimidine of the other chain. Similarly, cytosine (C), a pyrimidine lies opposite guanine (G), a purine. Three hydrogen bonds occur between cytosine and guanine $(C \equiv G)$ at positions 1′,2′, and 6′ and two hydrogen bonds between adenine and thymine (A= T) at positions 1′ and 6′.

20.(d) : DNA or deoxyribonucleic acid is the largest macromolecule made of the helically twisted two antiparallel polydeoxyribonucleotide strands held together by hydrogen bonds. The two strands of DNA are together called DNA duplex. It has a diameter of 20Å . One turn spiral has a distance of 34Å or 3.4 nm.

21.(d) : DNA is a type of nucleic acid that forms genetic material in many organisms. It consists of a long polymer of nucleotides which transcribes the coded information in the form of a triplet code of nucleotides in mRNA. It is a double helical molecule. The two strands of DNA run in opposite directions to one another with the hydrogen bonds between them. One strand of DNA has 5′–3′ direction and the other strand has 3′–5′ direction. So they are antiparallel. This direction is determined by the presence of a free phosphate or OH group at the end of the strand.

22. (c)

23.(c) : Endonucleases hydrolyse the internal phosphodiester bond. Exonucleases cleave the terminal nucleotides. Lipase digest fats and proteases break down proteins.

24. (c)

25.(c) : In a DNA, the percentage of thymine is 20%. So, as it pairs with adenine, it is also 20%. So, the guanine and cytosine together forms 60% of DNA and hence, guanine is 30%.

26.(a) : B-DNA is an antiparallel double helix. The double strand or duplex is coiled plectonemically in right handed fashion around a common axis like a rope stair case twisted in a spiral. The coiling produces alternate major and minor grooves. One turn of spiral has a distance between two adjacent nucleotides is 3.4 nm.

27.(b) : DNA is mainly found in nucleus. It is associated with RNA and proteins to form compact chromosomes. But some amount of DNA is also found in chloroplasts and mitochondria. This DNA is called extra-chromosomal DNA.

28.(b) : The genetic material of prokaryotes is circular and single stranded DNA. It has no association of histones. The eukaryotic genetic material is linear and double stranded DNA. It is associated with histone proteins to form nucleosome unit.

29.(a) : DNA molecule has four bases - adenine, guanine, cytosine and thymine. Adenine always pairs with thymine and guanine pairs with cytosine. Their association is A-T and G-C.

30.(b) : Genome refers to the total sets of chromosomes carried by each cell of the organism. In prokaryotes the genetic material is circular and single stranded DNA. It has no association of histones. The eukaryotic genetic material is linear and double stranded DNA. It is associated with histone proteins to form nucleosome unit.

31.(d) : In bacteria, DNA is highly charged molecule. The adjacent bases are linked by phosphate groups, each with an ionized hydroxyl group. It results in negative charges which are therefore balanced by an equivalent number of cationic groups. These charges are balanced by histones which are basic proteins in case of eukaryotes. Histones are absent in bacterial cells. In bacteria the charges are neutralised by polyamines such as spermine and spermidine and by Mg^{2+} ions.

32.(c) : ^{14}C and ^{3}H are incorporated in bases like thymidine, uridine and amino acids to study the structure of DNA and proteins. Radiotracer technique shows that DNA is in double helical form.

33.(d) : Nucleosome core is made up of H_2A, H_2B, H3 and H4. It is about 7–10 nm in diameter, consisting of histones around which a DNA strand, about 120 base pair long is wrapped in chromosomes.

34.(a) : A DNA with unequal nitrogen bases would most probably be single stranded. Nitrogenous bases are unequal in number in single stranded DNA, because they do not possess complementary base pairs.

35.(a) : Nucleotide arrangement in DNA can be seen

by X-ray crystallography. Watson and Crick, 1953 proposed the double helical model for DNA. They were awarded Nobel Prize in 1962. This model was developed by them on the basis of several previous observations including the d-helix of Pauling, 1951 and X-ray reflection studies of Franklin and Gosling, 1953.

36.(b) : An octamer of 4 histones complexed with DNA forms nucleosome. The association of histones with DNA is very characteristic. It involves the formation of linear array of spherical structures called nucleosomes. These structures contains four pairs of histones (H_2A, H_2B, H_3 and H4) in a ball; around which is wrapped a stretch of about 150 base pairs of DNA.

37.(c) : Both DNA and RNA are able to mutate. RNA being acatalyst is reactive and unstable and mutates at a faster rate. Consequently, viruses having RNA genome and having shorter life span mutate and evolve faster.

38.(d) : The unequivocal proof that DNA is the genetic material came from the experiments of Alfred Hershey and Martha Chase (1952). They worked with viruses that infect bacteria called bacteriophages.

39.(b) : Semi-conservative replication of DNA was proved by the work of Matthew Meselson and Franklin Stahl (1958) using bacterium Escherichia coli.

40. (a) : Ribozymes (ribonucleic acid enzymes) are RNA molecules that are capable of catalysing specific biochemical reactions similar to the action of protein enzymes.

41. (a)

42.(b) : Taylor et al. (1957) conducted experiment on Vicia faba (broad bean) to prove semi-conservative replication of DNA. He fed dividing cells of root tips of Vicia faba with radioactive 3H containing thymine instead of normal thymine and found that all the chromosomes became radioactive. Labelled thymine was then replaced with normal one. Next generation came to have radioactivity in one of the two chromatids of each chromosome while in subsequent generation radioactivity was present in 50% of the chromosomes. This is possible only if out of the two strands of a chromosome, one is formed afresh while the other is conserved at each replication.

43.(c) : Genetic material should be structurally and chemically stable otherwise its expression will change and lead to loss of several metabolic functions, etc.

44.(c) : Transformation was first studied by S.F. Griffith in 1928 while studying Streptococcus pneumoniae. He found that R-type non-virulent bacteria pick up virulence from heat killed virulent S-type bacteria and transform into virulent forms. It was this experiment which indicated presence of a 'transforming principle' which was later found out to be DNA, by Avery et al.

45.(d) : The unequivocal proof that DNA is the genetic material came from the experiments of Alfred Hershey and Martha Chase (1952). They worked with viruses that infect bacteria called bacteriophages.

46.(a) : Mathew Meselson and Franklin Stahl (1958) conducted various experiments using isotopically labelled DNA of Escherichia coli to provide evidence in favour of semiconservative mode of DNA replication.

47.(b) : Transformation involves transfer of genetic material of one bacterial cell into another bacterial cell by some unknown mechanism and it converts one type of bacterium into another type. This was first studied by Griffith

(1928) in Diplococcus pneumoniae and hence is known as Griffith effect.

48.(c) : Transformation was first discovered by Griffith (1928), in Pneumococcus (Streptococcus pneumoniae), that causes pneumonia. Griffith injected a group of mice with non-encapsulated, rough (R), pneumococci; a second group with heat-killed encapsulated pneumococci cells and a third group a mixture consisting of a few living non-encapsulated, rough pneumococci derived from a type S culture, and heat killed encapsulated cells (S type). Griffith observed that the mice in the first two groups were not infected, and the mice in the third group died within a few days. The mice of the third group should have survived as the organisms which could kill them had been killed and the cell of R type were incapable of causing disease. However, the mice died and living virulent encapsulated cells of the type S were recovered from their dead bodies. It was observed by Griffith, that killed encapsulated pneumococci had liberated some substance which favoured non-capsulated cells (R type) to produce a capsular substance This substance in later experiments was proved to be DNA. These experiments showed that DNA is the genetic material.

49.(a) : Autoradiography is the study of labelled precursors like 3H by knowing the movement of radioactivity with the help of photographic films and emulsions at short intervals. Radioactive material like tritiated thymidine which is formed by replacing normal hydrogen of thymidine with H3 (heavy isotope of hydrogen). Thymidine only is used for this purpose because RNA will not be labelled by this.

50.(b) : The transforming principle of Pneumococcus as found out by Avery, MacLeod and McCarty was DNA. In 1944, Avery, MacLeod and McCarty repeated Griffith's experiment successfully. They separated the proteins, carbohydrates and DNA of S III strains and separately mixed them in the pure cultures of R II. Only DNA could bring about transformation of R II type into S III and not the proteins or the carbohydrates.

51.(d) : Hershey and Chase proved that DNA is a basic genetic material. Hershey and Chase, 1952, by using ^{32}P and ^{35}S with a T–2 type phage concluded that DNA is the genetic material.

52.(a) : Experimental material in the study of DNA replication has been Escherichia coli. E. coli fully labelled with 15N is allowed to grow in ^{14}N medium. The two strands of DNA molecule of the first generation bacteria have different density and do not resemble parent DNA. Meselson and Stahl, 1958 by using 14N and 15N confirmed that the replication of DNA in E. coli is semi-conservative in nature.

53.(b) : Chargaff's rules are applicable only for double stranded DNA molecule. These are not applicable for single stranded DNA or RNA molecules. Chargaff's rules state that DNA helices contain equal molar ratios of A and T, G and C. This is because in a dsDNA molecule, complementary base pairing occurs between A and T, and C and G base pairs. This complementary base pairing is not possible in case of single stranded RNA molecule. Thus, Chargaff's rules are not applicable to RNA.

54.(a) : Deoxyribonucleic acid and ribonucleic acid as the name suggests are made up of several nucleotide monomers. Each nucleotide consists of pentose sugar, phosphate group and nitrogenous bases. DNA has deoxyribose sugar whereas RNA has ribose sugar. The bases in DNA molecule are A, T, G and C whereas in RNA, thymine is absent and instead uracil is found.

55.(c) : E. coli divides in 20 minutes. After 60 minutes, generation III would have 75% DNA completely free from ^{15}N and 25% of DNA would be hybrid $^{14}N/^{15}N$. So, out of 80 cells formed, 60 cells will be free from 15N DNA.

56.(c) : Lagging strand is a replicated strand of DNA which is formed in short segments called Okazaki fragments. Its growth is discontinuous. The direction of growth of the lagging strand is $3'\rightarrow5'$ though in each Okazaki fragment it is $5'\rightarrow3'$.

57.(d) : Prokaryotic DNA acts as a single replicating unit called replicon. Each replicon has a particular region where replication starts. It is called origin of replication or ori. In the region of ori, there is a particular nucleotide sequence called autonomic replicating sequence or ARS. Replication proceeds bidirectionally from each ori. A replication fork is produced on each side of ori. Replication will continue till a replication fork meets another replication fork.

58. (c) : The method of DNA replication is semiconservative. According to the semi-conservative model proposed by Watson and Crick, each strand of the two double helices formed would have one old and one new strand. So, the parental identity is conserved upto half extent and hence DNA replication is semi-conservative.

59.(b) : DNA is a double helical molecule and it opens to form a replication fork for its replication. The two strands of DNA are joined with the help of H-bonds between the strands. Topoisomerases are specialised to cause nicks or breaks in the double helix and helps separate the DNA stands. Helicase unwinds the DNA helix from that nick caused by the topoisomerase and this separates the two strands. DNA gyrase introduces negative supercoils in DNA strands of prokaryotes. DNA polymerase adds nucleotide units to the 3′ end of a DNA chain. DNA ligase joins the ends of DNA.

60.(c) : During DNA replication, the strands separate by unwindase/helicase. The molecule is unwound by DNA unwinding proteins called helicases. The helicases II and III get attached to lagging strand and protein to the leading strand. The formation of bands is avoided by single stranded DNA binding proteins (SSB).

61. (a)

62. (c)

63.(d) : RNA polymerase III is responsible for transcription of tRNA, 5S rRNA and snRNAs (small nuclear RNAs). RNA polymerase I transcribes rRNA (28S, 18S and 5.8S) whereas RNA polymerase II transcribes precursor of mRNA, the heterogeneous nuclear RNA (hnRNA).

64. (a)

65. (a)

66.(c) : Split gene arangement is a characteristic of eukaryotes. In capping, an unusual nucleotide (methyl guanosine triphosphate) is added to the 5^′-end of hnRNA. RNA polymerase binds with termination factor Rho (ρ) to terminate the process of transcription in bacteria. The coding strand does not code for anything.

67. (c): In bacteria, there is a single DNA dependent RNA polymerase that catalyses transcription of all types of RNA. It associates transiently with initiation factor (σ) and termination factor (ρ) to carry out initiation and termination of transcription respectively. It catalyses the elongation as its uses nucleoside triphosphates as substrates and polymerises in a template dependent fashion as rule of complementarity.

68. (d)

69. (b)

70. (c)

71.(b) : Franklin Stahl along with Matthew Meselson proved semi-conservative mode of replication in DNA. Punnett square was developed by a British geneticist, Reginald C. Punnett. Spliceosome formation is part of post-transcriptional change in eukaryotes. Transduction was discovered by Joshua Lederberg and Norton Zinder in the bacterium Salmonella.

72.(a) : Coding strand and mRNA have same nucleotide sequence except, 'T' - Thymine is replaced by 'U' – Uracil in mRNA.

73. (d) : rRNA (ribosomal RNA) is the most abundant of all types of RNA (70-88%). Hence, it will be present in highest amount. Percentage of tRNA and mRNA is 15% and 2-5% respectively. miRNA (micro RNA) are 21-22 bp long RNA that bring degeneration of m RNA.

74.(c) : Spliceosomes help in removal of introns. They will not occur in prokaryotes because prokaryotes do not have introns and thus, processing does not require splicing of mRNA.

75.(b) : Cistron (or gene) is a length of DNA that contains the information for coding a specific polypeptide chain or a functional RNA molecule (i.e. transfer RNA or ribosomal RNA). Hence cistron is a unit of function. Currently such a gene is called structural gene.

76.(c) : 23Sr RNA acts as structural RNA as well as ribozyme in bacteria.

77. (a): The strand of DNA on which RNA polymerase binds to catalyse transcription is called template strand. It is also known as master or antisense strand. It has the polarity of $3 \rightarrow 5$.

78.(a) : RNA polymerase initiates and extends the RNA (chain elongation) and functions always in 5 to 3 direction. The structural component of DNA has 3 to 5 polarity. It is also called template DNA strand or antisense (–) strand.

79.(d) : Introns, which occur principally in eukaryotes, are transcribed into messenger RNA (mRNA) but are subsequently removed from the transcription before translation. In certain cases, removal of the introns is an autocatalytic process (selfsplicing) whereby the RNA itself has the properties of an enzyme.

80.(b) : In RNA, thymine is substituted with uracil thus, the RNA strand complementary to DNA strand ATCTG will be UAGAC.

81.(b) : Nucleolus is the centre for synthesis of ribosomal RNA (r RNA) that form ribosomal subunits. Ribosomal proteins migrate to the nucleolus from their assembly sites in the cytoplasm and are packaged into ribonucleoproteins. These return to the cytoplasm where they become mature ribosome particles.

82.(a) : A transcription unit is a part of DNA that is able to transcribe a complete RNA. It consists of a promoter region (where RNA polymerase binds to start transcription), the structural gene (coding region) and the terminator region (that signals release of RNA polymerase and newly formed RNA strand).

83.(a) : In eukaryotes, RNA polymerase enzymes (Type I, II, III) catalyse the synthesis of RNA using as a template either an existing DNA strand or an RNA strand. Type I is responsible for synthesis of rRNA, type II for mRNA and type III for tRNA synthesis.

84.(d) : The 23 SrRNA is a component of the large prokaryotic (bacterial cell) subunit (50S). The ribosomal peptidyl transferase activity resides in this rRNA and acts as a ribozyme (catalytic RNA). In eukaryotic cells, the 60S (28S component) ribosome subunit contains the peptidyl transferase component and acts as the ribozyme.

85.(b) : Unlike in prokaryotes where transcription and translation take place in the same compartment, in eukaryotes primary transcript is first processed in the nucleus and then transported outside of the nucleus. Since the primary transcripts of the eukaryotes contains both the expressing genes (exons) and non-expressing genes (introns), it undergoes splicing of introns and later capping and tailing at 5-end and 3-end respectively.

86.(d) : Transfer RNA (tRNA) are types of RNA responsible for the transfer of specific amino acids to the growing end of a polypeptide chain during translation. R.Holly in 1965 gave clover leaf model of tRNA for yeast alanyl t RNA. It has four major sites - AA binding site, anticodon site, TΨC loop and DHU loop. The chain is having unpaired base sequence CCA at 3 end and G at 5 end.

87.(c) : During transcription RNA synthesis from a DNA template takes place. It involves rewriting of the code without a change in its language. In mRNA, adenine pairs with uracil because thymine is not present in m RNA. So the nucleotide sequence in mRNA would be-

DNA template	A	T	A	C	G
	|	|	|	|	|
*m*RNA	U	A	U	G	C

88.(a) : Promoter is region on a DNA molecule upstream from the coding sequence, area to which RNA polymerase initially binds prior to the initiation of transcription. The promoter, or at least part of it, determines the nature of the polymerase that associates with it. Certain consensus sequences within the promoter region seem to be particularly important in the binding of RNA polymerase and these are known as CAAT and TATA boxes. The promoter region extends from some 40 nucleotides to about five nucleotides upstream from the start of the gene-coding region, the CAAT and TATA boxes being located within the promoter region as short six or seven nucleotide sequence.

89.(c) : RNA polymerase enzyme catalyses the synthesis of RNA. It is single in prokaryotes. There are three types of RNA polymerases in eukaryotes-I for 28S, 18S and 5.8S RNA, II for m RNA and hnRNA and III for tRNA, 5S rRNA and snRNA. Primase is an RNA polymerase that is used to initiate DNA synthesis. RNA ligase reunites the exon segment after RNA splicing.

90.(a) : DNA transcribes to form mRNA. Its function is to carry coded information from DNA for the synthesis of proteins. The RNA consists of a coding region called exon and non-coding region called introns. The exons are thus the functional part that have code for proteins.

91.(a) : mRNA is synthesised on DNA template in 5→3 direction. Synthesis of m RNA exhibits several features that are synonymous with DNA replication. RNA synthesis requires accurate and efficient initiation, elongation proceeds in the 5→3 direction (i.e., the polymerase moves along the template strand of DNA in the 5→3 direction) and RNA synthesis requires distinct and accurate termination. Transcription exhibits several features that are distinct from replication.

92.(c) : A gene is a hereditary unit consisting of a sequence of DNA and occupying a specific position or locus within the genome. Gene activity ultimately affects the phenotype of the organism possessing the gene. Thus gene is a physical and functional unit of genetic information. A cistron is a unit of genetic function. In prokaryotes, there is one gene one enzyme correspondence. It means that in these organisms genes and cistrons are equivalent.

93. (c)

94. (a)

95. (a) : 3-D model of t RNA looks like flattened L-shaped molecule. tRNA acts as adapter molecule which carries amino acids to the site of protein synthesis (i.e., ribosomes). Most accepted model for tRNA structure is clover leaf model.

96.(d) : Operator genes are a region of DNA sequence capable of interacting with a specific repressor molecule and in doing so it affects the activity of other genes downstream from it.

97.(b) : Transposons are portable genetic elements which can insert themselves at random into a plasmid or any chromosome independently of the host cell recombination system. It was discovered by Barbara Mc Clintock (1940) in maize and termed as jumping genes. Later Hedges and Jacob termed them as transposons. Introns are nontranslated sequences within the coding sequence of a gene. Such sequences are transcribed into hnRNA but are then spliced out and are not represented in the message. The non-intron sequences of the gene are referred to as exons. Cistron sequence of nucleotides in a DNA molecule code for one particular polypeptide chain.

98.(a) : The codon 'AUG' codes for methionine only and it act as an initiator codon. The codon 'UUU' and 'UUC' code for phenylalanine. 'AAA' and 'AAG' both codons code for the amino acid lysine.

99.(a) : Insertion or deletion of three or its multiple bases insert or delete one or multiple codon hence one or multiple amino acids, and reading frame remains unaltered from that point onwards.

100.(d) : As genetic code is nearly universal means almost all organisms (from a virus, bacteria to a tree or human being) will have amino acids coded by same kind of codons as given in checkerboard. So, this property is utilised to produce human insulin using bacteria.

101.(b) : 1 codon consists of 3 bases. Therefore, a deletion on 901 position will affect 33 codons.

102.(c) : Polypeptide synthesis is signalled by two initiator codons or start codons i.e., AUG (methionine codon) and rarely by GUG (valine codon).

103.(b) : Genetic code is non-ambiguous. Non-ambiguous code means that there is no ambiguity about a particular code. One codon specifies only one amino acid and not any other. There are 64 codons. Out of 64,3 are stop codons or non-sense codons, i.e., these do not code for any amino acid and rest 61 code for one of the 20 amino acids. Neither of them code for more than one amino acids except GUG which normally code for valine but in certain conditions it also codes for N-formyl methionine as initiation codon.

104.(b) : As genetic code is nearly universal means almost all organisms (from a virus, bacteria to a tree or human being) will have amino acids coded by same kind of codons as given in checkerboard. So, this property is utilised to produce human insulin using bacteria

105.(d) : Genetic code was deciphered in 1960's by Crick, Ochoa, Nirenberg, Mathaei and Khorana.

106.(d) : The relationship between the sequence of amino acids in a polypeptide and nucleotide sequence of DNA or m RNA is called genetic code. The genetic code is continuous and does not possess pause after the triplets. So, a codon in m RNA is present in contiguous fashion. If a nucleotide is deleted or added, the whole genetic code will read differently.

107.(d) : AUG codes for methionine and is initiation or start codon which starts the synthesis of polypeptide. UAA (ochre), UAG (amber) and UGA (opal) do not specify any amino acid so they are called termination codons. CUU, CUC, CUA and CUG codes for leucine whereas GCU, GCC, GCA and GCG codes for alanine.

108.(a) : A mutation involves a change in the sequence of nucleotides in a nucleic acid molecule. This change will express itself in the form of a change in the sequence of amino acids in the protein molecule synthesised through the information, encoded in nucleic acid segment. Therefore, mutations at molecule level can be studied both by the study of the sequence of amino acids in a protein and also by the study of sequence of nucleotides in a segment of nucleic acid.

109.(c) : Transition mutation is one in which a purine is substituted by a different purine, or a pyrimidine by a different pyrimidine. Such a change involves a base pair change between a G-C pair and an A-T pair in the DNA whereas transversion results when one nitrogen base is replaced by another different type, e.g., C-G and A-T. Transcription is the formation of m RNA on DNA template.

110.(a) : UGA, UAG and UAA are three non-sense (or termination) codon which do not code for any amino acid. If in a gene encoding a polypeptide of 50 aminoacid, 25th codon is mutated to UAA or any of the termination codon, then the chain will be terminated at that place because it will become difficult for tRNA to bring amino acid from amino acid pool. So in that case a polypeptide of 24 amino acids will be formed.

111.(d) : Codon UAC is correctly matched as it codes for amino acid tyrosine. UCG codes for serine, UUU codes for phenylalanine and UGU codes for cysteine. Start codon is AUG and stop codons are UAA, UAG and UGA.

112.(d) : In a triplet, for a particular amino acid more than one word (synonyms) can be used. This phenomenon is described by saying that the code is degenerate. A degenerate code would be one where there is one to one relation between amino acids and the codons that 44 codons out of 64 will be useless or non-sense codons. A code is degenerate because of the third base of the codon. It has been shown that the same tRNA can recognize more than one codons differing only at the third position, For example GCU, GCC and GCA all code for alanine amino acids.

113. (c)

114. (a)

115.(b) : A mutation involves a change in the sequence of nucleotides in a nucleic acid molecule. This change will express itself in the form of a change in the sequence of amino acids in the protein molecule synthesised through the information, encoded in nucleic acid segment. Therefore mutations at molecule level can be studied both by the study of the sequence of amino acids in a protein and also by the study of sequence of nucleotides in a segment of nucleic acid.

116. (c)

117. (c)

118. (b)

119. (a)

120.(a) : Non-sense mutation is a mutation which interconverts a nonsense to or from a sense-coding triplet, resulting in an abnormally foreshortened or elongated polypeptide chain. But in this example cytosine is added at the beginning so CAT GAT GAT G will result.

121.(a) : Anticodon is the sequence of three nucleotides in a transfer RNA molecule that pairs with a complementary sequence of three nucleotides (codon) on a molecule of messenger RNA. t RNA has clove like shape or L shape (three dimensional). It has G at 5′ end CCA at 3′ end. CCA at 3′ end is meant for attaching to a specific amino acid (AA-binding site). On the opposite side lies an anticodon that is complementary to a specific codon of mRNA. The two are called recognition sites.

122. (d)

123. (d)

124.(d) : The genetic information is transferred from DNA to m RNA to protein. The proteins are made up of some 20 amino acids whose sequence is hidden in the sequence of nucleotides of m RNA. Hence, genetic code consists of all 20 amino acids. Thus genetic code is the relationship of amino acids sequence in a polypeptide and nucleotide/base sequence in mRNA antisense strand and DNA.

125.(a) : Ribosome is responsible for synthesising proteins. The ribosome consists of structural RNAs and about 80 different proteins. In its inactive state, it exists as two subunits; large subunit and a small subunit when the small subunit encounters mRNA, the process of translation of the mRNA to protein begins.

126.(a) : siRNA is not required for protein synthesis. Instead there are highly specific and interfere with the expression of specific genes with complementary nucleotide sequences by degrading m RNA after transcription, thus preventing translation.

127.(c) : Translation is the process of polymerisation of amino acids to form a polypeptide. The order and sequence of amino acids are defined by the sequence of bases in the m RNA. The amino acids are joined by a bond that is known as a peptide bond. Formation of a peptide bond requires energy. So, in the first phase itself amino acids are activated in the presence of ATP and linked to their cognate tRNA-a process commonly called as charging of tRNA or aminoacylation of t RNA.

128.(a) : The association of many ribosomes with single mRNA leads to formation of polyribosomes or polysomes. It occurs during translation process of protein synthesis.

129. (c)

130. (c)

131.(a) : Ribosomes are very small organelles having a diameter of 150Å–250Å. Each ribosome is made up of two subunits, a smaller subunit and another larger subunit. These two subunits are associated with the help of Mg^{2+} ions (at 0.001 M concentration). If the Mg^{2+} ions concentration is less in cytoplasm, the two units of ribosome separate but when the Mg^{2+} ions concentration is increased ten times, the two unites and form a dimer.

132.(c) : Neomycin is a broad spectrum antibiotic which was first isolated from a strain of Streptomyces fradiae. It is effective against Gram positive as well as Gram negative bacteria. Its mechanism of action is by selective inhibition of protein synthesis on the 70S (prokaryotic) ribosome by inhibiting the interaction of m RNA and t RNA during translation process.

133.(c) : Messenger RNA or mRNA has been named so because it carries the coded information from DNA for the synthesis of proteins. It carries the coded information in a number of base triplets called codons. It is transcribed on DNA by the enzyme RNA polymerase. Hence, its base sequence is complementary to DNA on which it has been synthesised. In eukaryotes, each gene transcribes its own mRNA, therefore the number of mRNAs corresponds to the number of genes. rRNA is a type of RNA that forms structural and functional components of ribosomes. tRNA is a class of RNA having structures with triplet nucleotide sequences that are complementary to the triplet nucleotide coding sequences of m RNA. It binds with amino acids and transfers them to ribosomes.

134.(c) : Streptomycin is broad spectrum (active against both Gram-positive and Gram-negative bacteria) and was the first really effective drug against tuberculosis, but its use is limited by the development of resistant strains and by toxic side-effects. The bactericidal action of streptomycin, as with other aminoglycoside antibiotics (e.g., neomycin) is through selective inhibition of protein synthesis on 70S ribosomes. To check resistance of mutants against streptomycin they must be grown on plates with streptomycin. Only those bacterial colonies will propagate from the master that are resistant to the antibiotic.

135.(d) : The mitochondria contains its own set of ribosomes which synthesise proteins, so protein synthesis occurs both in mitochondria and cytoplasm.

136.(c) : The initiation of polypeptide chain in prokaryotes is always brought about by the amino acid methionine but it has to be formylated to form tRNA f^{met}. Then methionine binds with tRNA f^{met} to form f^{-met} -tRNA f^{met}. This f^{met} tRNA f^{met} complex binds with the mRNA-30S subunit complex using initiation factors IF-2 and IF-1 and GTP.

137.(d) : Transfer RNA or tRNA help in transfer of amino acids to ribosomes. mRNA complex to form the polypeptide chain. It has four key regions a carrier and recognition end, enzyme site and ribosome site. This recognition end has three anticodons with the help of which amino acids are identified. rRNA forms 67% of 70S ribosomes and 50% of 80S ribosomes. mRNA carries the coded information from DNA for the synthesis of proteins.

138.(d) : Protein synthesis in an animal cell, takes place in the nucleolus as well as in the cytoplasm. Main part of protein synthesis (transcription and translation) occurs in nucleolus. Chain elongation occurs in cytoplasm.

139.(d) : Transcription is the mechanism of copying the message of DNA on RNA with the help of enzyme RNA polymerase. It is meant for taking the coded information from DNA to the site where it is required for protein synthesis. Translation or protein synthesis is a complicated process involving several steps such as - activation of amino acid, transfer of amino acid to tRNA, initiation of polypeptide synthesis, elongation of polypeptide chain and termination of polypeptide chain.

140.(c) : Certain amino acids are identified by more than one codons. This phenomenon is called as degeneracy, e.g., phenylalanine is code by UUU and UUC.

141.(b) : The process of translation is protein synthesis. Emil Fischer, a German chemist established that the proteins are polymers of amino acids. There are some twenty amino acids involved in protein synthesis. In translation, the message coded by DNA on m RNA is translated into a specific protein.

142. (d)

Gene 'a' $\rightarrow$ Transacetylase

Gene 'y' $\rightarrow$ Permease

Gene 'i' $\rightarrow$ Repressor protein

Gene 'z' $\rightarrow$ β-galactosidase

143.(c) : In lac operon, lactose is an inducer. It binds with repressor and inactivates it.

144. (d)

145. (d) : Alec Jeffreys (1984) invented the DNA fingerprinting technique. Alfred Hershey and Martha Chase proved that DNA is genetic material using T_2 bacteriophages in an experiment. Matthew Meselson and F. Stahl proved semiconservative mode of replication in bacterium E. coli.

146.(c) : Operon concept is for prokaryotes that consist of operator gene, promoter gene, regulator gene and structural gene. Structural, operator and regulator genes are also present in eukaryotic gene expression along with enhancer gene but enhancer gene is present only in eukaryotic gene expression. It changes the rate of transcription of structural genes.

147.(a) : In Lac operon, lactose is an inducer. It binds with repressor and inactivates it. It allows RNA polymerase access to the promoter and transcription proceeds.

148.(d) : The control of expression of lac operon is negative (as it is turned off normally) and inducible. Inducible operon is an operon which remains switched off normally but becomes operational in the presence of an inducer (lactose, actually allolactose a metabolite of lactose, in case of lac operon). The inducible operon generally functions in catabolic pathways. In the presence of an inducer, the repressor has a higher affinity for the inducer than for the operator gene. When lactose is added, a few lactose molecules are carried into the cell by the enzyme lactose permease as small amount of this enzyme is present in the cell even when the operon is not working. These few lactose molecules are converted into allolactose molecules which act as an inducer and bind to the repressor (a product of regulator gene). The repressor-inducer complex fails to join with the operator gene, thus it is turned on.

149. (a,d) : Transcription is the process in living cells in which the genetic information of DNA is transferred to m RNA as first step of gene expression. An operon consists of structural genes, promoter, operator and regulator gene.

150.(c) : A non-sense mutation is the one which stops polypeptide synthesis due to the formation of termination or non-sense codon. In lac operon, sequence of structural genes is Z, Y and A, which respectively code for β-galactosidase, lactose permease and transacetylase. If the gene Y has nonsense mutation, gene expression will stop at it, resulting in non-expression of both gene Y and successive gene A. Thus, only β-galactosidase enzyme will be produced.

151.(a) : The control of expression of lac operon is negative (as it is turned off normally) and inducible. Inducible operon is an operon which remains switched off normally but becomes operational in the presence of an inducer (lactose, actually allolactose a metabolite of lactose, in case of lac operon). The inducible operon generally functions in catabolic pathways. In the presence of an inducer, the repressor has a higher affinity for the inducer than for the operator gene. When lactose is added, a few lactose molecules are carried into the cell by the enzyme lactose permease as small amount of this enzyme is present in the cell even when the operon is not working. These few lactose molecules are converted into allolactose molecules which act as an inducer and bind to the repressor (a product of regulator gene). The repressor-inducer complex fails to join with the operator gene, thus it is turned on.

152.(c) : The two French scientists, Jacob and Monod proposed the lac operon of E. coli. The lac operon (an inducible operon) contains a promoter, an operator, a regulator gene and three structural genes z, y and a, coding for the enzymes β-galactosidase, β-galactoside permease and β-galactoside transacetylase, respectively. β-galactoside permease "pumps" lactose into the cell, where β-galactosidase cleaves it into glucose and galactose. The function of the transacetylase is still not clear. The lac regulator gene, designated the i gene, codes for a repressor. In the absence of the inducer (i.e., lactose, actually allolactose), the repressor binds to the lac operator sequence, preventing RNA polymerase from binding to the promoter and transcribing the structural genes. The inducer of the operon, allolactose, is derived from lactose in a reaction that is catalysed by β-galactosidase. Once formed, allolactose binds to the repressor, causing it to be released from the operator; in doing so, it Induces transcription of the z, y and a structural genes. CAP is activator called catabolic activator protein. It exerts a positive control in lac operon because in its absence RNA polymerase is unable to recognise promotor gene. CAP activates lac genes only when glucose is absent. Such enzymes whose synthesis can be induced by adding the substrate are known as inducible enzymes and the genetic systems responsible for the synthesis of such an enzyme are known as inducible operons.

153. (b)

154. (b)

155.(a) : In lac operon, lac refers to lactose. The lac operator is a part of the structural genes (lac Z, lac Y, lac A and lac I). It is responsible for the uptake and initial catabolism of lactose.

$$\text{Lactose} \xrightarrow{\beta\text{-galactosidase}} \text{Glucose} + \text{Galactose}$$

156.(b) : Operon model was given by Jacob and Monod (1961) for regulation of protein synthesis in prokaryotes and some eukaryotes. In bacteria, the genes that contain the information for assembling the enzymes for a metabolic pathway are usually clustered together on the chromosome in a functional complex called an operon. Regulation of protein synthesis in eukaryotes is explained by gene battery model given by Britten and Davidson.

157.(b) : In the lac operon of E.coli, due to the activity of regulator gene synthesis of repressor molecules occurs. These repressor molecules get attached to the operator gene and thus check m RNA synthesis and because of this no protein synthesis occurs.

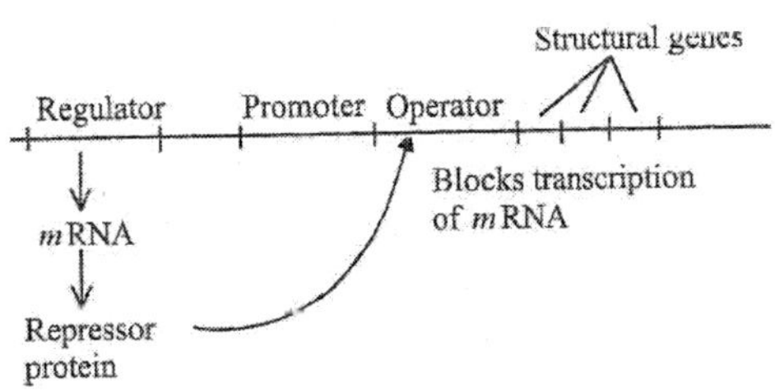

158.(a) : The tryptophan operon (trp operon) in bacteria is a repressible operon. Here, repressor is inactive and it becomes active as DNA binding protein only when complexed with a co-repressor (tryptophan). In absence of tryptophan, the operator site is open to binding by RNA polymerase, which transcribes the structural genes of tryptophan operon, leading to production of enzymes that synthesise tryptophan. When tryptophan becomes available, the enzymes of tryptophan synthetic pathway are no longer needed and tryptophan (co-repressor)-repressor complex blocks transcription. The regulation of this operon is also a negative control.

159.(a) : When E.coli bacteria are transferred to medium containing lactose, then the lac operon is induced. The lac operon consists of 3 structural gene (lac Z, lac Y and lac A). It involves the synthesis of β-galactosidase enzyme in E.coli, which hydrolyses lactose into glucose and galactose.

160. (d)

161.(c) : Expressed sequence tag is one of the major approach of human genome project methodology. It is focused on identifying all the genes that are expressed as RNA.

162.(a) : In sequence annotation the geneticist used the blind approach of simple sequencing the whole set of genome that contained all the coding and non-coding sequence and later assigning different regions in the sequence with functions.

163.(b) : Expressed Sequence Tags (ESTs) are genes that are expressed as RNA. It is used in sequencing of human genome.

164.(a) : In genome all the genes are contained in a single set of chromosomes. The instructions in our genome are present in the form of DNA. DNA has a complicated structure in the form of a double helix. Single strands of DNA are coiled up into structures called chromosomes. Within the chromosomes, segments of DNA are "read" together to form genes. 'Thus, a gene is a segment of DNA or chromosome situated at a specific locus (gene locus) which carries coded information associated with a specific function and can undergo crossing over as well as mutation. A nucleotide is the basic unit of DNA made up of a pentose sugar, phosphoric acid and a nitrogenous base.

165.(d) : Satellite DNA is that part of repetitive DNA which has long repetitive nucleotide sequences in tandem that forms a separate fraction on density ultracentrifugation. DNA fingerprinting involves identifying differences in some specific regions in DNA sequence called as repetitive DNA, because in these sequences, a small stretch of DNA is repeated many times. These repetitive DNA sequences are separated from bulk genomic DNA as different peaks during density gradient centrifugation. The bulk DNA forms a major peak and the other small peaks are referred to as satellite DNA. Depending on base composition (A:T rich or G:C rich), length of segment, and number of repetitive units, the satellite DNA is classified into many categories, such as micro-satellites, mini-satellites, etc. These sequences normally do not code for any proteins, but they form a large portion of human genome. These sequences show high degree of polymorphism and form the basis of DNA fingerprinting. Since DNA from every tissue (such as blood, hair-follicle, skin, bone, saliva, sperm, etc.) from an individual show the same degree of polymorphism, they become very useful identification tool in forensic applications.

166.(c) : Polymorphism (variation at genetic level) arises due to mutation. Polymorphism in DNA sequence is the basis of genetic mapping of human genome as well as of DNA fingerprinting.

167.(c) : DNA fingerprinting involves identifying differences in some specific regions in DNA sequence called as repetitive DNA, as in these sequences a small stretch of DNA is repeated many times.

168.(d) : Any small, functional, freely folded domain in which coordination of one or more zinc ions is required to stabilise its structure is known as zinc finger. The zinc finger domains are widely dispersed in eukaryotic genomes and are actively involved in sequence specific binding to DNA/RNA and contribute in protein-protein recognitions.

169. (a)

170.(d) : DNA fingerprinting is a technique of determining nucleotide sequences of certain areas of DNA which are unique to each individual. The difference of about 0.1% or 3 × 106 base pairs (out of 3×109 bp) provides individuality to each human being. Human genome possesses numerous small noncoding but inheritable sequences of bases which are repeated many times. These sequences occur near telomere, centromeres, Y chromosome and heterochromatic area. The area with same sequence of bases repeated several times is called repetitive DNA. It is separated as satellite from the bulk DNA during density gradient centrifugation and hence called satellite DNA where, repetition of bases is in tandem. Satellite DNAs show polymorphism (the occurrence of mutations in a population at high frequency), which is the basis of genetic mapping of human genome as well as DNA fingerprinting. While mutations in genes produce alleles with different expressions, mutations in non-coding repetitive DNA have no immediate impact. These mutations which have piled up with time form the basis of polymorphism.

171. (a)

Chapter : 25

EVOLUTION

ORIGIN OF LIFE

1. From his experiments, S.L. Miller produced amino acids by mixing the following in a closed flask. **(2020)**
(a) CH_4, H_2, NH_3 and water vapor at 800°C
(b) CH_3, H_2, NH_4 and water vapor at 800°C
(c) CH_4, H_2, NH_3 and water vapor at 600°C
(d) CH_3, H_2, NH_3 and water vapor at 600°C

2. Which of the following is the correct sequence of events in the origin of life? ***(NEET-II 2016)***

I. Formation of protobionts

II. Synthesis of organic monomers

III. Synthesis of organic polymers

IV. Formation of DNA-based genetic systems
(a) I, II, III, IV (b) I, III, II, IV
(c) II, III, I, IV (d) II, III, IV, I

3. Following are the two statements regarding the origin of life. ***(NEET-I 2016)***

(A) The earliest organisms that appeared on the earth were non-green and presumably anaerobes.

(B) The first autotrophic organisms were the chemoautotrophs that never released oxygen.

Of the above statements which one of the following options is correct?
(a) Both (A) and (B) are correct.
(b) Both (A) and (B) are false.
(c) (A) is correct but (B) is false.
(d) (B) is correct but (A) is false.

4. Which one of the following is incorrect about the characteristics of protobionts (coacervates and microspheres) as envisaged in the abiogenic origin of life? ***(2008)***
(a) They were partially isolated from the surroundings.
(b) They could maintain an internal environment.
(c) They were able to reproduce.
(d) They could separate combinations of molecules from the surroundings.

5. The concept of chemical evolution is based on ***(2007)***
(a) interaction of water, air and clay under intense heat
(b) effect of solar radiation on chemicals
(c) possible origin of life by combination of chemicals under suitable environmental conditions
(d) crystallisation of chemicals.

6. Which of the following amino acids was not found to be synthesised in Miller's experiment? ***(2006)***
(a) Alanine (b) Glycine
(c) Aspartic acid (d) Glutamic acid

7. Which one of the following experiments suggests that simplest living organisms could not have originated spontaneously from non-living matter? ***(2005)***
(a) Larvae could appear in decaying organic matter.
(b) Microbes did not appear in stored meat.
(c) Microbes appeared from unsterilised organic matter.
(d) Meat was not spoiled, when heated and kept sealed in a vessel.

8. According to Oparin, which one of the following was not present in the primitive atmosphere of the earth? ***(2004)***
(a) Methane (b) Oxygen
(c) Hydrogen (d) Water vapour

9. There is no life on moon due to the absence of ***(2002)***

(a) O_2 (b) water
(c) light (d) temperature.

10. Most abundant organic compound on earth is ***(2001)***

(a) protein (b) cellulose
(c) lipids (d) steroids.

11. 1st life on earth was ***(2001)***

(a) cyanobacteria
(b) chemoheterotrophs
(c) autotrophs
(d) photoautotrophs.

12. The correct sequence for the manufacture of molecules/organic compounds on the primitive earth is ***(1996)***

(a) NH_3, nucleic acid, protein and carbohydrate
(b) protein, carbohydrate, water and nucleic acid
(c) NH_3, protein, carbohydrate and nucleic acid
(d) NH_3, water, nucleic acid and protein.

13. The first organisms were ***(1992)***

(a) chemoautotrophs (b) chemoheterotrophs
(c) autotrophs (d) eukaryotes.

14. Which was absent in the atmosphere at the time of origin of life? ***(1991)***

(a) NH_3 (b) H_2
(c) O_2 (d) CH_4

EVOLUTION OF LIFE FORMS - A THEORY

15. Which one of the following sequences was proposed by Darwin and Wallace for organic evolution? ***(2003)***

(a) Overproduction, variations, constancy of population size, natural selection
(b) Variations, constancy of population size, overproduction, natural selection
(c) Overproduction, constancy of population size, variations, natural selection
(d) Variations, natural selection, overproduction, constancy of population size

WHAT ARE EVIDENCES FOR EVOLUTION?

16. Which of the following statement is not true? ***(2022)***

(a) Analogous structures are a result convergent evolution.
(b) Sweet potato and potato is an example of analogy.
(c) Homology indicates common ancestry.
(d) Flippers of penguins and dolphins are a pair of homologous organs.

17. Which of the following refer to correct example(s) of organisms which have evolved due to changes in environment brought about by anthropogenic action? ***(2020)***

(1) Darwin's Finches of Galapagos islands.

(2) Herbicide resistant weeds.

(3) Drug resistant eukaryotes.

(4) Man-created breeds of domesticated animals like dogs.

(a) only (1) (b) (1) and (3)
(c) (2), (3) and (4) (d) only (4)

18. Embryological support for evolution was disapproved by ***(2020)***

(a) Karl Ernst von Baer (b) Alfred Wallace
(c) Charles Darwin (d) Oparin.

19. Flippers of penguins and dolphins are examples of ***(2020)***

(a) adaptive radiation
(b) convergent evolution
(c) industrial melanism
(d) natural selection.

20. The similarity of bone structure in the forelimbs of many vertebrates is an example of ***(2018)***

(a) homology
(b) analogy
(c) convergent evolution
(d) adaptive radiation.

21. Among the following sets of examples for divergent evolution, select the incorrect option. ***(2018)***
(a) Forelimbs of man, bat and cheetah
(b) Heart of bat, man and cheetah
(c) Brain of bat, man and cheetah
(d) Eye of octopus, bat and man

22. Which of the following structures is homologous to the wing of a bird? ***(NEET-I 2016)***
(a) Hindlimb of rabbit (b) Flipper of whale
(c) Dorsal fin of a shark (d) Wing of a moth

23. Analogous structures are a result of ***(NEET-I 2016)***
(a) shared ancestry
(b) stabilising selection
(c) divergent evolution
(d) convergent evolution.

24. The wings of a bird and the wings of an insect are ***(2015)***
(a) phylogenetic structures and represent divergent evolution
(b) homologous structures and represent convergent evolution
(c) homologous structures and represent divergent evolution
(d) analogous structures and represent convergent evolution.

25. Industrial melanism is an example of ***(2015)***
(a) mutation (b) Neo-Lamarckism
(c) Neo-Darwinism (d) natural selection.

26. Forelimbs of cat, lizard used in walking; forelimbs of whale used in swimming and forelimbs of bats used in flying are an example of ***(2014)***
(a) analogous organs
(b) adaptive radiation
(c) homologous organs
(d) convergent evolution.

27. Which one of the following are analogous structures? ***(2014)***
(a) Wings of bat and wings of pigeon
(b) Gills of prawn and lungs of man
(c) Thorns of Bougainvillea and tendrils of Cucurbita
(d) Flippers of dolphin and legs of horse

28. The process by which organisms with different evolutionary history evolve similar phenotypic adaptations in response to a common environmental challenge, is called ***(2013)***
(a) non-random evolution
(b) adaptive radiation
(c) natural selection
(d) convergent evolution.

29. The eye of octopus and eye of cat show different patterns of structure, yet they perform similar function. This is an example of ***(2013)***
(a) analogous organs that have evolved due to convergent evolution
(b) analogous organs that have evolved due to divergent evolution
(c) homologous organs that have evolved due to convergent evolution
(d) homologous organs that have evolved due to divergent evolution.

30. Which one of the following options gives one correct example each of convergent evolution and divergent evolution? (2012)

	Convergent evolution	**Divergent evolution**
(a)	Eyes of octopus and mammals	Bones of forelimbs of vertebrates
(b)	Thorns of Bougainvillea and tendrils of Cucurbita	Wings of butterflies and bird
(c)	Bones of forelimbs of vertebrates	Wings of butterfly and birds
(d)	Thorns of Bougainvillea and tendrils of Cucurbita	Eyes of octopus and mammals

31. Given below are four statements (A-D) each with one or two blanks. Select the option which correctly fills up the blanks in two statements. ***(Mains 2010)***

Statements:

(A) Wings of butterfly and birds look alike and are the results of __(i)__ evolution.

(B) Miller showed that CH_4,H_2,NH_3 and __(i) when exposed to electric discharge in a flask resulted in formation of __(ii)__.

(C) Vermiform appendix is a __(i)__ organ and an __(ii)__ evidence of evolution.

(D) According to Darwin evolution took place due to __(i)__ and __(ii)__ of the fittest.

(a) (D) - (i) small variations, (ii) survival, (A) - (i) convergent
(b) (A) - (i) convergent, (B) - (i) oxygen, (ii) nucleosides
(c) (B) - (i) water vapour, (ii) amino acids (C) - (i) rudimentary, (ii) anatomical (d)
(d) (C) - (i) vestigial, (ii) anatomical (D) - (i) mutations, (ii) multiplication

32. *Peripatus* is a connecting link between ***(2009)***
(a) mollusca and echinodermata
(b) annelida and arthropoda
(c) coelenterata and porifera
(d) ctenophora and platyhelminthes.

33. In the case of peppered moth (Biston betularia) the black-coloured form became dominant over the light-coloured form in England during industrial revolution. This is an example of ***(2009)***
(a) appearance of the darker coloured individuals due to very poor sunlight
(b) protective mimicry
(c) inheritance of darker colour character acquired due to the darker environment
(d) natural selection whereby the darker forms were selected.

34. Thorn of Bougainvillea and tendril of Cucurbita are examples of ***(2008)***
(a) vestigial organs
(b) retrogressive evolution
(c) analogous organs
(d) homologous organs.

35. Which one of the following pairs of items correctly belongs to the category of organs mentioned against it? ***(2008)***
(a) Nephridia of earthworm and Malpighian tubules of cockroach - excretory organs
(b) Wings of honeybee and wings of crow homologous organs
(c) Thorn of Bougainvillea and tendrils of Cucurbita - analogous organs
(d) Nictitating membrane and blind spot in human eye - vestigial organs

36. Which one of the following statements is correct? ***(2007)***
(a) There is no evidence of the existence of gills during embryogenesis of mammals.
(b) All plant and animal cells are totipotent.
(c) Ontogeny repeats phylogeny.
(d) Stem cells are specialised cells.

37. When two species of different genealogy come to resemble each other as a result of adaptation, the phenomenon is termed ***(2007)***
(a) microevolution
(b) co-evolution
(c) convergent evolution
(d) divergent evolution.

38. An important evidence in favour of organic evolution is the occurrence of ***(2006)***
(a) homologous and analogous organs
(b) homologous and vestigial organs
(c) analogous and vestigial organs
(d) homologous organs only.

39. Which one of the following is not a living fossil? ***(2006)***
(a) Peripatus (b) King crab
(c) Sphenodon (d) Archaeopteryx

40. Which of the following is the relatively most accurate method for dating of fossils? ***(2005)***
(a) Radio-carbon method
(b) Potassium-argon method
(c) Electron-spin resonance method
(d) Uranium-lead method

41. Age of fossils in the past was generally determined by radio-carbon method and other methods involve radioactive elements found in the rocks. More precise methods, which were used recently and led to the revision of the evolutionary periods for different groups of organisms, includes ***(2004)***
(a) study of carbohydrates/proteins in fossils
(b) study of the conditions of fossilisation
(c) electron spin resonance (ESR) and fossil DNA
(d) study of carbohydrates/proteins in rocks.

42. Convergent evolution is illustrated by ***(2003)***
(a) rat and dog
(b) bacterium and protozoan
(c) starfish and cuttle fish
(d) dogfish and whale.

43. Industrial melanism is an example of ***(2003)***
(a) drug resistance
(b) darkening of skin due to smoke from industries
(c) protective resemblance with the surroundings
(d) defensive adaptation of skin against ultraviolet radiations.

44. Which one of the following describes correctly the homologous structures? ***(2003)***
(a) Organs with anatomical similarities, but performing different functions
(b) Organs with anatomical dissimilarities, but performing same function
(c) Organs that have no function now, but had an important function in ancestor
(d) Organs appearing only in embryonic stage and disappearing later in the adult

45. Which of the following are homologous organs? ***(2002)***
(a) Wings of birds and locust
(b) Wings of birds and pectoral fins of fish
(c) Wings of bat and butterfly
(d) Legs of frog and cockroach

46. Phenomenon of 'Industrial melanism' demonstrates ***(1999)***
(a) geographical isolation
(b) reproductive isolation
(c) natural selection
(d) induced mutation.

47. Which of the following are homologous organs? ***(1999)***
(a) Wings of bird and hands of human
(b) Nails of human being and claws in animals
(c) Wings of bird and wings of insect
(d) Wings of bat and wings of cockroach

48. Study of fossils is ***(1991)***
(a) palaeontology (b) herpetology
(c) saurology (d) organic evolution.

WHAT IS ADAPTIVE RADIATION?

49. Select the correct group/set of Australian Marsupials exhibiting adaptive radiation. ***(2023)***
(a) Mole, Flying squirrel, Tasmanian tiger cat
(b) Lemur, Anteater, Wolf
(c) Tasmanian wolf, Bobcat, Marsupial mole
(d) Numbat, Spotted cuscus, Flying phalanger

50. Match List-I with List-II. ***(2021)***

List-I	List-II
(p) Adaptive radiation	(i) Selection of resistant varieties due to excessive use of herbicides and pesticides
(q) Convergent evolution	(ii) Bones of forelimbs in man and whale
(r) Divergent evolution	(iii) Wings of butterfly and bird
(s) by anthropogenic action	(iv) Darwin finches

Choose the correct answer from the options given below.

	p	q	r	s
(a)	(i)	(iv)	(iii)	(ii)
(b)	(iv)	(iii)	(ii)	(i)
(c)	(iii)	(ii)	(i)	(iv)
(d)	(ii)	(i)	(iv)	(iii)

51. The finch species of Galapagos islands are grouped according to their food sources. Which of the following is not a finch food? ***(Karnataka NEET 2013)***

(a) Carrion (b) Insects
(c) Tree buds (d) Seeds

52. Evolution of different species in a given area starting from a point and spreading to other geographical areas is known as ***(2012)***

(a) adaptive radiation
(b) natural selection
(c) migration
(d) divergent evolution.

53. Darwin's finches are a good example of ***(2010,2008)***

(a) industrial melanism
(b) connecting link
(c) adaptive radiation
(d) convergent evolution.

54. The Finches of Galapagos islands provide an evidence in favour of ***(2007)***

(a) evolution due to mutation
(b) retrogressive evolution
(c) biogeographical evolution
(d) special creation.

55. Adaptive radiation refers to ***(2007)***

(a) evolution of different species from a common ancestor
(b) migration of members of a species to different geographical areas
(c) power of adaptation in an individual to a variety of environments
(d) adaptations due to geographical isolation.

56. Which evidence of evolution is related to Darwin's finches? ***(2000)***

(a) Evidences from biogeographical distribution
(b) Evidences from comparative anatomy
(c) Evidences from embryology
(d) Evidences from paleontology

BIOLOGICAL EVOLUTION

57. Which one of the following scientist's name is correctly matched with the theory put forth by him? ***(2008)***

(a)	De Vries	Natural selection
(b)	Mendel	Theory of Pangenesis
(c)	Weismann	Theory of continuity of germplasm
(d)	Pasteur	Inheritance of acquired characters

58. Which one of the following phenomena supports Darwin's concept of natural selection in organic evolution? ***(2005)***

(a) Development of transgenic animals
(b) Production of 'Dolly', the sheep by cloning
(c) Prevalence of pesticide resistant insects
(d) Development of organs from 'stem cells' for organ transplantation

59. Darwin in his "Natural Selection Theory" did not believe in any role of which one of the following in organic evolution? ***(2003)***

(a) Parasites and predators as natural enemies
(b) Survival of the fittest
(c) Struggle for existence
(d) Discontinuous variations

60. Species occurring in different geographical area are called as ***1998)***

(a) sympatric (b) allopatric
(c) sibling (d) neopatric.

61. Weismann cut off tails of mice generation after generation but tails neither disappeared nor shortened showing that ***(1993)***
(a) Darwin was correct
(b) tail is an essential organ
(c) mutation theory is wrong
(d) Lamarckism was wrong in inheritance of acquired characters.

62. "Continuity of germplasm" theory was given by ***(1989)***
(a) De Vries (b) Weismann
(c) Darwin (d) Lamarck.

63. Theory of inheritance of acquired characters was given by ***(1989)***
(a) Wallace (b) Lamarck
(c) Darwin (d) De Vries.

64. 'Origin of Species' was written by ***(1989)***
(a) Oparin (b) Weismann
(c) Lamarck (d) Darwin.

MECHANISM OF EVOLUTION

65. Variations caused by mutation, as proposed by Hugo de Vries, are ***(2019)***
(a) small and directionless
(b) random and directional
(c) random and directionless
(d) small and directional.

66. According to Hugo de Vries, the mechanism of evolution is ***(2018)***
(a) multiple step mutations
(b) saltation
(c) phenotypic variations
(d) minor mutations.

67. The idea of mutations was brought forth by ***(Mains 2012)***
(a) Hugo de Vries who worked on evening primrose
(b) Gregor Mendel who worked on Pisum sativum
(c) Hardy-Weinberg who worked on allele frequencies in a population
(d) Charles Darwin who observed a wide variety of organisms during sea voyage.

68. De Vries gave his mutation theory on organic evolution while working on ***(2005)***
(a) Pisum sativum
(b) Drosophila melanogaster
(c) Oenothera lamarckiana
(d) Althea rosea.

HARDY-WEINBERG PRINCIPLE

69. Natural selection where more individual acquire specific character value other than the mean character value, leads to ***(2022)***
(a) stabilising change
(b) directional change
(c) disruptive change
(d) random change.

70. The factor that leads to Founder effect in a population is ***(2021)***
(a) genetic drift
(b) natural selection
(c) genetic recombination
(d) mutation.

71. A gene locus has two alleles A, a. If the frequency of dominant allele A is 0.4 , then what will be the frequency of homozygous dominant, heterozygous and homozygous recessive individuals in the population? ***(2019)***
(a) 0.16(AA);0.36(Aa);0.48(aa)
(b) 0.36(AA);0.48(Aa);0.16(aa)
(c) 0.16(AA);0.24(Aa);0.36(aa)
(d) 0.16(AA);0.48(Aa);0.36(aa)

72. In a species, the weight of newborn ranges from 2 to 5 kg. 97% of the newborn with an average weight between 3 to 3.3 kg survive whereas 99% of the infants born with weights from 2 to 2.5 or 4.5 to 5 kg die. Which type of selection process is taking place? ***(2019)***
(a) Cyclical selection
(b) Directional selection
(c) Stabilising selection
(d) Disruptive selection

73. Artificial selection to obtain cows yielding higher milk output represents ***(2017)***

(a) directional as it pushes the mean of the character in one direction

(b) disruptive as it splits the population into two, one yielding higher output and the other lower output

(c) stabilising followed by disruptive as it stabilises the population to produce higher yielding cows

(d) stabilising selection as it stabilises this character in the population.

74. Genetic drift operates in ***(NEET-II 2016, 2002)***

(a) small isolated population

(b) large isolated population

(c) non-reproductive population

(d) slow reproductive population.

75. In Hardy-Weinberg equation, the frequency of heterozygous individual is represented by ***(NEET-II 2016)***

(a) p^2 (b) 2pq

(c) pq (d) q^2.

76. In a population of 1000 individuals 360 belong to genotype AA, 480 to Aa and the remaining 160 to aa. Based on this data, the frequency of allele A in the population is ***(2014)***

(a) 0.4 (b) 0.5

(c) 0.6 (d) 0.7

77. The tendency of population to remain in genetic equilibrium may be disturbed by ***(2013)***

(a) lack of mutations

(b) lack of random mating

(c) random mating

(d) lack of migration.

78. Variation in gene frequencies within populations can occur by chance rather than by natural selection. This is referred to as ***(2013)***

(a) random mating (b) genetic load

(c) genetic flow (d) genetic drift.

79. Random unidirectional change in allele frequencies that occurs by chance in all populations and especially in small populations is known as

(Karnataka NEET 2013)

(a) migration (b) natural selection

(c) genetic drift (d) mutation.

80. Genetic variation in a population arises due to ***(Karnataka NEET 2013)***

(a) recombination only

(b) mutation as well as recombination

(c) reproductive isolation and selection

(d) mutations only.

81. At a particular locus, frequency of A allele is 0.6 and that of a is 0.4 . What would be the frequency of heterozygotes in a random mating population at equilibrium? ***(2005)***

(a) 0.36 (b) 0.16

(c) 0.24 (d) 0.48

82. Which of the following is not true for a species? ***(2005)***

(a) Members of a species can interbreed.

(b) Gene flow does not occur between the populations of a species.

(c) Each species is reproductively isolated from every other species.

(d) Variations occur among members of a species.

83. Random genetic drift in a population probably results from ***(2003)***

(a) highly genetically variable individuals

(b) interbreeding within this population

(c) constant low mutation rate

(d) large population size.

84. In which condition, the gene ratio remains constant for any species population? ***(2002)***

(a) Sexual selection (b) Random mating

(c) Mutation (d) Gene flow

85. In the developmental history of mammalian heart, it is observed that it passes through a two chambered fish like heart, three chambered frog like heart and finally four chambered stage. To which hypothesis can this above cited statement be approximated? ***(1998)***
(a) Lamarck's principle
(b) Mendelian principles
(c) Biogenetic law
(d) Hardy-Weinberg law

86. Genetic drift operates only in ***(1998)***
(a) larger populations
(b) Mendelian populations
(c) island populations
(d) smaller populations.

A BRIEF ACCOUNT OF EVOLUTION

87. Dinosaurs dominated the world in which of the following geological eras?

(Karnataka NEET 2013)

(a) Cenozoic (b) Jurassic
(c) Mesozoic (d) Devonian

88. Jurassic period of the Mesozoic era is characterised by
(a) flowering plants and first dinosaurs appear
(b) gymnosperms are dominant plants and first birds appear
(c) radiation of reptiles and origin of mammal like reptiles
(d) dinosaurs become extinct and angiosperms appear.

89. Diversification in plant life appeared ***(2004)***
(a) due to long periods of evolutionary changes
(b) due to abrupt mutations
(c) suddenly on earth
(d) by seed dispersal.

90. In which era reptiles were dominant? ***(2002)***
(a) Coenozoic era (b) Mesozoic era
(c) Palaeozoic era (d) Archaeozoic era

91. Correct order is
(a) Palaeozoic → Archaeozoic → Coenozoic
(b) Archaeozoic → Palaeozoic → Proterozoic
(c) Palaeozoic → Mesozoic → Coenozoic
(d) Mesozoic → Archaeozoic → Proterozoic.

ORIGIN AND EVOLUTION OF MAN

92. Match the hominids with their correct brain size. ***(2019)***

(A) *Homo habilis*	(i) 900cc
(B) *Homo neanderthalensis*	(ii) 1350cc
(C) *Homo erectus*	(iii) 650-800cc
(D) *Homo sapiens*	(iv) 1400cc

Select the correct option.

(A) (B) (C) (D)
(a) (iv) (iii) (i) (ii)
(b) (iii) (i) (iv) (ii)
(c) (iii) (ii) (i) (iv)
(d) (iii) (iv) (i) (ii)

93. Which of the following statements is correct about the origin and evolution of men?

(Odisha NEET 2019)

(a) Agriculture came around 50,000 years back.
(b) The Dryopithecus and Ramapithecus primates existing 15 million years ago, walked like men.
(c) Homo habilis probably ate meat.
(d) Neanderthal men lived in Asia between 1,00,000 and 40,000 years back.

94. The chronological order of human evolution from early to the recent is ***(NEET-II 2016)***
(a) Australopithecus → Ramapithecus → Homo habilis → Homo erectus
(b) Ramapithecus → Australopithecus → Homo habilis → Homo erectus
(c) Ramapithecus → Homo habilis → Australopithecus → Homo erectus
(d) Australopithecus → Homo habilis → Ramapithecus → Homo erectus

95. Which of the following had the smallest brain capacity? ***(2015 Cancelled)***
(a) Homo neanderthalensis
(b) Homo habilis
(c) Homo erectus (d) Homo sapiens

96. What was the most significant trend in the evolution of modern man (*Homo sapiens*) from his ancestors? ***(2012,2011)***
(a) Shortening of jaws
(b) Binocular vision
(c) Increasing cranial capacity
(d) Upright posture

97. The extinct human who lived 1,00,000 to 40,000 years ago, in Europe, Asia and parts of Africa, with short stature, heavy eye brows, retreating fore heads, large jaws with heavy teeth, stocky bodies, a lumbering gait and stooped posture was ***(2012)***
(a) Homo habilis
(b) Neanderthal human
(c) Cro-magnon human
(d) Ramapithecus.

98. The most apparent change during the evolutionary history of Homo sapiens is traced in ***(Mains 2010)***
(a) loss of body hair
(b) walking upright
(c) shortening of the jaws
(d) remarkable increase in the brain size

99. There are two opposing views about origin of modern man. According to one view *Homo erectus* in Asia were the ancestors of modern man. A study of variation of DNA however suggested African origin of modern man. What kind of observation on DNA variation could suggest this? ***(2005)***
(a) Greater variation in Asia than in Africa
(b) Greater variation in Africa than in Asia
(c) Similar variation in Africa and Asia
(d) Variation only in Asia and no variation in Africa

100. What kind of evidence suggested that man is more closely related with chimpanzee than with other hominoid apes? **(2004)**
(a) Evidence from DNA extracted from sex chromosomes only
(b) Comparison of chromosomes morphology only
(c) Evidence from fossil remains, and the fossil mitochondrial DNA alone
(d) Evidence from DNA extracted from sex chromosomes, autosomes.

101. In recent years, DNA sequences (nucleotide sequence) of mtDNA and Y chromosomes were considered for the study of human evolution, because ***(2003)***
(a) they are small and therefore, easy to study
(b) they are uniparental in origin and do not take part in recombination
(c) their structure is known in greater detail
(d) they can be studied from the samples of fossil remains.

102. According to fossils discovered up to present time origin and evolution of man started from ***(2002)***
(a) France (b) Java
(c) Africa (d) China.

103. Which of the following is closest relative of man? ***(2001)***
(a) Chimpanzee (b) Gorilla
(c) Orangutan (d) Gibbon

104. Character which is closely related to human evolution is ***(2000)***
(a) disappearance of tail
(b) reduction in size of jaws
(c) binocular vision (d) flat nails.

105. Which of the following statements is correct regarding evolution of mankind? ***(1997)***
(a) Homo erectus is preceded by Homo habilis.
(b) Neanderthal man and cro-magnon man were living at the same time.
(c) Australopithecus was living in Australia.
(d) None of these

106. Common origin of man and chimpanzee is best shown by *(1997)*

(a) binocular vision (b) chromosome number

(c) dental formula (d) cranial capacity.

107. Which of the following is the direct ancestor of Homo sapiens? *(1996)*

(a) Australopithecus

(b) H. sapiens neanderthals

(c) Homo erectus

(d) Homo sapiens fossilis

ANSWER KEY

1.	(a)	2.	(c)	3.	(a)	4.	(c)	5.	(c)	6.	(d)	7.	(d)
8.	(b)	9.	(b)	10.	(b)	11.	(b)	12.	(d)	13.	(b)	14.	(c)
15.	(c)	16.	(d)	17.	(c)	18.	(a)	19.	(b)	20.	(a)	21.	(d)
22.	(b)	23.	(d)	24.	(d)	25.	(d)	26.	(c)	27.	(a,b)	28.	(d)
29.	(a)	30.	(a)	31.	(a)	32.	(b)	33.	(d)	34.	(d)	35.	(a)
36.	(c)	37.	(c)	38.	(b)	39.	(d)	40.	(c)	41.	(c)	42.	(d)
43.	(c)	44	(a)	45.	(b)	46.	(c)	47.	(a)	48.	(a)	49.	(d)
50.	(b)	51.	(a)	52.	(a)	53.	(c)	54.	(c)	55.	(a)	56.	(a)
57.	(c)	58.	(c)	59.	(d)	60.	(b)	61.	(d)	62.	(b)	63.	(b)
64.	(d)	65.	(c)	66.	(b)	67.	(a)	68.	(c)	69.	(b)	70.	(a)
71.	(d)	72.	(c)	73.	(a)	74.	(a)	75.	(b)	76.	(c)	77.	(b)
78.	(d)	79.	(c)	80.	(b)	81.	(d)	82.	(b)	83.	(b)	84.	(b)
85.	(c)	86.	(d)	87.	(c)	88.	(b)	89.	(a)	90.	(b)	91.	(c)
92.	(d)	93.	(d)	94.	(b)	95.	(b)	96.	(c)	97.	(b)	98.	(d)
99.	(b)	100.	(d)	101.	(b)	102.	(c)	103.	(a)	104.	(a)	105.	(a)
106.	(d)	107.	(d)										

HINTS & EXPLANATIONS

1.(a) : In 1953, S.L. Miller, an American scientist created imilar conditions in a laboratory scale. He created electric lischarge in a closed flask containing CH4, H2, NH3 and water apour at 800° C and observed formation of amino acids

2. (c)

3. (a)

4.(c) : The condition for origin of life, partial isolation, has been attained within aggregates of artificially formed prebiotic molecules. These aggregates are called protobionts which can separate combinations of molecules from the surroundings. they maintain an internal environment but are unable to reproduce. Two important protobionts are coacervates and microspheres.

5.(c) : Chemical evolution has two meanings and uses. The first refers to the theories of evolution of the chemical elements in the universe through nucleosynthesis. The second use of chemical evolution or chemosynthesis is as a hypothesis to explain how life might possibly have developed or evolved from non-life.

6.(d) : Stanley Miller in 1953, who was then a grad student of Harold Urey at the University of Chicago, circulated four gases - methane, ammonia, hydrogen and water vapour in an air tight apparatus and passed electrical discharges from electrodes. He passed the mixture through a condenser. He circulated the gases continuously in this way for one week and then analysed the chemical composition of the liquid inside the apparatus. He found a large number of simple organic compounds including some amino acid such as alanine, glycine and aspartic acid. Glutamic acid was not found.

7.(d) : Microbes were killed by heating the meat and the sealed vessel formed a closed system wherein the new microbes could not come in contact with the nutrient medium and hence no spoilage of meat.

8.(b) : The first scientific explanation of origin of life was put forward by a Russian Scientist, A.I. Oparin in 1923. J.B.S. Haldane (1928), England-born Indian Scientist, also made similar observations regarding the origin of life. According to them primitive atmosphere was reducing atmosphere because hydrogen atoms (most numerous and most reactive) combined with all available oxygen atoms to form water and leaving no free oxygen.

9.(b) : Water is the most essential material to survive. One can thrive without O_2 (anaerobic bacteria) and light and in a wide range of temperature but one cannot live without water which is the most important component of the body (about 90% of plasma consists of water) and life was originated from abiogenetic materials in water.

10. (b)

11.(b) : The first living beings were prokaryotic, like bacteria. They were single-celled. Nucleic acid core consisted of naked DNA. These living beings were present in the environment of soupy sea having abundant organic molecules. Nutritionally they were chemoheterotrophs. They absorbed the organic materials from outside both for body building and liberation of energy. Respiration was anaerobic since free oxygen was absent in the environment.

12.(d) : Hydrogen atoms were most numerous and most reactive in primitive atmosphere. First hydrogen atoms combined with all oxygen atoms to form water and leaving no free oxygen. Hydrogen atoms also combined with nitrogen, forming ammonia (NH3). So water and ammonia were probably the first compound molecules of primitive earth. Later methane, water and NH3 join to form amino acids which gets converted into proteins while hydrogen bases, sugars and phosphates combine to form nucleic acids.

13. (b)

14.(c) : The primitive atmosphere was reducing atmosphere, i.e., without free oxygen.

15.(c) : The gist (in brief) of Darwin - Wallace theory is as follows.

(i) Individuals within species show considerable but continuous variation in the form and physiology.

(ii) This variation arises in a random fashion and is heritable.

(iii) The potential for increase within population of animals and plants is considerable.

(iv) Since resources are limited, so individuals in a population struggle for their own existence.

(v) Only some survive and leave offspring with the same trait through this natural selection of the fittest species become represented by individuals which are better adapted.

16.(d) : Flippers of penguins and dolphins are pair of analogous organs.

17.(c) : Herbicide resistant weeds, drug resistant eukaryotes and man-created breeds of domesticated animals like dogs are examples of evolution by anthropogenic action. Darwin's Finches of Galapagos islands are example of natural selection, adaptive radiation and Founder's effect.

18.(a) : Embryological support for evolution was disapproved by Karl Ernst von Baer. He noted that embryos never pass through the adult stages of other animals.

19.(b) : Analogous structures are result of convergent evolution, i.e., different structures evolving for the same function and hence having similarity. For example, the eye of the octopus and of mammals, the flippers of penguins and dolphins.

20.(a) : Homologous organs are those organs which have the same fundamental structure but are different in functions. Wings of birds and forelimbs of horse show homology because skeletal parts of their forelimbs are similar in structure and arrangement but have different functions.

21.(d) : Eye of octopus, bat and man are examples of analogous organs showing convergent evolution.

22.(b) : Homologous organs have same fundamental structure but different functions. The wing of a bird and flipper of a whale are structurally forelimbs, which consist of humerus, radio-ulna, carpals, metacarpals and digits but they perform different functions. The wings of birds help them to fly while flipper helps the whale to swim.

23.(d) : The organs which have similar functions but are different in their structural details and origin are called analogous organs. The analogous structures are the result of convergent evolution.

24.(d) : Analogous organs are the organs which have similar function but are different in their structural details and origin. The analogous structures are the result of convergent evolution. The wings of an insect are analogous to wings of a bird because the basic structure of the wings of the insects is different from the wings of bird. However, their function is similar.

25.(d) : Natural selection is the most widely accepted theory concerning the principal causal mechanism of evolutionary change profounded by Charles Darwin and Alfred Russel Wallace. It results from the differential reproduction (some members of a population produce abundant offspring, some only a few and still others none), one phenotype as compared with other phenotypes in the same population. This determines the relative share of different genotypes which individuals possess and propagate in a population. Industrial melanism supports evolution by natural selection. It is an adaptation where the moths living in the industrial areas developed melanin pigments to match their bodies to the tree trunks.

26. (c) : The organs which have the same fundamental structure but are different in functions are called homologous organs. These organs follow the same basic plan of organisation during their development. But in the adult condition, these organs are modified to perform different functions as an adaptation to different environments. The forelimbs of cat, lizard, whale and bat have the same basic structural plan. In each case the forelimb consists of humerus, radio-ulna, carpals, metacarpals and digits. The skeletal parts of the forelimbs of all these vertebrates are similar in structure and arrangement. But the forelimbs of these animals have different shapes and functions. In lizard they are used for walking, in cat for running, in whale for swimming and in bat for flying.

27. (a, b) : The organs which have similar functions but are different in their structural details and origin are called analogous organs. The wings of bat are analogous to wings of pigeon. It is due to the fact that the basic structure of the wings of the mammal is different from the wings of bird. However, their function is similar. Similarly, gills of prawn and lungs of man, both are respiratory organs yet they have very different basic structure.

28.(d) : Convergent evolution is the development of superficially similar structures in unrelated organisms, usually because the organisms live in the same kind of environment. Examples are the wings of insects and birds and the streamlined bodies of whales and fish. One can say that it is the similar habitat that has resulted in selection of similar adaptive features in different groups of organisms but toward the same function. An example of convergent evolution is the similar nature of the flight/wings of insects, birds, pteridosaurs and bats. All four serve the same function and are similar in structure, but each evolved independently. Some species of the lens of eyes also evolved independently in various animals.

29.(a)

30.(a) : Development of similar adaptive functional structures in unrelated groups of organisms is called convergent evolution. It shows analogy. Examples are wings of butterfly and birds, eye of the octopus and the mammals, flippers of penguins and dolphins, etc. On the other hand, divergent evolution involves development of different functional structures along different directions due to adaptations to different needs from a common ancestral form. For example, forelimbs of vertebrates (whales, bat, cheetah, human). Though these perform different functions, they have similar anatomical structures.

31. (a)

32. (b): Peripatus belongs to Phylum Onychophora. It shows characters of annelids as well as arthropods. Owing to its resemblance with two different phyla, Peripatus is often referred to as connecting link between them. This shows an important morphological and anatomical evidence of evolution.

33.(d) : During post industrialisation period, the tree trunk became dark due to industrial smoke and soots. White winged moths did not survive due to predators and dark winged moths survived because they were less easily seen by them against a dark background. Thus industrial melanism supports evolution by natural selection that favours the establishment of one particular advantageous mutation within a population.

34. (d): The organs which have the same fundamental structure but are different in function are called homologous organs. Thorn of Bougainvillea and tendril of Cucurbita both arises in the axillary position, but have different functions.

35. (a): Nephridia are excretory organs of earthworm which consist of a simple or branched tube formed by the ingrowth of ectoderm with cilia at the inner end. Excretory products diffuse into the nephridium and are wafted to the exterior by ciliary action. Malpighian tubules are the organs that are involved in the excretion of nitrogenous wastes in cockroach. It open into the intestine; selectively extract from the blood uric acid, which together with water and salts - is deposited into the hindgut and excreted in the faeces.

36.(c) : Haeckel (1810) proposed that developing animal embryo passes through stages resembling adult forms of its ancestors. Ernst Haeckel (1868,1874) formulated biogenetic law or recapitulation theory which states that ontogeny (developmental history of an individual) repeats phylogeny (development history of races).

37.(c) : Convergent evolution is the development of superficially similar structures in unrelated organisms, usually because the organisms live in the same kind of environment. Examples are the wings of insects and birds and the streamlined bodies of whales and fish. One can say that it is the similar habitat that has resulted in selection of similar adaptive features in different groups of organisms but towards the same function. An example of convergent evolution is the similar nature of the flight/wings of insects, birds, pteridosaurs and bats. All four serve the same function and are similar in structure, but each evolved independently.. Some species of the lens of eyes also evolved independently in various animals.

38.(b) : Homologous organ and vestigial organs provide an important evidence in favour of organic evolution (process by which changes in the genetic composition of populations of organisms occur in response to environmental changes). For example, human appendix is a developmental derivative and evolutionary vestige of the end of the much larger herbivorous caecum found in our primate ancestors. They both are structurally homologous and have different functions. In most vertebrates, the caecum is a large, complex gastrointestinal organ, enriched in mucosal lymphatic tissue and specialised for digestion of plants. The caecum varies in size among species, but in general the size of the caecum is proportional to the amount of plant matter in a given organism's diet. It is largest in obligate herbivores, animals whose diets consist entirely of plant matter. However, even though humans are herbivorous, the small human caecum does not house cellulose-digesting bacteria and lost an essential function of cellulose digestion. This shows the close evolutionary relationships between homologous and vestigial organs.

39.(d) : Living fossil is a term for any living species of organism which closely resembles species otherwise only known from fossils and has no close living relatives. These species have all survived major extinction events and generally retain low taxonomic diversities.

Some examples of living fossils in animals are - coelacanth, coral (polyp), crocodylia (crocodiles, gavials and alligators), horseshoe crab (*Limulus polyphemus*), monotremes (*Platypus* and *Echidna*), snout-nosed frog (*Nasikabatrachus sahyadrensis*). Archaeopteryx is the earliest and most primitive known bird. It lived in the Jurassic Period around 150-155 million years ago. It has feathers and wings but it also had teeth and a skeleton similar to a small carnivorous dinosaur, therefore, it had both bird and theropod dinosaur features. Archaeopteryx is a powerful piece of evidence that shows that birds have evolved from dinosaurs.

40.(c) : Electron spin resonance (ESR) measures the

number of charges occupying deep traps in the crystal bandgap. By measuring the change in absorption of microwave energy within a continuously varying strong magnetic field, this method detects the number of "unpaired spins" of electronic charges trapped at various defects in the mineral lattice.

41.(c) : Electron spin resonance (ESR) measures the number of charges occupying deep traps in the crystal bandgap. By measuring the change in absorption of microwave energy within a continuously varying strong magnetic field, this method detects the number of "unpaired spins" of electronic charges trapped at various defects in the mineral lattice.

42.(d) : Convergent evolution is the formation of similar traits by unrelated groups of organisms. Dogfish and whale are the interesting examples of convergent evolution in animals as both of them have more or less similar body organisation.

43.(c) : Industrial melanism is an adaptation where the moths living in the industrial areas developed melanin pigments to match their body to the soot-covered surroundings. These melanic forms are mainly distributed in and around large industrial cities, where the environment has been altered by the pollution of the atmosphere; and is manifested by the appearance of dark colour of lichen-covered tree trunks, on which the moths rest during the day time. The peppered moth exists in two strains (forms) : light coloured (white) and melanic (black). In the past, bark of trees was covered by whitish lichens, so white moths escaped unnoticed from predatory birds. After industrialisation barks got covered by smoke, so the white moths were selectively picked up by birds. But black moths escaped unnoticed so they managed to survive resulting in more population of black moths and less population of white moths.

44 (a)

45. (b)

46. (c)

47.(a) : Wings of birds and hands of human have the same structure but different functions. Birds use their wings for flying while humans use their hands for grasping. Other options show examples of analogous organs. Analogous organs are those organs which have similar functions but different structural details.

48.(a) : Palaeontology is the study of extinct organisms, including their structure, environment, evolution, and distribution, as revealed by their fossil remains. Herpetology is the study of reptiles and amphibians. Saurology is the study of snakes. Organic evolution deals with study of origin of life and origin of new species.

49.(d) : Adaptive radiation is the process of evolution of different species in given geographical area starting from a point and radiating to other areas of geography. Example; Australian marsupials where a number of marsupials each different from other evolved from an ancestral stock, but all within Australian island continent. Marsupial mole, numbat, spotted cuscus, flying phalanger, tasmanian wolf, tasmanian tiger cat are examples of Australian marsupials.

50. (b)

51.(a) : Darwin's finches show adaptive radiation. This radiation occurred in response to various food resources available. These finches feed on insects, tree buds, seeds, cactus, etc. Carrion are dead bodies and no finches feed on them.

52.(a) : Adaptive radiation (divergent evolution) is the evolution from one species of animals or plants of a number of different forms. As the original population increases in size it spreads out from its centre of origin to exploit new habitats and food sources. In time, this results in a number of populations each adapted to its particular habitat, eventually these populations will differ from each other sufficiently to become new species.

53. (c)

54.(c) : Biogeographical evolution is a process in which gene pool of a population gradually changes in response to environmental pressures, natural selection and genetic mutations.

55. (a)

56.(a) : Galapagos Islands are a chain of 14 islands in the Pacific ocean on the west coast of South America. Charles Darwin visited these islands during his famous voyage on HMS Beagle (name of his ship) in 1835. The flora and fauna of these islands resemble with those of the South American mainland with which the Galapagos Islands were once connected. However, Darwin's finches (birds of Galapagos Islands) influenced Darwin to think about the evolutionary change. These birds designated as Darwins' finches by Dr. David Lack (1947) do not resemble the birds of the South American species. These finches were the first to reach the Galapagos Islands as migrants from the mainland (South America). When they reached the islands, they faced many problems for obtaining food. Thus, they had to change their feeding habits.

57.(c) : Theory of continuity of germplasm was put forward by August Weismann. According to this, the characters influencing the germ cells are only inherited. There is a continuity of germplasm but the somataplasm is not transmitted to the next generation hence it does not carry characters to next generation.

58.(c) : According to Darwin's theory of survival of the fittest (Natural selection), the organisms which are provided with favourable variations would survive, because they are the fittest to face their surroundings, while the unfit are destroyed. Darwin considered that useful variations are transmitted to the offspring and appear more prominently in succeeding generations. After some generations these continuous and gradual variations in the possessor would be so distinct that they form a new species. This is proved by, the pesticide resistant insects that have the ability to survive as they have resistance genes and so they are selected by nature. Other insects lacking these genes will be killed by pesticides.

59. (d)

60.(b) : Allopatric species are those that could interbreed but do not because they are geographically isolated. Sympatric are groups of similar organisms that, although in close proximity and theoretically capable of interbreeding, do not interbreed because of differences in behaviour, flowering time, etc. Siblings are offspring of the same parents.

61.(d) : Lamarck gave theory of Lamarckism in which he explained inheritance of acquired characters which states that whatever an individual acquires characters in its life time due to internal vital force, effect of environment, new needs and use and disuse of organs, they are inherited to the next generations. The process continues. After several generations, the variations are accumulated upto such extent that they give rise to new species. This theory was proved wrong by August Weismann. Weismann cut off the tails of rats for as many as 22 generations and allowed them to breed, but tailless rats were never born.

62. (b)

63. (b)

64.(d) : Darwin published his observations and conclusions regarding evolution in the book "Origin of Species" in 1859. Darwin's this book became very popular and changed people's thinking about organic evolution.

65.(c) : Hugo de Vries (1901) put forward the theory of evolution called mutation theory. He believed that mutation causes evolution. Mutations are discontinuous variations that are random and directionless.

66.(b) : As per mutation theory given by Hugo de Vries, the evolution is a discontinuous phenomenon or saltatory phenomenon (single step large mutation).

67.(a) : The term mutation was coined by Hugo de Vries (1901) for large spontaneous inheritable changes which occur suddenly in naturally reproducing population. He also proposed mutation theory of evolution in his book "The Mutation Theory" published in 1903 in which he put forth that evolution occurred due to large discontinuous variations. He worked on Oenothera lamarckiana or evening primrose. During his experiments he found 834 mutations in a population of 54343 plants. It was later on found that the mutations observed by Hugo de Vries were actually chromosomal aberrations.

68.(c) : The term mutation was coined by Hugo de Vries (1901) for large spontaneous inheritable changes which occur suddenly in naturally reproducing population. He also proposed mutation theory of evolution in his book "The Mutation Theory" published in 1903 in which he put forth that evolution occurred due to large discontinuous variations. He worked on Oenothera lamarckiana or evening primrose. During his experiments he found 834 mutations in a population of 54343 plants. It was later on found that the mutations observed by Hugo de Vries were actually chromosomal aberrations.

69. (b)

70. (a)

71.(d) : Frequency of dominant allele (A) = 0.4

Applying Hardy-Weinberg equilibrium; $p + q = 1$

$q = 1-0.4 = 0.6; p^2 + q^2 + 2pq = 1$

Frequency of homozygous dominant genotype

$(p^2 \therefore AA) = (0.4)^2 = 0.16$

Frequency of heterozygous genotype

$(2pq \therefore Aa) = 2 \times 0.4 \times 0.6 = 0.48$

Frequency of homozygous recessive genotype

$(q^2 \therefore aa) = (0.6)^2 = 0.36$

72. (c) : Stabilising selection is a balancing type of natural selection which favours average sized individuals and eliminates extreme individuals.

73. (a)

74.(a) : The random changes in gene frequencies in a population occurring by chance alone rather than by natural selection are called genetic drift or Sewall Wright effect. The effects of genetic drift are most marked in very small isolated population, although it occurs in all populations.

75.(b) : In a stable population, for a gene with two alleles, 'A' (dominant) and 'a' (recessive), if the frequency of 'A' is p and the frequency of 'a' is q, then the frequencies of the three possible genotypes (AA, Aa and aa) can be expressed by the Hardy Weinberg equation:

where

$p^2 + 2pq + q^2 = 1$

p^2 = Frequency of AA (homozygous dominant) individuals

q^2 = Frequency of aa (homozygous recessive) individuals

2pq = Frequency of Aa (heterozygous) individuals

76.(c) : According to Hardy-Weinberg principle

$p^2 + 2pq + q^2 = 1; (p + q)^2 = 1$

(AA) $p^2 = 360$ out of 1000 individual

or $p^2 = 0.36$

Therefore, $p = 0.6$

77.(b) : Hardy-Weinberg law states that allele frequencies in a population are stable and remain constant from generation to generation when there is random and non-selective mating. In case of lack of random mating, genetic equilibrium may be disturbed.

78.(d) : Genetic drift (Sewall Wright effect) is the random change in the frequency of alleles in a population over successive generations in the gametes. Each new generation differs from its parental generation with regard to allele frequencies simply because of random variation in the distribution of gametes. This process is more rapid in smaller populations, or when the alleles concerned confer no apparent benefit compared to their counterparts.

79. (c)

80.(b) : The genetic variations exist due to reshuffling of genes caused by recombinations or by mutations. The recombinations are produced by the routine reshuffling of genes during independent assortment of chromosomes, reciprocal crossing of genes during crossing over and random fertilisation of gametes. Mutation is the sudden inheritable discontinuous variation which appears in an organism due to permanent changes in its genotype. Mutation can occur at any stage during the development. Mutations are heritable changes, that is, if they appear in somatic cells they are inherited to daughter cells by mitosis but if they appear in gamete cells they are inherited to the offspring. The former are known as somatic mutations and latter as germ mutations. They bring about a change in the genetic message and cause variation.

81.(d) : In a stable population, for a gene with two alleles, A (dominant) and a (recessive), if the frequency of A is p and the frequency of a is q, then the frequencies of the three possible genotypes (AA,Aa, and aa) can be expressed by the given Hardy-Weinberg equation :

$p^2 + 2pq + q^2 = 1$

where p^2 = frequency of AA (homozygous dominant) individuals, 2pq = frequency of Aa (heterozygous) individuals, and q^2 = frequency of aa (homozygous recessive) individuals. The equation can be used to calculate allele frequencies if the numbers of homozygous recessive individuals in the population is known. The equation and the equilibrium are named after British mathematician G.H. Hardy and German physician W. Weinberg.

So $p = 0.6$ and $q = 0.4$ (given)

$\therefore$ 2pq (frequency of heterozygote)

$= 2 \times 0.6 \times 0.4 = 0.48$

82.(b) : Species may be defined as an uniform interbreeding population or group of individuals which freely interbreed among themselves. Gene flow occurs between populations of a species by gene migration i.e., emigration and immigration.

83. (b)

84.(b) : Allele frequency in a population can remain

constant only if individuals of the population randomly interbreed. Generally it never happens in nature and species populations exist in small groups of randomly breeding subpopulations. Thus allele frequency between two subpopulations may differ but allele frequency within the subpopulation will remain constant. Such subpopulations are termed Mendelian populations or deme. Exchange of genes between demes takes place occasionally. Mutation, gene flow (due to migration), etc. may tend to change the allele frequency of the subpopulation.

85.(c) : Haeckel's biogenetic law states that "Ontogeny repeats phylogeny". Ontogeny is the life history of an organism while phylogeny is the evolutionary history of the race of that organism. In other words an organism repeats its ancestral history during development. Therefore, during embryonic development the mammalian heart first takes the form of fish, then frog and at last mammal.

86.(d) : The random changes in gene frequencies in a population occurring by chance alone rather than by natural selection are called genetic drift or Sewall Wright effect. The effects of genetic drift are most marked in very small isolated population, although it occurs in all populations.

87.(c) : Dinosaurs dominated the world in Mesozoic era. There are three periods of this era:

(i) Dinosaurs originated in the Triassic period,

(ii) dominated in Jurassic period and

(iii) became extinct in cretaceous period.

88. (b): Jurassic period of Mesozoic era is characterised by gymnosperms as dominant plants and the appearance of first toothed bird. Conifers, cycads and ferns were widespread.

89.(a) : Diversification in plant life appeared due to long periods of evolutionary changes. Initially plants were thalloid. There were no differentiation among root, stem and leaves. Vascular tissues were absent.

90.(b) : Mesozoic era is the era during which reptiles were dominant. It includes three periods : Triassic (240 million years ago), Jurassic (195 million years ago) and Cretaceous (135 million years ago). Origin of dinosaurs occurred during Triassic period. During Jurassic period, lizards, crocodiles and alligators originated. Dinosaurs became large and reptiles were dominant during this period. During Cretaceous period, dinosaurs got extinct.

91.(c) : The first geological time scale was developed by Giovanni Avduina, Italian scientist in 1760. The history of the earth has been divided into a number of major divisions called eras. The eras are sub-divided into periods. The modern periods are further divided into epochs. There are four eras. The correct sequence is Precambrian Palaeozoic (era of ancient life) → Mesozoic (era of medieval life) → Coenozoic (era of modern life).

92. (d)

93.(d) : Agriculture came around 10,000 years back and human settlements started. About 15 mya primates called Dryopithecus and Ramapithecus were existing. They were hairy and walked like gorillas and chimpanzees. Homo erectus probably ate meat.

94. (b)

95. (b) : The brain capacity gradually increased from early human ancestors to modern man. Homo habilis had 650 - 800 cc brain capacity which increased around 900cc in Homo erectus. The Neanderthal man (Homo neanderthalensis) had 1400cc brain capacity which evolved to around 1450cc in Homo sapiens.

96. (c) : Binocular vision, smaller jaw and upright posture are the main adaptations that led to evolution of man from its ancestors. But, during human evolution major and most significant changes occurred in the cranial capacity of man. In living modern man it is about 1450cc compared to 500cc in Australopithecus. Increased cranial capacity accommodates larger brain and forms the basis of social, cultural and educational evolution of modern man.

97. (b)

98. (d) : The brain capacity gradually increased from early human ancestors to modern man. Homo habilis had 650 - 800 cc brain capacity which increased around 900cc in Homo erectus. The Neanderthal man (Homo neanderthalensis) had 1400cc brain capacity which evolved to around 1450cc in Homo sapiens.

99. (b)

100. (d): Apes are the members of the hominoidea superfamily of primates, which includes humans. Under the current classification system there are two families of hominoids:

• The family hylobatidae consists of 4 genera and 13 species of gibbons, including the Lar Gibbon and the Siamang, collectively known as the "lesser apes"

• The family hominidae consisting of orangutans, gorillas, chimpanzees, and humans, collectively known as the "great apes".

Within the Superfamily hominoidea, gibbons are the outgroup: this means that the rest of the hominoids are more closely related to each other than any of them are to gibbons.

Investigation showed orangutans to be the outgroup, but comparing humans to all three other hominid genera showed that African apes (chimpanzees and gorillas) and humans are more closely related to each other than any of them are to orangutans

However, DNA comparisons from sex chromosomes and autosomes provide convincing evidence that within the subfamily homininae, gorillas are the outgroup. This suggests that chimpanzees should be in hominini along with humans.

101. (b) : Sequence of both mtDNA and Y chromosomes are considered for the study of human evolution because they are uniparental in origin. mtDNA is inherited along with the maternal cytoplasm and Y chromosome is inherited from father. So they do not take part in recombination. In addition, mtDNA has a higher mutation rate than nuclear DNA so that it is more useful for short term evolutionary studies.

102. (c) : The common ancestor of both ape and man is Dryopithecus - a 20 million years old fossil discovered from Africa. Austroalopithecus also lived in Africa between 6 million to 1 million years ago. The Genus Homo evolved 2 million years ago from one of such Australopithecines in Africa and then only moved out of the continent.

The first such Homo lived throughout Asia, some parts of Europe and Africa. But obviously its evolution took place in Africa.

103. (a)

104. (a) : Humans differ from most primates in that they lack a tail. The lower primates have tails, and the apes, which are believed by many to be our closest relatives, likewise are tailless.

105. (a) : Homo habilis lived during Pleistocene. He lived in Africa about 2 million years ago.

He was about 1.2 to 1.5 metres tall. He had bipedal locomotion, moved erect and was omnivorous. Homo habilis (habilis = mentally able or skilful) was the first tool maker and used tools of chipped stones extensively. Homo erectus appeared about 1.7 million years ago in middle Pleistocene. H. erectus evolved from Homo habilis. He had erect posture, protruding jaws, projecting brow ridges and small canines and large molar teeth. He was omnivorous and made more elaborate tools of stones and bones, hunted big game and perhaps knew use of fire.

106. (d) : A close relationship of apes with man is revealed by their relatively larger brain and cranial capacity, efficient memory. Cranial capacity of apes is under 650 cc. Cranial capacity of man is 1350 to 1600cc.

107. (d) : Homo sapiens fossilis is also known by the name of Cro-magnon man. He was the direct ancestor of modern man (Homo sapiens). Cro-magnon man emerged about 34000 years ago in Holocene epoch. Thus, it is regarded as most recent ancestor of today's man. Its cranial capacity was, however, somewhat more than ours, being about 1650cc. It became extinct about 10000-11000 years ago.

Chapter : 26 HUMAN HEALTH AND DISEASES

COMMON DISEASES IN HUMANS

1. Match List I with List II. (2023)

List I	List II
A. Ringworm	I. *Haemophilus influenzae*
B. Filariasis	II. *Trichophyton*
C. Malaria	III. *Wuchereria bancrofti*
D. Pneumonia	IV. *Plasmodium vivax*

Choose the correct answer from the options given below.
(a) A-III, B-II, C-I, D-IV
(b) A-III, B-II, C-IV, D-I
(c) A-II, B-III, C-IV, D-I
(d) A-II, B-III, C-I, D-IV

2. Match List-I with List-II. ***(2021)***

List-I	List-II
(p) Filariasis	(i) *Haemophilus influenzae*
(q) Amoebiasis	(ii) *Trichophyton*
(r) Pneumonia	(iii) *bancrofti*
(s) Ringworm	(iv) *Entamoeba histolytica*

Choose the correct answer from the options given below

	p	q	r	s
(a)	(ii)	(iii)	(i)	(iv)
(b)	(iv)	(i)	(iii)	(ii)
(c)	(iii)	(iv)	(i)	(ii)
(d)	(i)	(ii)	(iv)	(iii)

3. The infectious stage of Plasmodium that enters the human body is ***(2020)***
(a) Trophozoites
(b) Sporozoites
(c) Female gametocytes
(d) Male gametocytes

4. Match the following diseases with the causative organism and select the correct option. ***(2020)***

Column-I	Column-II
A. Typhoid	(i) Wuchereria
B. Pneumonia	(ii) Plasmodium
C. Filariasis	(iii) Salmonella
D. Malaria	(iv) Haemophilus

	A	B	C	D
(a)	(i)	(iii)	(ii)	(iv)
(b)	(iii)	(iv)	(i)	(ii)
(c)	(ii)	(i)	(iii)	(iv)
(d)	(iv)	(i)	(ii)	(iii)

5. Identify the correct pair representing the causative agent of typhoid fever and the confirmatory test for typhoid. ***(2019)***
(a) Salmonella typhi / Widal test
(b) Plasmodium vivax / UTI test
(c) Streptococcus pneumoniae / Widal test
(d) Salmonella typhi / Anthrone test

6. In which disease does mosquito transmitted pathogen cause chronic inflammation of lymphatic vessels? ***(2018)***
(a) Elephantiasis (b) Ascariasis
(c) Ringworm disease (d) Amoebiasis

7. Which of the following sets of diseases is caused by bacteria? ***(NEET-II 2016)***
(a) Cholera and tetanus
(b) Typhoid and smallpox
(c) Tetanus and mumps
(d) Herpes and influenza

8. Which of the following diseases is caused by a protozoan? ***(2015)***
(a) Babesiosis (b) Blastomycosis
(c) Syphilis (d) Influenza

9. Match each disease with its correct type of vaccine. ***(2015 Cancelled)***

Column I	Column II
A. Tuberculosis	(i) Harmless virus
B. Whooping cough	(ii) Inactivated toxin
C. Diphtheria	(iii) Killed bacteria
D. Polio	(iv) Harmless bacteria

(a) A-(iv), B-(iii), C-(ii), D-(i)
(b) A-(i), B-(ii), C-(iv), D-(iii)
(c) A-(ii), B-(i), C-(iii), D-(iv)
(d) A-(iii), B-(ii), C-(iv), D-(i)

10. The active form of Entamoeba histolytica feeds upon ***(2015 Cancelled)***
(a) food in intestine
(b) blood only
(c) erythrocytes, mucosa and submucosa of colon
(d) mucosa and submucosa of colon only.

11. Infection of Ascaris usually occurs by ***(2013)***
(a) Tse-tse fly
(b) mosquito bite
(c) drinking water containing eggs of Ascaris
(d) eating imperfectly cooked pork.

12. Identify the site where Wuchereria bancrofti is normally found in human body. ***(Karnataka NEET 2013)***
(a) Muscles of the legs
(b) Blood vessels of the thigh region
(c) Skin between the fingers
(d) Lymphatic vessels of the lower limbs

13. Motile zygote of Plasmodium occurs in ***(2012)***
(a) gut of female Anopheles
(b) salivary glands of Anopheles
(c) human RBCs (d) human liver.

14. Widal test is carried out to test ***(2012)***
(a) malaria (b) diabetes mellitus
(c) HIV/AIDS (d) typhoid fever.

15. Common cold differs from pneumonia in that ***(2012)***
(a) pneumonia is a communicable disease whereas the common cold is a nutritional deficiency disease
(b) pneumonia can be prevented by a live attenuated bacterial vaccine whereas the common cold has no effective vaccine
(c) pneumonia is caused by a virus while the common cold is caused by the bacterium Haemophilus influenzae
(d) pneumonia pathogen infects alveoli whereas the common cold affects nose and respiratory passage but not the lungs.

16. Where will you look for the sporozoites of the malarial parasite? ***(2011)***
(a) Saliva of infected female Anopheles mosquito
(b) Red blood corpuscles of human suffering from malaria
(c) Spleen of infected humans
(d) Salivary glands of freshy moulted female Anopheles mosquito

17. Which one of the following options gives the correct match of a disease with its causative organism and mode of infection? (Mains 2011)

	Disease	Causative organism	Mode of infection
(a)	Typhoid	Salmonella typhi	With inspired air
(b)	Pneumonia	Streptococcus pneumoniae	Droplet infection
(c)	Elephantiasis	Wuchereria bancrofti	With infected water and food
(d)	Malaria	Plasmodium vivax	Bite of male Anopheles mosquito

18. Common cold is not cured by antibiotics because it is ***(Mains 2011)***
(a) caused by a virus
(b) caused by a Gram-positive bacterium
(c) caused by a Gram-negative bacterium
(d) not an infectious disease.

19. Ringworm in humans is caused by ***(2010)***
(a) bacteria (b) fungi
(c) nematodes (d) viruses.

20. Widal test is used for the diagnosis of ***(2010)***
(a) malaria (b) pneumonia
(c) tuberculosis (d) typhoid.

21. A person suffering from a disease caused by Plasmodium, experiences recurring chill and fever at the time when ***(Mains 2010)***
(a) the sporozoites released from RBCs are being rapidly killed and broken down inside spleen
(b) the trophozoites reach maximum growth and give out certain toxins
(c) the parasite after its rapid multiplication inside RBCs ruptures them, releasing the stage to enter fresh RBCs
(d) the microgametocytes and megagametocytes are being destroyed by the WBCs.

22. Which of the following is a pair of viral diseases? ***(2009)***
(a) Common cold, AIDS
(b) Dysentery, common cold
(c) Typhoid, tuberculosis
(d) Ringworm, AIDS

23. Match the disease in column I with the appropriate items (pathogen / prevention / treatment) in column II. ***(2008)***

Column I	**Column II**
A. Amoebiasis	(i) *Treponema pallidum*
B. Diphtheria	(ii) Use only sterilised food and water
C. Cholera	(iii) DPT vaccine
D. Syphilis	(iv) Use oral rehydration therapy

(a) A- (ii), B - (i), C - (iii), D - (iv)
(b) A- (ii), B - (iii), C - (iv), D - (i)
(c) A - (i), B - (ii), C - (iii), D - (iv)
(d) A - (ii), B - (iv), C - (i), D - (iii)

24. Which one of the following is not correctly matched? ***(2004)***
(a) Glossina palpalis - Sleeping sickness
(b) Culex pipiens - Filariasis
(c) Aedes aegypti - Dengue fever
(d) Anopheles culicifacies - Leishmaniasis

25. Salmonella is related with ***(2001)***
(a) typhoid (b) polio
(c) T.B. (d) tetanus.

26. Which is the most infectious disease? ***(2001)***
(a) Hepatitis-B (b) AIDS
(c) Amoebiasis (d) Malaria

27. Which is showing accurate pairing? ***(2000)***
(a) Syphilis - Treponema pallidum
(b) AIDS - Bacillus conjugalis
(c) Gonorrhoea - Leishmania donovani
(d) Typhoid - Mycobacterium leprae

28. Saline solution is given to patients of cholera because ***(2000)***
(a) Na^+ prevents water loss from body
(b) NaCl function as regulatory material
(c) NaCl produces energy
(d) NaCl is antibacterial.

29. Typhoid fever is caused by ***(1998)***
(a) Shigella (b) Escherichia
(c) Giardia (d) Salmonella.

30. Diphtheria is caused by ***(1997)***
(a) nematodes (b) bacteria
(c) virus (d) none of these.

31. Which of the following diseases is now considered completely eradicated from India? ***(1997)***
(a) Small pox (b) Poliomyelitis
(c) Plague (d) Kala-azar

32. Which of the following pair of diseases is caused by virus? ***(1996)***
(a) Rabies, mumps (b) Cholera, tuberculosis
(c) Typhoid, tetanus (d) AIDS, syphilis

33. Which one of the following pairs is not correctly matched? ***(1995)***
(a) Syphilis – Trichuris trichiura
(b) Sleeping sickness – Trypanosoma gambiense
(c) Dengue fever – Arbovirus
(d) Plague – Yersinia pestis

34. Which of the following causes plague? ***(1995)***
(a) Trichinella spiralis
(b) Salmonella typhimurium
(c) Yersinia pestis
(d) Leishmania donovani

35. Which one of the following does correctly match a sexually transmitted disease with its pathogen? ***(1994)***
(a) Syphilis-Treponema pallidum
(b) Gonorrhoea-Entamoeba histolytica
(c) Urethritis-Bacillus anthracis
(d) Softsore-Bacillus brevis

36. Give the correct matching of causative agent/ germ and disease. ***(1993)***
(a) Anopheles – Malaria
(b) Leishmania – Sleeping sickness
(c) Glossina – Kala-azar
(d) Wuchererla – Fllariasis

37. African sleeping sickness is due to ***(1991)***
(a) Plasmodium vivax transmitted by tse-tse fly
(b) Trypanosoma lewsii transmitted by bed bug
(c) Trypanosoma gambiense transmitted by Glossina palpalis
(d) Entamoeba gingivalis spread by housefly.

38. Malignant tertian malarial parasite, belongs to class ***(1991)***
(a) Plasmodium falciparum
(b) P. vivax
(c) P. ovale
(d) P. malariae.

39. The infective stage of malarial parasite, Plasmodium that enters human body is ***(1990)***
(a) merozoite (b) sporozoite
(c) trophozoite (d) minuta form.

40. A bite of tse-tse fly may pass to humans ***(1989)***
(a) Leishmania donovani
(b) Trypanosoma gambiense
(c) Entamoeba histolytica
(d) Plasmodium vivax.

41. The vector for sleeping sickness is ***(1989)***
(a) housefly (b) tse-tse fly
(c) sandfly (d) fruit fly.

IMMUNITY

42. Given below are two statements: ***(2022)***

Statement I : Autoimmune disorder is a condition where body defense mechanism recognizes its own cells as foreign bodies.

Statement II : Rheumatoid arthritis is a condition where body does not attack self cells.

In the light of the above statements, choose the most appropriate answer from the options given below:
(a) Both Statement I and Statement II are correct
(b) Both Statement I and Statement II are incorrect
(c) Statement I is correct but Statement II is incorrect
(d) Statement I is incorrect but Statement II is correct

43. Select the incorrect statement with respect to acquired immunity. ***(2022)***
(a) Primary response is produced when our body encounters a pathogen for the first time.
(b) Anamnestic response is elicited on subsequent encounters with the same pathogen.
(c) Anamnestic response is due to memory of first encounter.
(d) Acquired immunity is non-specific type of defense present at the time of birth.

44. Identify the wrong statement with reference to immunity. ***(2020)***

(a) When exposed to antigen (living or dead) antibodies are produced in the host's body. It is called "Active immunity".

(b) When ready-made antibodies are directly given, it is called "Passive immunity".

(c) Active immunity is quick and gives full response.

(d) Fetus receives some antibodies from mother, it is an example for passive immunity.

45. Which of the following immune responses is responsible for rejection of kidney graft? ***(2019)***

(a) Cell-mediated immune response

(b) Auto-immune response

(c) Humoral immune response

(d) Inflammatory immune response

46. Colostrum, the yellowish fluid, secreted by mother during the initial days of lactation is very essential to impart immunity to the new born infants because it contains ***(2019)***

(a) immunoglobulin A

(b) natural killer cells

(c) monocytes

(d) macrophages.

47. Which of the following is not an autoimmune disease? ***(2018)***

(a) Psoriasis (b) Rheumatoid arthritis

(c) Alzheimer's disease (d) Vitiligo

48. Transplantation of tissues/organs fails often due to non-acceptance by the patient's body. Which type of immune response is responsible for such rejections? ***(2017)***

(a) Cell-mediated immune response

(b) Hormonal immune response

(c) Physiological immune response

(d) Autoimmune response

49. MALT constitutes about lymphoid tissue in human body. ***(2017)***

(a) 20% (b) 70% (c) 10% (d) 50%

50. Antivenom injection contains preformed antibodies while polio drops that are administered into the body contain ***(NEET-I 2016)***

(a) gamma globulin

(b) attenuated pathogens

(c) activated pathogens

(d) harvested antibodies.

51. In higher vertebrates, the immune system can distinguish self-cells and non-self. If this property is lost due to genetic abnormality and it attacks selfcells, then it leads to ***(NEET-I 2016)***

(a) autoimmune disease

(b) active immunity

(c) allergic response

(d) graft rejection.

52. If you suspect major deficiency of antibodies in a person, to which of the following would you look for confirmatory evidence? ***(2015,2007)***

(a) Haemocytes

(b) Serum globulins

(c) Fibrinogen in plasma

(d) Serum albumins

53. Which of the following immunoglobulins does constitute the largest percentage in human milk? ***(2015)***

(a) IgA (b) IgG

(c) IgD (d) IgM

54. Grafted kidney may be rejected in a patient due to ***(2015)***

(a) passive immune response

(b) innate immune response

(c) humoral immune response

(d) cell-mediated immune response.

55. Increased asthmatic attacks in certain seasons are related to ***(2007)***

(a) eating fruits preserved in tin containers

(b) inhalation of seasonal pollen

(c) low temperature

(d) hot and humid environment.

56. Lysozyme that is present in perspiration, saliva and tears, destroys ***(2007)***
(a) certain types of bacteria
(b) all viruses
(c) most virus-infected cells
(d) certain fungi.

57. Antibodies in our body are complex ***(2006)***
(a) glycoproteins (b) lipoproteins
(c) steroids (d) prostaglandins.

58. Damage to thymus in a child may lead to ***(2005)***
(a) a reduction in haemoglobin content of blood
(b) a reduction in stem cell production
(c) loss of antibody mediated immunity
(d) loss of cell mediated immunity.

59. Short-lived immunity acquired from mother to fetus across placenta or through mother's milk to the infant is categorised as ***(2003)***
(a) active immunity
(b) passive immunity
(c) cellular immunity
(d) innate non-specific immunity.

60. Interferons are synthesized in response to ***(2001)***
(a) mycoplasma (b) bacteria
(c) viruses (d) fungi.

61. The antibodies are ***(1999)***
(a) proteins (b) carbohydrates
(c) lipids (d) germs.

62. The term 'active immunity' means ***(1999)***
(a) increasing rate of heart beat
(b) increasing quantity of blood
(c) resistance developed after disease
(d) resistance developed before disease.

63. If a person shows production of interferons in his body, the chances are that he has got an infection of ***(1997)***
(a) tetanus (b) malaria
(c) typhoid (d) measles.

64. Antibodies are produced by ***(1996)***
(a) leucocytes (b) monocytes
(c) lymphocytes (d) spleen.

65. The interferons are ***(1996)***
(a) antigen proteins (b) antiviral proteins
(c) antibiotic proteins (d) all of these.

66. Which one of the following diseases is due to an allergic reaction? ***(1995)***
(a) Enteric fever (b) Skin cancer
(c) Goitre (d) Hay fever

67. Antigens are present ***(1995)***
(a) inside the cytoplasm
(b) on nuclear membrane
(c) inside the nucleus
(d) on cell surface.

68. A cell-coded protein that is formed in response to infection, with most animal viruses, is called ***(1994)***
(a) histone(b) antibody
(c) interferon(d) antigen.

AIDS

69. In which blood corpuscles, the HIV undergoes replication and produces progeny viruses? ***(2023)***
(a) Basophils (b) Eosinophils
(c) TH cells (d) B-lymphocytes

70. Which of the following is correct regarding AIDS causative agent HIV? ***(NEET-II 2016)***
(a) HIV is enveloped virus containing one molecule of single-stranded RNA and one molecule of reverse transcriptase.
(b) HIV is enveloped virus that contains two identical molecules of single-stranded RNA and two molecules of reverse transcriptase.
(c) HIV is unenveloped retrovirus.
(d) HIV does not escape but attacks the acquired immune response.

71. HIV that causes AIDS, first starts destroying ***(2015 Cancelled, 2006)***
(a) helper T-lymphocytes
(b)thrombocytes
(c) B-lymphocytes (d) leucocytes.

72. At which stage of HIV infection does one usually show symptoms of AIDS? ***(2014)***
(a) Within 15 days of sexual contact with an infected person
(b) When the infected retro virus enters host cells
(c) When HIV damages large number of helper T lymphocytes
(d) When the viral DNA is produced by reverse transcriptase

73. Which one of the following statements is correct with respect to AIDS? ***(2010)***
(a) The HIV can be transmitted through eating food together with an infected person.
(b) Drug addicts are least susceptible to HIV infection.
(c) AIDS patients are being fully cured cent per cent with proper care and nutrition.
(d) The causative HIV retrovirus enters helper T-lymphocytes thus reducing their numbers.

74. Human immuno deficiency virus (HIV) has a protein coat and a genetic material which is ***(1998)***
(a) double stranded RNA
(b) double stranded DNA
(c) single stranded DNA
(d) single stranded RNA.

CANCER

75. Which of the following statements is not true for cancer cells in relation to mutations? ***(NEET-I 2016)***
(a) Mutations inactivate the cell control.
(b) Mutations inhibit production of telomerase.
(c) Mutations in proto-oncogenes accelerate the cell cycle.
(d) Mutations destroy telomerase inhibitor.

76. Which one of the following is not a property of cancerous cells, whereas the remaining three are?
(a) They compete with normal cells for vital nutrients.
(b) They do not remain confined in the area of formation.
(c) They divide in an uncontrolled manner.
(d) They show contact inhibition.

77. Which one of the following techniques is safest for the detection of cancers? ***(Mains 2010)***
(a) Magnetic resonance imaging (MRI)
(b) Radiography (X-ray)
(c) Computed tomography (CT)
(d) Histopathological studies

78. Carcinoma refers to ***(2003)***
(a) malignant tumours of the connective tissue
(b) malignant tumours of the skin or mucous membrane
(c) malignant tumours of the colon
(d) benign tumours of the connective tissue.

79. Cancerous cells can easily be destroyed by radiations due to ***(2002)***
(a) rapid cell division (b) lack of nutrition
(c) fast mutation (d) lack of oxygen.

80. Reason of lung cancer is ***(2001)***
(a) coal mining (b) calcium fluoride
(c) cement factory (d) bauxite mining.

81. The blood cancer is known as ***(1995)***
(a) haemolysis (b) haemophilia
(c) leukaemia (d) thrombosis.

DRUGS AND ALCOHOL ABUSE

82. Match List I with List II. ***(2023)***

List I	List II
A. Heroin	I. Effect on cardiovascular system
B. Marijuana	II. Slow down body function
C. Cocaine	III. Painkiller
D. Morphine	IV. Interfere with transport of dopamine

Choose the correct answer from the options given below.
(a) A-IV, B-III, C-II, D-I (b) A-III, B-IV, C-I, D-II
(c) A-II, B-I, C-IV, D-III (d) A-I, B-II, C-III, D-IV

83. Drug called 'Heroin' is synthesised by ***(2019)***
(a) nitration of morphine
(b) methylation of morphine
(c) acetylation of morphine
(d) glycosylation of morphine.

84. Which part of poppy plant is used to obtain the drug "smack"? ***(2018)***

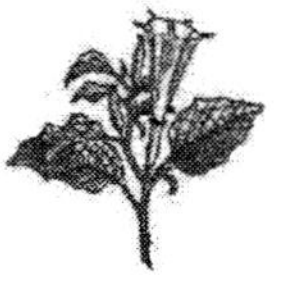

(a) Flowers (b) Latex
(c) Roots (d) Leaves

85. Which is the particular type of drug that is obtained from the plant whose one flowering branch is shown here? ***(2014)***
(a) Hallucinogen (b) Depressant
(c) Stimulant (d) Pain killer

86. Which one of the following is a hallucinogenic drug? ***(Karnataka NEET 2013)***
(a) Caffeine
(b) Morphine
(c) Lysergic acid diethylamide
(d) Opium

87. Cirrhosis of liver is caused by the chronic intake of ***(2012)***
(a) opium (b) alcohol
(c) tobacco (chewing) (d) cocaine.

88. Identify the molecules (A) and (B) shown below and select the right option giving their source and use. ***(Mains 2012)***

(A) 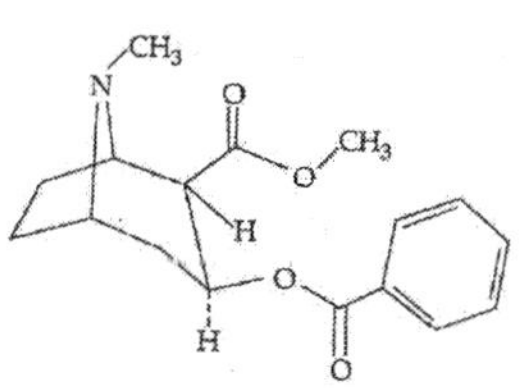

(B) 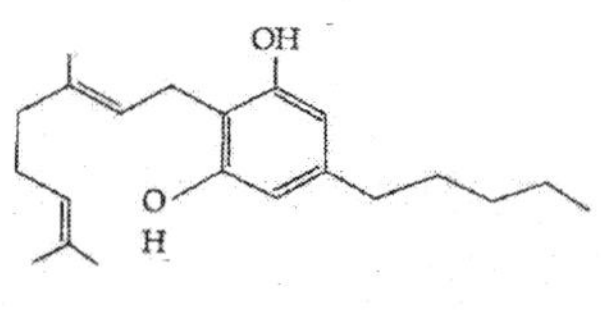

	Molecule	Source	Use
(a)	(A) Cocaine	*Erythroxylum coca*	Accelerates the transport of dopamine
(b)	(B) Heroin	*Cannabis sativa*	Depressant and slows down body functions
(c)	(B) Cannabinoid	*Atropa belladonna*	Produces hallucinations
(d)	(A) Morphine	*Papaver somniferum*	Sedative and pain killer

89. Select the correct statement from the ones given below. ***(2010)***
(a) Barbiturates, when given to criminals, make them tell the truth.
(b) Morphine is often given to persons, who have undergone surgery, as a pain killer.
(c) Chewing tobacco lowers blood pressure and heart rate.
(d) Cocaine is given to patients after surgery as it stimulates recovery.

90. Which one of the following statements is correct? ***(2009)***
(a) Benign tumours show the property of metastasis.
(b) Heroin accelerates body functions.
(c) Malignant tumours may exhibit metastasis.
(d) Patients who have undergone surgery are given cannabinoids to relieve pain.

91. Which one of the following is the correct statement regarding the particular psychotropic drug specified? ***(2008)***
(a) Morphine leads to delusions and disturbed emotions.
(b) Barbiturates cause relaxation and temporary euphoria.
(c) Hashish causes after thought perceptions and hallucinations.
(d) Opium stimulates nervous system and causes hallucinations.

92. A person showing unpredictable moods, outbursts of emotion, quarrelsome behaviour and conflicts with others is suffering from ***(2006)***

(a) addictive disorders
(b) schizophrenia
(c) borderline personality disorder (BPD)
(d) mood disorders.

93. Which one of the following depresses brain activity and produces feelings of calmness, relaxation and drowsiness? ***(2005)***

(a) Morphine (b) Valium
(c) Amphetamines (d) Hashish

94. Which one of the following is correct match? ***(2001)***

(a) Reserpine – tranquilliser
(b) Cocaine – opiatic narcotic
(c) Morphine – hallucinogenic
(d) Bhang – analgesic

95. L.S.D. is ***(2001)***

(a) hallucinogenic (b) sedative
(c) stimulant (d) tranquilliser.

96. Which of the following is an opiate narcotic? **(1997)**

(a) Amphetamines (b) LSD
(c) Barbiturates (d) Morphine

97. Nicotine acts as a stimulant, because it mimics the effect of ***(1995)***

(a) testosterone (b) dopamine
(c) thyroxine (d) acetylcholine.

98. Opiate narcotic is ***(1993)***

(a) bhang (b) charas
(c) heroin (d) nicotine.

99. Analgesic drugs ***(1990)***

(a) form tissues (b) relieve pain
(c) relieve fatigue (d) cause pain.

ANSWER KEY

1.	(c)	2.	(c)	3.	(b)	4.	(b)	5.	(a)	6.	(a)	7.	(a)
8.	(a)	9.	(a)	10.	(c)	11.	(c)	12.	(d)	13.	(a)	14.	(d)
15.	(d)	16.	(a)	17.	(b)	18.	(a)	19.	(b)	20.	(d)	21.	(c)
22.	(a)	23.	(b)	24.	(d)	25.	(a)	26.	(a)	27.	(a)	28.	(a)
29.	(d)	30.	(b)	31.	(a)	32.	(a)	33.	(a)	34.	(c)	35.	(a)
36.	(d)	37.	(c)	38.	(a)	39.	(b)	40.	(b)	41.	(b)	42.	(c)
43.	(d)	44.	(c)	45.	(a)	46.	(a)	47.	(c)	48.	(a)	49.	(d)
50.	(b)	51.	(a)	52.	(b)	53.	(a)	54.	(d)	55.	(b)	56.	(a)
57.	(a)	58.	(d)	59.	(b)	60.	(c)	61.	(a)	62.	(c)	63.	(d)
64.	(c)	65.	(b)	66.	(d)	67.	(d)	68.	(c)	69.	(c)	70.	(b,d)
71.	(a)	72.	(c)	73.	(d)	74.	(d)	75.	(b)	76.	(d)	77.	(a)
78.	(b)	79.	(a)	80.	(a)	81.	(c)	82.	(c)	83.	(c)	84.	(b)
85.	(a)	86.	(c)	87.	(b)	88.	(d)	89.	(b)	90.	(c)	91.	(c)
92.	(c)	93.	(b)	94.	(a)	95.	(a)	96.	(d)	97.	(d)	98.	(c)
99.	(b)												

HINTS & EXPLANATIONS

1.(c) : Ringworm → Trichophyton

Filariasis → Wuchereria bancrofiti

Malaria → *Plasmodium vivax*

Pneumonia → *Haemophilus influenzae*

2. (c)

3.(b) : Plasmodium enters the human body as sporozoites (infectious form) through the bite of infected female Anopheles mosquito.

4. (b)

5. (a) : Typhoid is caused by bacteria Salmonella typhi, transmitted through fecal oral route. It results in high fever, abdominal pain and frequent stools and is confirmed by Widal test.

6.(a) : Elephantiasis is caused by the parasitic filarial worm, Wuchereria bancrofti which is transmitted from an infected person to a healthy person via the bite of mosquito (especially Culex). It is characterised by gross enlargement of the skin and underlying connective tissues caused by lymphatic obstruction of lymph vessels by these worms which prevent drainage of lymph from the surrounding tissues. The parts commonly affected are legs, feet, thighs but scrotum, breasts and vulva may also be involved.

7.(a) : Cholera is caused by bacterium Vibrio cholerae, tetanus is caused by bacterium Clostridium tetani, typhoid is caused by bacterium Salmonella typhi, small pox is caused by Variola virus, mumps is caused by Paramyxo virus, Herpes is caused by Herpes simplex virus and influenza is caused by Orthomyxovirus.

8.(a) : Babesiosis is a malaria-like parasitic disease caused by infection with Babesia, a parasitic protozoan. Babesiosis has been recognised as a disease of cattle and other domestic animals, until human forms of babesiosis had been discovered. Babesia parasites reproduce in red blood cells of mammals and cause haemolytic anaemia, quite similar to malaria. The parasite is transmitted by ticks.

9. (a)

10.(c) : Entamoeba histolytica is the causative organism of amoebic dysentery or amoebiasis in man. It is a microscopic endoparasite of man. It is commonly found in the upper part of the large intestine (colon) and is very often lodged in the liver, lungs, brain and testes. In its life cycle, it occurs in three distinct forms (i) trophozoite or magna form, (ii) precystic or minuta form, and (iii) cystic form. Trophozoite is the most active, motile and feeding form which is pathogenic to man. It lives in the mucosa and submucosa layers of the colon and feeds on these layers and erythrocytes.

11.(c) : Man acquires infection of Ascaris by directly ingesting Ascaris eggs, containing the infective second stage larva, with contaminated food or water. Life cycle of Ascaris is monogenetic. There is no vector or intermediate host.

12.(d) : Elephantiasis is caused by the parasitic filarial worm, Wuchereria bancrofti which is transmitted from an infected person to a healthy person via the bite of mosquito (especially Culex). It is characterised by gross enlargement of the skin and underlying connective tissues caused by lymphatic obstruction of lymph vessels by these worms which prevent drainage of lymph from the surrounding tissues. The parts commonly affected are legs, feet, thighs but scrotum, breasts and vulva may also be involved.

13.(a) : Plasmodium, a tiny protozoan parasite causes malaria in humans, and is transmitted through the bite of infected female Anopheles mosquito. When female Anopheles sucks the blood of infected human it takes up gametocytes (sexual stages of parasite) with blood meal. The gametocytes come out of the RBCs into the lumen (cavity) of the stomach of the mosquito. In the stomach, the male gametocyte divides and forms 6 to 8 long, motile, whip-like microgametes (male gametes). The female gametocyte does not divide but undergoes a process of maturation to become the macrogamete (female gamete). A microgamete penetrates a macrogamete and fertilisation (syngamy) takes place, resulting in the formation of a zygote. The zygote elongates and becomes worm like motile organism called ookinete. Ookinete further changes into sporozoites (mature infective stage of Plasmodium).

14.(d) : Typhoid is caused by bacteria Salmonella typhi, transmitted through fecal oral route. It results in high fever, abdominal pain and frequent stools and is confirmed by Widal test.

15.(d) : Common cold or rhinitis is one of the most infectious diseases caused by Rhino viruses. It affects nose and respiratory passage but not lungs. It spreads by droplet infection or contaminated objects. Pneumonia, caused by bacteria Streptococcus pneumoniae and Haemophilus influenzae is a serious disease of lungs, in which fluid collects in the alveoli and bronchioles. The disease spreads by sputum of the patient.

16.(a) : Sporozoites represent the infective forms of malarial parasite. A healthy person acquires infection, when a female Anopheles mosquito, containing sporozoites, bites the person for sucking his blood. The mosquito punctures the host's skin by its proboscis and first introduces some saliva into the blood stream. Along with saliva, thousands of sporozoites are inoculated in the host also.

17. (b)

18. (a)

19.(b) : Ringworm (tinea) is a fungal infection of the skin, the scalp, or the nails. Ringworm is caused by the dermatophyte fungi-species of Microsporum, Trichophyton and Epidermophyton and also affects animals, a source of infection for humans. It can be spread by direct contact or via infected materials. The lesions of ringworm may form partial or complete rings and may cause intense itching. The disease is treated with antifungal agents taken by mouth or applied locally.

20. (d)

21.(c) : Plasmodium is a tiny protozoan which is responsible for malaria in the human. In malaria the patient experiences high fever which periodically rises and also experiences recurring chills with fever. Such symptoms are seen because when the RBCs carrying Plasmodium (one of the stage in the life cycle of the parasite) ruptures it releases a toxic substance called haemozoin which is chiefly responsible for the chill and high fever recurring every three to four days.

22.(a) : Common cold is a viral disease. It is caused by Rhino viruses. It causes fever and pain all over the body and affects the nose, throat and air passages. AIDS (Acquired immuno deficiency syndrome) is a disorder of cell mediated immune system of the body. It is caused by HIV (Human Immunodeficency Virus). HIV is a retrovirus that attacks helper T-cells.

23. (b)

24.(d) : All the options given are diseases with their associated vector which transmit the respective diseases.

Leishmaniasis, also called kala azar is caused by *Leishmania donovani*. It is spread by sand fly (Phlebotomus) and characterised by enlarged spleen and liver with high fever.

25.(a) : Typhoid is caused by Salmonella typhi. The organisms of the disease are present in the stool. They may be present in urine. They can, therefore, be carried by water and contaminated food. Their spread through water can give rise to severe epidemics.

Polio is caused by Enterovirus. TB is caused by *Mycobacterium tuberculosis*. Tetanus is caused by *Clostridium tetani*.

26.(a) : Hepatitis B (serum hepatitis) occurs at any age and mode of transmission is through contact or blood. Infection is severe, often fatal and is accompanied by loss of appetite, nausea, whitish stool (due to lack of bile) and jaundice. 0.0002% of hepatitis B infected blood contact is enough to transmit hepatitis B.

27. (a) : Syphilis is caused by a spirochete (spiral bacterium) Treponema pallidum. AIDS is a viral disease caused by Human Immuno deficiency Virus. Gonorrhoea is a sexual disease and its causative organism is Neisseria gonorrhoeae. Typhoid is caused by bacillus bacteria Salmonella typhi.

28.(a) : Cholera is an acute infection of the small intestine by the bacterium Vibrio cholerae, which causes severe vomiting and diarrhoea (known as ricewater stools) leading to dehydration. The disease is contracted from food or drinking water contaminated by faeces from a patient. The resulting dehydration and the imbalance in the concentration of body fluids can cause death within 24 hours. Since, a large quantity of fluid and salts are rapidly lost through stools and vomit, therefore, the most important treatment is to replace the lost fluid and salts equally rapidly. Rapid replacement of fluid and elecrolytes is needed by oral rehydration-therapy. The electrolytes consists of Na+ ions that prevents water loss from the body.

29. (d)

30.(b) : Diphtheria is caused by Corynebacterium diphtheriae (bacteria) usually affecting children upto five years of age. It may start as sore throat, chills with mild fever, sometimes vomiting and headache. The most important preventive measure-against this disease is that all babies should be immunised within the first six weeks of birth using DPT vaccine.

31.(a) : Small pox is an acute highly communicable disease. It is caused by virus named Variola virus. Now it is eradicated from world including India. It is highly infectious disease starting with high fever, chill, backache and headache, followed by appearance of rash on the third day of illness.

32.(a) : Mumps is an infectious disease causing fever, difficulty in opening the mouth and painful swelling of the parotid glands which lie just below the lobe of the ears. It is caused by a Paramyxovirus, which comes out in the saliva of the infected person.

Rabies (Hydrophobia) is caused by a virus named as rabies virus. It is introduced in the body by the bite of rabid (mad) dogs usually. Fear of water is the most important characteristic symptom of this disease. Other symptoms are saliva from the mouth, severe headache, high fever, alternating periods, of excitement and depression, inability to swallow even fluids due to choked throat. The virus destroys the brain and spinal cord. Rabies is 100% fatal.

Cholera and tuberculosis are bacterial diseases caused by Vibrio cholerae and Mycobacterium tuberculosis respectively. Typhoid and tetanius are bacterial diseases caused by Salmonella typhi and Clostridium tetani respectively. AIDS is caused by HIV (human immunodeficiency virus). Syphillis is caused by spirochaete Treponema pallidum.

33. (a)

34.(c) : Plague is an acute epidemic disease of rats and other wild rodents caused by the bacterium Yersinia pestis, which is transmitted to humans by rat fleas. Headache, fever, weakness, aching limbs, and delirium develop and are followed by acute painful swellings of the lymph nodes. Bleeding under the skin, producing black patches, can lead to ulcers, which may prove fatal. Treatment with tetracycline, streptomycin and chloramphenicol is effective.

35. (a)

36.(d) : Wuchereria bancrofti is a parasitic filarial nematode worm spread by a mosquito vector. It is one of the three parasites that cause lymphatic filariasis. Elephantiasis can result if the infection is left untreated. Limited treatment modalities exist and no vaccines have been developed. Malaria is caused by protozoan parasites of the genus Plasmodium. Malaria parasites are transmitted by female Anopheles mosquitoes. Sleeping sickness or African trypanosomiasis is a parasitic disease in people and animals, caused by protozoa of genus Trypanosoma and transmitted by the tse tse fly. Kala-azar is caused by Leishmania (protozoan) and is transmitted by sand fly.

37.(c) : Trypanosoma gambiense is the parasitic zooflagellate which causes one of the deadliest ailments in human beings called sleeping sickness or trypanosomiasis. The disease is common in humid and subhumid zones of the African continent. The disease is transmitted by shade loving tse-tse fly (Glossina palpalis) which acts as the vehicle that carries the culprit protozoan parasite.

38.(a) : Plasmodium falciparum is the greatest killer of human beings over most parts of Africa and else where in tropics. It causes malignant (or pernicious or cerebral or tropical) tertian malaria. This malaria is most harmful.

Plasmodium vivax causes benign tertian malaria.

Plasmodium malariae causes quartan malaria. Plasmodium ovale is the rarest of the four species which infect man and it causes mild tertian malaria.

39.(b) : The infective stage of Plasmodium is a minute organism called sporozoite. When the mosquito bites man, sporozoites present in the salivary gland of female Anopheles mosquito are injected into the blood of the man. These sporozoites are spindle-shaped or sickle-shaped uninucleate organisms capable of wrigging (worm-like) movements. Each sporozoite consists of elastic pellicle, cytoplasm and nucleus.

40. (b)

41. (b)

42.(c) : Rheumatoid arthritis (RA) is a result of autoimmune reaction. In RA, immune system mistakenly attacks healthy self cells in our body, causing inflammation, painful swelling in the affected parts of the body.

43.(d) : Acquired immunity is specific to pathogen. Innate immunity is non-specific type of defence present at the time of birth.

44.(c) : Active immunity is slow and takes time to give its full effective response.

45.(a) : Transplantation of tissue/organ often fails due to non-acceptance by the patient's body therefore, tissue matching and blood group matching are essential before undertaking any graft/transplant. When the immune system recognises the protein in the transplanted tissue or organ as foreign, it initiates cellular immunity. As a result of this, there is a rejection of transplanted organs. To suppress the immune response during transplantation, histocompatibility antigen and immunosuppressants play an important role.

46.(a) : Colostrum (Mother's first milk) rich in immunoglobulin A(IgA) antibodies are passed to newborn through the breast feed and provides natural passive immunity.

47.(c) : Autoimmune diseases are certain unrelated disorders caused by inflammation and destruction of tissues by the body's own immune response. These disorders include acquired hemolytic anaemia, pernicious anaemia, rheumatoid arthritis, myasthenia gravis, psoriasis, vitiligo, etc. Alzheimer's disease is a chronic neurodegenerative irreversible, progressive brain disorder that slowly destroys memory and thinking skills.

48. (a)

49. (d) : MALT are significant aggregations of lymphoid tissues which are seen in relation to the mucosa of the major tracts like respiratory, alimentary canal and urinogenital tracts. It constitutes about 50 percent of the lymphoid tissue in human body.

50.(b) : The Sabin vaccine or trivalent 'oral polio vaccine' consists of attenuated viral strains.

51.(a) : Autoimmunity is a disorder of the body's defence mechanisms in which an immune response is elicited against its own tissues, which are thereby damaged or destroyed. Autoimmunity may be caused due to genetic or environmental factors.

52.(b) : Serum globulins are proteins that include gamma globulins (antibodies) and a variety of enzymes and carrier/ transport proteins.

The specific profile of the globulins is determined by protein electrophoresis (SPEP), which separates the proteins according to size and charge. There are four major groups that can be identified : alpha-1 globulins, alpha-2 globulins, beta globulins and gamma globulins. Once the abnormal group has been identified, further studies can determine the specific protein excess or deficit. Since the gamma fraction usually makes up the largest portion of the globulins, therefore antibody deficiency is mainly related with the low level of serum globulins.

53.(a) : IgA immunoglobulins are the second most abundant class of immunoglobulins, which are mainly found in sweat, tears, saliva, mucus, colostrum and gastrointestinal secretions.

54.(d) : Cell-mediated immune response (CMIS) consists of T-lymphocytes. It reacts against transplants. Transplantation may result in the rejection of the transplanted organs. The immune system recognises the protein in the transplanted tissue or organ as foreign and initiates cellular immunity against it.

55.(b) : Increased asthmatic attacks in certain seasons are related to inhalation of seasonal pollen. Pollens are microscopic grains produced by plants in order to reproduce. Pollen allergy is a hypersensitive reaction to pollen. Pollen induced reactions include extrinsic asthma, rhinitis and bronchitis.

56.(a) : Lysozyme is an antibacterial enzyme with natural antibiotic properties. Normally excreted in the tears, nasal mucus, milk, and saliva in most animals, lysozyme is part of the body's first natural defence against bacteria and viruses.

57.(a) : Antibodies are members of a class of proteins known as immunoglobulins. Immunoglobulins are glycoproteins in the immunoglobulin superfamily. The terms antibody and immunoglobulin are often used interchangeably. They are found in the blood and tissue fluids, as well as many secretions. In structure, they are globulins (in the γ-region of protein electrophoresis). They are synthesized and secreted by plasma cells that are derived from the B cells of the immune system.

58.(d) : The thymus is the major gland of our immune system. The thymus is responsible for many immune system functions including the production of T-lymphocytes, a type of white blood cell responsible for cell mediated immunity. Cell mediated immunity is a type of immunity in which specialized cells carry out defensive activities. They protect the body against pathogens including the protists and fungi which have entered the host's cells.

59.(b) : Short-lived immunity acquired from mothers to fetus across placenta or through mother's milk to the infant is categorised as passive immunity. Passive immunity, an acquired immunity, is resistance based on antibodies performed in another host. In this case, the fetus is not directly responsible for its body immunity but it becomes immunised by mother's milk across placenta.

60.(c) : Interferons are proteins that increase the resistance of a cell to attack by viruses by unmasking genes that synthesize antiviral proteins. In humans, three groups of interferons have been discovered: α-interferons from white blood cells; β-interferons from connective tissue fibroblasts; and γ-interferons from lymphocytes.

61. (a)

62.(c) : Active immunity is the immune response generated in an individual due to contact with infectious pathogen or vaccination. In many cases, it is life long.

63.(d) : Interferons are antiviral proteins that increase the resistance of a cell to attack by viruses. As measles is a viral disease, so body produces interferons. Measles is an acute infectious eruptive viral disease of childhood, caused by an RNA containing Rubeola virus/ Polynosa morbillorum. Typhoid and tetanus are bacterial diseases caused by Salmonella typhi and Clostridium tetani respectively. Malaria is a protozoan disease caused by Plasmodium species.

64.(c) : Lymphocytes secrete antibodies to destroy microbes and their toxins, reject grafts and kill tumour cells. Antibodies are proteinaceous in nature. Monocytes (type of WBC) are phagocytic in nature and engulf bacteria and cellular debris. Spleen is an organ that produces lymphocytes.

65.(b) : Interferons are antiviral proteins that increase the resistance of a cell to attack by viruses. As measles is a viral disease, so body produces interferons. Measles is an acute infectious eruptive viral disease of childhood, caused by an RNA containing Rubeola virus/ Polynosa morbillorum. Typhoid and tetanus are bacterial diseases caused by Salmonella typhi and Clostridium tetani respectively. Malaria is a protozoan disease caused by Plasmodium species

66. (d): Hay fever is a form of allergy due to the pollen of grasses, trees, and other plants, characterized by inflammation of the membrane lining the nose and sometimes of the conjunctiva. The symptoms of sneezing, running or blocked nose and watering eyes are due to histamine released by the mast cells.

67.(d) : An antigen is any foreign substance like protein or polysaccaharide present on the external coating of pathogen, feathers, constituent of a vegetable, fruit, meat, drug, chemical, tissue or organ transplant which induces the immune system to produce antibodies.

68. (c)

69.(c) : HIV enters into helper T-lymphocytes (TH), replicates and produce progeny viruses. The progeny viruses released in the blood attack other helper T-lymphocytes. This is repeated, leading to a progressive decrease in number of helper T-lymphocytes in the body of infected person.

70. (b,d) : HIV is spherical virus with a diameter of about 90-120 nm. Its genome consists of a single-stranded RNA filament segmented into two identical filaments and associated with reverse transcriptase enzymes. The envelope consists of a lipid bilayer derived from host cell membrane and projecting knob like glycoprotein spikes. It contains two protein coats. HIV is a retrovirus that attacks helper T cells. Without an adequate supply of helper cells, the immune system cannot signal B cells to produce antibodies to kill infected cells, thus body becomes susceptible to infections. This immune deficiency is described by the name acquired immune deficiency syndrome or AIDS.

71.(a) : The AIDS retrovirus, called human immunodeficiency virus (HIV), mounts a direct attack on CD_4^+ T helper cells because it recognizes the CD_4^+ coreceptors associated with these cells.

HIV attack on CD_4^+T cells cripples the immune system in at least three ways. First, HIV-infected cells die only after releasing replicated viruses that infect other CD_4^+T cells, until the entire population of CD_4^+T cell is destroyed. Second, HIV causes infected CD_4^+T cells, to secrete a soluble suppressing factor that blocks other T cells from responding to the HIV antigen. Finally, HIV may block transcription of MHC genes, hindering the recognition and destruction of infected CD_4^+ T cells, and thus protecting those cells from any remaining vestiges of the immune system. The combined effect of these responses to HIV infection is to wipe out the human immune defense.

72.(c) : AIDS is a disorder of cell-mediated immune system of the body. Virus responsible for AIDS is HIV (Human Immunodeficiency virus). There is a reduction in the number of helper T-cells which stimulate antibody production by B-cells. This results in the loss of natural defence against viral infection.

73.(d) : AIDS (acquired immuno deficiency syndrome) a syndrome, is caused by the retrovirus HIV (human immunodeficiency virus). The virus destroys a subgroup of lymphocytes, the helper T-cells (or CD_4 lymphocytes), resulting in suppression of the body's immune response. HIV is transmitted in blood, semen and vaginal fluid; the major routes of infection are unprotected vaginal and anal intercourse, intravenous drug abuse, and the administration of contaminated blood and blood products. A combination of antiviral drugs can delay the development of full-blown AIDS for many years but cannot fully care the disease.

74.(d) : HIV is a retrovirus, which contains single stranded RNA, surrounded by protein coat (core shell) as genetic material. It causes AIDS. HIV is different in structure from other retroviruses. It is around 120 nm in diameter (around 60 times smaller than a red blood cell) and roughly spherical.

75. (b)

76.(d) : Contact inhibition is a property of normal cells by virtue of which contact with other cells inhibits their uncontrolled growth. Cancerous cells lack this property.

77.(a) : Histopathological study is the invasive technique. Radiography and CT involves X-rays which are harmful.

In MRI strong magnetic fields and non-ionising radiations are used to detect any physiological changes in the concerned tissue. Hence it is safest for the detection of cancers.

78.(b) : Carcinoma is a cancer that arises in epithelium, the tissue that lines the skin and internal organs of the body. It may occur in any tissue containing epithelial cells. It includes cervical cancer, breast cancer, skin cancer, stomach cancer etc.

79.(a) : Cancerous cells are the cells that undergo rapid cell division. These cells are destroyed by X-ray radiation. During cell division, the DNA double helix opens up and undergo various other processes. Such processes are disrupted when exposed to radiation and the cancerous cells die selectively when radiated.

80.(a) : Lung cancer is a disease where tissue in the lung grows out of control. This may lead to metastasis, invasion of adjacent tissue and infiltration beyond the lungs. The vast majority of primary lung cancers are carcinomas of the lung, resulting from epithelial cells. One of the causes of lung cancer is exposure to coal dust. Exposure to coal dust can cause some coal mine workers to develop pneumoconiosis, or "black lung." This occurs when inhaled coal dust becomes embedded in the lungs, causing them to harden and making breathing difficult.

81.(c) : The normal count of WBCs is 5000 to 10000 per cubic millimeter of blood. Leukaemia or blood cancer is characterized by abnormal increase of WBCs count, 200001000000/mm3 due to their increased formation in the bone marrow. Haemolysis is breakdown of RBCs. Haemophilia is a disease in which blood clots slowly. Thrombosis is a clot formation inside the blood vessels.

82.(c) : Heroin → Slow down body function

Marijuana → Effect on cardiovascular system

Cocaine → Interfere with transport of dopamine

Morphine → Painkiller

83.(c) : Heroin (smack) is chemically diacetylmorphine which is white, odourless, bitter crystalline compound. It is obtained by acetylation of morphine, extracted from latex of poppy plant.

84. (b)

85.(a) : The plant illustrated in the diagram is Datura. Seeds of Datura stramonium are misused for their hallucinogenic properties because of the presence of anticholinergic alkaloids atropine, hyoscyamine and scopolamine (= hyoscine). However, even in slight excess, they can cause death.

86. (c) : LSD is a psychedelic drug since it causes optical and auditory hallucinations and induces behavioural abnormalities. Opium and morphine are opiate narcotics that suppress brain activity and relieve pain. Caffeine is a stimulant that temporarily stimulates the nervous system.

87.(b) : Cirrhosis is a condition in which the liver responds to injury or death of some of its cells by producing interlacing strands of fibrous tissue between which are nodules of regenerating cells. The liver becomes tawny and characteristically knobbly (due to the nodules). One of the causes include alcoholism (alcoholic cirrhosis).

88.(d) : The given chemical structures (A) and (B) are of morphine and cannabinoid respectively. Morphine is the principal opium alkaloid. It is a strong analgesic. It also has sedative and calming effect. Morphine depresses respiratory centre, it contributes to the fall in blood pressure. Morphine is a very effective sedative and painkiller. It is very useful in patients who have undergone surgery. Natural cannabinoids are obtained from the inflorescence of hemp plant Cannabis sativa, family Cannabinaceae. They affect the cardiovascular system of the body.

89.(b) : Morphine is a potent opioid analgesic used mainly to relieve severe and persistent pain, particularly in terminally ill patients or who have undergone surgery. It also induces feelings of euphoria. It is administered by mouth, injection, or in suppositories. Common side-effects are nausea and vomiting, constipation, and drowsiness. With regular use, tolerance develops and dependence may occur.

90.(c) : Tumour is of two types : benign and malign. Malign or malignant tumour exhibit metastasis. It is the phenomenon in which cancer cells spread to distant sites through body fluids to develop secondary tumour.

91.(c) : Hashish or charas is a pure resin obtained from female flowers and leaves of selected varieties of Cannabis sativa. It is the most potent hemp product (cannabinoids), and is usually smoked with tobacco. Its use may lead to euphoria, hallucination, drowsiness and continuous laughing. The hallucinogens act mainly on CNS and greatly alter one's thought, feelings and perceptions.

92.(c) : Borderline personality disorder (BPD) is a serious mental illness characterized by persuasive instability in moods, interpersonal relationships, self-image, and behaviour. This instability often disrupts family and work life, long-term planning, and the individual's sense of self-identity. Originally thought to be at the "borderline" of psychosis, people with BPD suffer from a disorder of emotion regulation.

Schizophrenia is a group of severe mental disorders characterized by disturbances of language and communication; thought disturbances that may involve distortion of reality, misperceptions, delusions and hallucinations; mood changes and withdrawn, regressive, or bizarre behaviour, lasting longer than six months. A mood disorder is a condition where the prevailing emotional mood is distorted or inappropriate to the circumstances. Addiction is a state of dependence produced by the habitual taking of drugs, alcohol etc.

93.(b) : Valium is a benzodiazephine (sedative) that gives a feeling of relaxation, calmness or drowsiness in the body. Morphine is the main opium alkaloid that depresses respiratory centre and contributes to the fall in blood pressure. Amphetamines are synthetic drugs and are stimulant in nature. Hashish is a hallucinogen.

94.(a) : Tranquillisers are drugs that have good effect in all types of psychosis, especially in schizophrenia. In a psychotic patient, these drugs reduce aggressiveness, thoughts and behaviour are gradually normalized and anxiety is relieved, e.g., reserpine which is an alkaloid extracted from the roots of Rauwolfia serpentina. Higher doses of it can cause sedation and mental depression. Cocaine is a stimulant. Morphine is an opiate narcotic. Bhang is a hallucinogenic.

95.(a) : Hallucinogens are drugs that change thoughts, feelings and perceptions of individuals. They cause hallucinations. LSD (Lysergic acid diethylamide) is one such hallucinogen that causes horrible dreams, chronic psychosis and severe damage to the central nervous system. Sedatives give a feeling of calmness, relaxation or drowsiness in the body. Their high doses induce sleep. Tranquillisers lower tension and anxiety without inducing sleep. Stimulants are the drugs that stimulate the nervous system, make a person more wakeful, alert and active; and cause excitement.

96.(d) : Opiates are derived from opium along with their synthetic relatives. Opiates have narcotic, analgesic, sedative and astringent effects. Narcotic is a drug that induces stupor and relieves pain. Morphine is the main opium alkaloid, which is a strong analgesic and also has sedative and calming effect. It depresses respiratory centre and contributes to the fall in blood pressure. It can cause release of ADH, reduction in urine output, constipation and mild hyperglycemia, etc. It causes addiction.

97.(d) : Nicotine is the major stimulatory component of tobacco products including cigarettes. Nicotine has a number of effects on the human body similar to acetylcholine. It stimulates passage of nerve impulses, causes muscles to relax and causes the release of adrenaline, increasing both blood pressure and heart beat rate.

98.(c) : The drugs derived from opium alongwith their synthetic relatives are called opioids or opiates. Opiates have narcotic, analgesic, astringent (that causes contraction of body parts), and sedative effect, i.e., heroin.

99.(b) : A substance that reduces pain without causing unconsciousness, either by reducing the pain threshold or by increasing pain tolerance. There are several categories of analgesic drugs, including morphine and its derivatives which produce analgesia by acting on the central nervous system; nonsteroidal anti-inflammatory drugs (e.g. aspirin); and local anaesthetics.

Chapter : 27

MICROBES IN HUMAN WELFARE

MICROBES IN HOUSEHOLD PRODUCTS

1. Conversion of milk to curd improves its nutritional value by increasing the amount of **(2018)**

(a) vitamin D (b) vitamin A
(c) vitamin B12 (d) vitamin E.

2. Dough kept overnight in warm weather becomes soft and spongy because of **(2004)**

(a) absorption of carbon dioxide from atmosphere
(b) fermentation
(c) cohesion
(d) osmosis.

3. During the formation of bread it becomes porous due to release of CO_2 by the action of **(2002)**

(a) yeast (b) bacteria
(c) virus (d) protozoans.

4. In cheese manufacture, the microorganisms are important for **(1994)**

(a) the ripening only
(b) the souring of milk only
(c) the development of resistance to spoilage only
(d) both the souring and the ripening processes.

MICROBES IN INDUSTRIAL PRODUCTS

5. Identify the microorganism which is responsible for the production of an immunosuppressive molecule cyclosporin A. **(2022)**

(a) Trichoderma polysporum
(b) Clostridium butylicum
(c) Aspergillus niger
(d) Streptococcus cerevisiae

6. Match List - I with List - II **(2021)**

List - I	List - II
(p) *Aspergillus niger*	(i) Acetic acid
(q) *Acetobacter aceti*	(ii) Lactic Acid
(r) *Clostridium butylicum*	(iii) Citric Acid
(s) *Lactobacillus*	(iv) Butyric Acid

Choose the correct answer from the option given below.

	p	q	r	s
(a)	(iv)	(ii)	(i)	(iii)
(b)	(iii)	(i)	(iv)	(ii)
(c)	(i)	(ii)	(iii)	(iv)
(d)	(ii)	(iii)	(i)	(iv)

7. Match the following columns and select the correct option.

Column-I	Column-II
(A) *Clostridium butylicum*	(i) Cyclosporin-A
(B) *Trichoderma polysporum*	(ii) Butyric acid
(C) *Monascus purpureus*	(iii) Citric acid
(D) *Aspergillus niger*	(iv) Blood cholesterol lowering agent

	A	B	C	D
(a)	(iii)	(iv)	(ii)	(i)
(b)	(ii)	(i)	(iv)	(iii)
(c)	(i)	(ii)	(iv)	(iii)
(d)	(iv)	(iii)	(ii)	(i)

8. Which of the following is a commercial blood cholesterol lowering agent? **(2019)**

(a) Lipases (b) Cyclosporin A
(c) Statin (d) Streptokinase

9. Match the following organisms with the products they produce. ***(2019)***

Column-I	Column-II
(A) *Lactobacillus*	(i) Cheese
(B) *Saccharomyces* cerevisiae	(ii) Curd
(C) *Aspergillus niger*	(iii) Citric acid
(D) *Acetobacter aceti*	(iv) Bread
	(v) Acetic acid

Select the correct option.

	A	B	C	D
(a)	(ii)	(i)	(iii)	(v)
(b)	(ii)	(iv)	(v)	(iii)
(c)	(ii)	(iv)	(iii)	(v)
(d)	(iii)	(iv)	(v)	(i)

10. Which of the following is correctly matched for the product produced by them? ***(2017)***
(a) Methanobacterium : Lactic acid
(b) Penicillium notatum: Acetic acid
(c) Sacchromyces cerevisiae : Ethanol
(d) Acetobacter aceti : Antibiotics

11. Match column I with column II and select the correct option using the codes given below. ***(NEET-II 2016)***

Column-I	Column-II
A. Citric acid	(i) *Trichoderma*
B. Cyclosporin A	(ii) *Clostridium*
C. Statins	(iii) *Aspergillus*
D. Butyric acid	(iv) *Monascus*

(a) A-(iii), B-(i), C-(ii), D-(iv)
(b) A-(iii), B-(i), C-(iv), D-(ii)
(c) A-(i), B-(iv), C-(ii), D-(iii)
(d) A-(iii), B-(iv), C-(i), D-(ii)

12. Which of the following is wrongly matched in the given table? ***(NEET-I 2016)***

	Microbe	Product	Application
(a)	Streptococcus	Streptokinase	Removal of clot from blood vessel
(b)	Clostridium butylicum	Lipase	Removal of oil stains
(c)	Trichoderma polysporum	Cyclosporin A	Immuno-suppressive drug
(d)	Monascus purpureus	Statins	Lowering of blood cholesterol

13. Match the following list of microbes and their importance. ***(2015)***

Column-I	Column-II
A.Saccharomyces cerevisiae	(i) Production of immuno-suppressive agent
B.Monascus purpureus	(ii) Ripening of Swiss cheese
C.Trichoderma polysporum	(iii) Commercial production of ethanol
D.Propionibacterium shermanii	(iv) Production of blood-cholesterol lowering agents

(a) A-(iv), B-(ii), C-(i), D-(iii)
(b) A-(iii), B-(i), C-(iv), D-(ii)
(c) A-(iii), B-(iv), C-(i), D-(ii)
(d) A-(iv), B-(iii), C-(ii),D-(i)

14. A good producer of citric acid is ***(2013)***
(a) Clostridium (b) Saccharomyces
(c) Aspergillus (d) Pseudomonas.

15. Monascus purpureus is a yeast used commercially in the production of ***(2012)***
(a) ethanol
(b) streptokinase for removing clots from the blood vessels
(c) citric acid
(d) blood cholesterol lowering statins.

16. A patient brought to a hospital with myocardial infarction is normally immediately given ***(2012)***
(a) penicillin (b) streptokinase
(c) cyclosporin-A (d) statins.

17. Read the following four statements (A-D). ***(Mains 2012)***

(A) Colostrum is recommended for the new born because it is rich in antigens.

(B) Chikungunya is caused by a Gram negative bacterium.

(C) Tissue culture has proved useful in obtaining virus-free plants.

(D) Beer is manufactured by distillation of fermented grape juice.

How many of the above statements are wrong?
(a) Two (b) Three
(c) Four (d) One

18. The most common substrate used in distilleries for the production of ethanol is ***(2011)***
(a) corn meal (b) soya meal
(c) ground gram (d) molasses.

19. Ethanol is commercially produced through a particular species of ***(2011)***
(a) Saccharomyces (b) Clostridium
(c) Trichoderma (d) Aspergillus.

20. Continuous addition of sugars in 'fed batch' fermentation is done to ***(2011)***
(a) produce methane (b) obtain antibiotics
(c) purify enzymes (d) degrade sewage.

21. Read the following statement having two blanks (A and B). ***(Mains 2011)***

A drug used for __A__ patients is obtained from a species of the organism __B__.

The one correct option for the two blanks is

	A	B
(a)	heart	*Penicillium*
(b)	organ-transplant	*Trichoderma*
(c)	swine flu	*Monascus*
(d)	AIDS	*Pseudomonas.*

22. Which one of the following is a wrong matching of a microbe and its industrial product, while the remaining three are correct? ***(Mains 2011)***
(a) Yeast - Statins
(b) Acetobacter aceti - Acetic acid
(c) Clostridium butylicum - Lactic acid
(d) Aspergillus niger - Citric acid

23. Which one of the following pairs is wrongly matched? ***(2009)***
(a) Alcohol - Nitrogenase
(b) Fruit juice - Pectinase
(c) Textile - Amylase
(d) Detergents - Lipase

24. Probiotics are ***(2007)***
(a) cancer inducing microbes
(b) new kind of food allergens
(c) live microbial food supplement
(d) safe antibiotics.

25. Which of the following is used to manufacture ethanol from starch? ***(2000)***
(a) Penicillium (b) Saccharomyces
(c) Azotobacter (d) Lactobacillus

26. Yeast (Saccharomyces cerevisiae) is used in the industrial production of ***(1998)***
(a) tetracyline (b) ethanol
(c) butanol (d) citric acid.

27. Which of the following microorganisms is used for production of citric acid in industries? ***(1998)***
(a) Aspergillus niger
(b) Rhizopus nigricans
(c) Lactobacillus bulgaris
(d) Penicillium citrinum

28. Which of the following is the false statement about antibiotics? ***(1996)***
(a) Some persons have allergy from antibiotics.
(b) Antibiotics are capable of curing any disease.
(c) This term was given by Waksman in 1942.
(d) Antibiotics is produced by microorganisms.

29. The citric acid is produced by ***(1995)***
(a) Candida utilis
(b) Azotobacter suboxydans
(c) Aspergillus niger
(d) Streptococcus lactis.

30. The organism, used for alcohol fermentation, is ***(1995)***
(a) Aspergillus (b) Saccharomyces
(c) Pseudomonas (d) Penicillium.

31. The main reason why antibodies could not solve all the problems of bacteria mediated disease is ***(1994)***
(a) decreased efficiency of the immune system
(b) insensitivity of the individual following prolonged exposure to antibiotics
(c) development of mutant strains resistant to antibodies
(d) inactivation of antibiotics by bacterial enzymes.

MICROBES IN SEWAGE TREATMENT

32. Which of the following is put into anaerobic sludge digester for further sewage treatment? ***(2020)***
(a) Primary sludge
(b) Floating debris
(c) Effluents of primary treatment
(d) Activated sludge

33. Which of the following in sewage treatment removes suspended solids? ***(2017)***
(a) Secondary treatment
(b) Primary treatment
(c) Sludge treatment
(d) Tertiary treatment

34. What gases are produced in anaerobic sludge digesters? ***(2014)***
(a) Methane and CO_2 only
(b) Methane, Hydrogen sulphide and CO_2
(c) Methane, Hydrogen sulphide and O_2
(d) Hydrogen sulphide and CO_2

35. The domestic sewage in large cities ***(Mains 2012)***
(a) has a high BOD as it contains both aerobic and anaerobic bacteria
(b) is processed by aerobic and then anaerobic bacteria in the secondary treatment in Sewage Treatment Plants (STPs)
(c) when treated in STPs does not really require the aeration step as the sewage contains adequate oxygen
(d) has very high amount of suspended solids and dissolved salts.

36. Secondary sewage treatment is mainly a ***(2011)***
(a) physical process
(b) mechanical process
(c) chemical process
(d) biological process.

37. Which of the following is mainly produced by the activity of anaerobic bacteria on sewage? ***(2011)***
(a) Laughing gas (b) Propane
(c) Mustard gas (d) Marsh gas

MICROBES IN PRODUCTION OF BIOGAS

38. The guts of cow and buffalo possess ***(2015 Cancelled)***
(a) methanogens (b) cyanobacteria
(c) Fucus sp. (d) Chlorella sp.

39. In gobar gas, the maximum amount is that of ***(Mains 2012)***
(a) butane (b) methane
(c) propane (d) carbon dioxide.

40. Organisms called methanogens are most abundant in a ***(2011)***
(a) sulphur rock (b) cattle yard
(c) polluted stream (d) hot spring.

41. Select the correct statement from the following. ***(2010)***
(a) Biogas is produced by the activity of aerobic bacteria on animal waste.
(b) Methanobacterium is an aerobic bacterium found in rumen of cattle.
(c) Biogas, commonly called gobar gas, is pure methane.
(d) Activated sludge-sediment in settlement tanks of sewage treatment plant is a rich source of aerobic bacteria.

42. Which one of the following pairs is wrongly matched? ***(2007)***
(a) Yeast - Ethanol
(b) Streptomycetes - Antibiotic
(c) Coliforms - Vinegar
(d) Methanogens - Gobar gas

43. A major component of gobar gas is ***(2004)***
(a) ammonia (b) methane
(c) ethane (d) butane.

44. During anaerobic digestion of organic waste, such as in producing biogas, which one of the following is left undegraded? ***(2003)***
(a) Lipids (b) Lignin
(c) Hemi-cellulose (d) Cellulose

45. Which bacteria is utilized in gobar gas plant? ***(2002)***
(a) Methanogens
(b) Nitrifying bacteria
(c) Ammonifying bacteria
(d) Denitrifying bacteria

46. Gobar gas contains mainly ***(1997)***
(a) $CO_2 + H_2$ (b) $CO_2 + H_2O$
(c) CH_4 only (d) $CH_4 + CO_2$

MICROBES AS BIOCONTROL AGENTS

47. Which of the following can be used as a biocontrol agent in the treatment of plant disease? ***(2019)***
(a) Lactobacillus (b) Trichoderma
(c) Chlorella (d) Anabaena

48. Select the correct group of biocontrol agents. ***(2019)***
(a) Nostoc, Azospirillium, Nucleopolyhedrovirus
(b) Bacillus thuringiensis, Tobacco mosaic virus, Aphids
(c) *Trichoderma, Baculovirus, Bacillus thuringiensis*
(d) Oscillatoria, Rhizobium, Trichoderma

49. A biocontrol agent to be a part of an integrated pest management should be ***Odisha NEET 2019)***
(a) species-specific and symbiotic
(b) free living and broad spectrum
(c) narrow spectrum and symbiotic
(d) species-specific and inactive on non-target organisms.

50. Microbe used for biocontrol of pest butterfly caterpillars is ***(Karnataka NEET 2013)***
(a) Saccharomyces cerevisiae
(b) Bacillus thuringiensis
(c) Streptococcus sp.
(d) Trichoderma sp.

51. Which one of the following is an example of carrying out biological control of pests/diseases using microbes? ***(2012)***
(a) *Trichoderma* sp. against certain plant pathogens.
(b) Nucleopolyhedrovirus against white rust in Brassica.
(c) Bt-cotton to increase cotton yield.
(d) Lady bird beetle against aphids in mustard.

52. A common biocontrol agent for the control of plant diseases is ***(2010)***
(a) Baculovirus (b) Bacillus thuringiensis
(c) Glomus (d) Trichoderma.

53. Which of the following is not used as a biopesticide? ***(2008)***
(a) Trichoderma harzianum
(b) Nucleopolyhedrovirus (NPV)
(c) Xanthomonas campestris
(d) Bacillus thuringiensis

54. Trichoderma harzianum has proved a useful microorganism for ***(2008)***
(a) gene transfer in higher plants
(b) biological control of soil-borne plant pathogens
(c) bioremediation of contaminated soils
(d) reclamation of wastelands.

55. Which one of the following proved effective for biological control of nematodal diseases in plants? ***(2008)***
(a) Gliocladium virens
(b) Paecilomyces lilacinus
(c) Pisolithus tinctorius
(d) Pseudomonas cepacia

56. A genetically engineered microorganism used successfully in bioremediation of oil spills is a species of ***(2007)***
(a) Trichoderma (b) Xanthomonas
(c) Bacillus (d) Pseudomonas.

57. When a natural predator (living being) is applied on the other pathogen organism to control them, this process is called
(a) artificial control (b) confusion technique
(c) biological control (d) genetic engineering.

58. One of the major difficulties in the biological control of insect pest is that ***(1995)***
(a) the method is less effective as compared with the use of insecticides
(b) the practical difficulty of introducing the predator to specific areas
(c) the predator develops a preference to other diets and may itself become a pest
(d) the predator does not always survive when transferred to a new environment.

MICROBES AS BIOFERTILISERS

59. Select the mismatch. ***(2017)***
(a) Rhodospirillum - Mycorrhiza
(b) Anabaena - Nitrogen fixer
(c) Rhizobium - Alfalfa
(d) Frankia - Alnus

60. A nitrogen-fixing microbe associated with Azolla in rice fields is ***(2012)***
(a) Spirulina (b) Anabaena
(c) Frankia (d) Tolypothrix.

61. Which one of the following microbes forms symbiotic association with plants and helps them in their nutrition? ***(2012)***
(a) Azotobacter (b) Aspergillus
(c) Glomus (d) Trichoderma

62. A prokaryotic autotrophic nitrogen fixing symbiont is found in ***(2011)***
(a) Alnus (b) Cycas
(c) Cicer (d) Pisum.

63. Which one of the following helps in absorption of phosphorus from soil by plants? ***(2011)***
(a) Glomus (b) Rhizobium
(c) Frankia (d) Anabaena

64. Which one of the following is not a biofertiliser? ***(2011)***
(a) Agrobacterium (b) Rhizobium
(c) Nostoc (d) Mycorrhiza

65. An organism used as a biofertilizer for raising soybean crop is ***(2011)***
(a) Azotobacter (b) Azospirillum
(c) Rhizobium (d) Nostoc.

66. Consider the following statements (A-D) about organic farming. ***(Mains 2011)***
(A) Utilizes genetically modified crops like Bt cotton
(B) Uses only naturally produced inputs like compost
(C) Does not use pesticides and urea
(D) Produces vegetables rich in vitamins and minerals Which of the above statements are correct?
(a) B, C and D (b) C and D only
(c) B and C only (d) A and B only

67. The common nitrogen-fixer in paddy fields is ***(2010)***
(a) Rhizobium (b) Azospirillum
(c) Oscillatoria (d) Frankia.

68. Which one of the following is not used in organic farming? ***(2010)***
(a) Glomus (b) Earthworm
(c) Oscillatoria (d) Snail

69. An example of endomycorrhiza is ***(Mains 2010)***
(a) Nostoc (b) Glomus
(c) Agaricus (d) Rhizobium.

70. Nitrogen fixation in root nodules of Alnus is brought about by ***(2008)***
(a) Frankia (b) Azorhizobium
(c) Bradyrhizobium (d) Clostridium.

71. Which one of the following pairs is not correctly matched? ***(2004)***
(a) Streptomyces - Antibiotic
(b) Serratia - Drug addiction
(c) Spirulina - Single cell protein
(d) Rhizobium - Biofertilizer

72. A free living nitrogen-fixing cyanobacterium which can also form symbiotic association with the water fern Azolla is ***(2004)***
(a) Tolypothrix (b) Chlorella
(c) Nostoc (d) Anabaena.

73. Which of the following is the pair of biofertilizers? ***(2001)***
(a) Azolla and BGA
(b) Nostoc and legume
(c) Rhizobium and grasses
(d) Salmonella and E.coli

74. Which aquatic fern is used to increase the yield in paddy crop? ***(2000)***
(a) Azolla (b) Salvinia
(c) Marsilea (d) Isoetes

75. Which of the following fern is an excellent biofertilizer? ***(1999)***
(a) Marsilea (b) Pteridium
(c) Azolla (d) Salvinia

76. Due to which of the following organism, yield of rice is increased? ***(1999)***
(a) Sesbania (b) Bacillus popilliae
(c) Anabaena (d) Bacillus subtilis

77. Which of the following is non-symbiotic biofertilizer? ***(1998)***
(a) Anabaena (b) Rhizobium
(c) VAM (d) Azotobacter

78. Farmers have reported over 50% higher yields of rice by using which of the following biofertilizer? ***(1998)***
(a) Cyanobacteria
(b) Legume-Rhizobium symbiosis
(c) Mycorrhiza
(d) Azolla pinnata

79. The biofertilizers are ***(1997)***
(a) Anabaena and Azolla
(b) cow dung, manure and farmyard waste
(c) quick growing crop ploughed under soil
(d) none of these.

80. Which of the following species does not have the ability to fix atmospheric nitrogen? ***(1994)***
(a) Azotobactor (b) Anabaena
(c) Nostoc (d) Spirogyra

81. Which one of the following statements is correct? ***(1994)***
(a) Legumes fix nitrogen only through the specialized bacteria that live in their roots.
(b) Legumes fix nitrogen independently of the specialized bacteria that live in their roots.
(c) Legumes fix nitrogen only through specialized bacteria that live in their leaves.
(d) Legumes are incapable of fixing nitrogen.

ANSWER KEY

1.	(c)	2.	(b)	3.	(a)	4.	(d)	5.	(a)	6.	(b)	7.	(b)
8.	(c)	9.	(c)	10.	(c)	11.	(b)	12.	(b)	13.	(c)	14.	(c)
15.	(d)	16.	(b)	17.	(b)	18.	(d)	19.	(a)	20.	(c)	21.	(b)
22.	(c)	23.	(a)	24.	(c)	25.	(b)	26.	(b)	27.	(a)	28.	(b)
29.	(c)	30.	(b)	31.	(c)	32.	(d)	33.	(b)	34.	(b)	35.	(b)
36.	(d)	37.	(d)	38.	(a)	39.	(b)	40.	(b)	41.	(d)	42.	(c)
43.	(b)	44.	(b)	45.	(a)	46.	(d)	47.	(b)	48.	(c)	49.	(d)
50.	(b)	51.	(a)	52.	(d)	53.	(c)	54.	(b)	55.	(b)	56.	(d)
57.	(c)	58.	(d)	59.	(a)	60.	(b)	61.	(c)	62.	(b)	63.	(a)
64.	(a)	65.	(c)	66.	(c)	67.	(b)	68.	(d)	69.	(b)	70.	(a)
71.	(b)	72.	(d)	73.	(a)	74.	(a)	75.	(c)	76.	(c)	77.	(d)
78.	(d)	79.	(a)	80.	(d)	81.	(a)						

HINTS & EXPLANATIONS

1.(c) : Lactobacillus bacteria convert milk into curd. It produces acids that coagulate and partially digest the milk proteins. A small amount of curd added to the fresh milk as inoculum or starter contains millions of Lactobacillus bacteria which at suitable temperature multiply, thereby converting milk to curd which also improves its nutritional value by increasing vitamin B12 content and a number of organic acids.

2. (b)

3.(a) : Saccharomyces converts starch or sugars to pyruvic acid through EMP pathway. Then this pyruvic acid is converted to acetaldehyde and finally to ethyl alcohol in the absence of oxygen. This entire process is called fermentation.

$$C_6H_{12}O_6 \rightarrow 2CH_2COCOOH \rightarrow 2C_2H_5OH + 2CO_2$$

This released carbon dioxide makes the dough to rise and gives spongy nature to bread.

4.(d) : Cheese is a protein rich nutritive preparation obtained after fermentation and curdling of milk. Cheese contains proteins (20-35%), fats (20-30%), minerals, vitamins and water. Milk is first curdled (soured) with the help of a lactic acid bacterium. Curd is gently heated to separate cheese from liquid called whey. Curd is placed in cloth-lined porous containers for draining out whey. The left out solidified material is called cottage cheese. For preservation and ripening, blocks of cottage cheese are salted and placed in brine solution. Salt solution is drained out. Cheese blocks are wiped and placed in sterilised rooms for ripening with the help of microorganisms.

5.(a) : Cyclosporin A is used as immuno-suppressant. This drug is derived from a fungus, Trichoderma polysporum and is used to prevent rejection of kidney, heart and liver transplants. Cyclosporin inhibits the activity of helper T-cells that acts against foreign bodies.

6. (b)

7. (b)

8. (c) : Statins are products of fermentation activity of yeast Monascus purpureus which resemble mevalovate and are competitive inhibitors of β-hydroxy- β-methylglutaryl or HMG CoA reductase. This inhibits cholesterol synthesis. Statins are, therefore, used in lowering blood cholesterol, e.g., lovastatin, pravastatin, simvastatin.

9. (c)

10.(c) : Methanobacterium is useful in the production of biogas. Penicillium notatum is used to produce penicillin, an antibiotic. Acetobacter aceti is used to obtain acetic acid.

11. (b)

12.(b) : Clostridium butylicum helps in the production of butyric acid. Candida lipolytica and Geotrichum candidum help in production of lipases that are added in detergents for removing oily stains from laundry.

13. (c)

14. (c) : Aspergillus niger produces citric acid, Clostridium butylicum produces butyric acid, Saccharomyces is used for commercial production of ethanol, Pseudomonas produces alkaline proteases.

15. (d) : Statins are produced by the yeast Monascus purpureus which have been commercialised as blood cholesterol lowering agents. It acts by competitively inhibiting the enzyme responsible for synthesis of cholesterol.

16. (b) : Streptokinase (Tissue Plasminogen Activator or TPA) is an enzyme obtained from the culture of some haemolytic bacterium Streptococcus which is modified genetically to function as clot buster. Therefore, it helps in clearing blood clots inside the blood vessels through dissolution of intravascular fibrin during myocardial infarction.

17.(b) : Chikungunya is caused by Chikungunya virus. Colostrum is the first breast milk of mother which contains antibodies (especially IgA) which protect the infant by the age of three months. Beer is manufactured by fermentation of barley malt by yeast species.

18. (d)

19.(a) : Ethanol is commercially produced through a particular species of yeast Saccharomyces (Saccharomyces cerevisiae)

20.(c) : A fed batch is a biotechnological batch process which is based on feeding of a growth limiting nutrient substrate to a culture. Continuous addition of sugars in fed batch fermentation is done to purify enzymes.

21.(b) : Cyclosporin A used as an immuno-suppressive agent in organ-transplant patients, is produced by the fungus Trichoderma polysporum.

22.(c) : Microbes are used for commercial and industrial production of certain chemicals like organic acids, alcohols and enzymes. Examples of acid producers are Aspergillus niger (a fungus) of citric acid, Acetobacter aceti (a bacterium) of acetic acid; Clostridium butylicum (a bacterium) of butyric acid and Lactobacillus (a bacterium) of lactic acid.

23.(a) : Yeast species are used in alcoholic fermentation due to the presence of zymase enzyme. It was known that the yeast extract contained an enzyme zymase, which is nondialyzable and a coenzyme which is dialyzable. It is now well known that the zymase is a complex mixture of many enzymes and that several coezymes are necessary for their function. The activity of this enzyme was lost because the main enzyme was separated from its coezyme during dialyzation. Thus, it was established later that extracellular enzyme zymase, secreted by yeast cells, carry out the process of fermentation.

24.(c) : Probiotics are dietary supplements containing potentially beneficial bacteria or yeast, with lactic acid bacteria (LAB) as the most common microbes used. LAB have been used in the food industry for many years because they are able to convert sugars (including lactose) and other carbohydrates into lactic acid. They not only provide the characteristic sour taste to fermented dairy foods such as yogurt, but also acts as a preservative, by lowering the pH and creating fewer opportunities for spoilage organisms to grow.

25. (b)

26. (b)

27. (a): Citric acid is obtained through the fermentation carried out by Aspergillus niger on sugary syrups. Citric acid is employed in dyeing, engraving, medicines, inks, flavouring and preservation of food and candies.

28.(b) : Antibiotics are not capable of curing any disease. Antibiotics are those substances that destroy or inhibit the growth of microorganisms, particularly disease producing bacteria and fungi. The term antibiotic was introduced by Waksman in 1942. Antibiotics are obtained form microorganisms (especially moulds) or synthesized. Common antibiotics include penicillins, streptomycin and tetracyclines. They are used to treat various infections but tend to weaken the body's natural defence mechanisms and can cause allergies. Overuse of antibiotic can lead to the development of resistant strains of microorganism.

29. (c)

30. (b)

31.(c) : Bacteria develop mutant strains that become resistant to antibodies, so these antibodies become incapable of removing bacteria mediated diseases.

32.(d) : The sediment in a settling tank is called activated sludge. A small part of it is pumped back into the aeration tank to serve as the inoculum. While the remaining major part of the sludge is pumped into large tanks called anaerobic sludge digesters.

33.(b) : Primary or physical treatment is the process of removal of small and large, floating and suspended solids from sewage through two processes of filtration and sedimentation.

34.(b) : The type of gases produced by microbial activity depend upon the microbes and the organic substrates they utilise. Certain bacteria, called methanogens, grow anaerobically on cellulosic material and produce large amount of methane along with carbon dioxide. These bacteria are commonly found in the anaerobic sludge during sewage treatment. Other anaerobic bacteria, involved in the process of anaerobic digestion produce other gases like ammonia and hydrogen sulphide.

35. (b) : Sewage water can be purified by passing it through sewage treatment plants with the action of heterotrophic microorganisms. There are three stages of this treatment - primary, secondary and tertiary. Primary treatment removes floating and suspended solids from sewage through two processes of filtration and sedimentation. First floating matter is removed through sequential filtration. The filtrate is kept in large open settling tanks where grit settles down. The sediment is called primary sludge while the supernatant is called effluent. The primary sludge traps a lot of microbes and debris. In secondary treatment, the primary effluent is taken to aeration tanks. A large number of aerobic heterotrophic microbes grow in the aeration tank. They form flocs. Flocs are masses of bacteria held together by slime and fungal filaments to form mesh like structures. The microbes digest a lot of organic matter, converting it into microbial biomass and releasing a lot of minerals. As the BOD of the waste matter is reduced to 10-15% of raw sewage, it is passed into settling tank. Thus secondary treatment is more or less biological. The sediment of settling tank is called activated sludge. The remaining is passed into a large tank called anaerobic sludge digester. It is designed for continuous operation. The aerobic microbes present in the sludge get killed. Anaerobic microbes digest the organic mass as well as aerobic microbes of the sludge. They are of two types, non-methanogenic and methanogenic. Methanogenic bacteria produce a mixture of gases containing methane, H_2S and CO_2.

36. (d)

37.(d) : Marsh gas or methane gas is mainly produced by the activities of anaerobic bacteria on sewage. Sewage contains large amounts of organic matter and microbes, many of which are pathogenic. These microbes (bacteria and fungi) are digested during secondary treatment process of sewage by anaerobic bacteria. During digestion, bacteria produce a mixture of gases such as methane, hydrogen sulphide and carbon dioxide. These gases are called biogas and can be easily used as a source of energy as it is inflammable.

38.(a) : Methanogens like Methanobacterium are found in the rumen (a part of the stomach) of cattle. A lot of cellulosic material is also available in the rumen. In rumen, these bacteria help in the breakdown of cellulose and play an important role in nutrition of cattle.

39.(b) : Biogas or gobar gas is a methane rich fuel gas produced by anaerobic breakdown or digestion of biomass with the help of methanogenic bacteria. It is made up of methane (50-70%), carbon dioxide (30-40%) with traces of nitrogen, hydrogen sulphide and hydrogen.

40.(b) : Methanogens are any of various archaebacteria that produce methane; they include genera such as Methanobacillus and Methanothrix. Methanogens are obligate anaerobes found in oxygen-deficient environments, such as marshes, swamps, sludge and the digestive systems of ruminants. They are also utilised in gobar gas plants.

41. (d)

42.(c) : Coliform bacteria are a commonly used bacterial indicator of sanitary quality of food and water. It is not involved in the production of vinegar.

43. (b)

44.(b) : Lignin is a complex polymer of phenylpropane units, which are cross-linked to each other with a variety of different chemical bonds. This complexity has thus far proven as resistant to microbial degradation.

45. (a)

46.(d) : Biogas or gobar gas is made up of methane (50-70%), carbon dioxide (30-40%) with traces of nitrogen, hydrogen sulphide and hydrogen.

47.(b) : Trichoderma species are free-living fungi that are very common in the root ecosystems. They are effective biocontrol agents of several plant pathogens.

48. (c)

49. (d)

50.(b) : Biopesticides are those biological agents that are used for control of weeds, insects and pathogens. The microorganisms used as biopesticides are viruses, bacteria, protozoa, fungi and mites. Some of the biopesticides are being used at a commercial scale. Most important example is the soil bacterium, Bacillus thuringiensis (Bt). Spores of this bacterium produce the insecticidal cry protein. Therefore, spores of this bacterium kill larvae of insects which eat them.

51.(a) : A biological control being developed for use in the treatment of plant disease is the fungus Trichoderma. Trichoderma species are free living fungi that are very common in the root ecosystems. They are effective biocontrol agents of several plant pathogens.

52.(d) : The natural method of pest and pathogen control involving use of viruses, bacteria and other insects (which are their natural predators and pests) is called biocontrol or biological control. For example, free living fungus Trichoderma exerts biocontrol over several plant pathogens for the control of plant diseases. Baculoviruses (mostly of genus Nucleopolyhedrovirus) are also used as biocontrol agents but they are used for the control of insects and arthropods. Bacillus thuringiensis is a soil bacterium which is used as biopesticide. Glomus species are the most common fungal partners of mycorrhiza residing in the roots of higher plants.

53.(c) : Xanthomonas campestris is a bacterial species that causes a variety of plant diseases. Rest all the others are used as a biopesticide.

54. (b)

55.(b) : Paecilomyces lilacinus proved effective for biological control of nematodal diseases in plant.

56.(d) : Bioremediation is the process of using living microorganisms to clean up a contaminated site. Microorganisms do this by removing toxins from materials. They decompose these compounds by using enzymes, specific proteins that control reactions in living cells. Organisms that produce enzymes capable of degrading petroleum are useful in cleaning up oil spills. Some common ones that break down oil are genetically engineered species of Pseudomonas and Azotobacter. Bioremediation accounts for 5 to 10 percent of all pollution treatment and has been used successfully in cleaning up leaking underground gasoline storage tanks. Bioremediation has many applications, from the ordinary garden compost to the removal of selenium and other toxic metals from waste. The best agents for bioremediation are the ones that can break down contaminants without becoming contaminated or harmful themselves.

57.(c) : The control of insect pests by the introduction, encouragment and artificial increase of biological agencies like predaceous and parasitic insects, other animals and diseases is termed as biological control. It is basically a natural control in which man plays significant role of making the biological agencies more effective. Of these agencies, insect enemies play important role in nature for managing the phytophagous insect pests and keep a balance e.g., lady bugs or praying mantis, frog, toads, lizard and birds are employed by man to eat up the insect pests like aphids. It is a self perpetuating method.

58.(d) : Insect enemies play an important role in nature for managing the phytophagous insect pests and keep a balance. It is just possible that predators of a particular plant pest are unable to get established and multiply in a particular environment. In such cases, the predators are reared in the laboratory and let off at a particular time when the pests are about to threaten the crops. And then this practice become expensive.

59.(a) : Rhodospirillum is a free-living nitrogen fixing bacteria. Mycorrhiza is the symbiotic association between fungi and roots of higher plants. The most common fungal partners of mycorrhiza are Glomus species.

60.(b) : Azolla plays a very important role in rice production. Azolla and its nitrogen-fixing partner, Anabaena, have been used as green manure to fertilise rice paddies and increase production. With the help of Azolla, rice can be grown year after year, several crops a year, with little or no decline in productivity; hence no rotation of crops is necessary. So, Azolla is an excellent biofertilizer.

61.(c) : Azotobacter, Aspergillus and Trichoderma all are free living microbes that help plants in their nutrition. Glomus is a fungus that symbiotically forms endomycorrhiza that helps in absorption of nutrition specially phosphorus from soil.

62.(b) : Cycas forms facultative symbiotic association with autotrophic nitrogen fixing cyanobacteria. Cycas provides carbon and a stable environment to the cyanobacteria in exchange for fixed nitrogen. These cyanobacteria are endosymbionts and live within the roots of Cycas. In addition to normal roots, Cycas develops specialised symbiotic organs at a young age called pre-coralloid roots which transform into coralloid roots upon successful colonisation by cyanobacteria.

63.(a) : Some fungi form symbiotic associations with plants (mycorrhiza). Many members of the genus Glomus form mycorrhiza. The fungal symbiont in these associations absorbs phosphorus from soil and passes it to the plant. Plants having such associations show other benefits also, such as resistance to root-borne pathogens, tolerance to salinity and drought, and an overall increase in plant growth and development.

64.(a) : Biofertilisers are organisms that enrich the nutrient quality of the soil. The main sources of biofertilisers are bacteria, fungi and cyanobacteria. Rhizobium bacteria is found in the nodules on the roots of leguminous plants by symbiotic association. These bacteria fix atmospheric nitrogen into organic forms, which is used by the plants as nutrient. Fungi are also known to form symbiotic associations with plants called mycorrhiza. Cyanobacteria are autotrophic microbes widely distributed in an aquatic and terrestrial environments. Many of which can fix atmospheric nitrogen, e.g., Anabaena, Nostoc, Oscillatoria, etc. Agrobacterium tumefaciens is a pathogen of several dicot plants. It causes gall tumour in the plants.

65.(c) : Rhizobium is used as a biofertilizer for raising leguminous crop. Rhizobium japonicum forms symbiotic association in the roots of the leguminous plant, soybean.

66.(c) : Organic farming is the form of agriculture that relies on techniques such as crop rotation, green manure, compost and biological pest control to maintain soil productivity and control pest on a farm. Organic farming excludes or strictly limited the use of manufactured fertilizers, pesticides (which include herbicides, insecticides and fungicides), plant growth regulators such as hormones, food additives and genetically modified organisms.

67.(b) : Azospirillum is an anaerobic nitrogen fixing bacteria which forms loose association with roots of some plants. Inoculation of paddy fields with these bacteria helps in increasing yield and saving of nitrogen fertilizers.

68.(d) : Organic farming is a method of farming system which primarily aimed to keep the soil alive and in good health by use of organic wastes and other biological material alongwith beneficial microbes (biofertilizers) to release nutrients to crops for increased sustainable production in an ecofriendly, pollution free environment.

Basic components of organic farming are green manures, farm yard manure, vermicompost, crop rotation, biopesticides and biofertilizers. *Glomus* being a mycorrhizal component, earthworm being a vermicompost and *Oscillatoria* being a nitrogen fixing blue green algae can be used in organic farming. Snail cannot be a component of organic farming.

69.(b) : The Genus Glomus form endomycorrhiza, a symbiotic associations with plants. The fungal symbiont in these associations absorbs phosphorus from soil and passes it to the plant. Plants having such associations show other benefits also, such as resistance to root-borne pathogens, tolerance to salinity and drought, and an overall increase in plant growth and development.

Nostoc is a blue green algae, *Agaricus* is a basidiomycetes *Rhizobium* is a eubacteria.

70. (a) : The most common symbiotic association of legume and bacteria on roots is as nodules, which are small outgrowth on the roots. The microbe Frankia is symbiont in root nodules of several non-legume plants like Casurina and Alnus. Both Rhizobium and Frankia are free living in soil but as symbiont can fix atmospheric nitrogen.

71.(b) : Serratia marcescens is considered a harmful human pathogen which has been known to cause urinary tract infections, wound infections and pneumonia. Serratia bacteria also have many antibiotic resistance properties which may become important if the incidence of Serratia infections dramatically increases.

72.(d) : Anabaena is a free living nitrogen fixing cyanobacterium which can form symbiotic association with the water fern Azolla.

73. (a)

74.(a) : Azolla plays a very important role in rice production. Azolla and its nitrogen-fixing partner, Anabaena, have been used as green manure to fertilise rice paddies and increase production. With the help of Azolla, rice can be grown year after year, several crops a year, with little or no decline in productivity; hence no rotation of crops is necessary. So, Azolla is an excellent biofertilizer.

75. (c)

76. (c)

77.(d) : Biofertilizers are organisms which bring about nutrient enrichment of the soil. Azotobacter is a free living, aerobic, nitrogen fixing bacteria. Anabena is a nitrogen fixing cyanobacteria that occurs in both free living and symbiotc associations with Azolla, Cycas roots, etc. Rhizobium lives symbiotically in root nodules of legumes and non-legumes. Vesicular-arbuscular mycorrhiza (VAM) is an example of endomycorrhiza in which fungal hyphae penetrate the cortical cells of grasses to form vesicles.

78.(d) : Azolla plays a very important role in rice production. Azolla and its nitrogen-fixing partner, Anabaena, have been used as green manure to fertilise rice paddies and increase production.

79. (a)

80.(d) : Members of Kingdom Monera - bacteria and cyanobacteria (blue green algae) have the ability to fix nitrogen. Azotobacter is a N2-fixing bacteria. Anabaena and Nostoc are heterocystous blue-green algae. The heterocysts are the sites of N2-fixation. Spirogyra is one of the commonest green algae. It has no function in nitrogen fixation.

81.(a) : The nitrogen-fixing ability of leguminous plants is not a property of the plants as such but results from infection of their roots by bacteria in the soil, infection leading to the formation of nodules. These organisms are Gram-negative motile rods that are classified in the genus Rhizobium.

Chapter : 28 BIOTECHNOLOGY: PRINCIPLES AND PROCESSES

PRINCIPLES OF BIOTECHNOLOGY

1. The DNA molecule to which the gene of interest is integrated for cloning is called **(2015)**
(a) template (b) carrier
(c) transformer (d) vector.

2. The cutting of DNA at specific locations became possible with the discovery of **(2015)**
(a) selectable markers (b) ligases
(c) restriction enzymes (d) probes.

3. Which one of the following is a case of wrong matching? **(2012)**
(a) Somatic hybridization – Fusion of two diverse cells
(b) Vector DNA – Site for tRNA synthesis
(c) Micropropagation – In vitro production of plants in large numbers
(d) Callus – Unorganised mass of cells produced in tissue culture

4. Which one of the following techniques made it possible to genetically engineer living organisms? **(Mains 2011)**
(a) Recombinant DNA techniques
(b) X-ray diffraction
(c) Heavier isotope labelling
(d) Hybridization

5. Which of the following are used in gene cloning? **(2010)**
(a) Nucleoids (b) Lomasomes
(c) Mesosomes (d) Plasmids

6. Manipulation of DNA in genetic engineering became possible due to the discovery of **(2002)**
(a) restriction endonuclease
(b) DNA ligase
(c) transcriptase
(d) primase.

7. The bacteria generally used for genetic engineering is **(2000)**
(a) Agrobacterium (b) Bacillus
(c) Pseudomonas (d) Clostridium

8. Which of the following is related to genetic engineering? **(1999)**
(a) Heterosis (b) Mutation
(c) Plastid (d) Plasmid

9. Genetic engineering is possible, because **(1998)**
(a) we can cut DNA at specific sites by endonucleases like DNase I
(b) restriction endonucleases purified from bacteria can be used in vitro
(c) the phenomenon of transduction in bacteria is well understood
(d) we can see DNA by electron microscope.

10. When scientists make an animal superior by view of genotype, introducing some foreign genes in it, is called **(1996)**
(a) immunization (b) genetic engineering
(c) tissue culture (d) biotechnology.

11. Which of the following organelles is related with genetic engineering? **(1994)**
(a) Mitochondria (b) Plasmids
(c) Golgi bodies (d) Lysosomes

TOOLS OF RECOMBINANT DNA TECHNOLOGY

12. Upon exposure to UV radiation, DNA stained with ethidium bromide will show **(2023)**
(a) bright yellow colour (b) bright orange colour
(c) bright red colour (d) bright blue colour.

13. In gene gun method used to introduce alien DNA into host cells, microparticles of _____ metal are used. **(2023)**
(a) tungsten or gold (b) silver
(c) copper (d) zinc

14. Which of the following is not a cloning vector? ***(2023)***

(a) pBR322 (b) Probe
(c) BAC (d) YAC

15. Which one of the following statement is not true regarding gel electrophoresis technique? ***(2022)***

(a) The process of extraction of separated DNA strands from gel is called elution.
(b) These parated DNA fragment sarestained by using ethidium bromide.
(c) The presence of chromogenic substrate gives blue coloured DNA bands on the gel.
(d) Bright orange coloured bands of DNA can be observed in the gel when exposed to UV light.

16. In the following palindromic base sequences of DNA, which one can be cut easily by particular restriction enzyme? ***(2022)***

(a) 5′G A T A C T 3′; 3′C T A T G A 5′
(b) 5′G A A T T C 3′; 3′C T T A A G 5^′
(c) 5′C T CAGT 3′; 3′G A G T C A 5′
(d) 5′G T A T C 3′; 3′C A T A A G 5′

17. Given below are two statements: ***(2022)***

Statement I: Restriction endonucleases recognise specific sequence to cut DNA known as palindromic nucleotide sequence.

Statement II: Restriction endonucleases cut the DNA strand a little away from the centre of the palindromic site.

In the light of the above statements, choose the most appropriate answer from the options given below:

(a) Both Statement I and Statement II are correct.
(b) Both Statement I and Statement II are incorrect.
(c) Statement I is correct but Statement II is incorrect.
(d) Statement I is incorrect but Statement II is correct.

18. Which of the following is not a desirable feature of a cloning vector? ***(2021)***

(a) Presence of origin of replication
(b) Presence of a marker gene
(c) Presence of single restriction enzyme site
(d) Presence of two or more recognition sites

19. DNA strands on a gel stained with ethidium bromide when viewed under UV radiation, appear as ***(2021)***

(a) bright blue bands
(b) yellow bands
(c) bright orange bands
(d) dark red bands.

20. Plasmid pBR322 has PstI restriction enzyme site within gene amp^R that confers ampicillin resistance. If this enzyme is used for inserting a gene for β-galactosidase production and the recombinant plasmid is inserted in an E.coli strain. ***(2021)***

(a) It will be able to produce a novel protein with dual ability.
(b) It will not be able to confer ampicillin resistance to the host cell.
(c) The transformed cells will have the ability to resist ampicillin as well as produce β-galactosidase.
(d) It will lead to lysis of host cell.

21. A specific recognition sequence identified by endonucleases to make cuts at specific positions within the DNA is ***(2021)***

(a) poly (A) tail sequences
(b) degenerate primer sequence
(c) okazaki sequences
(d) palindromic nucleotide sequences.

22. Identify the wrong statement with regard to restriction enzymes. ***(2020)***

(a) Each restriction enzyme functions by inspecting the length of a DNA sequence.
(b) They cut the strand of DNA at palindromic sites.
(c) They are useful in genetic engineering.
(d) Sticky ends can be joined by using DNA ligases.

23. Choose the correct pair from the following. ***(2020)***

(a) Ligases – Join the two DNA molecules
(b) Polymerases – Break the DNA into fragments
(c) Nucleases – Separate the two strands of DNA
(d) Exonucleases - Make cuts at specific positions within DNA

24. The specific palindromic sequence which is recognised by EcoRI is ***(2020)***

(a) 5′ - GAATTC - 3′
3′ - CTTAAG - 5′
(b) 5′ - GGAACC - 3′
3′ - CCTTGG - 5′
(c) 5′ - CTTAAG - 3′
3′ - GAATTC - 5
(d) 5′ - GGATCC - 3′
3′ - CCTAGG - 5′

25. The sequence that controls the copy number of the linked DNA in the vector, is termed ***(2020)***

(a) selectable marker
(b) Ori site
(c) palindromic sequence
(d) recognition site.

26. In gel electrophoresis, separated DNA fragments can be visualized with the help of ***(2020)***

(a) acetocarmine in bright blue light
(b) ethidium bromide in UV radiation
(c) acetocarmine in UV radiation
(d) ethidium bromide in infrared radiation.

27. Following statements describe the characteristics of the enzyme restriction endonuclease. Identify the incorrect statement. ***(2019)***

(a) The enzyme recognises a specific palindromic nucleotide sequence in the DNA.
(b) The enzyme cuts DNA molecule at identified position within the DNA.
(c) The enzyme binds DNA at specific sites and cuts only one of the two strands.
(d) The enzyme cuts the sugar-phosphate backbone at specific sites on each strand.

28. A selectable marker is used to ***(Odisha NEET 2019)***

(a) help in eliminating the non-transformants, so that the transformants can be regenerated
(b) identify the gene for a desired trait in an alien organism
(c) select a suitable vector for transformation in a specific crop
(d) mark a gene on a chromosome for isolation using restriction enzyme.

29. Given below are four statements pertaining to separation of DNA fragments using gel electrophoresis. Identify the incorrect statements. ***(Odisha NEET 2019)***

(i) DNA is negatively charged molecule and so it is loaded on gel towards the anode terminal.

(ii) DNA fragments travel along the surface of the gel whose concentration does not affect movement of DNA.

(iii) Smaller the size of DNA fragment larger is the distance it travels through it.

(iv) Pure DNA can be visualized directly by exposing UV radiation.

Choose correct answer from the options given below.

(a) (i), (iii) and (iv) (b) (i), (ii) and (iii)
(c) (ii), (iii) and (iv) (d) (i), (ii) and (iv)

30. Which of the following is commonly used as a vector for introducing a DNA fragment in human lymphocytes? ***(2018)***

(a) Retrovirus (b) Ti plasmid
(c) I phage (d) pBR322

31. The DNA fragments separated on an agarose gel can be visualised after staining with ***(2017)***

(a) acetocarmine (b) aniline blue
(c) ethidium bromide (d) bromophenol blue.

32. DNA fragments are ***(2017)***
(a) negatively charged
(b) neutral
(c) either positively or negatively charged depending on their size
(d) positively charged.

33. A gene whose expression helps to identify transformed cell is known as ***(2017)***
(a) vector (b) plasmid
(c) structural gene (d) selectable marker.

34. What is the criterion for DNA fragments movement on agarose gel during gel electrophoresis? ***(2017)***
(a) The smaller the fragment size, the farther it moves.
(b) Positively charged fragments move to farther end.
(c) Negatively charged fragments do not move.
(d) The larger the fragment size, the farther it moves.

35. A foreign DNA and plasmid cut by the same restriction endonuclease can be joined to form a recombinant plasmid using ***(NEET-II 2016)***
(a) EcoRI (b) Taq polymerase
(c) polymerase III (d) ligase.

36. Which of the following restriction enzymes produces blunt ends? ***(NEET-II 2016)***
(a) SalI (b) EcoRV
(c) XhoI (d) HindIII

37. Which of the following is not a feature of the plasmids? ***(NEET-I 2016)***
(a) Transferable
(b) Single-stranded
(c) Independent replication
(d) Circular structure

38. Which of the following is a restriction endonuclease? ***(NEET-I 2016)***
(a) DNase I (b) RNase
(c) Hind II (d) Protease

39. The introduction of T-DNA into plants involves ***(2015)***
(a) exposing the plants to cold for a brief period
(b) allowing the plant roots to stand in water
(c) infection of the plant by Agrobacterium tumefaciens
(d) altering the pH of the soil, then heat-shocking the plants.

40. Which vector can clone only a small fragment of DNA? ***(2014)***
(a) Bacterial artificial chromosome
(b) Yeast artificial chromosome
(c) Plasmid
(d) Cosmid

41. Commonly used vectors for human genome sequencing are ***(2014)***
(a) T - DNA (b) BAC and YAC
(c) expression vectors (d) T/A cloning vectors.

42. The colonies of recombinant bacteria appear white in contrast to blue colonies of non-recombinant bacteria because of ***(2013)***
(a) insertional inactivation of alpha galactosidase in recombinant bacteria
(b) inactivation of glycosidase enzyme in recombinant bacteria
(c) non-recombinant bacteria containing beta galactosidase
(d) insertional inactivation of alpha galactosidase in non-recombinant bacteria.

43. DNA fragments generated by the restriction endonucleases in a chemical reaction can be separated by ***(2013)***
(a) electrophoresis
(b) restriction mapping
(c) centrifugation
(d) polymerase chain reaction.

44. The given figure is the diagrammatic representation of the E. coli vector pBR322. Which one of the given options correctly identifies its certain component(s)? ***(2012)***

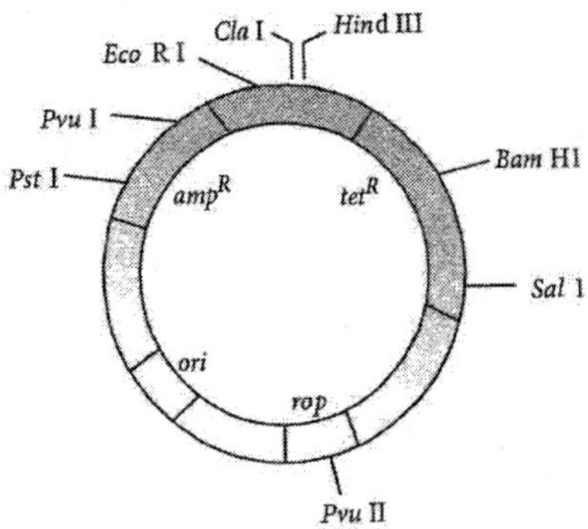

(a) ori-original restriction enzyme
(b) rop-reduced osmotic pressure
(c) HindIII, EcoRI - selectable markers
(d) amp^R, tet^R-antibiotic resistance genes

45. A single strand of nucleic acid tagged with a radioactive molecule is called ***(2012)***
(a) vector (b) selectable marker
(c) plasmid (d) probe.

46. For transformation, micro-particles coated with DNA to be bombarded with gene gun are made up of ***(2012)***
(a) silver or platinum (b) platinum or zinc
(c) silicon or platinum (d) gold or tungsten.

47. Biolistics (gene-gun) is suitable for ***(Mains 2012)***
(a) disarming pathogen vectors
(b) transformation of plant cells
(c) constructing recombinant DNA by joining with vectors
(d) DNA fingerprinting.

48. In genetic engineering, the antibiotics are used ***(Mains 2012)***
(a) as selectable markers
(b) to select healthy vectors
(c) as sequences from where replication starts
(d) to keep the cultures free of infection.

49. Which one of the following represents a palindromic sequence in DNA? ***(Mains 2012)***
(a) 5′- GAATTC - 3′
3′- CTTAAG - 5′
(b) 5′- CCAATG - 3′
3′- GAATCC - 5′
(c) 5′- CATTAG - 3′
3′- GATAAC - 5′
(d) 5′- GATACC - 3′
3′- CCTAAG - 5′

50. Given below is a sample of a portion of DNA strand giving the base sequence on the opposite strands. What is so special shown in it? ***(Mains 2012)***

5′___ GAATTC_____ 3′
3′____TTAAG _____ 5′
(a) Replication completed
(b) Deletion mutation
(c) Start codon at the 5′ end
(d) Palindromic sequence of base pairs

51. There is a restriction endonuclease called EcoRI. What does "co" part in it stand for? ***(2011)***
(a) colon (b) coelom
(c) coenzyme (d) coli

52. Agarose extracted from sea weeds is used in ***(2011)***
(a) spectrophotometry (b) tissue culture
(c) PCR (d) gel electrophoresis.

53. Which one of the following palindromic base sequencesin DNA can beeasily cutataboutthe middle by some particular restriction enzyme? ***(2010)***
(a) 5′____ CGTTCG ____3′
3′_____ATGGTA____5′
(b) 5′____ GATATG ____3′
3′_____CTACTA____5′
(c) 5′_____ GAATTC ____3′
3_____ CTTAAG ____5
(d) 5′_____ CACGTA ____3′
3′_____CTCAGT_____5′

54. Which one of the following is used as vector for cloning genes into higher organisms? ***(2010)***
(a) Baculovirus
(b) Salmonella typhimurium
(c) Rhizopus nigricans
(d) Retrovirus

55. DNA or RNA segment tagged with a radioactive molecule is called ***(2010)***
(a) vector (b) probe
(c) clone (d) plasmid.

56. Restriction endonucleases are enzymes which ***(2010)***
(a) make cuts at specific positions within the DNA molecule
(b) recognize a specific nucleotide sequence for binding of DNA ligase
(c) restrict theaction of theenzymeDNA polymerase
(d) remove nucleotides from the ends of the DNA molecule.

57. In genetic engineering, a DNA segment (gene) of interest, is transferred to the host cell through a vector. Consider the following four agents (i-iv) in this regard and select the correct option about which one or more of these can be used as a vector/vectors. ***(Mains 2010)***
(i) Bacterium
(ii) Plasmid
(iii) *Plasmodium*
(iv) Bacteriophage
(a) (i), (ii) and (iv) (b) (i) only
(c) (i) and (iii) (d) (ii) and (iv)

58. Polyethylene glycol method is used for ***(2009)***
(a) biodiesel production
(b) seedless fruit production
(c) energy production from sewage
(d) gene transfer without a vector.

59. Which one of the following is commonly used in transfer of foreign DNA into crop plants? **(2009)**
(a) Meloidogyne incognita
(b) Agrobacterium tumefaciens
(c) Penicillium expansum
(d) Trichoderma harzianum

60. Gel electrophoresis is used for ***(2008)***
(a) construction of recombinant DNA by joining with cloning vectors
(b) isolation of DNA molecules
(c) cutting of DNA into fragments
(d) separation of DNA fragments according to their size.

61. The linking of antibiotic resistance gene with the plasmid vector became possible with ***(2008)***
(a) DNA polymerase (b) exonucleases
(c) DNA ligase (d) endonucleases.

62. Restriction endonuclease ***(2006)***
(a) synthesizes DNA
(b) cuts the DNA molecule randomly
(c) cuts the DNA molecule at specific sites
(d) restricts the synthesis of DNA inside the nucleus.

63. Two microbes found to be very useful in genetic engineering are ***(2006)***
(a) crown gall bacterium and *Caenorhabditis elegans*
(b) *Escherichia coli* and *Agrobacterium tumefaciens*
(c) Vibrio cholerae and a tailed bacteriophage
(d) Diplococcus sp. and Pseudomonas sp.

64. Restriction endonucleases ***(2004)***
(a) are present in mammalian cells for degradation of DNA when the cell dies
(b) are used in genetic engineering for ligating two DNA molecules
(c) are used for in vitro DNA synthesis
(d) are synthesized by bacteria as part of their defense mechanism.

65. The Ti plasmid, is often used for making transgenic plants. The plasmid is found in ***(2004)***
(a) Azotobacter
(b) Rhizobium of the roots of leguminous plants
(c) Agrobacterium
(d) Yeast as a 2 mm plasmid.

66. The most thoroughly studied of the known bacteria plant interactions is the ***(2004)***
(a) cyanobacterial symbiosis with some aquatic ferns
(b) gall formation on certain angiosperms by Agrobacterium
(c) nodulation of Sesbania stems by nitrogen fixing bacteria
(d) plant growth stimulation by phosphate solubilising bacteria.

67. Which one of the following bacteria has found extensive use in genetic engineering work in plants? ***(2003)***
(a) Clostridium septicum
(b) Xanthomonas citri
(c) Bacillus coagulans
(d) Agrobacterium tumefaciens

68. Which of the following enzymes are used to join bits of DNA? ***(2002)***
(a) Ligase (b) Primase
(c) DNA polymerase (d) Endonuclease

69. Which of the following cut the DNA from specific places? ***(2001)***
(a) E.coli restriction endonuclease I
(b) Ligase
(c) Exonuclease
(d) Alkaline phosphate

70. Maximum number of bases in plasmids discovered so far ***(2001)***
(a) 50 kilo base (b) 500 kilo base
(c) 5000 kilo base (d) 5 kilo base.

71. Plasmid has been used as vector because ***(2000)***
(a) it is circular DNA which have capacity to join to eukaryotic DNA
(b) it can move between prokaryotic and eukaryotic cells
(c) both ends show replication
(d) it has antibiotic resistance gene.

72. Two bacteria found to be very useful in genetic engineering experiments are ***(1998)***
(a) Nitrobacter and Azotobacter
(b) Rhizobium and Diplococcus
(c) Nitrosomonas and Klebsiella
(d) Escherichia and Agrobacterium.

73. Restriction endonucleases are ***(1998)***
(a) used for in vitro DNA synthesis
(b) used in genetic engineering
(c) synthesized by bacteria
(d) present in mammalian cells for degradation of DNA.

74. The restriction enzymes are used in genetic engineering, because ***(1995)***
(a) they can cut DNA at specific base sequence
(b) they are nucleases that cut DNA at variable sites
(c) they can degrade harmful proteins
(d) they can join different DNA fragments.

PROCESSES OF RECOMBINANT DNA TECHNOLOGY

75. Main steps in the formation of recombinant DNA are given below. Arrange these steps in a correct sequence. ***(2023)***

A. Insertion of recombinant DNA into the host cell.

B. Cutting of DNA at specific location by restriction enzyme.

C. Isolation of desired DNA fragment.

D. Amplification of gene of interest using PCR.

Choose the correct answer from the options given below :
(a) C, B, D, A (b) B, D, A, C
(c) B, C, D, A (d) C, A, B, D

76. During the purification process for recombinant DNA technology, addition of chilled ethanol precipitates out ***(2023)***
(a) histones (b) polysaccharides
(c) RNA (d) DNA.

77. Given below are two statements: one is labelled as Assertion (A) and the other is labelled as Reason (R).

Assertion (A) : Polymerase chain reaction is used in DNA amplification.

Reason (R) : The ampicillin resistant gene is used as a selectable marker to check transformation.

In the light of the above statements, choose the correct answer from the options given below. ***(2022)***

(a) Both (A) and (R) are correct and (R) is the correct explanation of (A).
(b) Both (A) and (R) are correct but (R) is not the correct explanation of (A).
(c) (A) is correct but (R) is not correct.
(d) (A) is not correct but (R) is correct.

78. Which of the following is a correct sequence of steps in a PCR (Polymerase Chain Reaction)? ***(2021)***

(a) Annealing, Denaturation, Extension
(b) Denaturation, Annealing, Extension
(c) Denaturation, Extension, Annealing
(d) Extension, Denaturation, Annealing

79. During the purification process for recombinant DNA technology, addition of chilled ethanol precipitates out ***(2021)***

(a) polysaccharides (b) RNA
(c) DNA (d) histones.

80. Which of the following is not an application of PCR (Polymerase Chain Reaction)? ***(2021)***

(a) Detection of gene mutation
(b) Molecular diagnosis
(c) Gene amplification
(d) Purification of isolated protein

81. During the process of gene amplification using PCR, if very high temperature is not maintained in the beginning, then which of the following steps of PCR will be affected first? ***(2021)***

(a) Ligation (b) Annealing
(c) Extension (d) Denaturation

82. Match the organism with its use in biotechnology. ***(2020)***

(A) Bacillus	(i) Cloning vector thuringiensis
(B) Thermus	(ii) Construction of first aquaticus rDNA molecule
(C) Agrobacterium	(iii) DNA polymerase tumefaciens
(D) Salmonella	(iv) Cry proteins typhimurium

Select the correct option from the following.

	A	B	C	D
(a)	(ii)	(iv)	(iii)	(i)
(b)	(iv)	(iii)	(i)	(ii)
(c)	(iii)	(ii)	(iv)	(i)
(d)	(iii)	(iv)	(i)	(ii)

83. DNA precipitation out of a mixture of biomolecules can be achieved by treatment with ***(2019)***

(a) chilled chloroform
(b) isopropanol
(c) chilled ethanol
(d) methanol at room temperature.

84. Which one of the following equipments is essentially required for growing microbes on a large scale, for industrial production of enzymes? ***(2019)***

(a) Bioreactor (b) BOD incubator
(c) Sludge digester (d) Industrial oven

85. The correct order of steps in Polymerase Chain Reaction (PCR) is ***(2018)***

(a) extension, denaturation, annealing
(b) annealing, extension, denaturation
(c) denaturation, extension, annealing
(d) denaturation, annealing, extension.

86. The process of separation and purification of expressed protein before marketing is called ***(2017)***
(a) downstream processing
(b) bioprocessing
(c) postproduction processing
(d) upstream processing

87. Stirred-tank bioreactors have been designed for ***(NEET-II 2016)***
(a) purification of product
(b) addition of preservatives to the product
(c) availability of oxygen throughout the process
(d) ensuring anaerobic conditions in the culture vessel.

88. Which of the following is not a component of downstream processing? ***(NEET-II 2016)***
(a) Separation (b) Purification
(c) Preservation (d) Expression

89. The Taq polymerase enzyme is obtained from ***(NEET-I 2016)***
(a) Bacillus subtilis
(b) Pseudomonas putida
(c) Thermus aquaticus
(d) Thiobacillus ferrooxidans.

90. An analysis of chromosomal DNA using the Southern hybridization technique does not use ***(2014)***
(a) electrophoresis (b) blotting
(c) autoradiography (d) PCR.

91. In vitro clonal propagation in plants is characterized by ***(2014)***
(a) PCR and RAPD
(b) Northern blotting
(c) electrophoresis and HPLC
(d) microscopy.

92. Which of the following is not correctly matched for the organism and its cell wall degrading enzyme? ***(2013)***
(a) Algae - Methylase
(b) Fungi - Chitinase
(c) Bacteria - Lysozyme
(d) Plant cells - Cellulase

93. During the process of isolation of DNA, chilled ethanol is added to ***(Karnataka NEET 2013)***
(a) precipitate DNA
(b) break open the cell to release DNA
(c) facilitate action of restriction enzymes
(d) remove proteins such as histones.

94. PCR and restriction fragment length polymorphism are the methods for ***(2012)***
(a) study of enzymes
(b) genetictransformation
(c) DNA sequencing
(d) genetic fingerprinting.

95. Which one is a true statement regarding DNA polymerase used in PCR? ***(2012)***
(a) It is used to ligate introduced DNA in recipient cells.
(b) It serves as a selectable marker.
(c) It is isolated from a virus.
(d) It remains active at high temperature.

96. The figure below shows three steps (A, B, C) of Polymerase Chain Reaction (PCR). Select the option giving correct identification together with what it represents? ***(Mains 2012)***

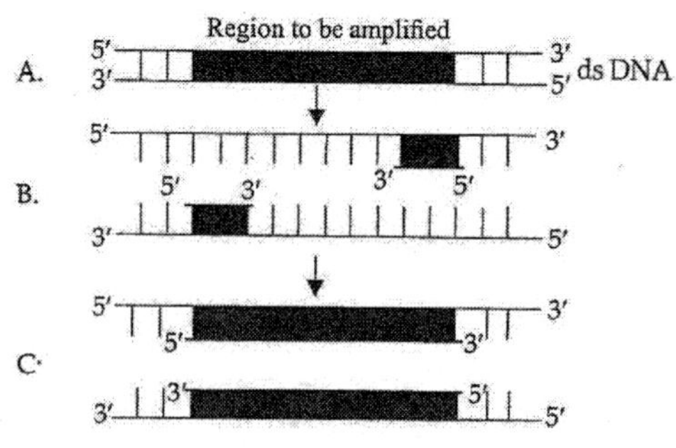

(a) B - denaturation at a temperature of about 98° C separating the two DNA strands
(b) A - denaturation at a temperature of about 50° C
(c) C - extension in the presence of heat stable DNA polymerase
(d) A - annealing with two sets of primers

97. Stirred-tank bioreactors have been designed for *(2010)*
(a) addition of preservatives to the product
(b) purification of the product
(c) ensuring an aerobic condition sin the culture vessel
(d) availability of oxygen throughout the process.

ANSWER KEY

1.	(d)	2.	(c)	3.	(b)	4.	(a)	5.	(d)	6.	(a)	7.	(a)
8.	(d)	9.	(b)	10.	(b)	11.	(b)	12.	(b)	13.	(a)	14.	(b)
15.	(c)	16.	(a)	17.	(a)	18.	(d)	19.	(c)	20.	(b)	21.	(d)
22.	(d)	23.	(a)	24.	(a)	25.	(b)	26.	(b)	27.	(c)	28.	(a)
29.	(d)	30.	(a)	31.	(c)	32.	(a)	33.	(d)	34.	(a)	35.	(d)
36.	(b)	37.	(b)	38.	(c)	39.	(c)	40.	(c)	41.	(b)	42.	(c)
43.	(a)	44.	(d)	45.	(d)	46.	(d)	47.	(b)	48.	(a)	49.	(a)
50.	(d)	51.	(d)	52.	(d)	53.	(c)	54.	(d)	55.	(b)	56.	(a)
57.	(d)	58.	(d)	59.	(b)	60.	(d)	61.	(c)	62.	(c)	63.	(b)
64.	(d)	65.	(c)	66.	(b)	67.	(d)	68.	(a)	69.	(a)	70.	(b)
71.	(a)	72.	(d)	73.	(d)	74.	(a)	75.	(a)	76.	(d)	77.	(b)
78.	(b)	79.	(c)	80.	(d)	81	(d)	82.	(b)	83.	(c)	84.	(a)
85.	(d)	86.	(a)	87.	(c)	88.	(d)	89.	(c)	90.	(d)	91.	(a)
92.	(a)	93.	(a)	94.	(d)	95.	(d)	96.	(c)	97.	(d)		

HINTS & EXPLANATIONS

1.(d) : Vector is a DNA molecule that carries a foreign DNA segment and replicates inside a host cell. The vector DNA and foreign DNA carrying gene of interest are cut by the same restriction endonuclease enzyme to produce complementary sticky ends. With the help of DNA ligase enzyme, the complementary sticky ends of the two DNAs are joined to produce a recombinant DNA (rDNA), which is then introduced into the host cell.

2.(c) : Restriction enzymes recognise specific base sequences in a DNA molecule and cut its strands, e.g., EcoRI cuts DNA strands in the base sequence GAATTC.

3.(b) : Vectors are DNA molecules that can carry a foreign DNA segment and replicate inside the host cell. They are used in recombinant DNA technology.

4.(a)

5.(d) : Plasmid is a small circular double stranded DNA molecule present in the cytoplasm of the bacterial cell. It can replicate independently of bacterial chromosome. Due to this characteristic of plasmid, it is used as the vector (vectors are for the transferring of a piece of DNA to target gene) in gene cloning.

6.(a) : DNA restriction endonuclease are important,

which cut double-stranded DNA molecules only at sites characterized by a specific nucleotide sequence. Restriction enzymes are isolated from bacterial cells and are tools for molecular biologists.

7. (a)

8. (d)

9. (b)

10.(b) : Genetic engineering is an experimental manipulation of genetic material, especially for industrial or medical uses. It encompasses the techniques of gene cloning, the DNA modification by changes in sequence arrangement or deletion, and the introduction of novel genes into cells and organisms. It may prove possible to advantageously modify the genes of farmed animals, to correct genetic deficiencies of the human by inserting novel genes. This can be done by breakage of a DNA molecule at two desired places into another DNA molecule of the desired animal.

11.(b) : Plasmids are extrachromosomal genetic element found in many bacteria and in a few eukaryotic cells. Plasmids are closed circles of double-stranded DNA ranging in size from 1 to 200 kilobases. They frequently carry genes conferring antibiotic resistance. Plasmids are becoming important tools for genetic engineering since they have the ability to replicate and migrate to daughter cells. Plasmids are widely used as carriers of cloned genes, for example the E. coli plasmid pBR322. When plasmids are used as cloning vectors and carry a novel DNA sequence they are referred to as chimeric plasmids.

12.(b) : The DNA fragments separated by gel electrophoresis can be visualised after staining the DNA with ethidium bromide followed by exposure to UV radiations. Bands of DNA are seen as bright orange coloured bands in ethidium bromide stained gel exposed to UV light.

13.(a) : In biolistics or gene gun method, cells are bombarded with high velocity micro-particles of gold or tungsten coated with DNA.

14.(b): Cloning vectors are DNA molecules into which foreign DNA can be introduced and transmitted to host cell for use in cloning. Different types of cloning vectors are plasmids, bacteriophages, BAC, YAC. A probe is single stranded sequence of DNA or RNA use to identify complementary sequence in genome.

15.(c) : In gel electrophoresis, the DNA fragments separate according to their size through the agarose gel, with smaller fragments moving farther away as compared to larger ones. The orange coloured bands of DNA can be visualised by staining them with ethidium bromide followed by exposure to UV radiations. The separated bands of DNA are cut out from the agarose gel is called elution.

16. (a)

17. (a)

18.(d) : In order to link alien DNA, the vector needs to have preferable single recognition site for commonly used restriction enzyme. Presence of more than one recognition sites within vector will generate several fragments and will complicate the gene cloning.

19.(c) : In the process of gel electrophoresis, the separated DNA fragments can be seen after staining the DNA with a compound like ethidium bromide (EtBr) followed by exposure to UV radiation as bright orange coloured bands.

20. (b)

21. (d) : A restriction endonuclease recognises a specific palindromic nucleotide sequence to make a cut at specific position within the DNA.

22. (d)

23. (a)

24.(a) : The palindromes in DNA are base pair sequences that are same when read forward (left to right) or backward (right to left) from a central axis of symmetry.

Thus, $\frac{\text{GAATTC}}{\text{CTTAAG}}$ is a palindromic sequence which is recognised by EcoRI.

25.(b) : Ori site is a sequence from where replication starts and any piece of DNA when linked to this sequence can be made to replicate within the host cells. This sequence is also responsible for controlling the copy number of the linked DNA in the vector. So, if one wants to recover many copies of the target DNA it should be cloned in a vector whose origin support high copy number.

26.(b) : In gel electrophoresis, separated DNA fragments can be visualised only after staining the DNA with a compound i.e., ethidium bromide and followed by exposure to UV radiation as bright orange coloured bands.

27.(c) : The restriction endonuclease enzyme inspects the length of a DNA sequence. Once it recognises specific sequence, it binds to the DNA and cuts each of the two strands of the double helix at specific points in their sugar phosphate backbone. Special sequence in the DNA recognised by restriction endonuclease is called palindromic nucleotide sequence.

28. (a)

29.(d) : DNA is a negatively charged molecule, so they can be separated by forcing them to move towards the anode under an electric field. DNA fragments separate according to size through the pores of agarose gel. The separated DNA fragments can be visualised only after staining the DNA with a compound known as ethidium bromide then followed by exposure to UV radiation.

30.(a) : Retroviruses cause cancer in animals including humans. So modified retroviruses are used to transfer desirable genes into animal cells. It is used in gene therapy, in which lymphocytes from blood of patient are taken and grown in culture medium outside the body, a functional gene is introduced by using a retroviral vector into these lymphocytes which are again reintroduced into the patient body.

31.(c) : The separated DNA fragments can be seen only after staining them with a compound known as ethidium bromide (EtBr) followed by exposure to UV radiation as bright orange coloured bands.

32. (a)

33.(d) : Some genes called "selectable markers". help in selecting those host cells which contain the vectors (transformants) and eliminating the non-transformants.

34.(a) : Electrophoresis is a technique used for the separation of substances of different ionic properties. Since the DNA fragments are negatively charged molecules, they can be separated by allowing them to move towards the anode. DNA fragments move towards the anode according to their molecule size through the pores of agarose gel. Thus, the smaller fragments move farther away as compared to larger fragments.

35. (d) : Ligase is a class of enzymes that catalyse the formation of covalent bonds using the energy released by the cleavage of ATP. Ligases are important in the synthesis and repair of many biological molecules, including DNA ligase and used in genetic engineering to insert foreign DNA into cloning vectors.

36.(b) : EcoRV is a type II restriction endonuclease isolated from certain strains of E.coli. It creates blunt ends. It recognises the palindromic sequence of 6 bases. SalI, XhoI and HindIII restriction enzymes produce sticky ends.

37.(b) : Plasmids are extra-chromosomal, self-replicating, usually circular, double-stranded DNA molecules that serve as vectors which carry foreign DNA segment and replicate inside host cell.

38.(c) : Hind II is the first restriction endonuclease. It was isolated from Haemophilus influenzae Rd. It always cut DNA at specific position producing blunt ends. DNase I is an endonuclease that cleaves DNA preferentially at phosphodiester linkages adjacent to a pyrimidine nucleotide. RNase is a type of nuclease that catalyses the degradation of RNA into smaller components. It can be endoribonuclease or exoribonuclease. A protease is an enzyme that perform proteolysis, i.e., protein catabolism by hydrolysis of the peptide bonds.

39.(c) : Ti plasmid (tumor inducing) from the soil bacterium Agrobacterium tumefaciens is effectively used as vector for gene transfer to plant cells. The part of Ti plasmid transferred into plant cell DNA, is called the T-DNA. This T-DNA with desired DNA spliced into it, is inserted into the chromosomes of the host plant where it produces copies of itself. Such plant cells are then cultured, induced to multiply and differentiate to form plantlets. By transferring into soil, the plantlets grow into mature plants, carrying the foreign gene, expressed throughout the new plant.

40.(c) : Plasmids have been modified to be used as vectors. They can clone DNA fragments of about 10kbp size while cosmid can carry upto 45 kb, YAC can carry upto 1000 2500kbp and BAC can carry around 300-350Kbp long DNA fragments.

41.(b) : Bacterial artificial chromosome (BAC) vectors are based on natural, extra-chromosomal plasmid of E. coli. BAC vector contains genes for replication and maintenance of the F-factor, a selectable marker and 'cloning site. These vectors can accommodate upto 300-350 kb of foreign DNA and are also being used in genome sequencing project. Yeast artificial chromosome (YAC) vectors are used to clone DNA fragments of more than 1Mb in size. Therefore, they have been exploited extensively in mapping the large genomes, e.g., in the Human Genome Project. These vectors contain the telomeric sequence, the centromere and the autonomously replicating sequence from yeast chromosomes.

42.(c) : The presence of restriction sites within the markers tet^r and amp^r of plasmid permits an easy selection for cells transformed with recombinant plasmid. Insertion of the DNA fragment into the plasmid makes antibiotic resistance genes nonfunctional, for example, insertion of the DNA fragment into the plasmid (pBR322) using Pst I or Pvu I makes ampr non-functional. Bacterial cells containing such a recombinant pBR322 will be unable to grow in the presence of ampicillin, but will grow on tetracycline. This process, however, becomes burdensome because it requires simultaneous plating on two plates having different antibiotics. Thus, alternative selectable marker is developed to differentiate recombinants and non-recombinants on the basis of their ability to produce colour in the presence of a chromogenic substance. Here, a recombinant DNA is inserted in the coding sequence of an enzyme β-galactosidase. pUC 18 plasmid contains this gene which allows it to produce β-galactosidase which degrades certain sugars and produces a blue pigment when exposed to specific substrate analog. If the plasmid in the bacterium does not have an insert, i.e., is non-recombinant, the presence of chromogenic substrate gives blue coloured colonies. Presence of insert in the plasmid in recombinant bacterium does not produce any colour, such bacterial colonies are marked as recombinant colonies.

43. (a)

44.(d) : In pBR322, ori-represents site or origin of replication, rop-codes for proteins that take part in the replication of plasmid. Hind III, EcoRI-recognition sites of restriction endonucleases. ampR and tetR - antibiotic resistance genes.

45.(d) : Probes are single stranded, radiolabelled molecules of nucleic acids with known sequence. The probes having sequence complementary to the gene to be identified are supplied. They bind with the particular gene segment. Radiation imaging identifies the location of that particular segment which bind with probe. Probes are used as identification tool.

46.(d) : A gene or a biolistic particle delivery system, originally designed for plant transformation, is a device for injecting cells with genetic information. The payload is an elemental particle of a heavy metal such as gold or tungsten coated with plasmid DNA. The device is used to transform almost any type of cell including plants, and is not limited to genetic material of the nucleus. It can also transform organelles, including plastids.

47.(b) : Biolistics is a technique for introducing genetic material into living cells, especially plant cells, in which DNAcoated microscopic particles (tungsten or gold particles) are bombarded with a very high velocity into the target cell using a special gun. The microprojectiles, typically 1 mm in diameter, are accelerated to high velocity by a specially modified small calibre gun and penetrate the cell walls and plasma membrane with minimal damage. Hence, the novel DNA can be inserted into intact plant cells ultimately transforming it without using a vector.

48.(a) : Selectable markers are those genes which help in selecting those host cells which contain vectors (i.e., transformants) and eliminating the non-transformants. The genes encoding resistance to antibiotics such as tetracycline, ampicillin, kanamycin, etc., are useful selectable markers for E.coli. Plasmid pBR322 has two resistance genes - ampicillin resistance (amp^r) and tetracycline resistance (tt^r) which are considered useful for selectable markers. The presence of restriction sites within the markers tet^r and amp^r permits an easy selection for cells transformed with the recombinant pBR322. Insertion of the DNA fragment into the plasmid using enzyme Pst I or Pvu I places the DNA insert within the gene amp^r; this makes amp^r nonfunctional. Bacterial cells containing such a recombinant pBR322 will be unable to grow in the presence of ampicillin, but will grow on tetracycline. Similarly, when restriction enzyme Bam HI or SalI is used, the DNA insert is placed within the gene tet t^r aking it nonfunctional. Bacterial cells possessing such a recombinant pBR322 will, therefore, grow on ampicillin but not on tetracycline.

49.(a) : Palindromes are groups of letters that form the same words when read both forward and backward, e.g., "MALAYALAM". As against a word-palindrome where the same word is read in both directions, the palindrome in DNA is a sequence of base pairs that reads same on the two strands when orientation of reading is kept the same. For example, the following sequences read the same on the two strands in 5′→ 3′ direction. This is also true if read in the 3′→5′ direction. In this case, it is

5′ – GAATTC – 3′

3′ – CTTAAG –5′

50. (d)

51.(d) : The enzyme restriction endonuclease EcoRI is found in the colon bacteria E. coli. So, here 'co' stands for coli. According to nomenclature of restriction enzyme, the first letter used for the enzyme is the first letter of the genus name (in italics) of the bacterium, then comes the first two letters of its species (also in italics), next is the strain of the organism. At last is a Roman numeral signifying the order of discovery. Here, the enzyme EcoRI was isolated from the bacterium Escherichia coli (co), strain RY13(R) and it was first endonuclease (I) isolated from E.coli.

52.(d) : In gel electrophoresis, DNA fragments separate (resolve) according to their size through sieving effect provided by the agarose gel. Agarose is a natural polymer extracted from sea weeds and is commonly used as a matrix.

53.(c) : Palindromic nucleotide sequences in the DNA molecule are groups of bases that form the same sequence when read in both forward and backward direction. In the given question, only option (c) represents a palindromic sequence, that can be easily cut at about the middle by some particular restriction enzyme.

54.(d) : Retroviruses in animals have the ability to transform normal cells into cancerous cells. We have transformed these pathogens into useful vectors for delivering genes of interest to humans. Retroviruses have been disarmed and are now used to deliver desirable genes into animal cells. So, once a gene or a DNA fragment has been ligated into a suitable retroviral vector it is transferred into a bacterial, plant or animal host (where it multiplies).

55. (b)

56.(a) : Restriction endonucleases were found by Arber in 1962 in bacteria. They act as "molecular scissors" or chemical scalpels. They recognize the specific base sequence at palindrome sites in DNA duplex and cut its strands. For example, restriction endonuclease EcoRI found in the colon bacteria E. coli recognizes the base sequence GAATTC in DNA duplex and cuts its strands between G and A.

57.(d) : Plasmid and bacteriophage are used as vectors in genetic engineering. Plasmid is an autonomously replicating circular extra-chromosomal DNA found in bacteria. They can be transferred from cell to cell in a bacterial colony. This characteristic is being used in biotechnology for transferring desirable gene into target gene of the host. Bacteriophage is a bacterial virus which can infect it, quickly multiply within and destroy (lyse) their host (virus) cells. During infection bacteriophages inject their DNA into these cells. The injected DNA selectively replicate and are expressed in the host that results in a multiplication of phages that ultimately burst out of the cell (by lysis). This ability of transferring DNA from the phage genome to specific host during infection process gave scientists the idea that specially designed phage vectors could be used for gene cloning.

58. (d) : Direct gene transfer is the transfer of naked DNA into plant cells, but the presence of rigid plant cell wall acts as a barrier to uptake. Therefore, protoplasts are the favoured target for direct gene transfer. Polyethylene glycol mediated DNA uptake is a direct gene transfer method that utilizes the interaction between PEG, naked DNA, salts and the protoplast membrane to effect transport of the DNA into the cytoplasm.

59. **(b)** : Agrobacterium tumefaciens has been extensively used in genetic engineering experiments. It is the causative agent of crown gall, an important disease of many commercial crops. This disease has come to be recognized in recent years as being caused by a DNA plasmid (Ti plasmid) carried by bacterium and transferred to the plant cells. Following the discovery of the relationship between crown gall and the Ti plasmid, this plasmid has come to be widely used in plant genetic engineering as a vector in order to inject a novel gene in host plant to form a transgenic plant.

60. **(d)** : Electrophoresis is a technique used for the separation of substances of different ionic properties. Since the DNA fragments are negatively charged molecules, they can be separated by allowing them to move towards the anode. DNA fragments move towards the anode according to their molecule size through the pores of agarose gel. Thus, the smaller fragments move farther away as compared to larger fragments.

61. **(c)** : The construction of the first recombinant DNA emerged from the possibility of linking a gene encoding antibiotic resistance with a native plasmid. The cutting of DNA at specific locations became possible with the discovery of the so called 'molecular scissors' - restriction enzymes. The cut piece of DNA was then linked with the plasmid DNA. This plasmid DNA acts as vector to transfer the piece of DNA attached to it. The linking of antibiotic resistance gene with the plasmid vector became possible with the enzyme DNA ligase, which acts on cut DNA molecules and joins their ends. This makes a new combination of circular autonomously replicating DNA created in vitro and is known as recombinant DNA.

62. **(c)**

63. **(b)** : E.coli contains many important standard cloning vectors widely used in gene cloning experiments like pBR322 contains origin of replication (ori). Other cloning vectors like PACYC177, pBR324, contain ampicillin resistance gene are also found in E.coli. Among higher plants, Ti plasmid of Agrobacterium tumefaciens and Ri plasmid of A. rhizogenes is the best known vector. T-DNA from Ti or Ri plasmid of Agrobacterium is considered to be a very potential vector for cloning experiments with higher plants.

64. **(d)** : Restriction endonucleasses are enzymes that digest double stranded DNA following recognition of specific nucleotide sequences. This is achieved by cleaving the two phosphodiester bonds, one within each strand of the DNA duplex. They are found in bacteria and their function in bacteria is to cut up any invading virus as a part of its defense mechanism, thus restricting the multiplication of viruses in the bacterial cell. Different species of bacteria produce different restriction endonucleases.

65. **(c)**

66. **(b)** : Agrobacterium tumefaciens is the causative agent of crown gall, an important disease of many commercial crops. This disease has come to be recognized in recent years as being caused by a DNA plasmid (Ti plasmid) carried by bacterium and transferred to the plant cells.

67. **(d)** : Agrobacterium tumefaciens has been

extensively used in genetic engineering experiments. It is the causative agent of crown gall, an important disease of many commercial crops. This disease has come to be recognized in recent years as being caused by a DNA plasmid (Ti plasmid) carried by bacterium and transferred to the plant cells. Following the discovery of the relationship between crown gall and the Ti plasmid, this plasmid has come to be widely used in plant genetic engineering as a vector in order to inject a novel gene in host plant to form a transgenic plant.

68. (a) : Ligases are used to join bits of DNA. Primase is an RNA polymerase, used to initiate DNA synthesis. DNA polymerase enzyme catalyses the synthesis of DNA. Endonuclease, causes the splicing of the intron carrying the coding sequence of the same endonuclease.

69. (a)

70. (b) : A plasmid is a DNA molecule separate from the chromosomal DNA and capable of autonomous replication. In many cases, it is typically circular and double-stranded. It usually occurs in bacteria and is sometimes found in eukaryotic organisms. The size of plasmids varies from 1 to over 400 kilobase pairs (kbp). There may be one copy, for large plasmids, to hundreds of copies of the same plasmid in a single cell.

71. (a)

72. (d)

73. (d)

74. (a) : DNA restriction endonuclease cut double-stranded DNA molecules only at sites characterised by a specific nucleotide sequence.

75. (a)

76. (d)

77. (b)

78. (b) : A single PCR cycle involves three basic steps.

(i) Denaturation (DNA is heated to high temperature, usually 94°–96° C

(ii) Primer annealing (two oligonucleotide primers anneal to each of the single stranded template DNA, temperature usually 40°–60° C) and

(iii) Extension (Taq DNA polymerase synthesises the DNA region between primers, optimum temperature 72° C).

79. (c)

80. (d) : Purification of isolated protein is one of the step used in downstream processing of recombinant DNA technology.

81. (d) : In PCR, the repeated amplification is achieved by the use of a thermostable DNA polymerase, which remain active during the high temperature induced denaturation of double stranded DNA. So, if high temperature is not maintained, denaturation will be affected first as it is carried out at a higher temperature 94° to 96° C.

82. (b)

83.(c) : In order to cut the DNA with restriction enzymes, it needs to be in pure form, free from other macromolecules. Since the DNA is enclosed by the membranes, we have to break the cell open to release DNA and other macromolecules like RNA, proteins, polysaccharides and lipids. It is obtained by treating the bacterial cells/plant or animal tissue with enzymes. Other molecules are removed by appropriate treatments and purified DNA ultimately precipitates out after the addition of chilled ethanol.

84. (a)

85.(d) : A single PCR amplification cycle involves three basic steps, denaturation heating of target DNA to high temperature resulting in separation of two strands, annealing two oligonucleotide primers anneal or hybridise to each single template DNA and extension. Taq DNA polymerase synthesises DNA between primers and primers extend towards each other such that DNA stranded segment lying between the two is copied.

86.(a) : After the formation of the product in the bioreactor it undergoes some processes before a finished product is ready for marketing. The process includes separation and purification of products which are collectively called downstream processing.

87.(c) : A stirred-tank reactor is usually cylindrical or with a curved base to facilitate the mixing of the reactor contents. The stirrer facilitates, even mixing and oxygen availability throughout the bioreactor.

88.(d) : After the formation of the product in bioreactor, it undergoes some processes before a finished product to be ready for marketing. Downstream processing includes separation and purification process. The product obtained is subjected to quality control, testing and kept in suitable preservatives.

89.(c) : Taq polymerase, generally used in PCR is isolated from thermophilic bacterium Thermus aquaticus.

90.(d) : PCR is used only for amplification of DNA. It is not directly involved in Southern hybridisation technique.

91.(a) : Clonal propagation can be characterized by PCR and RAPD. The polymerase chain reaction (PCR) technique, generates microgram (μg) quantities of DNA copies (upto billion copies) of the desired DNA (or RNA) segment, present even as a single copy in the initial preparation, in a matter of few hours. RAPD stands for Random Amplification of Polymorphic DNA. It is a type of PCR, but the segments of DNA that are amplified are random. No knowledge of the DNA sequence for the targeted gene is required, as the primers will bind somewhere in the sequence, but it is not certain exactly where. Its resolving power is much lower than targeted, species specific DNA comparison methods, such as short tandem repeats.

92.(a) : Cell wall of algae is made up of cellulose, pectin and mucilage. These substances cannot be degraded by methylase. Methylase is a type of transferase enzyme that transfers a methyl group from a donor to an acceptor.

93.(a) : Ethanol is much less polar than water. Adding it to the solution disrupts the screening charges exerted by water. The electrical attraction between phosphate and any positive ions (Na+) present in solution becomes strong enough to form a stable ionic bond and DNA precipitates. Ethanol precipitation is a widely used technique to purify, or concentrate nucleic acid.

94. (d)

95.(d) : In PCR, Taq polymerase is used which is obtained from Thermus aquaticus bacteria. It is a relatively thermostable enzyme thus used in PCR as during the process the step involving denaturation of DNA strands requires high temperature.

96. (c)

97. (d)

Chapter : 29 BIOTECHNOLOGY AND ITS APPLICATIONS

BIOTECHNOLOGICAL APPLICATIONS IN AGRICULTURE

1. Transposons can be used during which one of the following? ***(2022)***
(a) Polymerase Chain Reaction
(b) Gene silencing
(c) Autoradiography
(d) Gene sequencing

2. Bt cotton variety that was developed by the introduction of toxin gene of Bacillus thuringiensis (Bt) is resistant to ***(2020)***
(a) insect pests (b) fungal diseases
(c) plant nematodes (d) insect predators.

3. What triggers activation of protoxin to active toxin of Bacillus thuringiensis in bollworm? ***(2019)***
(a) Acidic pH of stomach
(b) Body temperature
(c) Moist surface of midgut
(d) Alkaline pH of gut

4. Which of the following is true for Golden rice? ***(2019)***
(a) It has yellow grains, because of a gene introduced from a primitive variety of rice.
(b) It is vitamin A enriched, with a gene from daffodil.
(c) It is pest resistant, with a gene from Bacillus thuringiensis.
(d) It is drought tolerant, developed using Agrobacterium vector.

5. In RNAi, the genes are silenced using ***(Odisha NEET 2019)***
(a) ds-RNA (b) ss-DNA
(c) ss-RNA (d) ds-DNA.

6. Which part of the tobacco plant is infected by Meloidogyne incognitia? ***(NEET-I 2016)***
(a) Stem (b) Root
(c) Flower (d) Leaf

7. Golden rice is a genetically modified crop plant where the incorporated gene is meant for biosynthesis of ***(2015)***
(a) omega 3 (b) vitamin A
(c) vitamin B (d) vitamin C

8. In Bt cotton, the Bt toxin present in plant tissue as protoxin is converted into active toxin due to ***(2015 Cancelled)***
(a) action of gut microorganisms
(b) presence of conversion factors in insect gut
(c) alkaline pH of the insect gut
(d) acidic pH of the insect gut.

9. The crops engineered for glyphosate are resistant/ tolerant to ***(2015 Cancelled)***
(a) insects (b) herbicides
(c) fungi (d) bacteria.

10. Which of the following Bt crops is being grown in India by the farmers? ***(2013)***
(a) Brinjal (b) Soybean
(c) Maize (d) Cotton

11. RNA interference involves ***(Karnataka NEET 2013)***
(a) synthesis of cDNA and RNA using reverse transcriptase
(b) silencing of specific mRNA due to complementary RNA
(c) interference of RNA in synthesis of DNA
(d) synthesis of mRNA from DNA.

12. Consumption of which one of the following foods can prevent the kind of blindness associated with vitamin 'A' deficiency? ***(2012)***
(a) 'Flavr Savr' tomato (b) Canolla
(c) Golden rice (d) Bt-Brinjal

13. Tobacco plants resistant to a nematode have been developed by the introduction of DNA that produces (in the host cells) ***(Mains 2012)***
(a) both sense and anti-sense RNA
(b) a particular hormone
(c) an antifeedant
(d) a toxic protein.

14. The process of RNA interference (RNAi) has been used in the development of plants resistant to ***(2011)***
(a) nematodes (b) fungi
(c) viruses (d) insects.

15. Bacillus thuringiensis forms protein crystals which contain insecticidal protein. This protein ***(Mains 2011)***
(a) binds with epithelial cells of midgut of the insect pest ultimately killing it
(b) is coded by several genes including the gene cry
(c) is activated by acid pH of the foregut of the insect pest
(d) does not kill the carrier bacterium which is itself resistant to this toxin.

16. Silencing of m RNA has been used in producing transgenic plants resistant to ***(Mains 2011)***
(a) boll worms (b) nematodes
(c) white rusts (d) bacterial blights.

17. The genetically-modified (GM) brinjal in India has been developed for ***(2010)***
(a) insect-resistance
(b) enhancing shelf life
(c) enhancing mineral content
(d) drought-resistance.

18. Some of the characteristics of Bt cotton are ***(2010)***
(a) long fibre and resistance to aphids
(b) medium yield, long fibre and resistance to beetle pests
(c) high yield and production of toxic
(d) high yield and resistance to bollworms.

19. An improved variety of transgenic basmati rice ***(2010)***
(a) does not require chemical fertilizers and growth hormones
(b) gives high yield and is rich in vitamin A
(c) is completely resistant to all insect pests and diseases of paddy
(d) gives high yield but has no characteristic aroma.

20. What is true about Bt toxin? ***(2009)***
(a) Bt protein exists as active toxin in the Bacillus.
(b) The activated toxin enters the ovaries of the pest to sterilise it and thus prevent its multiplication.
(c) The concerned Bacillus has antitoxins.
(d) The inactive protoxin gets converted into active form in the insect gut.

21. Transgenic plants are the ones ***(2009)***
(a) generated by introducing foreign DNA into a cell and regenerating a plant from that cell
(b) produced after protoplast fusion in artificial medium
(c) grown in artificial medium after hybridization in the field
(d) produced by a somatic embryo in artificial medium.

22. The bacterium Bacillus thuringiensis is widely used in contemporary biology as ***(2009)***
(a) insecticide
(b) agent for production of dairy products
(c) source of industrial enzyme
(d) indicator of water pollution.

23. What is antisense technology? ***(2009)***
(a) When a piece of RNA that is complementary in sequence is used to stop expression of a specific gene
(b) RNA polymerase producing DNA
(c) A cell displaying a foreign antigen used for synthesis of antigens
(d) Production of somaclonal variants in tissue cultures

24. Cry I endotoxins obtained from Bacillus thuringiensis are effective against ***(2008)***
(a) nematodes (b) bollworms
(c) mosquitoes (d) flies.

25. A transgenic food crop which may help in solving the problem of night blindness in developing countries is ***(2008)***
(a) Bt soybean (b) Golden rice
(c) Flavr Savr tomatoes(d) Starlink maize.

26. Main objective of production/use of herbicide resistant GM crops is to ***(2006)***
(a) encourage eco-friendly herbicides
(b) reduce herbicide accumulation in food articles for health safety
(c) eliminate weeds from the field without the use of manual labour
(d) eliminate weeds from the field without the use of herbicides.

27. Golden rice is a promising transgenic crop. When released for cultivation, it will help in ***(2006)***
(a) producing a petrol-like fuel from rice
(b) alleviation of vitamin A deficiency
(c) pest resistance
(d) herbicide tolerance.

28. Bacillus thuringiensis (Bt) strains have been used for designing novel ***(2005)***
(a) biofertilizers
(b) bio-metallurgical techniques
(c) bio-mineralization processes
(d) bioinsecticidal plants.

29. Golden rice is a transgenic crop of the future with the following improved trait ***(2005)***
(a) insect resistance
(b) high lysine (essential amino acid) content
(c) high protein content
(d) high vitamin-A content.

30. The first transgenic crop was ***(1999)***
(a) tobacco (b) cotton
(c) pea (d) flax.

BIOTECHNOLOGICAL APPLICATIONS IN MEDICINE

31. Which one of the following techniques does not serve the purpose of early diagnosis of a disease for its early treatment? ***(2023)***
(a) Polymerase Chain Reaction (PCR) technique
(b) Enzyme Linked Immuno-Sorbent Assay (ELISA) technique
(c) Recombinant DNA Technology
(d) Serum and Urine analysis

32. In gene therapy of Adenosine Deaminase (ADA) deficiency, the patient requires periodic infusion of genetically engineered lymphocytes because ***(2022)***
(a) retroviral vector is introduced into these lymphocytes.
(b) gene isolated from marrow cells producing ADA is introduced into cells at embryonic stages
(c) lymphocytes from patient's blood are grown in culture, outside the body,
(d) genetically engineered lymphocytes are not immortal cells.

33. Statements related to human insulin are given below. Which statement(s) is/are correct about genetically engineered insulin? ***(2022)***
(A) Pro-hormone insulin contain extra stretch of C-peptide
(B) A-peptide and B-peptide chains of insulin were produced separately in E.coli, extracted and combined by creating disulphide bond between them.
(C) Insulin used for treating diabetes was extracted from cattle and pigs.
(D) Pro-hormone insulin needs to be processed for converting into a mature and functional hormone.
(E) Some patients develop allergic reactions to the foreign insulin.

Choose the most appropriate answer from the options given below:

(a) (A), (B) and (D) only
(b) (B) only
(c) (C) and (D) only
(d) (C), (D) and (E) only

34. When gene targeting involving gene amplification is attempted in an individual's tissue to treat disease, it is known as ***(2021)***
(a) safety testing (b) biopiracy
(c) gene therapy (d) molecular diagnosis.

35. Now a days it is possible to detect the mutated gene causing cancer by allowing radioactive probe to hybridise its complimentary DNA in a clone of cells, followed by its detection using autoradiography because ***(2021)***
(a) mutated gene does not appear on photographic film as the probe has complementarity with it
(b) mutated gene partially appears on a photographic film
(c) mutated gene completely and clearly appears on a photographic film
(d) mutated gene does not appear on a photographic film as the probe has no complementarity with it.

36. For effective treatment of the disease, early diagnosis and understanding its pathophysiology is very important. Which of the following molecular diagnostic techniques is very useful for early detection? ***(2021)***
(a) Hybridization Technique
(b) Western Blotting Technique
(c) Southern Blotting Technique
(d) ELISA Technique

37. With regard to insulin choose correct options. ***(2021)***
(A) C-peptide is not present in mature insulin.
(B) The insulin produced by rDNA technology has C-peptide.
(C) The pro-insulin has C-peptide.
(D) A-peptide and B-peptide of insulin are interconnected by disulphide bridges.

Choose the correct answer from the options given below.
(a) (A) and (D) only (b) (B) and (D) only
(c) (B) and (C) only (d) (A), (C) and (D) only

38. The Adenosine deaminase deficiency results into ***(2021)***
(a) addison's disease
(b) dysfunction of immune system
(c) parkinson's disease
(d) digestive disorder.

39. Match the following columns and select the correct option. ***(2020)***

Column-I	Column-II
(A) Bt cotton	(i) Gene therapy
(B) Adenosine deaminase deficiency	(ii) Cellular defence
(C) RNA i	(iii) Detection of HIV infection
(D) PCR	(iv) Bacillus thuringiensis

	A	B	C	D
(a)	(iv)	(i)	(ii)	(iii)
(b)	(iii)	(ii)	(i)	(iv)
(c)	(ii)	(iii)	(iv)	(i)
(d)	(i)	(ii)	(iii)	(iv)

40. Which of the following statements is not correct? ***(2020)***
(a) In man insulin is synthesised as a proinsulin.
(b) The proinsulin has an extra peptide called C-peptide.
(c) The functional insulin has A and B chains linked together by hydrogen bonds.
(d) Genetically engineered insulin is produced in E.coli.

41. Which kind of therapy was given in 1990 to a four year-old girl with adenosine deaminase (ADA) deficiency? ***(NEET-II 2016)***
(a) Gene therapy (b) Chemotherapy
(c) Immunotherapy (d) Radiation therapy

42. The two polypeptides of human insulin are linked together by ***(NEET-I 2016)***
(a) covalent bond
(b) disulphide bridges
(c) hydrogen bonds
(d) phosphodiester bond.

43. The first human hormone produced by recombinant DNA technology is ***2014)***
(a) insulin (b) estrogen
(c) thyroxin (d) progesterone.

44. Which one of the following vectors is used to replace the defective gene in gene therapy? ***(Karnataka NEET 2013)***
(a) Adenovirus (b) Cosmid
(c) Ri plasmid (d) Ti plasmid

45. The first clinical gene therapy was given for treating ***(Mains 2012)***
(a) diabetes mellitus
(b) chicken pox
(c) rheumatoid arthritis
(d) adenosine deaminase deficiency.

46. Which one of the following is now being commercially produced by biotechnological procedures? ***(Mains 2010)***
(a) Nicotine (b) Morphine
(c) Quinine (d) Insulin

47. The genetic defect-adenosine deaminase (ADA) deficiency may be cured permanently by ***(2009)***
(a) administering adenosine deaminase activators
(b) introducing bone marrow cells producing ADA into cells at early embryonic stages
(c) enzyme replacement therapy
(d) periodic infusion of genetically (engineered lymphocytes having functional ADA cDNA.

48. Human insulin is being commercially produced from a transgenic species of ***(2008)***
(a) Rhizobium (b) Saccharomyces
(c) Escherichia (d) Mycobacterium.

49. ELISA is used to detect viruses where the key reagent is ***(2004,2003)***
(a) alkaline phosphatase
(b) catalase
(c) DNA probe
(d) RNase.

50. Maximum application of animal cell culture technology today is in the production of ***(2003)***
(a) insulin (b) interferons
(c) vaccines (d) edible proteins.

51. The term 'humulin' is used for ***(1999)***
(a) hydrolytic enzyme (b) powerful antibiotic
(c) human insulin (d) isoenzyme.

52. Hybridoma cells are ***(1999)***
(a) only cells having oncogenes
(b) product of spore formation in bacteria
(c) nervous cells of frog
(d) hybrid cells resulting from myeloma cells.

TRANSGENIC ANIMALS

53. Maximum number of existing transgenic animals is of ***(2011)***
(a) fish (b) mice (c) cow (d) pig.

54. Read the following four statements (A-D) about certain mistakes in two of them. ***(Mains 2011)***
(A) The first transgenic buffalo, Rosie produced milk which was human alpha-lactalbumin enriched.
(B) Restriction enzymes are used in isolation of DNA from other macromolecules.
(C) Downstream processing is one of the steps of r DNA technology.
(D) Disarmed pathogen vectors are also used in transfer of r DNA into the host.

Which of the two statements have mistakes?
(a) B and C (b) C and D
(c) A and C (d) A and B

55. Genetic engineering has been successfully used for producing ***(2010)***
(a) transgenic mice for testing safety of polio vaccine before use in humans
(b) transgenic models for studying new treatments for certain cardiac diseases
(c) transgenic cow-Rosie which produces high fat milk for making ghee
(d) animals like bulls for farm work as they have super power

56. Production of a human protein in bacteria by genetic engineering is possible because ***(2005)***
(a) the human chromosome can replicate in bacterial cell
(b) the mechanism of gene regulation is identical in humans and bacteria
(c) bacterial cell can carry out the RNA splicing reactions
(d) the genetic code is universal.

57. In transgenics, expression of transgene in target tissue is determined by ***(2004)***
(a) enhancer (b) transgene
(c) promoter (d) reporter

58. The transgenic animals are those which have ***(1995)***
(a) foreign RNA in all its cells
(b) foreign DNA in some of its cells
(c) foreign DNA in all its cells
(d) both (a) and (b)

ETHICAL ISSUES

59. A 'new' variety of rice was patented by a foreign company, though such varieties have been present in India for a long time. This is related to ***(2018)***
(a) Co-667 (b) Sharbati Sonora
(c) Lerma Rojo (d) Basmati.

60. In India, the organisation responsible for assessing the safety of introducing genetically modified organisms for public use is ***(2018)***
(a) Indian Council of Medical Research (ICMR)
(b) Council for Scientific and Industrial Research (CSIR)
(c) Research Committee on Genetic Manipulation (RCGM)
(d) Genetic Engineering Appraisal Committee (GEAC).

61. Use of bioresources by multinational companies and organisations without authorisation from the concerned country and its people is called ***(2018)***
(a) bio-infringement (b) biopiracy
(c) biodegradation (d) bioexploitation.

62. Which body of the Government of India regulates GM research and safety of introducing GM organisms for public services? ***(2015 Cancelled)***
(a) Genetic Engineering Approval Committee
(b) Research Committee on Genetic Manipulation
(c) Bio-safety committee
(d) Indian Council of Agricultural Research

ANSWER KEY

1.	(b)	2.	(a)	3.	(d)	4.	(b)	5.	(a)	6.	(b)	7.	(b)
8.	(c)	9.	(b)	10.	(d)	11.	(b)	12.	(c)	13.	(a)	14.	(a)
15.	(a)	16.	(b)	17.	(a)	18.	(d)	19.	(b)	20.	(d)	21.	(a)
22.	(a)	23.	(a)	24.	(b)	25.	(b)	26.	(b)	27.	(b)	28.	(d)
29.	(d)	30.	(a)	31.	(d)	32.	(d)	33.	(b)	34.	(c)	35.	(d)
36.	(d)	37.	(d)	38.	(b)	39.	(a)	40.	(c)	41.	(a)	42.	(b)
43.	(a)	44.	(a)	45.	(d)	46.	(d)	47.	(b)	48.	(c)	49.	(a)
50.	(c)	51.	(c)	52.	(d)	53.	(b)	54.	(d)	55.	(a)	56.	(d)
57.	(d)	58.	(c)	59.	(d)	60.	(d)	61.	(b)	62.	(a)		

SOLUTION

1.(b) : Transposons or mobile genetic elements are used in gene silencing for the source of the complementary RNA

2.(a) : Bt cotton is resistance to cotton bollworm infestation. The genes cry I Ac and cry II Ab control cotton bollworms, thus acts as bio-pesticide.

3.(d) : Some strains of Bacillus thuringiensis produce proteins that kill certain insects such as lepidopterans and dipterans. B. thuringiensis forms protein crystals during a particular phase of their growth. These crystals contain a toxic insecticidal protein which exists as inactive protoxins but once an insect ingest the inactive toxin, it is converted into an active form of toxin due to the alkaline pH of the gut which solubilise the crystals.

4.(b) : Rice is a staple food in many countries, particularly in Asia, but does not contain vitamin A or its immediate precursors. By inserting two genes from daffodil and one gene from a bacterial species into rice plants, Swiss researchers have produced rice capable of synthesising β-carotene, the precursor of vitamin A. Vitamin A is required by all individuals as it is present in retina of eyes. Deficiency of vitamin A causes night blindness and skin disorders. This rice is called 'Golden rice' because of yellow colour of rice grains due to the presence of β-carotene.

5. (a)

6.(b) : Meloidogyne incognitia is a nematode which infects the roots of the tobacco plants and causes a great reduction in the yield.

7.(b) : Golden rice is a transgenic variety of rice (Oryza sativa) which contains good quantities of β-carotene (provitamin A - inactive state of vitamin A). β-carotene is a principal source of vitamin A. Since the grains of this rice is yellow in colour due to β-carotene, it is commonly called golden rice.

8. (c) : Soil bacterium Bacillus thuringiensis produces proteins that kill certain insects like lepidopterans (tobacco budworm, armyworm), coleopterans (beetles) and dipterans (flies, mosquitoes). B. thuringiensis forms some protein crystals. These crystals contain a toxic insecticidal protein. This toxin does not kill the Bacillus (bacterium) because it exists as inactive protoxins in them. But, once an insect ingests it, it is converted into an active form of toxin due to the alkaline pH of the alimentary canal. The activated toxin binds to the surface of midgut epithelial cells and create pores that cause swelling and lysis and finally cause death of the insect.

9.(b) : Glyphosate is a broad spectrum herbicide which especially kills broad leaved herbs. Crop plants may also get affected by the herbicide, thus now crop plants are genetically engineered for glyphosate resistance. So, when glyphosate herbicide is applied, only weeds and no crop plants get harmed.

10.(d) : Bt toxin genes were isolated from Bacillus thuringiensis and incorporated into the several crop plants such as cotton. The choice of genes depends upon the crop and targeted pest, as most Bt toxins are insect-group specific. The toxin is coded by a gene named cry. There are numerous genes. Two cry genes cry I Ac and cry II Ab have been incorporated in cotton. The genetically modified crop is called Bt cotton as it contains Bt toxin genes against cotton bollworms.

11.(b) : RNA interference (RNAi) is the phenomenon of inhibiting activity of a gene through production of both sense and antisense RNA. RNAi takes place in all eukaryotic organisms as a method of cellular defense. This method involves a specific m RNA silencing. It is due to a complementary RNA molecule which binds to and prevents translation of the mRNA causing its silencing.

12. (c)

13.(a) : Many nematodes live in plants and animals including human beings. A nematode Meloidogyne incognitia infests the roots of tobacco plants and causes a great reduction in yield. A novel strategy was adopted to prevent this infection that was based on the process of RNA interference (RNAi). RNA interference (RNAi) is the phenomenon of inhibiting activity of a gene by synthesis of RNA molecules complementary to the m RNA. The normal (in vivo synthesized) m RNA of a gene is said to be "sense" because it carries the codons that are "read" during translation. Normally, the complement to the mRNA "sense" strand will not contain a sequence of codons that can be translated to produce a functional protein; thus, this complementary strand is called "anti-sense RNA". The antisense RNA and m RNA molecules will anneal to form duplex RNA molecules (or double stranded RNA) and the duplex RNA molecules can not be translated. Thus, the presence of antisense RNA will block translation of the mRNA of the affected gene.

14. (a)

15.(a) : B. thuringiensis forms some protein crystals. These crystals contain a toxic inactive insecticidal protein. When an insect ingests it, it is converted into an active form of toxin. The activated toxin binds to the surface of midgut epithelial cells and create pores that cause swelling and lysis and finally cause death of the insect.

16. (b)

17.(a) : The genetically modified (GM) Bt brinjal in India has been developed mainly for insect resistance. Through genetic engineering Bt toxin genes were isolated from Bacillus thuringiensis and incorporated into the several crop plants such as cotton, brinjal, etc.

18.(d) : Bt toxin genes were isolated from Bacillus thuringiensis and incorporated into cotton plant. The genetically modified crop is called Bt cotton. Bt cotton has the following useful characteristics: pest resistance, herbicide tolerance, high yield and resistance to boll worm infestation.

19. (b)

20. (d)

21.(a) : The plants produced through genetic engineering contain gene or genes usually from an unrelated organism. Such genes are called transgenes and the plants having transgenes are called transgenic plants. Recombinant DNA techniques are being used to improve crop plants by increasing their productivity, by making them more nutritious and by developing disease resistance. Transgenic plants may have resistance to herbicides, pests and abiotic stresses.

22.(a) : Some strains of Bacillus thuringiensis produce proteins that kill certain insects such as lepidopterans and dipterans.

23. (a)

24. (b)

25. (b)

26.(b) : Genetic engineering has helped to develop such transgenic crop plants which are resistant to herbicides so that they are not damaged when farmers spray herbicides in the fields. Herbicide resistant plants have been developed in such a way that they continue to produce normal crop yield and at the same time remain unaffected by the activity of herbicides. These plants also reduces the use of weeding labour, farmer's cost and increases yield.

27.(b) : Golden rice is a transgenic variety of rice (Oryza sativa) which contains good quantities of β-carotene. β-carotene is a principal source of vitamin A, so it will help in alleviation of vitamin A deficiency.

28.(d) : Bacillus thuringiensis strains have been used for designing bio-insecticidal plants. A gene from this bacteria have insecticidal property which is transferred to cotton plants to produce Bt cotton which is resistant to bollworm insect which is a major pest of cotton. Similarly, insects affecting maize; cabbage, sunflower, etc., are also controlled by mutant strains of Bacillus thuringiensis bacteria.

29.(d) : Golden rice is a transgenic crop rice with high vitamin A content. It has been developed by transferring beta carotene synthesizing gene into the transgenic rice. Beta carotene is the precursor of vitamin A. This transgenic rice has been crossed with the already adapted varieties of rice to make them grow well in a particular area. It is very useful for the people suffering from vision impairment due to vitamin A deficiency.

30.(a) : Transgenic plants are those plants in which a foreign gene has been introduced and stably integrated into host DNA. The first transgenic plants were produced in tobacco (Nicotiana tabacum). A gene resistant to PPT (L-phosphinothricin), an active ingredient of herbicide 'Basta', was isolated from Medicago sativa. It inhibits the enzyme GS (glutamine synthase) which is involved in ammonia assimilation. This gene resistant to PPT was incorporated into tobacco, as a result of which transgenic tobacco was produced which was resistant to PPT.

31.(d) : Serum and urine analysis are conventional methods of diagnosis, through which early detection is not possible.

32.(d) : In gene therapy for ADA deficiency, lymphocytes from patient's blood are grown in culture outside the body. A functional ADA cDNA is then introduced into these lymphocytes, which are subsequently returned to patient. As these cells are not immortal, thus patient requires periodic infusion of genetically engineered lymphocytes.

33. (b)

34.(c) : Gene therapy is a collection of methods which allows genes to be inserted into a person's cells and tissues to treat a disease.

35.(d) : PCR is used to detect mutations in gene in suspected cancer patients. A single stranded DNA or RNA tagged with a radioactive molecule (probe) is allowed to hybridise to its complementary DNA in a clone of cells followed by detection using autoradiography. The clone having the mutated gene will hence not appear on the photographic film, because the probe will not have complementarity with the mutated gene.

36.(d) : Enzyme Linked Immuno-Sorbent Assay (ELISA) is one of the techniques that serve the purpose of early diagnosis of disease.

37.(d) : The insulin produced by rDNA technology does not contain C peptide.

38.(b) : Adenosine deaminase deficiency (ADA) caused due to deletion of the gene for enzyme adenosine deaminase causes SCID which results in dysfunctioning of immune system.

39. (a)

40.(c) : Insulin consists of two short polypeptide chains : Chain A and chain B, that are linked together by disulphide bridges.

41.(a) : Gene therapy is a technique of genetic engineering which involves replacement of a faulty/disease causing gene by a normal healthy functional gene. The first clinical gene therapy was given in 1990 to a 4-year old girl with adenosine deaminase (ADA) deficiency. This enzyme is very important for the immune system to function. The deficiency of this enzyme can lead to severe combined immune deficiency (SCID).

42.(b) : Human insulin is made up of 51 amino acids arranged in two polypeptide chains. Chain A has 21 amino acids and chain B has 30 amino acids. The two polypeptide chains are interconnected by disulphide bridges or S-S-linkages.

43.(a) : The recombinant DNA technological processes have made great impact in the area of health care by mass production of safe and more effective therapeutic drugs. In 1983, Eli Lily, an American company, first prepared two DNA sequences corresponding to A and B chains of human insulin and introduced them in plasmids of Escherichia coli to produce insulin chains. Chains A and B were produced separately, extracted and combined by creating disulphide bonds to form human insulin (humulin).

44.(a) : Gene therapy is a corrective therapy that is given to patients with diseases caused by some gene defects. Here, genes are inserted into a person's cells and tissues to treat disease by replacing the defective gene. The normal gene delivered into the individual or embryo takes over the function and compensate for the non-functional gene. Viral vectors like adenovirus are generally used to deliver the normal gene.

45.(d) : Gene therapy is a collection of methods that allows correction of a gene defect that has been diagnosed in a child/ embryo. Here genes are inserted into a person's cells and tissues to treat a disease. Correction of a genetic defect involves delivery of a normal gene into the individual or embryo to take over the function of and compensate for the non-functional gene. The first clinical gene therapy was given in 1990 to a 4 - year old girl with adenosine deaminase (ADA) deficiency. This enzyme is very important for the immune system to function. SCID is caused due to defect in the gene for the enzyme adenosine deaminase. In some children ADA deficiency can be cured by bone marrow transplantation. Here, the isolated gene from bone marrow cells producing ADA is introduced into cells at early embryonic stages; it can be a permanent cure.

46.(d) : Insulin is now being commercially produced by genetic engineering. Insulin consists of two short polypeptide chains: chain A and chain B, that are linked together by disulphide bonds. Insulin, in mammal is synthesised as a prohormone which contains an extra stretch called the C-peptide. During maturation this C-peptide is removed. The major problem for production of insulin using rDNA technique was getting insulin assembled in mature form.

This problem was solved in 1988 by Eli Lilly, an American company which prepared functionable insulin from two DNA sequences corresponding to A and B chains of human insulin and introduced them in plasmids of *E.coli* to produce insulin chains. In this way, chains A and B were produced separately which was extracted and combined by creating disulphide bonds to get human insulin.

47.(b) : ADA deficiency can be permanently cured if the isolated gene from bone marrow cells producing ADA is introduced into cells at early embryonic stages.

48.(c) : Insulin is now being commercially produced by genetic engineering with the help of E.coli bacteria.

49.(a) : ELISA (enzyme linked immunosorbent assay) screening test is the initial test to diagnose. AIDS. The test works by detecting antibodies/ substances or protein which are produced in the blood when virus is present. Alkaline phosphatase and peroxidases are commonly used enzymes as key reagent to perform the ELISA test. These enzymes are used to provide antibody-antigen complex in a specialised ELISA plate or tray. In ELISA test for detecting a particular antigen, its antibody is buffered and a drop of serum (supernatant of centrifuged blood) poured over it. If the latter contains antigen, it will produce antigen-antibody complex. A second enzyme labelled antibody is added. It forms enzyme antigen-antibody complex, if the antigen is present. Substrate is now added. It produces a stain if the antigen is present.

50.(c) : Maximum application of animal cell culture technology is in the production of vaccines. Vaccines are chemical substances prepared from the proteins of other animals which confer immunity to a particular virus. Some of the vaccines synthesized biologically through genetic engineering are vaccines for hepatitis-B virus, vaccines for rabies virus, vaccines for poliovirus and vaccines for small pox virus, etc.

51.(c) : Human insulin (humulin) is the first therapeutic product produced by means of recombinant DNA technology by Eli lily and Co. on July 5, 1983

52. (d) : Hybridoma is hybrid cell resulting from the artificial fusion of an antibody-producing lymphocyte and a myeloma cell from a lymphoid tumour. Such cells can produce a clone that may be maintained in tissue culture and used for the continuing production of monoclonal antibody.

53. (b)

54.(d) : In 1997, the first transgenic cow, Rosie, produced human protein enriched milk. The milk contained the human alpha-lactalbumin and was nutritionally a more balanced product for human babies than natural cow-milk.

Isolation of DNA from other macromolecule is achieved by treating the bacterial cells/plant or animal tissue with enzymes such as lysozyme (bacteria), cellulase (plant cells), chitinase (fungus).

55.(a) : Many transgenic animals are designed to increase our understanding of how genes contribute to the development of diseases. These are specially made to serve as models for human diseases so that investigation of new treatments for diseases is made possible. Today transgenic models exist for many human diseases such as cancer, cystic fibrosis, rheumatoid arthritis and Alzheimer's. Transgenic mice are being developed for use in testing the safety of vaccines before they are used on humans. Transgenic mice are being used to test the safety of the polio vaccine.

56.(d) : Genetic code may be defined as the sequence of nucleotides in polynucleotide chain which determines the sequence of amino acids in a polypeptide chain. The genetic code is universal. It means that each codon codes for the same amino acid in all organisms including bacteria, plants and animals.

57.(d) : The plants, in which a functional foreign gene has been incorporated by any biotechnological methods that generally is not present in plant, are called transgenic plants. When plant cell are transformed by any of the transformation methods it is necessary to isolate the transformed cells/tissue. There are certain selectable marker genes present in vectors that facilitate the selection process. In transformed cells the selectable marker genes are introduced through vector. There is a number of marker genes which are commonly described as reporter genes screenable genes. Some of the reporter genes which are most commonly used in plant transformation are : cat, gus, lux, nptII., etc.

58.(c) : Transgenic organism is one that has become transformed following the introduction of novel genes into its genome. It is most frequently achieved by integration of cloned DNA sequences following their injection into the fertilized egg. This fertilized egg divides mitotically to form the whole organism so that all the cells of the organism will carry the transferred gene. The transferred genes are known as transgenes. Transgenesis can be done by microinjection and somatic cell nuclear transfer or cloning. Transgenic animals produced by this technology include mice, Drosophila, Xenopus and some of the fish species.

59.(d) : In 1997, a Texas company got patent rights on Basmati rice through the US Patent and Trademark Office. This allowed the company to sell a 'new' variety of Basmati, in the US and abroad. This new variety of Basmati had actually been derived from Indian farmers' varieties. Indian Basmati was crossed with semi-dwarf varieties and claimed as an invention or a novelty. It caused a brief diplomatic crisis between India and United States with India threatening to take the matter to WTO (World Trade Organisation) as a violation of TRIPS (Trade Related Aspects of Intellectual Property Rights). Both voluntarily and due to review decisions by United States patent office, Rice Tec lost most of the claims of the patent.

60.(d) : Indian government has set up organisation such as GEAC (Genetic Engineering Appraisal Committee) which makes decisions regarding the validity of GM research and safety of introducing GM organisms for public services.

61.(b) : Some organisations and multinational

companies exploit or patent biological resources or bioresources of other nations without proper authorisation from the countries concerned. This is called biopiracy.

62.(a) : Genetic modification of organisms can have unpredictable results, when such organisms are introduced into the ecosystem. Therefore, the Indian Government has set up organizations such as GEAC (Genetic Engineering Approval Committee), (now, changed as Genetic Engineering Appraisal Committee) which makes decisions regarding the validity of GM research and the safety of introducing GM-organisms for public services.

Chapter : 30

ORGANISMS AND POPULATIONS

ORGANISM AND ITS ENVIRONMENT

1. Match List-I with List- II. ***(2021)***

List - I	List - II
(p) Allen's Rule	(i) Kangaroo rat
(q) Physiological adaptation	(ii) Desert lizard
(r) Behavioural adaptation	(iii) Marine fish at depth
(s) Biochemical adaptation	(iv) Polar seal

Choose the correct answer from the options given below.

	p	q	r	s
(a)	(iv)	(iii)	(ii)	(i)
(b)	(iv)	(ii)	(iii)	(i)
(c)	(iv)	(i)	(iii)	(ii)
(d)	(iv)	(i)	(ii)	(iii)

2. Assertion (A) : A person goes to high altitude and experiences 'altitude sickness' with symptoms like breathing difficulty and heart palpitations.

Reason (R) : Due to low atmospheric pressure at high altitude, the body does not get sufficient oxygen. ***(2021)***

In the light of the above statements, choose the correct answer from the options given below.
(a) (A) is false but (R) is true.
(b) Both (A) and (R) are true and (R) is the correct explanation of (A).
(c) Both (A) and (R) are true but (R) is not the correct explanation of (A).
(d) (A) is true but (R) is false.

3. Niche is ***(2018)***
(a) all the biological factors in the organism's environment
(b) the physical space where an organism lives
(c) the range of temperature that the organism needs to live
(d) the functional role played by the organism where it lives.

4. Pneumatophores occur in ***(2018)***
(a) halophytes
(b) free-floating hydrophytes
(c) carnivorous plants
(d) submerged hydrophytes.

5. Plants which produce characteristic pneumatophores and show vivipary belong to ***(2017)***
(a) halophytes (b) psammophytes
(c) hydrophytes (d) mesophytes.

6. Presence of plants arranged into well defined vertical layers depending on their height can be seen best in ***(2017)***
(a) tropical rainforest (b) grassland
(c) temperate forest (d) tropical savannah.

7. It is much easier for a small animal to run uphill than for a large animal, because ***(NEET-I 2016)***
(a) small animals have a lower O_2 requirement
(b) the efficiency of muscles in large animals is less than in the small animals
(c) it is easier to carry a small body weight
(d) smaller animals have a higher metabolic rate.

8. An association of individuals of different species living in the same habitat and having functional interactions is ***(2015)***
(a) ecosystem (b) population
(c) ecological niche (d) biotic community.

9. Most animals are tree dwellers in a **(2015 Cancelled)**

(a) temperate deciduous forest
(b) tropical rainforest
(c) coniferous forest
(d) thorn woodland.

10. Just as a person moving from Delhi to Shimla to escape the heat for the duration of hot summer, thousands of migratory birds from Siberia and other extremely cold northern regions move to **(2014)**

(a) Western Ghat
(b) Meghalaya
(c) Corbett National Park
(d) Keoladeo National Park.

11. Which one of the following is not a parasitic adaptation? **(Karnataka NEET 2013)**

(a) Development of adhesive organs
(b) Loss of digestive organs
(c) Loss of reproductive capacity
(d) Loss of unnecessary sense organs

12. Benthic organisms are affected the most by **(Karnataka NEET 2013)**

(a) light reaching the forest floor
(b) surface turbulence of water
(c) sediment characteristics of aquatic ecosystems
(d) water-holding capacity of soil.

13. People who have migrated from the planes to an area adjoining Rohtang Pass about six months back **(2012)**

(a) have more RBCs and their haemoglobin has a lower binding affinity to O_2
(b) are not physically fit to play games like football
(c) suffer from altitude sickness with symptoms like nausea, fatigue, etc.
(d) have the usual RBC count but their haemoglobin has very high binding affinity to O_2.

14. Large woody vines are more commonly found in **(2011)**

(a) temperate forests (b) mangroves
(c) tropical rainforests (d) alpine forests.

15. Consider the following four conditions (1–4) and select a correct pair of them as adaptations to environment in desert lizards. **(2011)**

Conditions:

1. Burrowing in soil to escape high temperature.
2. Losing heat rapidly from the body during high temperature.
3. Bask in sun when temperature is low.
4. Insulating body due to thick fatty dermis.

(a) 3,4 (b) 1, 3 (c) 2,4 (d) 1,2

16. The figure given below is a diagrammatic representation of response of organisms to abiotic factors. What do (i), (ii) and (iii) represent respectively? **(2010)**

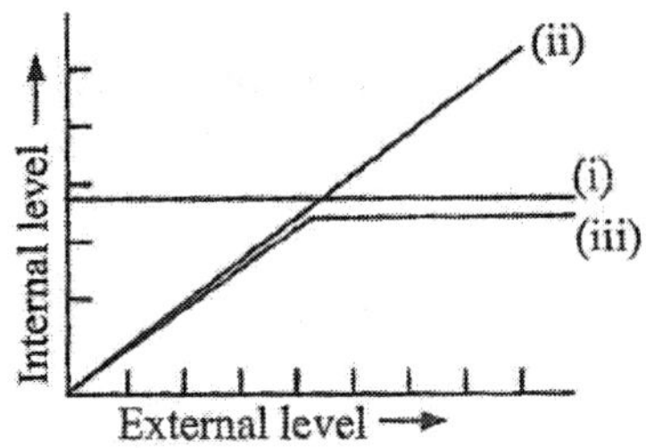

	(i)	(ii)	(iii)
(a)	Conformer	Regulator	Partial regulator
(b)	Regulator	Partial regulator	Conformer
(c)	Partial regulator	Regulator	Conformer
(d)	Regulator	Conformer	Partial regulator

17. Reduction in vascular tissue, mechanical tissue and cuticle is characteristic of **(2009)**

(a) mesophytes (b) epiphytes
(c) hydrophytes (d) xerophytes.

18. Consider the following four statements (1-4) about certain desert animals such as kangaroo, rat. ***(2008)***
(1) They have dark colour and high rate of reproduction and excrete solid urine.
(2) They do not drink water, breathe at a slow rate to conserve water and have their body covered with thick hairs.
(3) They feed on dry seeds and do not require drinking water.
(4) They excrete very concentrated urine and do not use water to regulate body temperature.

Which two of the above statements for such animals are true?
(a) 3 and 1 (b) 1 and 2
(c) 3 and 4 (d) 2 and 3

19. Quercus species are the dominant component in ***(2008)***
(a) scrub forests
(b) tropical rainforests
(c) temperate deciduous forests
(d) alpine forests.

20. Niche overlap indicates ***(2006)***
(a) mutualism between two species
(b) active cooperation between two species
(c) two different parasites on the same host
(d) sharing of one or more resources between the two species.

21. People living at sea level have around 5 million RBC per cubic millimeter of their blood whereas those living at an altitude to 5400 metres have around 8 million. This is because at high altitude ***(2006)***
(a) people eat more nutritive food, therefore more RBCs are formed
(b) people get pollution-free air to breath and more oxygen is available
(c) atmospheric O_2 level is less and hence more RBCs are needed to absorb the required amount of O_2 to survive
(d) there is more UV radiation which enhances RBC production.

22. Annual migration does not occur in the case of ***(2006)***
(a) arctic tern (b) salmon
(c) siberian crane (d) salamander.

23. Praying mantis is a good example of ***(2006)***
(a) camouflage
(b) mullerian mimicry
(c) warning colouration
(d) social insects

24. More than 70% of world's freshwater is contained in ***(2005)***
(a) polar ice
(b) glaciers and mountains
(c) Antarctica (d) Greenland.

25. Animals have the innate ability to escape from predation. Examples for the same are given below. Select the incorrect example. ***(2005)***
(a) Colour change in Chamaeleon
(b) Enlargement of body size by swallowing air in puffer fish
(c) Poison fangs in snakes
(d) Melanism in moths

26. Which one of the following pairs is mismatched? ***(2005)***
(a) Tundra – Permafrost
(b) Savanna – Acacia trees
(c) Prairie – Epiphytes
(d) Coniferous forest- Evergreen trees

27. In which one of the following habitats does the diurnal temperature of soil surface vary most? ***(2004)***
(a) Shrub land (b) Forest
(c) Desert (d) Grassland

28. What is true for individuals of same species? ***(2002)***
(a) Live in same niche
(b) Live in same habitat
(c) Interbreeding
(d) Live in different habitat

29. Cause of mimicry is ***(2002)***
(a) concealment (b) offence
(c) defence (d) both (b) and (c).

30. Which part of the world has a high density of organisms? ***(1999)***
(a) Deciduous forests
(b) Tropical rainforests
(c) Grasslands
(d) Savannah

31. In desert grasslands, which type of animals are relatively more abundant? ***(1998)***
(a) Aquatic (b) Fossorial
(c) Diurnal (d) Arboreal

32. Plants such as *Prosopis*, *Acacia* and *Capparis* represent examples of tropical ***(1998)***
(a) deciduous forests (b) evergreen forests
(c) grasslands (d) thorn forests.

33. Which of the following communities is more vulnerable to invasion by outside animals and plants? ***(1998)***
(a) Temperate forests
(b) Oceanic island communities
(c) Mangroves
(d) Tropical evergreen forests

34. Benthic animals are those, which ***(1996)***
(a) are submerged in area
(b) float on the sea surface
(c) are deep dweller in sea
(d) are floating (free) organisms.

35. The 'niche' of a species is meant for ***(1996)***
(a) habitat and specific functions of a species
(b) specific place where an organism lives
(c) specific species function and its competitive power
(d) none of these.

36. The animals of cold countries have relatively shorter and poorly developed ears, eyes, hairs and other phenotypic characters. This is known by which law? ***(1996)***
(a) Cope's Law (b) Dollo's Law
(c) Allen's Law (d) Bergamann's Law

37. Study of inter-relationships between organisms and their environment is ***(1993)***
(a) ecology (b) ecosystem
(c) phytogeography (d) ethology.

38. The sum total of the populations of the same kind of organisms constitute ***(1993)***
(a) colony (b) genus
(c) community (d) species.

39. Homeostasis is ***(1991)***
(a) tendency of biological systems to change with change in environment
(b) tendency of biological systems to resist change
(c) disturbance of self regulatory system and natural controls
(d) biotic materials used in homeopathic medicines.

40. Deep black soil is productive due to high proportion of ***(1991)***
(a) sand and zinc
(b) gravel and calcium
(c) clay and humus
(d) silt and earthworm.

POPULATIONS

41. Match List I with List II : ***(2023)***

List I (Interaction)	List II (Species A and B)
A. Mutualism	I. + (A), 0 (B)
B. Commensalism	II. – (A), 0 (B)
C. Amensalism	III. + (A), – (B)
D. Parasitism	IV. + (A), + (B)

Choose the correct answer from the options given below :
(a) A-IV, B-III. C-I. D-II
(b) A-III, B-I, C-IV, D-II
(c) A-IV, B-II C-I, D-III
(d) A-IV, B-I, C-II, D-III

42. Given below are two statements : ***(2023)***

Statement I : Gause's 'Competitive Exclusion Principle' states that two closely related species competing for the same resources cannot co-exist indefinitely and competitively inferior one will be eliminated eventually.

Statement II : In general, carnivores are more adversely affected by competition than herbivores.

In the light of the above statements,choose the correct answer from the options given below:
(a) Statement I is correct but Statement II is false.
(b) Statement I is incorrect but Statement II is true.
(c) Both Statement I and Statement II are true.
(d) Both Statement I and Statement II are false.

43. Match List I with List II. ***(2023)***

List I	**List II**
A. Logistic growth	I. Unlimited resource availability condition
B. Exponential growth	II. Limited resource availability condition
C. Expanding age pyramid	III. The percent individuals growth of prereproductive age is largest followed by reproductive and post reproductive age groups
D. Stable age pyramid	IV. The percent individuals of pre-reproductive and reproductive age group are same

Choose the correct answer from the options given below:
(a) A-II, B-IV, C-I, D-III
(b) A-II, B-IV, C-III, D-I
(c) A-II, B-I, C-III, D-IV
(d) A-II, B-III, C-I, D-IV

44. Match List I with List II ***(2023)***

List I (Interacting species)	**List II (Name of Interaction)**
A. A Leopard and a lion in a forest/ grassland	I. Competition
B. A cuckoo laying egg in a Crow's nest	II. Brood parasitism
C. Fungi and root of a higher plant in mycorrhizae	III. Mutualism
D. A cattle egret and a IV Commensalism cattle in a field	IV. Commensalism

Choose the correct answer from the options given below:
(a) A-III, B-IV, C-I, D-II
(b) A-II, B-III, C-I, D-IV
(c) A-I, B-II, C-III, D-IV
(d) A-I, B-II, C-IV, D-III

45. Which one of the following statements cannot be connected to predation? ***(2022)***
(a) It helps in maintaining species diversity in a community
(b) It might lead to extinction of a species.
(c) Both the interacting species are negatively impacted.
(d) It is necessitated by nature to maintain the ecological balance.

46. While explaining interspecific interaction of population, (+) sign is assigned for beneficial interaction, (-) sign is assigned for detrimental interaction and (0) for neutral interaction. Which of the following interactions can be assigned (+) for one species and (-) for another species involved in the interaction? ***(2022)***
(a) Predation (b) Amensalism
(c) Commensalism (d) Competition

47. If '8' *Drosophila* in a laboratory population of '80' died during a week, the death rate in the population is ____ individuals per Drosophila per week. ***(2022)***
(a) 0.1 (b) 10 (c) 1.0 (d) zero

48. Inspite of interspecific competition in nature, which mechanism the competing species might have evolved for their survival? ***(2021)***
(a) Predation
(b) Resource partitioning
(c) Competitive release
(d) Mutualism

49. Amensalism can be represented as ***(2021)***
(a) Species A (+); Species B (0)
(b) Species A (-); Species B (0)
(c) Species A (+); Species B (+)
(d) Species A (-) ; Species B (–).

50. In the exponential growth equation $N_t = N_0e^{rt}$, e represents ***(2021)***
(a) the base of geometric logarithms
(b) the base of number logarithms
(c) the base of exponential logarithms
(d) the base of natural logarithms.

51. Which of the following is not an attribute of a population? ***(2020)***
(a) Sex ratio (b) Natality
(c) Mortality (d) Species interaction

52. Carnivorous animals lions and leopards, occupy the same niche but. lions predate mostly larger animals and leopards take smaller ones. This mechanism of competition is referred to as ***(Odisha NEET 2019)***
(a) character displacement
(b) altruism
(c) resource partitioning
(d) competitive exclusion.

53. Between which among the following, the relationship is not an example of commensalism? ***(Odisha NEET 2019)***
(a) Orchid and the tree on which it grows
(b) Cattle Egret and grazing cattle
(c) Sea Anemone and Clown fish
(d) Female wasp and fig species

54. Natality refers to ***(2018)***
(a) death rate
(b) birth rate
(c) number of individuals leaving the habitat
(d) number of individuals entering a habitat.

55. Which one of the following plants shows a very close relationship with a species of moth, where none of the two can complete its life cycle without the other? ***(2018)***
(a) Hydrilla (b) Yucca
(c) Banana (d) Viola

56. In a growing population of a country, ***(2018)***
(a) pre-reproductive individuals are more than the reproductive individuals
(b) reproductive individuals are less than the postreproductive individuals
(c) reproductive and pre-reproductive individuals are equal in number
(d) pre-reproductive individuals are less than the reproductive individuals.

57. Which one of the following population interactions is widely used in medical science for the production of antibiotics? ***(2018)***
(a) Commensalism (b) Mutualism
(c) Parasitism (d) Amensalism

58. Asymptote in a logistic growth curve is obtained when ***(2017)***
(a) $K = N$
(b) $K > N$
(c) $K < N$
(d) the value of 'r' approaches zero.

59. Mycorrhizae are the example of ***(2017)***
(a) amensalism (b) antibiosis
(c) mutualism (d) fungistasis.

60. Which of the following is correct for r-selected species? ***(NEET-II 2016)***
(a) Large number of progeny with small size
(b) Large number of progeny with large size
(c) Small number of progeny with small size
(d) Small number of progeny with large size

61. If '+' sign is assigned to beneficial interaction, '–' sign to detrimental and 'O' sign to neutral interaction, then the population interaction represented by '+''–' refers to ***(NEET-II 2016)***

(a) mutualism (b) amensalism
(c) commensalism (d) parasitism.

62. The principle of competitive exclusion was stated by ***(NEET-II 2016)***

(a) C. Darwin (b) G.F. Gause
(c) Mac Arthur (d) Verhulst and Pearl.

63. When does the growth rate of a population following the logistic model equal zero? The logistic model is given as dN/dt = rN(1-N/K) ***(NEET-I 2016)***

(a) when N/K equals zero
(b) when death rate is greater than birth rate
(c) when N/K is exactly one
(d) when N nears the carrying capacity of the habitat.

64. Gause's principle of competitive exclusion states that ***(NEET-I 2016)***

(a) no two species can occupy the same niche indefinitely for the same limiting resources
(b) larger organisms exclude smaller ones through competition
(c) more abundant species will exclude the less abundant species through competition
(d) competition for the same resources exclude species having different food preferences.

65. In which of the following interactions both partners are adversely affected? ***(2015)***

(a) Parasitism (b) Mutualism
(c) Competition (d) Predation

66. The following graph depicts changes in two populations (A and B) of herbivores in a grassy field. A possible reason for these changes is tha t ***(2015 Cancelled)***

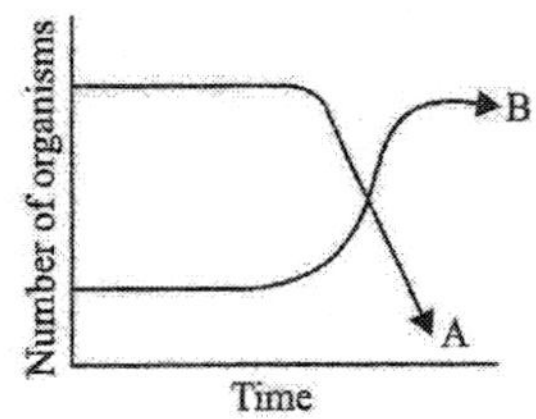

(a) population A produced more offspring than population B
(b) population A consumed the members of population B
(c) both plant populations in this habitat decreased
(d) population B competed more successfully for food than population A.

67. According to Darwin, the organic evolution is due to ***(2013)***

(a) competition within closely related species
(b) reduced feeding efficiency in one species due to the presence of interfering species
(c) intraspecific competition
(d) interspecific competition.

68. Besides paddy fields, cyanobacteria are also found inside vegetative part of ***(2013)***

(a) Equisetum (b) Psilotum
(c) Pinus (d) Cycas.

69. A sedentary sea anemone gets attached to the shell lining of hermit crab. The association is ***(2013)***

(a) commensalism (b) amensalism
(c) ectoparasitism (d) symbiosis.

70. A biologist studied the population of rats in a barn. He found that the average natality was 250, average mortality 240, immigration 20 and emigration 30. The net increase in population is ***(2013)***

(a) 05 (b) zero (c) 10 (d) 15

71. The age pyramid with broad base indicates ***(Karnataka NEET 2013)***

(a) high percentage of old individuals
(b) low percentage of young individuals
(c) a stable population
(d) high percentage of young individuals.

72. Cuscuta is an example of ***(Mains 2012)***
(a) ectoparasitism (b) brood parasitism
(c) predation (d) endoparasitism.

73. What type of human population is represented by the following age pyramid? ***(2011)***

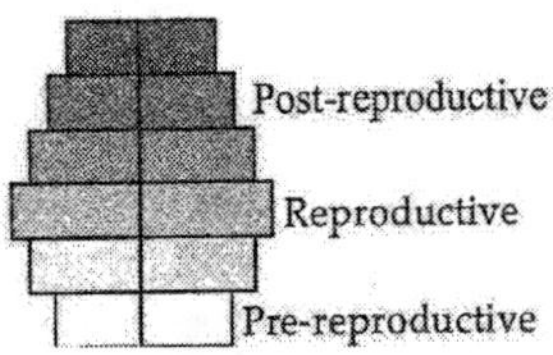

(a) Vanishing population
(b) Stable population
(c) Declining population
(d) Expanding population

74. Which one of the following is categorised as a parasite in true sense? ***(2011)***
(a) The female Anopheles bites and sucks blood from humans.
(b) Human fetus developing inside the uterus draws nourishment from the mother.
(c) Head louse living on the human scalp as well as laying eggs on human hair.
(d) The cuckoo (koel) lays its eggs in crow's nest.

75. The logistic population growth is expressed by the equation **(Mains 2011)**
(a) dt/dN=Nr((K-N)/K) (b) dN/dt=rN((K-N)/K)
(c) dN/dt=rN (d) dN/dt=rN((N-K)/N).

76. Which one of the following is most appropriately defined? ***(Mains 2010)***
(a) Host is an organism which provides food to another organism.
(b) Amensalism is a relationship in which one species is benefitted whereas the other is unaffected.
(c) Predator is an organism that catches and kills other organism for food.
(d) Parasite is an organism which always lives inside the body of other organism and may kill it.

77. A country with a high rate of population growth took measures to reduce it. The figure below shows age-sex pyramids of populations A and B twenty years apart. Select the correct interpretation about them. ***(2009)***

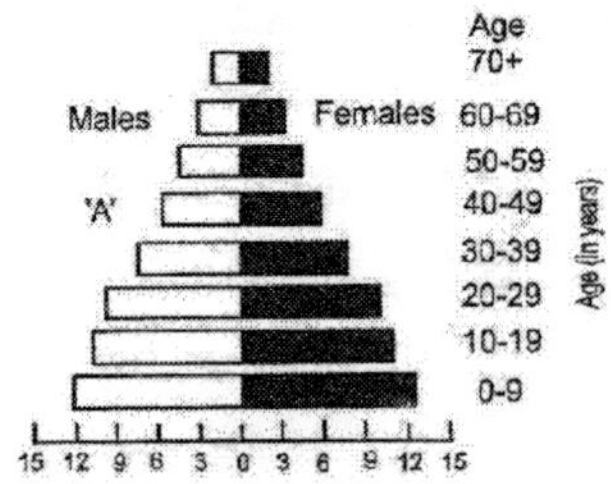

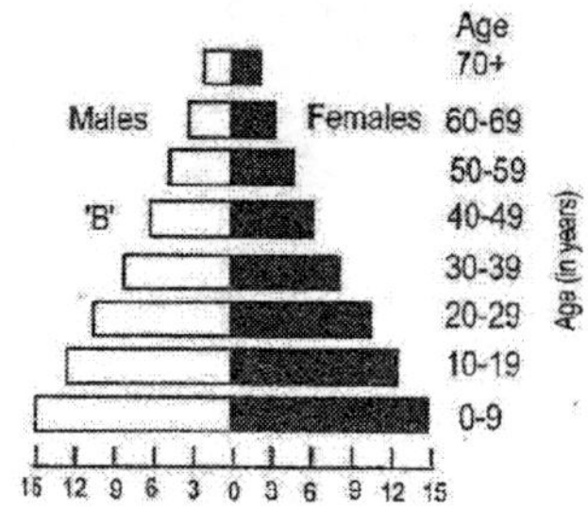

Interpretations:
(a) "B" is earlier pyramid and shows stabilized growth rate.
(b) "B" is more recent showing that population is very young.
(c) "A" is the earlier pyramid and no change has occurred in the growth rate.
(d) "A" is more recent and shows slight reduction in the growth rate.

78. Geometric representation of age structure is a characteristic of ***(2007)***
(a) population (b) landscape
(c) ecosystem (d) biotic community.

79. The population of an insect species shows an explosive increase in numbers during rainy season followed by its disappearance at the end of the season. What does this show? ***(2007)***
(a) The food plants mature and die at the end of the rainy season.
(b) Its population growth curve is of J-type.
(c) The population of its predators increases enormously.
(d) S-shaped or sigmoid growth of this insect.

80. If the mean and the median pertaining to a certain character of a population are of the same value, the following is most likely to occur ***(2007)***
(a) a bi-modal distribution
(b) a T-shaped curve
(c) a skewed curve
(d) a normal distribution.

81. A high density of elephant population in an area can result in ***(2007)***
(a) intraspecific competition
(b) interspecific competition
(c) predation on one another
(d) mutualism.

82. Certain characteristic demographic features of developing countries are ***(2004)***
(a) high fertility, low or rapidly falling mortality rate, rapid population growth and a very young age distribution
(b) high fertility, high density, rapidly rising mortality rate and a very young age distribution
(c) high infant mortality, low fertility, uneven population growth and a very young age distribution
(d) high mortality, high density, uneven population growth and a very old age distribution.

83. What is a keystone species? ***(2004)***
(a) A species which makes up only a small proportion of the total biomass of a community, yet has a huge impact on the community's organization and survival.
(b) A common species that has plenty of biomass, yet has a fairly low impact on the community's organization.
(c) A rare species that has minimal impact on the biomass and on other species in the community
(d) A dominant species that constitutes a large. proportion of the biomass and which affects many other species.

84. The maximum growth rate occurs in ***(2004)***
(a) stationary phase (b) senescent phase
(c) lag phase (d) exponential phase.

85. Mycorrhiza is an example of ***(2003)***
(a) symbiotic relationship
(b) ectoparasitism
(c) endoparasitism
(d) decomposers.

86. Which type of association is found in between entomophilous flower and pollinating agent? ***(2002)***
(a) Mutualism (b) Commensalism
(c) Co-operation (d) Co-evolution

87. Two different species cannot live for long duration in the same niche or habitat. This law is ***(2002)***
(a) Allen's law (b) Gause's hypothesis
(c) Dollo's rule (d) Weismann's theory.

88. In a population, unrestricted reproductive capacity is called as ***(2002)***
(a) biotic potential (b) fertility rate
(c) carrying capacity (d) birth rate.

89. In which of the following plant sunken stomata are found? ***(2001)***
(a) Nerium (b) Hydrilla
(c) Mango (d) Guava

90. An interesting modification of flower shape for insect pollination occurs in some orchids in which a male insect mistakes the pattern on the orchid flower for the female species and tries to copulate with it, thereby pollinating the flower. This phenomenon is called ***(1998)***
(a) pseudopollination
(b) pseudoparthenocarpy
(c) mimicry
(d) pseudocopulation.

91. Which one of the following pairs is correctly matched? ***(1995)***
(a) Parasitism - intraspecific relationship
(b) Uricotelism - aquatic habitat
(c) Excessive perspiration - xeric adaptation
(d) Streamlined body - aquatic adaptation

92. Mycorrhiza exhibits the phenomenon of ***(1994)***
(a) parasitism (b) symbiosis
(c) antagonism (d) endemism.

93. Association of animals when both partners are benefitted ***(1993)***
(a) colony (b) mutualism
(c) commensalism (d) ammensalism.

94. Which one is true? ***(1991)***
(a) Commensalism when none of the interacting populations affect each other.
(b) Symbiosis when the interaction is useful to both the populations.
(c) Symbiosis when neither populations affects each other.
(d) Commensalism when the interaction is useful to both the populations.

95. The relation between algae and fungi in a lichen is ***(1989)***
(a) symbiosis (b) parasitism
(c) commenalism (d) protocooperation.

96. A mutually beneficial association necessary for survival of both partners is ***(1988)***
(a) mutualism/symbiosis
(b) commensalism
(c) amensalism
(d) both (a) and (b).

97. Competition for light, nutrients and space is most severe between ***(1988)***
(a) closely related organism growing in different niches
(b) closely related organisms growing in the same area/niche
(c) distantly related organisms growing in the same habitat
(d) distantly related organisms growing in different niches.

ANSWER KEY

1.	(d)	2.	(b)	3.	(d)	4.	(a)	5.	(a)	6.	(a)	7.	(d)
8.	(d)	9.	(b)	10.	(d)	11.	(c)	12.	(c)	13.	(a)	14.	(c)
15.	(b)	16.	(d)	17.	(c)	18.	(c)	19.	(c)	20.	(d)	21.	(c)
22.	(d)	23.	(a)	24.	(a)	25.	(c)	26.	(c)	27.	(c)	28.	(c)
29.	(d)	30.	(b)	31.	(b)	32.	(d)	33.	(d)	34.	(c)	35.	(a)
36.	(c)	37.	(a)	38.	(d)	39.	(b)	40.	(c)	41.	(d)	42.	(a)
43.	(c)	44.	(c)	45.	(c)	46.	(a)	47.	(a)	48.	(b)	49.	(b)
50.	(d)	51.	(d)	52.	(c)	53.	(d)	54.	(b)	55.	(b)	56.	(a)
57.	(d)	58.	(a)	59.	(c)	60.	(a)	61.	(d)	62.	(b)	63.	(c)
64.	(a)	65.	(c)	66.	(d)	67.	(c)	68.	(d)	69.	(a)	70.	(b)
71.	(d)	72.	(a)	73.	(c)	74.	(c)	75.	(b)	76.	(c)	77.	(d)
78.	(a)	79.	(b)	80.	(d)	81.	(a)	82.	(a)	83.	(a)	84.	(d)
85.	(a)	86.	(d)	87.	(b)	88.	(a)	89.	(a)	90.	(d)	91.	(d)
92.	(b)	93.	(b)	94.	(b)	95.	(a)	96.	(a)	97.	(b)		

HINTS & EXPLANATIONS

1. (d)

2. (b) : A person going to high altitude experiences 'altitude sickness' with symptoms like breathing difficulty and heart palpitations because of low atmospheric pressure at high altitude, due to which body does not get enough oxygen.

3. (d) : Niche is specific part of habitat occupied by individuals of a species which is circumscribed by its range of tolerance, range of movement, microclimate, etc. Hence, niche refers to the functional role played by the organism where it lives.

4. (a) : Pneumatophores are breathing or respiratory roots which are found in plants growing in mangroves or water logged soil or saline swamps. Such plants are called halophytes.

5. (a) : Presence of pneumatophores, i.e., small negatively geotropic vertical roots and vivipary or seed germination while attached to plant are adaptations of halophytes, i.e., plants growing in saline habitat.

6. (a)

7. (d) : The small animals have smaller surface area to body volume ratio. They have higher metabolic rates than larger animals. Therefore, it is much easier for small animals to move uphill than large animals.

8. (d) : Biological or biotic community is an assemblage of populations of different species of plants, animals, bacteria and fungi which live in a particular area and interact with one another through competition, predation, mutualism, etc. Each biotic community has a specific composition and structure, e.g., pond community.

9. (b) : Tropical rainforests have a very dense plant cover. They also experience a large amount of precipitation, thus the forest floor is always damp. Thus, the conditions there have led animals to get adapted to arboreal habitats. Most animals found there are tree dwellers as almost every space on the forest floor is occupied by the vegetation.

10. (d)

11. (c) : Parasitism is a relationship between two living organisms of different species in which one organism called parasite obtains its food directly from another living organism called host. The parasite spends a part or whole of its life either on or inside the body of the host. The general parasitic adaptations are (i) anaerobic respiration in internal parasites, (ii) loss of certain organs, (iii) presence of adhesive organs, (iv) excessive multiplication, (v) resistant cysts and eggs for safe transfer of their progeny to new hosts and (vi) well developed and complicated reproductive organs.

12. (c) : Benthic organisms are bottom dwelling forms found crawling or attached to the bottom. The sediment characteristics often determine the type of benthic animals that can thrive there.

13. (a) : Tourists visiting high altitude areas such as Rohtang Pass or Mansarovar, experience altitude sickness. Its symptoms include nausea, fatigue and heart palpitations. This is because in the low atmospheric pressure of high altitudes, the body does not get enough oxygen. But, gradually we get acclimatized and stop experiencing altitude sickness. The body compensates low oxygen availability by increasing red blood cell production, decreasing the binding affinity of haemoglobin and by increasing breathing rate.

14. (c) : Lianas are large climbing woody vines that drape tropical rainforest trees. They have adapted to life in rainforest by having their roots in the ground and climbing high onto the tree canopy to reach available sunlight. Many lianas start life in the rainforest canopy and send roots down to the ground.

15. (b) : Desert lizards lack the physiological ability that mammals have to deal with the high temperature of their habitat, but manage to keep their body temperature fairly constant by behavioural means. They bask in the sun and absorb heat when their body temperature drops below the comfort zone, but move into shade when the ambient temperature starts increasing. Some species are capable of borrowing into the soil to hide and escape from the above-ground heat.

16. (d) : Some organisms are able to maintain homeostasis by physiological (sometimes behavioural also) means which ensures constant body temperature, constant osmotic concentration, etc. They are known as regulators. A majority of animals and plants cannot maintain a constant internal environment. Their body temperature changes with the ambient temperature. These animals and plants are simply conformers. During the course of evolution, the costs and benefits of maintaining a constant internal environment are taken into consideration. Some species have evolved the ability to regulate, but only over a limited range of environmental conditions, beyond which they simply conform. They are known as partial regulators.

17. (c) : In hydrophytes mechanical tissue, i.e., sclerenchyma, conducting tissue xylem, absorbing tissues are in reduced form or absent. Cuticle is either completely absent or if present it is thin and poorly developed.

18. (c) : Kangaroo rat (Dipodomys merriami) feeds on dry seeds. It seldom drinks water. The requirement of water is met by food (10%) and metabolic water (90%). Water loss is prevented by living in burrows during the day, concentration of urine and solidification of faeces. It has a thick coat to minimise evaporative desiccation.

19. (c) : Temperate broad leaf (deciduous) forests have warm summer and moderately cool winter. Rainfall is 100-250 cm. Dominant trees are oak, elm, birch, maple ash, chestnut, hickory, beech, poplar and Magnolia. Indian temperate broad leaves forests are dominated by oak like Quercus semecarpifolia (Brown oak of Himalayas, Khrsu oak), Q. floribunda (Tilonaj oak), Q. lanuginose (Rianj oak) and Q. leucotrichophora (Banj oak). Fauna of latitudinal temperate broad leaf forests consists of deer, fox, beaver, wild cat, racoon, etc.

20. (d) : Niche/ecological niche is specific part of habitat occupied by individuals of a species which is circumscribed by its range of tolerance, range of movement, microclimate, type of food and its availability, shelter, type of predator and timing of activity. A habitat has several ecological niches and supports a number of species. An ecological niche is used by a single species. Two or more species cannot use the same niche despite having a mutualistic association. Organisms or populations in competition have a niche overlap of a limited resource for which they compete. Both owl and cat feed on shrews and mice. They occupy the same niche because of being ecological equivalents though their habitats are different.

21. (c) : At high altitudes composition of air remains almost same as at sea level, but density (barometric pressure) of air gradually decreases due to which arterial pO2 is also decreased (hypoxemia). High altitudes has complex conditions to which human body has to acclimatize. Number of red blood cells per unit volume of blood is likely to be higher in a person living at high altitudes. This is in response to the air being less dense at high altitude. More number of red blood cells are needed to trap O2 from rarefied air having low pO2 (partial pressure of oxygen).

22. (d) : Migration is the seasonal movement of complete populations of animals to a more favourable environment. It is common in mammals (e.g., porpoises), fish (e.g., eels and salmon) and some insects but is most marked in birds. The arctic tern, for example, migrates annually from its breeding ground in the Arctic circle to the Antarctic. Salmon usually migrate from marine to fresh water to spawn. The siberian crane, breeds in arctic Russia in Yakutia and Western Siberia. It is a long distant migrant. Salamander is an amphibian with slender body, short legs and long tail. Outside the breeding season they are seldom seen as they spend most of their time underground.

23. (a) : Praying mantis shows the phenomenon of camouflage by blending itself into the background. This enables it to elude predators.

24. (a) : Nearly about 97% of the earth's water is saline in the oceans and seas. 3% of the earth's water is locked up on the polar ice caps. 85% of the frozen freshwater is in the Antarctic is ice cap, 15% of the frozen freshwater is in the northern polar ice cap and glaciers.

25.(c) : Colour change in Chameleon and melanism in moths are examples of camouflage in animals adapted to prevent predation from prey. As a defence mechanism puffers have the ability to inflate rapidly, filling their extremely elastic stomach with water (or air) until they are almost spherical. This prevents them from being identified by the predator. But poison fangs in snakes are a method adopted for preying and not escaping predation.

26.(c) : A biome is a major terrestrial community characterized by a distinct climate and inhabited by a particular species of plants and animals. Tundra is characterized by precipitation of less than 25 cm annually. Permafrost or permanent ice is found about a meter down from the surface, it never melts and is impenetrable to both water and roots. Savannahs are open grasslands with scattered shrubs and trees. Coniferous forest contain evergreen trees. In these forests all plants do not shed their leaves at the same time hence forest remains always evergreen. But Prairies is a grassland and epiphytes and ephemerals are found in deserts.

27.(c) : Deserts are places where the diurnal temperatures vary greatly. It is extremely hot during the day time and very cold at night. This change in temperature also affects the temperature condition of the soil.

28.(c) : Species may be defined as the uniform interbreeding population of individuals which freely interbreed among themselves. Niche represents the habitat and functions of a species. Habitat is a specific place where an organisms lives.

29.(d) : Mimicry is defined as the resemblance of one organism to another or to any natural object. It is specially evolved primarily for concealment and protection. Concealment itself may prove to be defensive and may also help in offence.

30.(b) : Tropical forests are found in tropical zone of the world and are characterized by very high temperature with rainfall in abundance. The flora of tropical rain forest is very rich and highly diversified. The tropical forests have a very rich fauna both in density as well as in varieties. The reason for this high diversity and variety of flora and fauna is the occurrence of suitable conditions in these forests.

31.(b) : Desert animals prefer to live under the surface. The animal residing either permanently or for most of life inside the burrows or under the earth surface are known as burrowing or fossorial animals and their mode of existence is described as subterranean or underground.

32.(d) : Tropical shrubs or thorn forests are found in places where moisture conditions are intermediate between desert and savanna on one hand and seasonal or rainforests on the other hand. Acacia and Prosopis are non-succulent perennial plants and Capparis is a xerophytic shrub.

33.(d) : Tropical forests are found in tropical zone of the world and are characterised by very high temperature with rainfall in abundance. The flora of tropical rain forest is very rich and highly diversified. The tropical forests have a very rich fauna both in density as well as in varieties. The reason for this high diversity and variety of flora and fauna is the occurrence of suitable conditions in these forests. So these are more vulnerable to invasion by outside plants and animals.

34.(c) : Benthic organisms are attached or rest on the bottom sediments. Benthic animal may be divided into filter feeders, e.g., clams and deposit feeders, e.g., snails.

35. (a)

36.(c) : Allen's law states, animals that live in very cold climates, their extremities such as ears, tails, etc., become progressively smaller. Cope's law states that there is a tendency for animals to increase in size during the long course of evolution. Dollo's law states that evolution is irreversible. Bergmann's law states that warm blooded animals become larger in the northern and colder parts of their range.

37.(a) : Ecology is the branch of science which deals with the study of inter-relationship between organisms and their environment. The scope of ecology is very vast as it treats the organisms at the level of population, community and ecosystem.

38.(d) : The sum total of the populations of the same kind of organisms constitute species. A species is a group of individuals of same kind of phenotypic characters and can interbreed.

39.(b) : The ability to maintain a steady state within constantly changing environment is essential for the survival of living systems. The maintenance of a constant internal environment is called homeostasis.

40.(c) : Deep black soil is productive due to high proportion of clay and humus. The organic matter present in the soil is contributed by the death and decay of living organisms. These are the richest in nutrients and therefore these soils are the most fertile.

41. (d)

List I (Interaction)	**List II (Species A and B)**
Mutualism	+ (A), + (B)
Commensalism	– (A), 0 (B)
Amensalism	– (A), 0 (B)
Parasitism	+ (A), – (B)

42.(a) : In general, herbivores and plants appear to be more adversely affected by competition than carnivores.

43. (c)

Logistic growth	Limited resource availability condition
Exponential growth	Unlimited resource availability condition
Expanding age pyramid	The percent individuals of pre-reproductive age is largest followed by reproductive and post reproductive age groups
Stable age pyramid	The percent individuals of pre-reproductive and reproductive age group are same

44.(c) : A leopard and a lion in a forest/grassland → Competition A cuckoo laying egg in a crow's nest → Brood parasitism Fungi and root of higher plant in mycorrhizae → Mutualism A cattle egret and a cattle in a field → Commensalism

45.(c) : In predation one species derives benefit while the other one is harmed. So, in this type of population interaction one species is positively impacted, whereas another one is negatively impacted.

46.(a) : In predation only one species benefits and other is harmed.

47.(a) : Death rate in the given population of Drosophila during given time interval is $\frac{8}{80} = 0.1$

48.(b) : If two species compete for the same resource, they could avoid competition by choosing different times for feeding or different foraging patterns. This is called resource partitioning.

49.(b) : Amensalism is an interaction in which one species is harmed and other is unaffected.

50.(d) : In the exponential growth equation, $N_t = N_0$ ert. Here e is base of natural logarithms (2.71828).

51. (d)

52. (c)

53.(d) : Female wasp and fig species shows example of mutualism.

54.(b) : Natality refers to the number of births during a given period in the population that are added to the initial density. Death rate or mortality is the number of deaths in the population during a given time period. Immigration is the number of individuals entering a habitat. Emigration is the number of individuals of the population that left the habitat and had gone elsewhere during a time period.

55.(b) : Yucca has an obligate mutualism with a species of moth, i.e., Pronuba. The only pollinator of this plant is the Yucca moth. The Yucca moth is likewise dependent upon the Yucca plant as Yucca moth caterpillars need to eat Yucca seed only or starve.

56.(a) : In a population where the number of pre-reproductive individuals or the younger individual is larger than the reproductive individuals, the population will increase.

57. (d) : Amensalism is a relationship between organisms of different species in which an organism does not allow other organism to grow or live near it. Inhibition is achieved through the secretion of chemicals called allochemics. Antibiotics are a kind of allochemics produced by some microbes which in small concentration can kill or retard growth of harmful microbes without adversely affecting the host.

58.(a) : Asymptote in a logistic growth curve is obtained when carrying capacity (K) reaches the population density (N), i.e., K – N.

59.(c) : Mycorrhiza is a mutualistic interaction between a fungus and roots of higher plants.

60.(a) : Organisms that are r-selected (r-strategists) able to colonise a habitat rapidly, utilising the food and other resources before other organisms are established and begin to compete. The r-strategists tend to be relatively small organisms with short life spans (e.g., bacteria) and often live in temporary or unstable environments; characteristically their survival depends on their ability to produce large numbers of offspring rather than on their ability to compete.

61.(d) : Parasitism is an association in which one organism (the parasite) lives on (ectoparasitism) or in (endoparasitism) the body of another organism (host), from which it obtains its nutrients. This association is beneficial for the parasites as they get continuous supply of nutrients from their host and are able to rapidly multiply their numbers. But it is detrimental for the host organism as parasitic infection leads to various complications and diseases in the host body may also be fatal to the host under certain circumstances.

62.(b)

63. (c)

64.(a) : Two or more species with closely similar niche requirements cannot exist indefinitely in the same area as sooner or later they come into competition for possession of it. This is called as Gause's principle of competitive exclusion, which states that an ecological niche cannot be simultaneously and completely occupied by established populations of more than one species. Two species can live in same habitat but not in the same niche. More similar the two niches are, severe the competition is.

65.(c) : Competition is the rivalry between two or more organisms for obtaining the same resources such as food, light, water, space, shelter, mate, etc. Competitors adversely affect each other.

66.(d) : Both the populations are herbivorous, thus they cannot affect each other. If the food sources for these populations A and B have decreased, then both the populations A and B would have declined. If population A have produced more offspring then the graph A should have increased. Based on the graph, population B is more successful in competing with population A, that is why number of organisms in population B increased while that in population A decreased, as they get access to limited resources.

67.(c) : Intraspecific competition leads to evolution. Variations arise naturally in a growing population due to crossing over, etc. Organisms with variations better suited to their environment are favoured by natural selection, while less fitted ones are eliminated. Gradually this continued process of natural selection leads to evolution. Interspecfic struggle also plays a role in evolution but intraspecific struggle is more intense and prominent one.

68.(d) : Coralloid roots of Cycas have symbiotic association with blue-green algae like Nostoc and Anabaena. Coralloid roots are irregular, negatively geotropic, dichotomously branched coral like roots which do not possess root hairs and root caps.

69. (a)

70.(b) : Natality and immigration positively contribute to the population growth while mortality and emigration are negative factors. In the given question.

The net increase in population is

natality + immigration =250 + 20 = 270

The net decrease in population is

mortality + emigration = 240 + 30 = 270

Thus, net increase in population =270-270=0

71.(d) : Age pyramid is a graphic representation of abundance of individuals of different age groups with pre-reproductive individuals at the base, reproductive individuals in the middle and post-reproductive individuals at the top. Triangular age pyramid has high proportion of pre-reproductive individuals, moderate number of reproductive individuals and fewer post-reproductive individuals. It represents young or rapidly growing population. In bell-shaped age pyramid, the number of pre-reproductive and reproductive individuals is almost equal. Post-reproductive individuals are comparatively fewer. It represents stable or stationary population where growth rate is nearly zero. In urnshaped age pyramid, the number of reproductive individuals is higher than the number of pre-reproductive individuals. It represents declining or diminishing population.

72.(a) : Cuscuta is a total stem parasite which is a good example of ectoparasitism. It is commonly found growing on hedge plants. It has lost chlorophyll and leaves in the course of evolution. It attaches and wraps itself around the stem of host plant and produces haustoria that gets inserted into the vascular system of host. The parasitic plant sucks all the nutrients from the host plant with the help of haustoria. Cuscuta is known to receive even the flower inducing hormone or florigen from the host.

73. (c)

74.(c) : Parasitism is an association in which one organism (the parasite) lives on (ectoparasitism) or in (endoparasitism) the body of another (the host), from which it obtains its nutrients. They also produce vast numbers of eggs there, e.g., head louse living on the human scalp.

75.(b) : Logistic population growth is expressed by following equation:

$$\frac{dN}{dt} = rN\left(\frac{K-N}{K}\right)$$

Where, N = population density at time t

r = intrinsic rate of natural increase

K = carrying capacity

76.(c) : Predation is an interaction between members of two species in which members of one species capture, kill and eat up members of other species. Host is a term which is specifically related to parasitism. Amensalism is an interspecies interaction in which one species is harmed whereas the other one is unaffected. Parasitic organism can live both over the surface of their host or inside their body.

77.(d) : "A" is more recent and shows slight reduction in growth rate.

78.(a) : Population has several characteristics or attributes which are a function of the whole group and not of an individual. Age distribution is one of them that is the number or the percentage of individuals in a population in different age groups. This is represented geometrically in the form of age pyramid.

79.(b) : J-shape of growth pattern can be easily observed in algae blooms, some insects, annual plants and the lemmings of Tundra. In the beginning density of the population increases rapidly in compound interest fashion and then stops abruptly as the environmental resistance or other limiting factors become effective. These factors may be food, space, seasonal (frost, excessive rain, etc.) or the termination of reproduction session.

80.(d) : If the mean and the median pertaining to a certain character of a population are of the same value, a normal distribution is most likely to occur.

81.(a) : Competition is rivalry for obtaining the same resource. Competition is of two types, intraspecific and interspecific. Intraspecific competition is the competition amongst members of the same species for a common resource. It may be for food, space and mate. So if the density of elephant population in an area increases, it will lead to intraspecific competition. This will lead to the establishment of territories in elephants which will result in pushing out of the extra number securing shelter, mate and food for the rest.

82.(a) : In developing countries, the conditions are becoming better for survival of human beings. So the mortality rate or the number of individuals dying per unit of time is low. Mortality or the average number of individuals produced by a population in a unit of time is high. So that there is rapid population growth and there are more individuals in the prereproductive age group. So there is young age distribution.

83.(a) : Keystone species are those species which has significant and disproportionately large influence on the community structure and characteristics. It has often considerably low abundance and biomass as compared to dominant species. Removal of such species causes serious disruption in structure and function of community.

84.(d) : Maximum growth rate occurs in exponential or acceleration or log phase. The point at which the exponential growth begins to slow down is known as inflexion point.

85.(a) : In mutalism or symbiosis both the organisms in association are mutually benefitted and further this association is obligatory, i.e., necessary for existence of both organisms. Mycorrhiza is a example of symbiosis. It is association between roots of higher plants and fungal hyphae. The fungal hyphae supply water and nutrients to the plant and in turn get food form the plant. So both the organism are mutually benefitted.

86.(d) : Co-evolution can occur in any interspecific relationship like symbiosis or mutualism. The relation between an entomophilous flower and pollinating insect shows co-evolved mutualism. In this the plant depends exclusively on the insect for pollination and the insect relies on the plant for food.

87.(b) : Interspecific competition is rivalry amongst members of different species. The severity of competition depends upon similarity in the requirement of food and shelter. Every type of organism has a particular niche, no two organisms can live in same niche. One of the two is eliminated. This phenomenon is called Gause hypothesis of competitive exclusion.

88.(a) : Biotic potential is defined as the physiological capacity of organisms to produce their offspring under natural conditions. It is also called reproductive potential. In nature, the biotic potential of organisms is enormous but all the organisms do not survive due to the lack of food and space. There are also a number of diseases and the predatory organisms, that feed upon other organisms. The carrying capacity is the maximum number of individuals which the environment can support or sustain.

89.(a) : Usually the stomata are placed at the same level as the adjoining epidermal cells (e.g., Helianthus, Mangifera). In xerophytes the stomata are sunken as they are located in a cupshaped depression (e.g., Nerium). It is an adaptation to reduce the loss of water in xerophytic plants.

90.(d) : In an orchid Ophrys speculum, there is most interesting and unique mechanism of pollination. Here pollination occurs by a wasp called Colpa aurea. In this orchid, pollination occurs by act of pseudocopulation. The appearance and odour of Ophrys is similar to female wasp and are mistaken by male wasps and they land on Ophrys flowers to perform act of pseudocopulation and thus pollination takes place. This plant-insect relationship is useful only to plant.

91.(d) : Streamlined body is a secondary aquatic adaptation. It is found in animals that live permanently in water but most of them are amphibious in nature. The streamlined body consists of compression of head, body and tail into a curved streamlined form. There is no protruberance over the body so that the animal can move easily through water. Parasitism is a relationship between two organisms of different species in which one organism called parasite obtains its food directly from another living organism called host. In xeric adaptation perspiration is reduced to conserve water. Uricotelism is characteristic of terrestrial animals which excrete uric acid.

92.(b) : Association between roots of higher plants, e.g., pine, birch and fungal hyphae is called mycorrhiza. It exhibits the phenomenon of symbiosis. Here both the organisms in association are mutually benefitted. In this, fungal hyphae

take nutrition from the plant and in return increase surface area for absorption of water and minerals for the plant. Parasitism is a phenomenon that involves a parasite which lives in constant association of the host and gets its food directly or indirectly without killing the host. Antagonism is the inhibition of growth of one organism by another. Endemism is the permanent occurrence of an organism inside another organism.

93.(b)

94. (b) : In mutalism or symbiosis both the organisms is association are mutually benefitted and further this association is obligatory, i.e., necessary for existence of both organisms.

95.(a) : Algae and fungi in a lichen show symbioti relationship. Fungi give support protection and help i absorption of water while algae provide food to fungi which : achlorophyllous. No one is harmed but both are benefitted t each other.

96. (a)

97. (b)

Chapter : 31

ECOSYSTEM

INTRODUCTION

1. The term ecosystem was coined by *(NEET-I 2016)*
   (a) E. Haeckel (b) E.Warming
   (c) E.P. Odum (d) A. G. Tansley.

ECOSYSTEM - STRUCTURE AND FUNCTION

2. Which one of the following is a characteristic feature of cropland ecosystem? *(NEET-I 2016)*
   (a) Absence of weeds
   (b) Ecological succession
   (c) Absence of soil organisms
   (d) Least genetic diversity

3. Vertical distribution of different species occupying different levels in a biotic community is known as *(2015 Cancelled)*
   (a) zonation (b) pyramid
   (c) divergence (d) stratification.

4. Which one of the following is not a functional unit of an ecosystem? *(2012)*
   (a) Energy flow (b) Decomposition
   (c) Productivity (d) Stratification

5. Which one of the following is one of the characteristics of a biological community? *(2010)*
   (a) Stratification (b) Natality
   (c) Mortality (d) Sex-ratio

6. Which of the following is the most stable ecosystem? *(1995)*
   (a) Mountain (b) Ocean
   (c) Forest (d) Desert

PRODUCTIVITY

7. In the equation *(2023)*
   GPP – R = NPP
   GPP is Gross Primary Productivity
   NPP is Net Primary Productivity
   R here is
   (a) respiratory loss
   (b) reproductive allocation
   (c) photosynthetically active radiation
   (d) respiratory quotient

8. In the equation, GPP – R = NPP *(2021)*
   R represents
   (a) respiration losses (b) radiant energy
   (c) retardation factor (d) environment factor

9. In relation to Gross primary productivity and Net primary productivity of an ecosystem, which one of the following statements is correct? *(2020)*
   (a) Gross primary productivity is always less than Net primary productivity.
   (b) Gross primary productivity is always more than Net primary productivity.
   (c) Gross primary productivity and Net primary productivity are one and same.
   (d) There is no relationship between Gross primary productivity and Net primary productivity.

10. The mass of living material at a trophic level at a particular time is called *(2015 Cancelled)*
    (a) net primary productivity
    (b) standing crop
    (c) gross primary productivity
    (d) standing state.

11. In an ecosystem the rate of production of organic matter during photosynthesis is termed as *(2015 Cancelled)*
    (a) secondary productivity
    (b) net productivity
    (c) net primary productivity
    (d) gross primary productivity.

12. Secondary productivity is rate of formation of new organic matter by ***(2013)***
(a) consumers (b) decomposers
(c) producers (d) parasites.

13. The rate of formation of new organic matter by rabbit in a grassland, is called ***(Mains 2013)***
(a) net productivity
(b) secondary productivity
(c) net primary productivity
(d) gross primary productivity.

14. Mass of living matter at a trophic level in an area at any time is called ***(2011)***
(a) standing crop (b) detritus
(c) humus (d) standing state.

15. The biomass available for consumption by the herbivores and the decomposers is called ***(2010)***
(a) net primary productivity
(b) secondary productivity
(c) standing crop
(d) gross primary productivity.

16. Which one of the following ecosystem types has the highest annual net primary productivity? ***(2007)***
(a) Tropical deciduous forest
(b) Temperate evergreen forest
(c) Temperate deciduous forest
(d) Tropical rainforest

17. Which of the following is expected to have the highest value ($gm/m^2/yr$) in a grassland ecosystem? ***(2004)***
(a) Secondary production
(b) Tertiary production
(c) Gross production (GP)
(d) Net production (NP)

18. The rate at which light energy is converted into chemical energy of organic molecules is the ecosystem's ***(1998)***
(a) net secondary productivity
(b) gross primary productivity
(c) net primary productivity
(d) gross secondary productivity.

19. Which of the following ecosystem has the highest gross primary productivity? **(1997)**
(a) Mangroves (b) Rainforest
(c) Grassland (d) Coral reef

DECOMPOSITION

20. Given below are two statements. ***(2022)***

Statement I : Decomposition is a process in which the detritus is degraded into simpler substances by microbes.

Statement II : Decomposition is faster if the detritus is rich in lignin and chitin.

In the light of the above statements, choose the correct answer from the options given below :
(a) Both Statement I and Statement II are correct
(b) Both Statement I and Statement II are incorrect
(c) Statement I is correct but Statement II is incorrect
(d) Statement I is incorrect but Statement II is correct.

21. Detritivores breakdown detritus into smaller particles.

This process is called: ***(2022)***
(a) Catabolism (b) Fragmentation
(c) Humification (d) Decomposition

22. Which one of the following processes during decomposition is correctly described? ***(2013)***
(a) Catabolism - Last step in the decomposition under fully anaerobic condition
(b) Leaching - Water soluble inorganic nutrients rise to the top layers of soil
(c) Fragmentation - Carried out by organisms such as earthworm
(d) Humification - Leads to the accumulation of a dark coloured substance humus which undergoes microbial action at a very fast rate.

23. The breakdown of detritus into smaller particles by earthworm is a process called ***(Mains 2011)***

(a) humification (b) fragmentation

(c) mineralisation (d) catabolism.

24. The slow rate of decomposition of fallen logs in nature is due to their ***(2008)***

(a) anaerobic environment around them

(b) low cellulose content

(c) low moisture content

(d) poor nitrogen content.

25. Plant decomposers are ***(2001)***

(a) monera and fungi

(b) fungi and plants

(c) protista and animalia

(d) animalia and monera.

26. Which of the following acts as "nature's scavengers"? ***(1997)***

(a) Insects (b) Microorganisms

(c) Man (d) Animals

27. If we completely remove the decomposers from an ecosystem, its functioning will be adversely affected, because ***(1995)***

(a) mineral movement will be blocked

(b) the rate of decomposition will be very high

(c) energy flow will be blocked

(d) herbivores will not receive solar energy.

ENERGY FLOW

28. Identify the correct statements : ***(2023)***

A. Detrivores perform fragmentation.

B. The humus is further degraded by some microbes during mineralization.

C. Water soluble inorganic nutrients go down into the soil and get precipitated by a process called leaching.

D. The detritus food chain begins with living organisms.

E. Earthworms break down detritus into smaller particles by a process called catabolism.

Choose the correct answer from the options given below:

(a) C, D, E only (b) D, E, A only

(c) A, B, C only (d) B, C, D only

29. The primary producers of the deep-sea hydrothermal vent ecosystem are ***(NEET-II 2016)***

(a) green algae

(b) chemosynthetic bacteria

(c) blue-green algae

(d) coral reefs.

30. Most animals that live in deep oceanic waters are ***(2015)***

(a) tertiary consumers

(b) detritivores

(c) primary consumers

(d) secondary consumers.

31. If 20 J of energy is trapped at producer level, then how much energy will be available to peacock as food in the following chain? ***(2014)***

Plant $\rightarrow$ Mice $\rightarrow$ Snake $\rightarrow$ Peacock

(a) 0.02 J (b) 0.002 J

(c) 0.2 J (d) 0.0002 J

32. Which of the following is a primary consumer in maize field ecosystem? ***(Karnataka NEET 2013)***

(a) Grasshopper (b) Wolf

(c) Phytoplankton (d) Lion

33. When man eats fish which feeds on zooplanktons which have eaten small plants, the producer in this chain is ***(Karnataka NEET 2013)***

(a) small plants (b) fish

(c) man (d) zooplankton.

34. Identify the possible link "A" in the following food chain. ***(2012)***

Plant $\rightarrow$ Insect $\rightarrow$ Frog $\rightarrow$"A" $\rightarrow$Eagle

(a) Rabbit (b) Wolf

(c) Cobra (d) Parrot

35. Identify the likely organisms (1), (2), (3) and (4) in the food web shown below. ***(Mains 2012)***

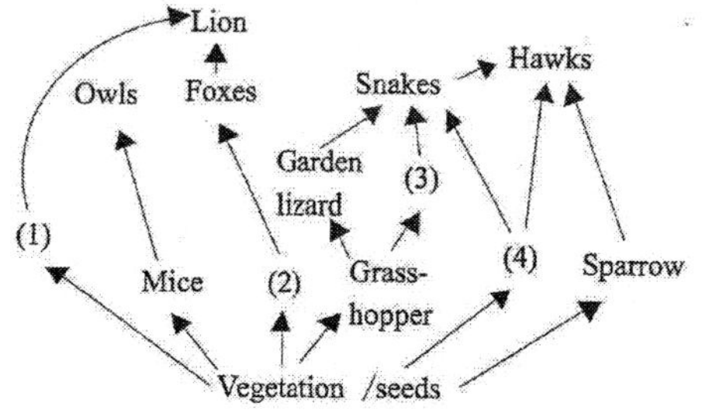

	(1)	(2)	(3)	(4)
(a)	Deer	Rabbit	Frog	Rat
(b)	Dog	Squirrel	Bat	Deer
(c)	Rat	Dog	Tortoise	Crow
(d)	Squirrel Cat	Cat	Rat	Pigeon

36. Of the total incident solar radiation the proportion of PAR is ***(2011)***

(a) about 70% (b) about 60%
(c) less than 50% (d) more than 80%.

37. Which one of the following animals may occupy more than one trophic levels in the same ecosystem at the same time? ***(Mains 2011)***

(a) Sparrow (b) Lion
(c) Goat (d) Frog

38. Which one of the following types of organisms occupy more than one trophic level in a pond ecosystem? ***(2009)***

(a) Fish (b) Zooplankton
(c) Frog (d) Phytoplankton

39. Consider the following statements concerning food chains. ***(2008)***

A. Removal of 80% tigers from an area resulted in greatly increased growth of vegetation.

B. Removal of most of the carnivores resulted in an increased population of deers.

C. The length of food chains is generally limited to 3–4 trophic levels due to energy loss.

D. The length of food chains may vary from 2 to 8 trophic levels.

Which two of the above statements are correct?

(a) A, D (b) A, B
(c) B, C (d) C, D

40. Bamboo plant is growing in a fir forest then what will be the trophic level of it? ***(2002)***

(a) First trophic level (T_1)
(b) Second trophic level (T_2)
(c) Third trophic level (T_3)
(d) Fourth trophic level (T_4)

41. Which is the reason for highest biomass in aquatic ecosystem? ***(2000)***

(a) Nano plankton, blue green algae and green algae
(b) Sea grass and slime moulds
(c) Benthic and brown algae
(d) Diatoms

42. Energy transfer from one trophic level to other, in a food chain, is ***(1999)***

(a) 10% (b) 20%
(c) 1% (d) 2%

43. In a terrestrial ecosystem such as forest, maximum energy is in which trophic level? ***(1998)***

(a) T_3 (b) T_4
(c) T_1 (d) T_2

44. The 10% energy transfer law of food chain was given by ***(1996)***

(a) Lindemann (b) Tansley
(c) Stanley (d) Weismann.

45. In a biotic community, the primary consumers are ***(1995)***

(a) detritivores (b) herbivores
(c) carnivores (d) omnivores.

46. The dominant second trophic level, in a lake ecosystem, is ***(1994)***

(a) phytoplankton (b) zooplankton
(c) benthos (d) plankton.

47. Food chain in which microorganisms breakdown the food formed by primary producers is ***(1991)***
(a) parasitic food chain
(b) detritus food chain
(c) consumer food chain
(d) predator food chain.

48. Pick up the correct food chain. ***(1991)***
(a) Grass $\rightarrow$ Chameleon $\rightarrow$ Insect $\rightarrow$ Bird
(b) Grass $\rightarrow$ Fox $\rightarrow$ Rabbit $\rightarrow$ Bird
(c) Phytoplankton $\rightarrow$ Zooplankton $\rightarrow$ Fish
(d) Fallen leaves $\rightarrow$ Bacteria $\rightarrow$ Insect larvae

ECOLOGICAL PYRAMIDS

49. Which of the following statements is not correct? ***(2021)***
(a) Pyramid of numbers in a grassland ecosystem is upright.
(b) Pyramid of biomass in sea is generally inverted.
(c) Pyramid of biomass in sea is generally upright.
(d) Pyramid of energy is always upright.

50. Match the trophic levels with their correct species examples in grassland ecosystem. ***(2020)***

(A) Fourth trophic level	(i) Crow
(B) Second trophic level	(ii) Vulture
(C) First trophic level	(iii) Rabbit
(D) Third trophic level	(iv) Grass

Select the correct option.

	A	B	C	D
(a)	(ii)	(iii)	(iv)	(i)
(b)	(iii)	(ii)	(i)	(iv)
(c)	(iv)	(iii)	(ii)	(i)
(d)	(i)	(ii)	(iii)	(iv)

51. Which of the following ecological pyramids is generally inverted? ***(2019)***
(a) Pyramid of biomass in a sea
(b) Pyramid of numbers in grassland
(c) Pyramid of energy
(d) Pyramid of biomass in a forest

52. What type of ecological pyramid would be obtained with the following data? ***(2018)***

Secondary consumer : 120 g

Primary consumer : 60 g

Primary producer : 10 g
(a) Inverted pyramid of biomass
(b) Pyramid of energy
(c) Upright pyramid of numbers
(d) Upright pyramid of biomass

53. Which ecosystem has the maximum biomass? ***(2017)***
(a) Grassland ecosystem
(b) Pond ecosystem
(c) Lake ecosystem
(d) Forest ecosystem

54. Given below is an imaginary pyramid of numbers. What could be one of the possibilities about certain organisms at some of the different levels? ***(2012)***

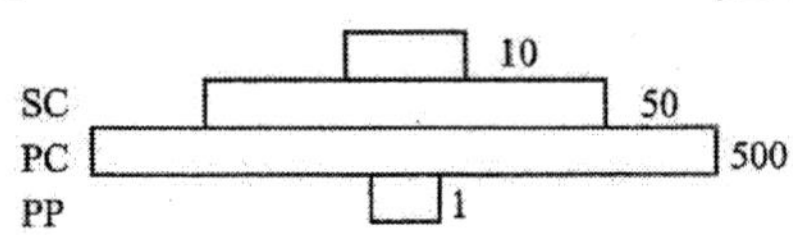

(a) Level PC is "insects" and level SC is "small insectivorous birds".
(b) Level PP is "phytoplanktons" in sea and "whale" on top level TC.
(c) Level one PP is "pipal trees" and the level SC is "sheep".
(d) Level PC is "rats" and level SC is "cats".

55. The upright pyramid of number is absent in ***(2012)***
(a) pond (b) forest
(c) lake (d) grassland.

56. Which one of the following statements for the pyramid of energy is incorrect? ***(2011)***
(a) Its base is broad.
(b) It shows energy content of different trophic level organisms.
(c) It is inverted in shape.
(d) It is upright in shape.

57. Which of the following representations shows the pyramid of numbers in a forest ecosystem? ***(Mains 2010)***

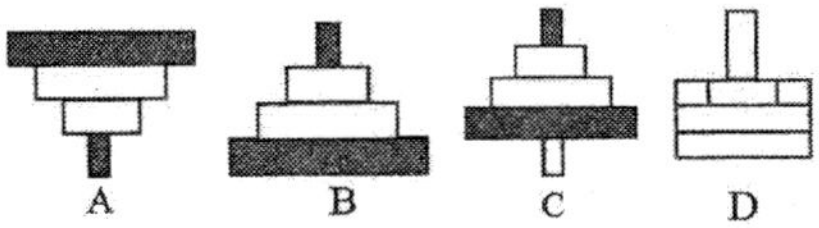

(a) D (b) A (c) B (d) C

58. Which one of the following is not used for construction of ecological pyramids? ***(2006)***

(a) Fresh weight
(b) Dry weight
(c) Number of individuals
(d) Rate of energy flow

59. Pyramid of numbers deals with number of ***(1993)***

(a) species in an area
(b) individuals in a community
(c) individuals in a trophic level
(d) subspecies in a community.

60. Pyramid of numbers in a pond ecosystem is ***(1993)***

(a) irregular (b) inverted
(c) upright (d) spindle shaped.

ANSWER KEY

1.	(d)	2.	(d)	3.	(d)	4.	(d)	5.	(a)	6.	(b)	7.	(a)
8.	(a)	9.	(b)	10.	(b)	11.	(d)	12.	(a)	13.	(b)	14.	(a)
15.	(a)	16.	(d)	17.	(c)	18.	(b)	19.	(b)	20.	(c)	21.	(b)
22.	(c)	23.	(b)	24.	(d)	25.	(a)	26.	(b)	27.	(a)	28.	(c)
29.	(b)	30.	(b)	31.	(a)	32.	(a)	33.	(a)	34.	(c)	35.	(a)
36.	(c)	37.	(a)	38.	(a)	39.	(c)	40.	(a)	41.	(c)	42.	(a)
43.	(c)	44.	(a)	45.	(b)	46.	(b)	47.	(b)	48.	(c)	49.	(c)
50.	(a)	51.	(a)	52.	(a)	53.	(d)	54.	(a)	55.	(b)	56.	(c)
57.	(b,d)	58.	(a)	59.	(c)	60.	(c)						

HINTS & EXPLANATIONS

1. (d) : The term ecosystem was coined by A.G. Tansley in 1935.

2. (d) : Cropland ecosystem is an artificial or man-made terrestrial ecosystem which is created and maintained by human beings for their maximum benefits. Therefore, they will have least genetic diversity.

3. (d)

4. (d) : Four important functional aspects of the ecosystem are productivity, decomposition, energy flow and nutrient cycling.

5. (a) : The characteristics of biological community are dominance, species diversity, trophic organisation, stratification, dynamism and stability. Organisms are not uniformly distributed throughout a community. They usually occur in definite zones. This spatial arrangement of populations is called stratification. Structurally a community may be divided horizontally into subcommunities. This horizontal division constitutes the zonation in the community. Natality, mortality, age structure and sex ratio are the basic characteristics of a population.

6. (b) : Of all the ecosystems, ocean is the largest and most stable ecosystem. Aquatic life is protected from vigorous climates and weather that are climatic conditions, problem of water supply, food, fire and artificial forces such as industrialization, farming and grazing are lacking in the oceans. The sea is continuous and not separated as land and freshwater habitats.

7. (a) : Gross primary productivity (GPP) of an ecosystem is the rate of production of organic matter during photosynthesis. A considerable amount of GPP is utilised by autotrophs in respiration. Gross primary productivity minus respiration losses (R) is the net primary productivity (NPP)

NPP = GPP – R

8. (a) : A considerable amount of GPP is utilised by plants in respiration (R). The energy left after respiration and stored as organic matter in the producers per unit time and area is NPP.

NPP = GPP – R

9. (b) : Gross primary productivity (GPP) is the rate of production of organic matter during photosynthesis. A considerable amount of GPP is utilised by plants in respiration. GPP minus respiration losses (R) is the net primary productivity GPP – R = NPP

Therefore, GPP is always more than NPP.

10. (b) : Standing crop is the total amount of living material in a specified population at a particular time, expressed as biomass (standing biomass) or its equivalent in terms of energy. The standing crop may vary at different times of the year; for example, in a population of deciduous trees between summer and winter.

11. (d) : The amount of energy accumulation in green plants as biomass or organic matter per unit area over a time period is known as primary productivity. The rate of total capture of energy, or the rate of total production of organic material (biomass), is known as gross primary productivity.

12. (a)

13. (b)

14. (a) : Standing crop is the total amount of living material in a specified population at a particular time, expressed as biomass (standing biomass) or its equivalent in terms of energy. The standing crop may vary at different times of the year; for example, in a population of deciduous trees between summer and winter.

15.(a) : The total organic matter synthesised by the producers in the process of photosynthesis per unit time and area is known as gross primary productivity. Net primary productivity is equal to the rate of organic matter created by photosynthesis minus the rate of respiration and other losses. It is actually the biomass available for consumption by the herbivores and the decomposers.

16.(d) : Net primary productivity is the total organic matter stored by producers per unit area per unit time. Gross primary productivity is the total organic matter synthesised by producers in the process of photosynthesis per unit area per unit time.

So, Net primary productivity = Gross productivity – Respiration and other losses

Tropical rainforests occur over equatorial/ subequatorial regions with abundant warmth and rainfall. Diversity and productivity are maximum as compared to other regions.

17.(c) : Productivity is rate of accumulation of energy containing organic matter by an ecosystem per unit area per unit time. It is of two types- primary and secondary.

Productivity at producer level is known as primary productivity. It is two types: Gross primary productivity is primary productivity including that amount which is utilized in respiration and other metabolic activities. Net primary productivity (NPP) is primary productivity in excess to that which is utilised in respiration and other metabolic activities.

NPP = GP – Respiration

Secondary productivity is productivity at consumer level. Since gross production includes total production including the amount utilized in respiration and other metabolic activities so it is more than other forms of productivity.

18. (b)

19.(b) : Gross primary productivity is the total rate of photosynthesis, including the organic matter used up in respiration during the measurement period. Tropical evergreen/rainforests occur over equatorial/subequatorial regions with abundant warmth and rainfall (200-350 cm/yr) almost throughout the year. The forests are impenetrable (= jungle) with maximum diversity, e.g., 200 types of trees in one hectare, 70-80% of all insects 80-85% of all birds. Productivity is maximum here, 12000kcal/m2/yr.

20.(c) : Decomposition rate is slower if the detritus is rich in lignin and chitin.

21. (b)

22.(c) : Decomposition is the process in which decomposers break down complex organic matter into inorganic substances like carbon dioxide, water and nutrients. The important steps in the process of decomposition are fragmentation, leaching catabolism, humification and mineralisation. Detritivores (e.g., earthworm) break down detritus into smaller particles. This process is called fragmentation. By the process of leaching water-soluble inorganic nutrients go down into the soil horizon and get precipitated as unavailable salts. Bacterial and fungal enzymes degrade detritus into simpler inorganic substances. This process is called as catabolism. Humification and mineralisation occur during decomposition in the soil. Humification leads to accumulation of a dark coloured amorphous substance called humus that is highly resistant to microbial action and undergoes decomposition at an extremely slow rate. The humus is further degraded by some microbes and release of inorganic nutrients occur by the process known as mineralisation.

23.(b) : Detritivores (e.g., earthworm) break down detritus into smaller particles. This process is called fragmentation.

24.(d) : Decomposition is largely an oxygen-requiring process. The rate of decomposition is controlled by chemical composition of detritus and climatic factors. In a particular climatic condition, decomposition rate is slower if detritus is rich in lignin and chitin, and quicker, if detritus is rich in nitrogen and water-soluble substances like sugar. Temperature and soil moisture are the most important climatic factors that regulate decomposition through their effects on the activities of soil microbes. Warm and moist environment favour decomposition whereas low temperature and anaerobiosis inhibit decomposition resulting in build up of organic materials.

25.(a) : Microorganisms (bacteria and fungi) are decomposers of the ecosystem. They feed upon dead decaying living organisms (both plant and animals) and break them into simpler compounds. These are released free in the atmosphere and are utilized by producers for the synthesis of their food materials. They mainly belong to Kingdom Monera and Fungi.

26.(b) : Microorganisms (bacteria and mould) are decomposers of the ecosystem. They feed upon dead decaying organisms (both plant and animals) and break them into simpler compounds. They are called nature's scavengers as they are consumers of dead matter.

27.(a) : Decomposers are saprotrophs which decompose the organic remains by secreting extracellular digestive enzymes. They are also known as mineralisers as they release minerals trapped in organic remains. So in the absence of microorganisms the flow of minerals will stop.

28.(c) : The detritus food chain begins with dead organic matter. It is comprises of decomposers which are heterotrophic organisms, mainly fungi and bacteria. Bacterial and fungal enzymes degrade detritus into simpler or smaller inorganic substances by a process called catabolism.

29.(b) : Hydrothermal vents are cracks in the ocean floor that emit jets of hot water loaded with minerals and chemosynthetic bacteria. These bacteria are autotrophs that oxidise hydrogen sulphide in vent water to obtain energy which is used to produce organic material. These chemosynthetic bacteria are the primary producers and form the base of vent food webs. All vent animals ultimately depend on bacteria for food.

30.(b) : Benthos is the community of organisms which live on, in, or near the sea bed, also known as the benthic zone. As no light is available at this zone of sea, the energy source for deep benthic ecosystems is often organic matter from higher up in the water column which drifts down to the depths. This dead and decaying matter sustains the benthic organisms, and therefore, most organisms in benthic zone, i.e:, in deep oceanic waters, are scavengers or detritivores.

31.(a) : Herbivores are eaten by primary carnivores. Only 10% of the herbivores productivity is utilized for raising productivity of primary carnivores. The rest is consumed in ingestion, respiration, maintenance of body heat and other activities. Higher carnivores similarly are able to retain only 10% of energy present in primary carnivores. It is called 10% law which was proposed by Lindemann. Accordingly, if plant trapped 20 J of energy, mice will have 2 J, snake will have 0.2 J and hence, peacock will have 0.02 J of energy.

32.(a) : Primary consumers are herbivorous organisms that feed on producers. Carnivores are termed secondary, tertiary, etc., consumers depending upon their position in food chain. In food chain on land, grasshopper is a herbivore (primary consumer) while wolf and lion are carnivores. Phytoplanktons are producers in aquatic food chains.

33.(a) : The transfer of food energy from producers to consumers through a series of organisms with repeated eating and being eaten is known as food chain. Green plants are always the first link of food chain because they alone are capable of synthesising organic food by using light energy by photosynthesis. The logical sequence of a food chain is :

Producer → Consumers → Decomposer

Small plants→	Zooplanktons →	Fish →	Man
(Primary producer)	(Primary consumer)	(Secondary consumer)	(Tertiary consumer)

34. (c)

35. (a)

36. (c) : The source of energy in all ecosystem is solar energy. About 50% of the solar energy incident over earth is present in PAR (Photosynthetically active radiation).

About 1-5% of incident solar radiation or 2-10% of PAR is captured by the photosynthetic organisms in the synthesis of organic matter (gross primary productivity). Roughly 20% of it is consumed in respiration so that net capture of energy (net primary productivity) is 0.8-4% of incident radiation or 1.6-8% of PAR.

37.(a) : Sparrow can be herbivorous (eating seeds and fruits) or carnivorous (eating insects).

38.(a) : A single species may occupy more than one trophic level. In pond, fish occupy more than one trophic level. Small fishes act as secondary consumer. They feed on primary consumer. Large fishes act as tertiary consumer. They feed on smaller fish.

39.(c) : Removal of 80% tigers (i.e., tertiary consumer) from an area resulted in decreased growth of vegetation because there will be increased numbers of primary consumers which feeds on green plant. Removal of most of the carnivores resulted in an increased population of deers on which carnivores depends. The length of food chain is generally limited to 3-4 trophic level due to energy loss because all the food available at one level is neither eaten nor used by animals at the next level and a lot of the energy is lost in respiration to drive the organisms metabolism, so less energy is left to support higher trophic level.

40.(a) : Trophic structure of ecosystem is a type of producer-consumer arrangement, in which each food level is called trophic level and the graphical representation of trophic structure of ecosystem constitutes ecological pyramids. The green plants are producers and represent the first trophic level (T_1). So bamboo plant is the first trophic level (T_1).

41.(c) : The benthic region includes all the sea floor from the wave-washed shore-line to the greatest depths. Depending upon the penetration of light it is subdivided into two main zones : the lighted or littoral zone and the deep sea system. Due to abundance of light, water, oxygen, carbon dioxide and less salinity of water, the tidal zone is characterized by exhorbitant growth of plants. The dense growth of vegetation, on the other hand, provides shelter and food for animals. A wide variety of algae, few grasses and animals of every phylum of animal kingdom are represented in this region.

42.(a) : Herbivores are eaten by primary carnivores. Only 10% of the herbivores productivity is utilized for raising productivity of primary carnivores. The rest is consumed in ingestion, respiration, maintenance of body heat and other activities. Higher carnivores similarly are able to retain only 10% of energy present in primary carnivores. It is called 10% law which was proposed by Lindemann. Accordingly, if plant trapped 20 J of energy, mice will have 2 J, snake will have 0.2 J and hence, peacock will have 0.02 J of energy.

43.(c) : In a terrestrial ecosystem maximum energy is in trophic level I because the organisms which trap solar energy are primary producers and they have got maximum energy. Only 10% energy is transferred from one trophic level to next trophic level.

44. (a)

45. (b)

46.(b) : Trophic level is a step or division of food chain which is characterized by the method of obtaining its food. The two fundamental trophic levels are producers and consumers. Producers belong to the first trophic level. In a lake the producers are mainly some rooted or floating plants and phytoplanktons.

Primary consumers form the second trophic level. They feed on living plants or plant parts. The primary consumers are zooplanktons.

47.(b) : The dead organic matter of plants or animals is called as detritus. While a part of it remains on the soil surface as litter, the other part enters the soil. Many. animals such as protozoans, nematodes, insects, etc., depend on detritus and hence they are called as detritivores. Even the human beings are detritivores when they eat cooked food. From detritus, the chain proceeds to detritivores, then to carnivores and finally to top carnivores.

48.(c) : The process of transfer of energy from producers through a series of organisms, i.e., from primary consumers to secondary consumers and from secondary consumers to tertiary consumers by process of eating and being eaten constitute a food chain. The correct food chain is :

Phytoplankton $\rightarrow$ Zooplankton $\rightarrow$ Fish

49.(c) : Pyramid of biomass in sea is generally inverted. In an aquatic system like sea, the producers are small organisms, their biomass is least and this value gradually shows an increase towards the apex of the pyramid, thus making the pyramid of biomass inverted in shape.

50. (a)

51.(a) : Pyramid of biomass in an aquatic ecosystem (e.g., pond, sea) is usually inverted because the biomass of fishes exceeds the biomass of phytoplanktons.

52.(a) : The given data depicts the inverted pyramid of biomass, usually found in aquatic ecosystem. This can be understood by taking an example of a pond in which phytoplankton (10 g) represents the producer. Small fishes (60 g) feeding upon these phytoplankton represent primary consumers which are further eaten by the big fishes (120g) representing secondary consumers.

53. (d)

54. (a)

55.(b) : In forest, a single tree can support a large number of birds thus base showing producers in a pyramid of number will be narrower than the next slab showing primary consumers. Hence an upright pyramid of number is not formed in a forest ecosystem.

56.(c) : Pyramid of energy is always upright, can never be inverted, because when energy flows from a particular trophic level to the next trophic level, some energy is always lost as heat at each step.

57. (b,d)

58.(a) : Ecological pyramids may be of three general types : pyramid of number, pyramid of biomass and pyramid of energy. Pyramid of number is graphic representation of number of individuals per unit area of various trophic levels stepwise with producers being kept at the base and top carnivores at the tip. The total amount of dry weight of living or organic matter in an ecosystem at any time is called biomass. The pyramid of biomass indicates the decrease or the gradual reduction in biomass at each trophic levels from base to apex. Fresh weight is not used in ecological pyramids. Pyramid of energy is the graphic representation of amount of energy trapped per unit time and area in different trophic levels of a food chain.

59.(c) : Pyramid of numbers is an ecological pyramid which employs the number of individuals per unit area at various trophic levels sequence wise with producers at the base and various consumers at successively higher levels. Pyramid of number assumes different shapes in different ecosystems. The pyramid of number in pond ecosystem is also upright. In forest ecosystem the pyramid of number is intermediate. Here, the number of primary consumers is more than producers as well as top consumers. In parasitic food chain the pyramid of number is inverted.

60. (c)

Chapter : 32

BIODIVERSITY AND CONSERVATION

BIODIVERSITY

1. Among 'The Evil Quartet', which one is considered the most important cause driving extinction of species? ***(2023)***
(a) Alien species invasions
(b) Co-extinctions
(c) Habitat loss and fragmentation
(d) Over exploitation for economic gain

2. Habitat loss and fragmentation, over exploitation, alien species invasion and co-extinction are causes for ***(2022)***
(a) population explosion
(b) competition
(c) biodiversity loss
(d) natality.

3. Which of the following regions of the globe exhibits highest species diversity? ***(2020)***
(a) Western Ghats of India
(b) Madagascar
(c) Himalayas
(d) Amazon forests

4. According to Robert May, the global species diversity is about ***(2020)***
(a) 1.5 million (b) 20 million
(c) 50 million (d) 7 million.

5. Which of the following is the most important for animals and plants being driven to extinction? ***(2019)***
(a) Alien species invasion
(b) Habitat loss and fragmentation
(c) Drought and floods
(d) Economic exploitation

6. Decline in the population of indian native fishes due to introduction of Clarias gariepinus in river Yamuna can be categoriesd as ***(Odisha NEET 2019)***
(a) co-extinction
(b) habitat fragmentation
(c) over-exploitation
(d) alien species invasion.

7. Alexander von Humboldt described for the first time ***(2017)***
(a) laws of limiting factor
(b) species area relationships
(c) population growth equation
(d) ecological biodiversity.

8. Which of the following is correctly matched? ***(NEET-II 2016)***
(a) Aerenchyma - Opuntia
(b) Age pyramid - Biome
(c) Parthenium - Threat to hysterophorus biodiversity
(d) Stratification - Population

9. Red list contains data or information on **(NEET-II 2016)**
(a) all economically important plants
(b) plants whose products are in international trade
(c) threatened species
(d) marine vertebrates only.

10. Which is the national aquatic animal of India? ***(NEET-I 2016)***
(a) Blue whale (b) Sea-horse
(c) Gangetic shark (d) River dolphin

11. Which of the following is the most important cause of animals and plants being driven to extinction? ***(NEET-I 2016)***
(a) Habitat loss and fragmentation
(b) Co-extinctions
(c) Over-exploitation
(d) Alien species invasion

12. A species facing extremely high risk of extinction in the immediate future is called **(2014)**
(a) vulnerable (b) endemic
(c) critically endangered
(d) extinct.

13. The organization which publishes the Red list of species is **(2014)**
(a) ICFRE (b) IUCN
(c) UNEP (d) WWF

14. Given below is the representation of the extent of global diversity of invertebrates. What groups the four portions (A-D) represent respectively? **(2014)**

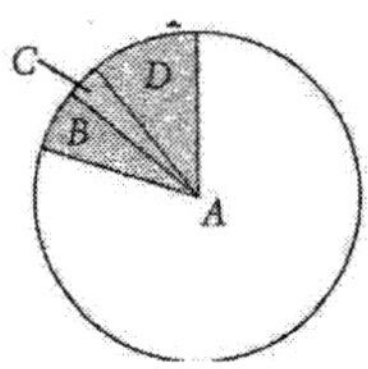

	A	B	C	D
(a)	Insects	Crustaceans	Other animal groups	Molluscs
(b)	Crustaceans	Insects	Molluscs	Other animal groups
(c)	Molluscs	Other animal groups	Crustaceans	Insects
(d)	Insects	Molluscs	Crustaceans	other animal groups

15. Which of the following represent maximum number of species among global biodiversity? **(2013,2012)**
(a) Fungi (b) Mosses and Ferns
(c) Algae (d) Lichens

16. Which of the following has maximum genetic diversity in India? ***(Karnataka NEET 2013, 2011)***
(a) Mango (b) Wheat
(c) Groundnut (d) Rice

17. Which organization publishes the 'Red Data Boo k'? ***(Karnataka NEET 2013)***
(a) IUCN (b) UNEP
(c) WWF (d) GEF

18. Which one of the following have the highest number of species in nature? **(2011)**
(a) Fungi (b) Insects
(c) Birds (d) Angiosperms

19. Biodiversity of a geographical region represents ***(Mains 2011)***
(a) endangered species found in the region
(b) the diversity in the organisms living in the region
(c) genetic diversity in the dominant species of the region
(d) species endemic to the region.

20. Study the four statements (i-iv) given below and select the two correct ones out of them. **(2010)**
(i) A lion eating a deer and a sparrow feeding on grains are ecologically similar in being consumers.
(ii) Predator star fish *Pisaster* helps in maintaining species diversity of some invertebrates.
(iii) Predators ultimately lead to the extinction of prey species.
(iv) Production of chemicals such as nicotine, strychnine by the plants are metabolic disorders.

The two correct statements are
(a) (ii) and (iii) (b) (iii) and (iv)
(c) (i) and (iv) (d) (i) and (ii)

21. The Indian rhinoceros is a natural inhabitant of which one of the Indian states? ***(Mains 2010)***
(a) Uttarakhand (b) Uttar Pradesh
(c) Himachal Pradesh (d) Assam

22. Which one of the following has maximum genetic diversity in India? **(2009)**
(a) Mango (b) Wheat
(c) Tea (d) Teak

23. The table gives the populations (in thousands) of ten species (A-J) in four areas (p-s) consisting of the number of habitats given within brackets against each. Study the table and answer the question which follows.

Area and No. of habitats in the areas	Species, and their populations (in thousands) in the areas									
	A	B	C	D	E	F	G	H	I	J
p (11)	2.3	1.2	0.52	6.0	–	3.1	1.1	9.0	–	10.3
q (11)	10.2	–	0.62	–	1.5	3.0	–	8.2	1.1	11.2
r (13)	11.3	0.9	0.48	2.4	1.4	4.2	0.8	8.4	2.2	4.1
s (12)	3.2	10.2	11.1	4.8	0.4	3.3	0.8	7.3	11.3	2.1

Which area out of p - s shows maximum species diversity? ***(2008)***

(a) s (b) p
(c) q (d) r

24. Which one of the following pairs of organisms are exotic species introduced in India? ***(2007)***

(a) Lantana camara, water hyacinth
(b) Water hyacinth, Prosopis cinereria
(c) Nile perch, Ficus religiosa
(d) Ficus religiosa, Lantana camara

25. One of the endangered species of Indian medicinal plants is that of ***(2007)***

(a) Ocimum (b) garlic
(c) Nepenthes (d) Podophyllum.

26. Occurrence of endemic species in South America and Australia is due to ***(2001)***

(a) these species has been extinct from other regions
(b) continental separation
(c) there is no terrestrial route to these places
(d) retrogressive evolution.

27. Which of the following is mainly responsible for the extinction of wildlife? ***(1999)***

(a) Pollution of air and water
(b) Hunting of flesh
(c) Destruction of habitats
(d) All of these

28. What is the major cause of diminishing wildlife number? ***(1998)***

(a) Felling of trees
(b) Paucity of drinking water
(c) Cannibalism
(d) Habitat destruction

BIODIVERSITY CONSERVATION

29. The historic convention on Biological Diversity, 'The Earth Summit' was held in Rio de Janeiro in the year ***(2023)***

(a) 1986 (b) 2002
(c) 1985 (d) 1992.

30. Which of the following is not a method of ex situ conservation? ***(2022)***

(a) In vitro fertilisation
(b) National parks
(c) Micropropagation
(d) Cryopreservation

31. In-situ conservation refers to ***(2022)***

(a) protect and conserve the whole ecosystem
(b) conserve only high risk species
(c) conserve only endangered species
(d) conserve only extinct species.

32. The Earth Summit held in Rio de Janeiro in 1992 was called ***(2019)***

(a) for immediate steps to discontinue use of CFCs that were damaging the ozone layer
(b) to reduce CO_2 emissions and global warming
(c) for conservation of biodiversity and sustainable utilisation of its benefits
(d) to assess threat posed to native species by invasive weed species.

33. Which one of the following is not a method of in situ conservation of biodiversity ? ***(2019)***

(a) Sacred grove (b) Biosphere reserve
(c) Wildlife sanctuary (d) Botanical garden

34. Western Ghats have a large number of plant and animal species that are not found anywhere else. Which of the following terms will you use to notify such species? ***(Odisha NEET 2019)***

(a) Endemic (b) Vulnerable
(c) Threatened (d) Keystone

35. All of the following are included in 'ex-situ conservation' except ***(2018)***
(a) wildlife safari parks
(b) sacred groves
(c) botanical gardens
(d) seed banks.

36. Which one of the following is related to ex-situ conservation of threatened animals and plants? ***(2017)***
(a) Biodiversity hotspots
(b) Amazon rainforest
(c) Himalayan region
(d) Wildlife safari parks

37. The region of biosphere reserve which is legally protected and where no human activity is allowed is known as ***(2017)***
(a) buffer zone (b) transition zone
(c) restoration zone (d) core zone.

38. How many hotspots of biodiversity in the world have been identified till date by Norman Myers? ***(NEET-II 2016)***
(a) 17 (b) 25 (c) 34 (d) 43

39. Which of the following national parks is home to the famous musk deer or hangul? ***(NEET-II 2016)***
(a) Keibul Lamjao National Park, Manipur
(b) Bandhavgarh National Park, Madhya Pradesh
(c) Eaglenest Wildlife Sanctuary, Arunachal Pradesh
(d) Dachigam National Park, Jammu and Kashmir

40. The species confined to a particular region and not found elsewhere is termed as ***(2015)***
(a) endemic (b) rare
(c) keystone (d) alien.

41. In which of the following, both pairs have correct combination? ***(2015 Cancelled)***
(a) In-situ conservation : Seed Bank
Ex-situ conservation : National Park
(b) In-situ conservation : Tissue culture
Ex-situ conservation : Sacred groves
(c) In-situ conservation : National Park
Ex-situ conservation : Botanical Garden
(d) In-situ conservation : Cryopreservation
Ex-situ conservation : Wildlife Sanctuary

42. Cryopreservation of gametes of threatened species in viable and fertile condition can be referred to as ***(2015 Cancelled)***
(a) in situ conservation by sacred groves
(b) in situ cryo-conservation of biodiversity
(c) in situ conservation of biodiversity
(d) advanced ex situ conservation of biodiversity.

43. An example of ex-situ conservation is ***(2014)***
(a) national park (b) seed bank
(c) wildlife sanctuary (d) sacred grove.

44. Which one of the following is not used for ex-situ plant conservation? ***(2013)***
(a) Shifting cultivation (b) Botanical gardens
(c) Field gene banks (d) Seed banks

45. The largest tiger reserve in India is ***(Karnataka NEET 2013)***
(a) Valmiki
(b) Nagarjunasagar-Srisailam
(c) Periyar (d) Nagarhole.

46. Which one of the following areas in India, is a hotspot of biodiversity? ***(2012)***
(a) Eastern Ghats (b) Gangetic Plain
(c) Sunderbans (d) Western Ghats

47. Select the correct statement about biodiversity ***(Mains 2012)***
(a) The desert areas of Rajasthan and Gujarat have a very high level of desert animal species as well as numerous rare animals.
(b) Large scale planting of Bt cotton has no adverse effect on biodiversity.
(c) Western ghats have a very high degree of species richness and endemism.
(d) Conservation of biodiversity is just a fad pursued by the developed countries.

48. Sacred groves are specially useful in ***(Mains 2012)***
(a) generating environmental awareness
(b) preventing soil erosion
(c) year-round flow of water in rivers
(d) conserving rare and threatened species.

49. Consider the following statements (A - D) each with one or two blanks. ***(Mains 2011)***
(a) Bears go into __(1)__ during winter to __(2)__ cold weather.
(b) A conical age pyramid with a broad base represents __(3)__ human population.
(c) A wasp pollinating a fig flower is an example of __(4)__ .
(d) An area with high levels of species richness is known as __(5)__.

Which one of the following options, gives the correct fill ups for the respective blank numbers from (1) to (5) in the statements ?
(a) (3) - stable (4) - commensalism, (5)-marsh
(b) (1) - aestivation, (2) - escape, (3) - stable, (4) - mutualism
(c) (3) - expanding, (4) - commensalism, (5) - biodiversity park
(d) (1) - hibernation, (2) - escape, (3) - expanding (5) - hotspot

50. Which one of the following is an example of ex-situ conservation? ***(2010)***
(a) Wildlife sanctuary (b) Seed bank
(c) Sacred groves (d) National park

51. Tiger is not a resident in which one of the following national parks? ***(2009)***
(a) Sunderbans (b) Gir
(c) Jim Corbett (d) Ranthambhor

52. Which one of the following is not observed in biodiversity hotspots? ***(2008)***
(a) Lesser inter-specific competition
(b) Species richness
(c) Endemism
(d) Accelerated species loss

53. World Summit on Sustainable Development (2002) was held in ***(2008)***
(a) Argentina (b) South Africa
(c) Brazil (d) Sweden.

54. Identify the odd combination of the habitat and the particular animal concerned. ***(2007)***
(a) Sunderbans – Bengal Tiger
(b) Periyar – Elephant
(c) Rann of Kutch – Wild Ass
(d) Dachigam National Park – Snow Leopard

55. Which of the following is considered a hotspot of biodiversity in India? ***(2006)***
(a) Aravalli hills
(b) Western ghats
(c) Indo-gangetic plain
(d) Eastern ghats

56. Which one of the following is not included under in situ conservation? ***(2006)***
(a) National park
(b) Sanctuary
(c) Botanical garden
(d) Biosphere reserve

57. Which one of the following is the correctly matched pair of an endangered animal and a national park? ***(2006)***
(a) Great Indian bustard : Keoladeo National Park
(b) Lion : Corbett National Park
(c) Rhinoceros : Kaziranga National Park
(d) Wild ass : Dudhwa National Park

58. Biodiversity Act of India was passed by the Parliament in the year ***(2005)***
(a) 1992 (b) 1996
(c) 2000 (d) 2002.

59. One of the most important functions of botanical gardens is that ***(2005)***
(a) they provide a beautiful area for recreation
(b) one can observe tropical plants there
(c) they allow ex situ conservation of germplasm
(d) they provide the natural habitat for wild life.

60. In your opinion, which is the most effective way to conserve the plant diversity of an area? ***(2004)***

(a) By tissue culture method
(b) By creating biosphere reserve
(c) By creating botanical garden
(d) By developing seed bank

61. Viable material of endangered species can be preserved by ***(2000)***

(a) gene bank (b) gene library
(c) herbarium (d) gene pool.

62. MAB stands for ***(1997)***

(a) mammals and biosphere
(b) mammals and biology programme
(c) man and biology programme
(d) man and biosphere programme.

63. Identify the correct match between tiger reserve and its state. ***(1995)***

(a) Manas - Assam
(b) Corbett - Madhya Pradesh
(c) Bandipur - Tamil Nadu
(d) Palamu - Odisha

64. Which of the following is the matching pair of a sanctuary and its main protected wild animal? ***(1995)***

(a) Kaziranga-Musk deer
(b) Gir-Lion
(c) Sunderban-Rhino
(d) All of these

ANSWER KEY

1.	(c)	2.	(c)	3.	(d)	4.	(d)	5.	(b)	6.	(d)	7.	(b)
8.	(c)	9.	(c)	10.	(d)	11.	(a)	12.	(c)	13.	(b)	14.	(d)
15.	(a)	16.	(d)	17.	(a)	18.	(b)	19.	(b)	20.	(d)	21.	(d)
22.	(a)	23.	(a)	24.	(a)	25.	(d)	26.	(b)	27.	(c)	28.	(d)
29.	(d)	30.	(b)	31.	(a)	32.	(c)	33.	(d)	34.	(a)	35.	(b)
36.	(d)	37.	(d)	38.	(c)	39.	(d)	40.	(a)	41.	(c)	42.	(d)
43.	(b)	44.	(a)	45.	(b)	46.	(d)	47.	(c)	48.	(d)	49.	(d)
50.	(b)	51.	(b)	52.	(a)	53.	(b)	54.	(d)	55.	(b)	56.	(c)
57.	(c)	58.	(d)	59.	(c)	60.	(b)	61.	(a)	62.	(d)	63.	(a)
64.	(b)												

HINTS & EXPLANATIONS

1.(c) : Habitat loss and fragmentation is the most important cause driving animals and plants to extinction. The most dramatic examples of habitat loss come from Amazon tropical rain forest.

2.(c) : There are four major causes (The Evil Quartet) of biodiversity losses : habitat loss and fragmentation, over exploitation, alien species invasion and co-extinctions.

3. (d)

4. (d)

5.(b) : Habitat loss and fragmentation is the most important cause of driving the animals and plants to extinction. When large habitats are broken into small fragments due to various human activities, mammals and birds requiring large territories and certain animals with migratory habitats are badly affected, leading to population declines. The same can be applicable to the plant (forest) loss and degradation as millions of species are being cut and cleared for the expansion of agricultural land, harvesting timber, forest fire, as well as overgrazing.

6. (d)

7.(b) : Alexander von Humboldt described species area relationship for the first time. He observed that within a region, species richness increases with increasing explored area, but vily upto a limit.

8.(c) : Parthenium hysterophorus is commonly known as congress grass or carrot weed. It is herbaceous annual plant of Family Asteraceae. It is a deadly invasive, noxious weed infesting cropped and non-cropped areas. It rapidly colonises area replacing the native vegetation and causes a number of human health related problems such as skin allergy, rhinitis and eye irritations. Also, being toxic and unpalatable it causes fodder scarcity. Hence, it is considered a threat to the biodiversity.

9.(c) : A red data book or red list is a catalogue of taxa facing risk of extinction. Red data book or red list was initiated in 1963.

10.(d) : River dolphin found in holy river Ganga, Brahmaputra, Indus and its tributaries is the National aquatic animal of India. Presence of river dolphin in Ganga indicates pure and freshwater.

11.(a) : Destruction of natural habitat causes the most serious threat to the biodiversity. Over-population, urbanisation and industrialisation lead to the destruction or fragmentation of natural habitats to fulfill the requirement of additional land. Loss of habitat results in annihilation of plants, microorganisms and forcing out of animals which in alien lands die out after some time. Fragmentation of habitats results in disruption of complex interactions amongst species, destruction of species in the cleared regions, annihilation of species restricted to deeper undisturbed parts of forests and decreased biodiversity in the habitat fragments.

12.(c) : The taxon under critically endangered category are facing very high risk of extinction in the wild and can become extinct at any moment in the immediate future.

13.(b) : IUCN is International Union of Conservation of Nature and Natural Resources which is now called World Conservation Union (WCU). It has its headquarters at Morges, Switzerland. It maintains a red data book or red list which is a catalogue of taxa facing risk of extinction. Red data book or red list was initiated in 1963. The Red list of year 2000 has made assessment of 18,000 species.

14. (d)

15.(a) : Fungi is a large kingdom of over 72,000 species. They are achlorophyllous, heterotrophic, spore forming, nonvascular, eukaryotic organisms which contain chitin or fungal cellulosc in their walls and possess glycogen as food reserve. They are major decomposers of many ecosystems and are associate of many organisms.

16.(d) : Genetic diversity is the diversity in the numbers and types of genes as well as chromosomes present in different species and the variations in the genes and their alleles in the same species. Oryza sativa (rice) has 32,000–50,000 genes.

17. (a)

18.(b) : Insects have highest number of species found in nature. The insecta is the largest class of animals. It has over 7,00,000 species. The insects are the most successful land invertebrates and the only major competitors with humans for dominance in the world.

19.(b) : Biodiversity (biological diversity) is the existence of a wide variety of species (species diversity) or other taxa of plants, animals and microorganisms in a natural community or habitat, or of communities within a particular environment (ecological diversity), or of genetic variation within a species (genetic diversity). The maintenance of a high level of biodiversity is important for the stability of ecosystems.

20.(d) : Predator and prey evolve together. The prey is part of the predator's environment, and the predator dies if it does to get food, so it evolves whatever is necessary in order to eat the prey. Likewise, the predator is part of the prey's environment, and the prey dies if it is eaten by the predator, so it evolves whatever is necessary to avoid being eaten. So, predators cannot lead to the extinction of prey species.

Nicotine is an alkaloid found in the night shade family of plants (Solanaceae) that constitutes approximately 0.6–3.0% of dry weight of tobacco, with biosynthesis taking place in the roots and accumulation occurring in the leaves. Strychnine is an alkaloid plant toxin extracted chiefly from Nux *vomica*; formerly used as a stimulant. These are not metabolic disorder products but are metabolic wastes.

21.(d) : The Indian rhinoceros is a endemic of north-east region of India. Kaziranga National Park (Assam) is famous for rhinoceros.

22. (a)

23.(a) : Species diversity is related to the variety in the number and richness of the species within a region and is measured at the level of 'species.' Thus, it is the product of species richness and species evenness. Species richness refers to the number of species per unit area. As the area of the site increases, the number of species also increases due to more availability of natural resources. Species evenness is the relative abundance with which each species is represented in an area. Thus, variation in the number of species, kinds of species as well as the number of individuals per species lead to greater diversity. In the given table, the area which shows maximum species diversity is 's'.

24.(a) : In India, large variety of exotic animal and plant species have been introduced from other parts of the world through the ages. Some exotic plants have turned into weeds, multiplying fast and causing harm to the ecosystem, e.g. water hyacinth and Luniunu cumara.

25.(d) : An endangered species is a population of an organism which are at risk of becoming extinct because it is either a few in number or threatened by changing environmental or predation parameters. Podophyllum is such an endangered species of Indian medicinal plants. They contain, podophyllotoxin and podophyllin that is used as a purgative and as a cytostatic. They are also grown as ornamental plants for their attractive foliage and flowers. Extracts of plants are used for genital warts and some skin cancers.

26.(b) : Occurrence of endemic species in South America and Australia is due to geographic isolation (continental separation). Animals occupy all diverse habitats. The distribution, continuous or discontinuous of a species or a group of organisms depends on many factors like evolutionary, climatic, physical or biological barriers, etc.

27. (c)

28. (d)

29.(d) : The historic convention on biological diversity. "The Earth Summit" held in Rio de Janeiro in 1992, called upon all nations to take appropriate measures for conservation of biodiversity and sustainable utilisation of its benefits.

30.(b) : National parks are the method of in-situ conservation (Conservation in natural habitat).

31.(a) : When we conserve and protect the whole ecosystem, its biodiversity at all levels is protected - we save the entire forest to save the tiger. This approach is called in situ (on site) conservation. However, when there are situations where an animal or plant is endangered or threatened (organisms facing a very high risk of extinction in the wild in the near future) and needs urgent measures to save it from extinction; ex situ (off site) conservation is the desirable approach.

32.(c) : 'The Earth Summit' held in Rio de Janeiro in 1992, called upon all nations to take appropriate measures for conservation of biodiversity and sustainable utilisation of its benefits.

33.(d) : Botanical garden comes under ex-situ method of conservation of biodiversity.

34. (a)

35.(b) : Sacred groves come under in-situ conservation and represent the pristine forest patches around places of worship which are held in high esteem by tribal communities. Cutting of trees and branches is prohibited due to religious reasons. Wildlife safari parks, botanical gardens and seed banks come under ex-situ conservation.

36. (d) : Ex-situ conservation is conservation of selected rare or threatened animals and plants in places outside their natural homes. It includes offsite collections like botanical gardens, zoological parks, wildlife safari parks, gene banks, etc.

37.(d) : Core zone or Natural zone area of a biosphere reserve is undisturbed and legally protected ecosystem. No human activity is allowed in this zone. Little human activity is allowed in the buffer zone whereas in transition zone, an active cooperation is present between reserve management and local people for activities like settlements, cropping, etc. Restoration region is degraded area which is selected for restoration to near natural form.

38.(c) : Biodiversity hotspots are a method to identify those regions of the world where attention is needed to address biodiversity loss and to guide investments in conservation. The idea was first developed by Norman Myers in 1988 to identify tropical forests hotspots characterised both by exceptional levels of plant endemism and serious habitat loss which he then expanded to a more global scope. Currently 34 biodiversity hotspots have been identified most of which occur in tropical forests.

39. (d)

40. (a)

41.(c) : In-situ (on site) conservation is conservation and protection of the whole ecosystem and its biodiversity at all levels, in order to protect the threatened species. Two in-situ methods are being used to save biodiversity viz., hotspots and protected areas. Protected areas include national parks, sanctuaries, biosphere reserves and sacred groves. Ex-situ (off site) conservation is conservation of selected rare plants/animals in places outside their natural homes. Ex-situ conservation includes offsite collections, seed banks, gene banks, in vitro fertilization, cryopreservation techniques and tissue culture.

42.(d) : Cryopreservation is an advanced method of exsitu conservation. It involves preservation at -196° C in liquid nitrogen. It can maintain tissue culture, embryos, animal cells/ tissues, spermatozoa indefinitely. The cryopreserved material is revived through special technique, when required.

43.(b) : Ex-situ (off site) conservation is conservation of selected rare plants/animals in places outside their natural homes. Ex-situ conservation includes offsite collections, seed banks, gene banks, in vitro fertilization, cryopreservation techniques and tissue culture.

44.(a) : Ex-situ conservation is conservation of selected rare plants/animals in places outside their natural homes. It includes botanical gardens or zoological parks, seed banks, cryopreservation, field gene banks and sacred plants. Many wild and domesticated species are well managed and collected in botanical gardens, zoological parks, wildlife safari parks, arboreta, etc. Most of these have capture breeding programmes to restore the decreasing number of animals and helping the survival of existing individuals of the species. Gene banks are institutes that maintain stocks of viable seeds (seed banks), live plants (orchards), tissue culture and frozen germplasm with the whole range of genetic viability.

45.(b) : Nagarjunasagar - Srisailam Tiger Reserve is the largest tiger reserve in India. It is present in Andhra Pradesh with a total area of 3568 km2. The core area of this reserve is 1200 km2.

46.(d) : Hotspots are areas with high density of biodiversity or megadiversity which are also the most threatened ones. Ecologically hotspots are determined by four factors - number of species/ species diversity, degree of endemism, degree of threat to habitat due to its degradation and fragmentation, and degree of exploitation. India has three hotspots : Indo-Burma, Himalayas and Western Ghats - Sri Lanka.

47. (c)

48.(d) : Sacred grove is an example of in situ conservation of forests and wildlife especially rare and threatened species. These forest patches are found around places of worship which are held in high esteem by tribal communities. They are the most undisturbed forest patches which are often surrounded by highly degraded landscapes. Not a single branch is allowed to be cut from these forests. As a result many endemic species which are rare or have become extinct elsewhere can be seen to flourish here. Such sacred groves are found in Khasi and Jaintia hills of Meghalaya, Aravalli hills of Rajasthan, Western ghat regions of Karnataka, Maharashtra, Sarguja, Chanda and

Bastar areas of Madhya Pradesh.

49. (d)

50.(b) : Seed bank is an example of ex-situ conservation, while wildlife sanctuary, sacred grove and national parks are examples of in-situ conservation.

51.(b) : Gir National Park is situated in district Junagarh of Gujarat. This national park is famous for Asiatic lion. Beside lion, panther, striped hyaena, sambhar, nilgai, cheetal are also conserved.

52. (a)

53.(b) : Conservation of biodiversity is a collective responsibility of all nations. The historic Convention on Biological Diversity ('The Earth Summit') held in Rio de Janeiro in 1992, called upon all nations to take appropriate measures for conservation of biodiversity and sustainable utilisation of its benefits. In a follow-up, the World Summit on Sustainable Development held in 2002 in Johannesburg, South Africa, 190 countries pledged their commitment to achieve by 2010 , a significant reduction in the current rate of biodiversity loss at global, regional and local levels.

54.(d) : Dachigam National Park is located only 22 kilometers from Srinagar, the capital city of the northern state of Jammu and Kashmir. Dachigam is considered home to some of the unique Himalayan range of flora and fauna. Primary amongst them is the hangul or Kashmiri stag, the most endangered species of red deer in the world. It was finally upgraded and declared a National Park in the year 1981.

55. (b)

56.(c) : In-situ conservation means "on-site conservation". In-situ conservation is the protection and management of important components of biological diversity through a network of protected areas e.g., National Park, sanctuary, biosphere reserve, etc. Botanical gardens come under ex-situ conservation.

57.(c) : Kaziranga National Park of Assam is known for the conservation of rhinoceros.

58.(d) : Biodiversity Act of India provides for conservation of biological diversity, substainable use of its components and fair and equitable sharing of the benefits arising out of the use of biological resources, knowledge and for matters connected therewith or incidental thereto. The biodiversity act of India was passed in 2002.

59.(c) : Ex situ conservation means "offsite conservation". It is the process of protecting endangered species of plants and animals by removing it from an unsafe or threatened habitat and placing it or part of it under the care of humans. Botanical garden serve as ex situ conservation of germplasm of different plants, to maintain rare and endemic plant species and also to provide recreation and knowledge about plants to a common man.

60.(b) : Biosphere reserves are multipurpose protected areas of different representative ecosystems which are meant for conservation of biodiversity or wildlife, traditional life style of tribals and their domesticated animals and also plant resources. Each biosphere reserve has a core zone (where no human activity is allowed), a buffer zone (with limited human activity) and manipulation zone (where human activity is allowed without degradation of ecology. Thus, the biosphere reserves protect not just wild varieties but also domesticated varieties of plants of an area.

61.(a) : Viable material of endangered species can be preserved by gene bank. Gene bank is an institute that maintains stocks of viable seeds (seed banks), live growing plants (orchards), tissue culture and frozen germplasm with the whole range of genetic variability.

62.(d) : Man and biosphere programme is an international biological programme of UNESCO (United Nations Educational Scientific and Cultural Organisation) which was started in 1971 but was introduced in India in 1986. MAB has studied human environment, impact of human interference and pollution on biotic and abiotic environment and conservation strategies for the present as well as future.

63.(a) : Manas biosphere reserve is located in Assam. Corbett National Park is located in district Nainital of Uttaranchal. Bandipur National Park is located in district Mysore of Karnataka. Palamu is located in Chhotanagpur, Jharkhand.

64. (b)